Practice Questions
for NCLEX-RN®

Practice Questions for NCLEX-RN®

DONNA F. GAUWITZ, RN, MS

Nursing Consultant
Former Senior Teaching Specialist
School of Nursing—
University of Minnesota, Twin Cities
Minneapolis, Minnesota

Former Nursing Education Specialist
Mayo Clinic
Rochester, Minnesota

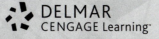

DELMAR
CENGAGE Learning™

Australia • Brazil • Japan • Korea • Mexico • Singapore • Spain • United Kingdom • United States

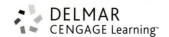

Practice Questions for NCLEX-RN®
Donna F. Gauwitz

Vice President, Health Care Business Unit:
William Brottmiller

Director of Learning Solutions:
Matthew Kane

Acquisitions Editor: Tamara Caruso

Project Manager: Patricia Gaworecki

Editorial Assistant: Tiffiny Adams

Editorial Intern: Jen Waters

Marketing Director: Jennifer McAvey

Marketing Channel Manager:
Michele McTighe

Marketing Coordinator: Danielle Pacella

Technology Director: Laurie Davis

Technology Project Managers:
Mary Colleen Liburdi,
Patricia Allen

Production Director: Carolyn Miller

Art Directors: Jack Pendleton,
Robert Plante

Content Project Managers: David Buddle,
Stacey Lamodi,
Jessica McNavich

Production Coordinator: Mary Ellen Cox

Library of Congress Control Number: 2006017453

ISBN-13: 978-1-4018-0590-6

ISBN-10: 1-4018-0590-6

Delmar
Executive Woods
5 Maxwell Drive
Clifton Park, NY 12065
USA

Cengage Learning is a leading provider of customized learning solutions with office locations around the globe, including Singapore, the United Kingdom, Australia, Mexico, Brazil, and Japan. Locate your local office at **international.cengage.com/region**

Cengage Learning products are represented in Canada by Nelson Education, Ltd.

For your course and learning solutions, visit **delmar.cengage.com**

Visit our corporate website at **www.cengage.com**

Notice to the Reader
Publisher does not warrant or guarantee any of the products described herein or perform any independent analysis in connection with any of the product information contained herein. Publisher does not assume, and expressly disclaims, any obligation to obtain and include information other than that provided to it by the manufacturer. The reader is expressly warned to consider and adopt all safety precautions that might be indicated by the activities described herein and to avoid all potential hazards. By following the instructions contained herein, the reader willingly assumes all risks in connection with such instructions. The publisher makes no representations or warranties of any kind, including but not limited to, the warranties of fitness for particular purpose or merchantability, nor are any such representations implied with respect to the material set forth herein, and the publisher takes no responsibility with respect to such material. The publisher shall not be liable for any special, consequential, or exemplary damages resulting, in whole or in part, from the readers' use of, or reliance upon, this material.

Printed in Canada
3 4 5 6 7 11 10 09 08

DEDICATION

This book is dedicated to my loving husband, William J. Gauwitz, Jr.,
who was always encouraging, supporting, and cheering me on.

CONTENTS

CONTRIBUTORS

Mary Mescher Benbenek, RN, MS, CPNP, CFNP
Teaching Specialist
School of Nursing, University of Minnesota
Twin Cities, Minnesota

Margaret Brogan, RN, BSN
Registered Nurse/Expert
Children's Memorial Hospital
Chicago, Illinois

Mary Lynn Burnett, RN, PhD
Assistant Professor of Nursing
Wichita State University
Wichita, Kansas

Corine K. Carlson, RN, MS
Assistant Professor
Department of Nursing, Luther College
Decorah, Iowa

Gretchen Reising Cornell, RN, PhD, CNE
Professor of Nursing
Utah Valley State College
Orem, Utah

Vera V. Cull, RN, DSN
Former Assistant Professor of Nursing
University of Alabama
Birmingham, Alabama

Laura DeHelian, RN, PhD, APRN, BC
Advanced Practice Nurse
Neighboring Mental Health Services
Mentor, OH

Lecturer
Case Western Reserve University
Cleveland, OH

Della J. Derscheid, RN, MS, CNS
Psychiatric Clinical Nurse Specialist
Department of Nursing, Mayo Clinic
Mayo Clinic College of Nursing
Rochester, Minnesota

Ann Garey, MSN, APRN, BC, FNP
Nurse Practitioner
OB Services
Carle Foundation Hospital
Urbana, Illinois

Beth Good, RN, MSN, BSN
Teaching Specialist
University of Minnesota
Minneapolis, Minnesota

Samantha Grover, RN, BSN, CNS
Psychiatric Mental Health Clinical Specialist
MeritCare Health System
Moorhead, Minnesota

Jeanne M. Harkness, RN, BA, MSN, BSN, AOCN
Clinical Practice Specialist
Jane Brattain Breast Center, Park Nicollet Clinic
St. Louis Park, Minnesota

Linda Irle, RN, MSN, APN, CNP
Coordinator, Maternal-Child Nursing
University of Illinois Chicago
Urbana, Illinois

Family Nurse Practitioner, Acute Care
Carle Clinic
Champaign, Illinois

Amy Jacobson, RN, BA
Staff Nurse
United Hospital
St. Paul, Minnesota

Nadine James, RN, PhD
Assistant Professor of Nursing
University of Southern Mississippi
Hattiesburg, Mississippi

Lisa Jensen, CS, MS, APRN
Associate Chief Nurse/Mental Health
George E. Whalen VA Medical Center
Salt Lake City, Utah

Ellen Joswiak, RN, MA
Assistant Professor of Nursing
Luther College
Decorah, Iowa

Staff Nurse
Mayo Medical Center
Rochester, Minnesota

Betsy Ann Skrha Kennedy, RN, MS, CS, LCCE
Nursing Instructor
Rochester Community and Technical College
Rochester, Minnesota

Robin M. Lally, PhD, RN, BA, AOCN, CNS
Teaching Specialist
School of Nursing, University of Minnesota
Minneapolis, Minnesota

Penny Leake, RN, PhD
Associate Professor
Luther College
Decorah, Iowa

Barbara Mandleco, RN, PhD
Associate Professor and Undergraduate Program
    Coordinator
College of Nursing, Brigham Young University
Provo, Utah

Gerry Matsumura, RN, PhD, MSN, BSN
Former Associate Professor of Nursing
Brigham Young University
Provo, Utah

Alberta McCaleb, RN, DSN
Associate Professor and Chair of Undergraduate
    Studies
University of Alabama School of Nursing, University
    of Alabama at Birmingham
Birmingham, Alabama

Deana Moinari, RN, PhD
Associate Professor
Idaho State University
Pocatello, Idaho

Director of Rural Internship
Washington University
Spokane, Washington

JoAnn Mulready-Shick, RN, MS
Dean, Nursing and Allied Health
Roxbury Community College
Boston, Massachusetts

Patricia Murdoch, RN, MS
Nurse Practitioner
University of Illinois, Chicago
Urbana, Illinois

Jayme S. Nelson, RN, MS, ARNP-C
Adult Nurse Practitioner and Assistant Professor of
    Nursing
Luther College
Decorah, Iowa

Janice Nuuhiwa, MSN, CPON, APN/CNS
Staff Development Specialist
Hematology/Oncology/Stem Cell Transplant
    Division, Children's Memorial Hospital
Chicago, Illinois

Kristen L. Osborn, MSN, CRNP
Pediatric Nurse Specialist
UAB School of Nursing
UAB Pediatric Hematology/Oncology
Birmingham, Alabama

Karen D. Peterson, RN, MSN, BSN, PNP
Pediatric Nurse Practitioner
Division of Endocrinology, Children's Memorial
    Hospital
Chicago, Illinois

Kristin Sandau, RN, PhD
Critical Care Education Coordinator
Abbott Northwest Hospital
Minneapolis, Minnesota

Elizabeth Sawyer, RN, BSN, CCRN
Registered Nurse
United Hospital
St. Paul, Minnesota

Lisa A. Seldomridge, RN, PhD
Associate Professor of Nursing
Salisbury University
Salisbury, Maryland

Janice L. Vincent, RN, DSN
Assistant Professor
University of Alabama School of Nursing, University
    of Alabama at Birmingham
Birmingham, Alabama

Margaret Vogel, RN, MSN, BSN
Former Nursing Instructor
Rochester Community & Technical College
Rochester, Minnesota

Wound, Ostomy, and Continence Nurse
Enterstomal Therapy
Mayo Clinic
Rochester, Minnesota

Mary Shannon Ward, RN, MSN
Director
Clinic Infectious Disease
Children's Memorial Hospital
Chicago, Illinois

REVIEWERS

Dr. Geri Beers, RN, EdD
Associate Professor of Nursing
Samford University
Birmingham, Alabama

Nancy D. Bingaman, RN, MS
Nursing Instructor
Maurine Church Coburn School of Nursing, Monterey
    Peninsula College
Monterey, California

Carol Boswell, EdD, RN
Associate Professor
College of Nursing, Texas Tech University Health
    Sciences Center
Odessa, Texas

Judy A. Bourrand, RN, MSN
Assistant Professor
Ida V. Moffett School of Nursing, Samford University
Birmingham, Alabama

Clara Willard Boyle, RN, BS, MS, EdD
Associate Professor
Salem State College
Salem, Massachusetts

Rebecca Gesler, MSN, RN
Assistant Professor
Spalding University
Louisville, Kentucky

Loretta J. Heuer, PhD, RN, FAAN
Associate Professor
College of Nursing, University of North Dakota
Grand Forks, North Dakota

Susan Hinck, PhD, RN, CS
Associate Professor
Department of Nursing, Missouri State University
Springfield, Missouri

Mary M. Hoke, PhD, APRN-BC
Academic Department Head
New Mexico State University
Las Cruces, New Mexico

Ann Putnam Johnson, EdD, RN
Professor of Nursing and Associate Dean, College of
    Applied Sciences
Western Carolina University
Cullowhee, North Carolina

Brenda P. Johnson, PhD, RN
Associate Professor
Department of Nursing, Southeast Missouri State
    University
Cape Girardeau, Missouri

Pat S. Kupina, RN, MSN
Professor of Nursing
Joliet Junior College
Joliet, Illinois

Mary Lashley, RN, PhD, APRN, BC
Associate Professor
Department of Nursing, Towson University
Towson, Maryland

Melissa Lickteig, EdD, RN
Assistant Professor
School of Nursing, Georgia Southern University
Statesboro, Georgia

Caron Martin, MSN, RN
Associate Professsor
School of Nursing and Health Professions, Northern
    Kentucky University
Highland Heights, Kentucky

**Darlene Mathis, MSN, RN, APRN, BC, NP-C,
CNE, CRNP**
Assistant Professor and Certified Nurse Educator
Ida V. Moffett School of Nursing, Samford University

Family Nurse Practitioner
Birmingham Health Care
Birmingham, Alabama

Carol E. Meadows, MNSc, RNP, APN
Instructor
Eleanor Mann School of Nursing, University of
    Arkansas
Fayetteville, Arkansas

Margaret A. Miklancie, PhD, RN
Assistant Professor
College of Nursing & Health Science, George Mason
    University
Fairfax, Virginia

Frances D. Monahan, PhD, RN
Professor of Nursing
SUNY Rockland Community College
Spring Valley, New York

Consultant, Excelsior College
Albany, New York

Deb Poling, MSN, APRN, BC, FNP, ANP
Assistant Professor
Regis University
Denver, Colorado

Case Manager
The Childrens Hospital
Denver, Colorado

Abby Selby, MNSc, RN
Faculty, Mental Health and Illness
Eleanor Mann School of Nursing, College of
    Education and Health Professions, University of
    Arkansas
Fayetteville, Arkansas

PRN Educator, Mental Health Topics
Northwest Health System
Springdale, Arkansas

Sarah E. Shannon, PhD, RN
Associate Professor, Biobehavioral Nursing and
    Health Systems
Adjunct Associate Professor, Medical History and
    Ethics
University of Washington
Seattle, Washington

Susan Sienkiewicz, MA, RN
Professor
Community College of Rhode Island
Warwick, Rhode Island

Maria A. Smith, DSN, RN, CCRN
Professor
School of Nursing, Middle Tennessee State University
Murfreesboro, Tennessee

Ellen Stuart, MSN, RN
Professor, Mental Health Nursing
Grand Rapids Community College
Grand Rapids, Michigan

Karen Gahan Tarnow, RN, PhD
Faculty
School of Nursing, University of Kansas
Kansas City, Kansas

Janice Tazbir, RN, MS, CCRN
Associate Professor of Nursing
School of Nursing, Purdue University—Calumet
Hammond, Indiana

Patricia C. Wagner, MSN, RNC
Clinical Assistant Professor
MCN Department, College of Nursing, University of
    South Alabama
Mobile, Alabama

PREFACE

Nursing is rapidly changing to meet the health care environment's needs and demands. Clients have very significant problems but due to the influx of technology have shorter hospital stays. To meet these needs, nurses must not only be more skilled practitioners but proficient in the areas of prioritization and delegation. In addition, they must become critical thinkers, decision makers, and leaders. As a result of the nursing profession's changing image and demands, the National Council of State Boards of Nursing has revised the National Council of Licensure Examination for Registered Nurses (NCLEX-RN®) to meet the challenges of health care in the 21st century. *Practice Questions for NCLEX-RN®* answers the challenge by providing the student with a powerful learning tool: a comprehensive practice text and CD to help you pass the NCLEX-RN® and launch your nursing career.

Practice Questions for NCLEX-RN® has 4400 questions that cover all of the topics included on the NCLEX examination. Each and every question is accompanied with a rationale for right and wrong choices as well as categories that identify the area of the nursing process, client need (from the current test plan), cognitive level, and subject area. This allows the student to pinpoint areas of further study and maximize his or her study time.

ACCOMPANYING MATERIALS

The CD-ROM included with this text holds 4400 test questions in an environment that simulates the test-taking experience. Students can test their knowledge and test-taking skills in two ways: learning mode and test mode. In learning mode, the rationale for correct and incorrect responses is immediately given after each question is answered. In test mode, the student will receive a score. Questions answered incorrectly may be reviewed after completing the exam.

In either mode, once the practice test is completed, the student has the option to view the results through bar-graph percentages that represent the areas of the test plan, cognitive levels, subject area, and client need. This element gives the student a clear and concise visual presentation of the enormous amounts of information that further enhance and maximize study time.

NATIONAL COUNCIL TEST PLAN FOR REGISTERED NURSES

The National Council of State Boards of Nursing (NCSBN) develops a licensure examination that is responsible for regulating the entrance of nursing practice in the United States.

Development of the Test Plan

Before presenting the actual test plan for the NCLEX-RN®, it is essential to understand the NCLEX-RN® test development procedure. It takes 18 months for each item to be taken through every step of the test development procedure to ensure a completely valid and reliable exam that measures the knowledge, skill, and ability to be a safe entry-level registered nurse.

The development of the NCLEX-RN® test plan goes through several steps. First, a job analysis is performed every 3 years by surveying new graduates of schools of nursing for what skills and procedures are most frequently performed. Hand washing and medication administration are two skills that, according to new graduates, are frequently performed. This job analysis serves as a guide in the test plan's development from which the items are developed according to the client need and the nursing process phase. Second, the test plan guides the development of the NCLEX-RN®. Although every candidate's exam is different, each exam is developed to equally assess the candidate's knowledge, skill, and ability to promote, maintain, or restore a client's health. In this way, the client is assessed to be a safe entry-level registered nurse.

COGNITIVE LEVELS

Each NCLEX-RN® item will be written to the cognitive level based on Bloom's taxonomy and both the Client Need category and subcategory. Although knowledge, comprehension, application, and analysis are cognitive levels, the majority of the items on the

NCLEX-RN® are written to the application and analysis level. Items written at the application and analysis level are more difficult and require critical thinking to answer.

CLIENT NEEDS AND CLIENT NEEDS SUBCATEGORIES

In addition to each NCLEX-RN® item being written to a cognitive level, each item is also written to Client Needs and Client Needs Subcategories. The Client Needs explain nursing tasks and competencies across the life span and in all client settings. There are four major categories of Client Needs (see Table 1).

Table 1   Categories of Client Needs

Client Needs I	Safe and Effective Care Environment
Client Needs II	Health Promotion and Maintenance
Client Needs III	Psychosocial Integrity
Client Needs IV	Physiological Integrity

The first Client Needs category, Safe and Effective Care Environment, ensures client outcomes by directly delivering or indirectly supervising nursing care while maintaining the safety of clients, their families, or health care individuals. The second Client Needs category, Health Promotion and Maintenance, provides care directly to or indirectly to clients and their families while considering principles of growth and development, in addition to preventing health problems and promoting an optimal health status. Psychosocial Integrity, the third Client Needs category, provides care to clients with chronic mental illness or facilitates emotional support to families of clients with varying degrees of physical or mental illness. The fourth and last Client Needs category, Physiological Integrity, provides basic and advanced nursing care including medications and parenteral therapies and decreases the potential for risks.

Two of the four Client Needs categories have subcategories (see Table 2).

Table 2   Client Needs Subcategories

Client Needs Category	Client Needs Subcategory
I. Safe and Effective Care Environment	Management of Care
	Safety and Infection Control
IV. Physiological Integrity	Basic Care and Comfort
	Pharmacological and Parenteral Therapies
	Reduction of Risk Potential
	Physiological Adaptation

The Client Needs categories of Health Promotion and Maintenance and Psychosocial Integrity do not have subcategories.

The percent of items under each Client Needs category and subcategory on each candidate's examination is constantly being evaluated through research. The total percent of items on any candidate's examination for the Client's Needs Safe and Effective Care Environment falls between 21%–36%. There are two subcategories under Safe and Effective Care Environment: Management of Care with 13%–19% of the total items, and Safety and Infection Control with 8%–14% of the total items. These subcategory percentages are very reflective of health care in the 21st century with delegation and the advent of new diseases such as severe acute respiratory syndrome (SARS), West Nile Virus, and the possibility of diseases such as anthrax and smallpox. Items coming from the Management of Care (see Table 3) and Safety and Infection Control subcategories (see Table 4) come from many content areas.

Table 3   Management of Care Subcategory Content Areas

Advanced directives and living wills
Case management
Collaboration
Confidentiality
Delegation
Ethical issues
Informed consent
Management of care
Priorities
Rights of clients
Staff development

Table 4   Safety and Infection Control Subcategory Content Areas

Asepsis (medical and surgical)
Bioterrorism and planning for disasters
Equipment safety
Prevention of accidents and injuries
Prevention of errors
Safety in the home
Precaution procedures (airborne, contact, droplet, and standard)
Restraints

The second Client Needs category, Health Promotion and Maintenance, does not have a subcategory. The possibility of items on any candidate's examination ranges from 6%–12%. Health Promotion and Maintenance provides direct and indirect care to clients and their families. This subcategory considers principles of growth and development while preventing health problems and promoting an optimal health status including development, obstetrics, health prevention, and promotion behaviors (see Table 5).

Table 5 Health Promotion and Maintenance Client Needs Content Areas

Aging
Body image changes (anticipated)
Concepts of growth and development
Concepts of health and wellness
Education of clients and families
Family planning high-risk behaviors
Newborn care (antepartum, intrapartum, and postpartum)
Physical assessment skills
Prevention of disease
Screening for health problems
Self-care
Vaccinations and immunizations

Like Health Promotion and Maintenance, Psychosocial Integrity does not have subcategories under the Client Needs category. Psychosocial Integrity provides care to clients with chronic mental illness and facilitates emotional support to families of clients with varying degrees of physical or mental illness. Many content areas are available from which items are asked (see Table 6).

Table 6 Psychosocial Integrity Client Needs Content Areas

Body image changes (unanticipated)
Changes in family or significant other roles
Chemical dependency
Concepts of death and dying
Coping strategies
Crisis management
Cultural issues
End-of-life issues
Family dynamics
Management of behavioral issues
Neglect and abuse
Spiritual issues
Stress
Therapeutic communication

The fourth and final Client Needs category, Physiological Integrity, encompasses the majority of items on the NCLEX-RN®, or 43%–67%. As previously defined, Physiological Integrity ranges from the most basic care to advanced nursing care including medication and parenteral therapies while decreasing potential risks. Because this Client Needs category makes up the largest percent of any candidate's examination, Table 7 breaks down the content areas into each subcategory to give you an overview of study items.

Table 7 Physiological Integrity Client Needs Content Areas

Subcategory 1: Basic Care and Comfort
Alternative and complementary therapies
Comfort interventions that are not pharmaceutical
Devices considered assistive
Elimination issues
Hygienic issues
Mobility and immobility issues
Nutritional issues
Palliative care
Rest and sleep issues

Subcategory 2: Pharmacological and Parenteral Therapies
Adverse effects, contraindications, nursing implications, interventions
Blood and blood products
Calculations
Central venous access devices
Intravenous therapy
Medication administration
Parenteral nutrition

Subcategory 3: Reduction of Risk Potential
Complications of health deviations and surgical procedures
Conscious sedation
Diagnostic procedures
Interpretation of diagnostic and laboratory tests
Laboratory test procedures
Vital signs

Subcategory 4: Physiological Adaptation
Body systems alterations
Emergencies
Imbalances of fluid and electrolytes
Hemodynamics
Pathophysiology
Radiation therapy

TEST-TAKING STRATEGIES

Always begin by reading the entire question and all of the answers carefully before selecting a response. If the answer is not immediately known, use test-taking strategies to help maximize your success.

Analyze the Stem

A good stem will not have a lot of extraneous information in it that is not necessary for answering the item. For example, names are never used on the NCLEX exam. They have no bearing on the item. Other biographical data such as age, sex, race, and occupation are never used unless they are necessary for answering the item. For example, some conditions occur more frequently in women or men, certain races, certain ages, or in certain types of occupations. In these cases, it is essential to present this information to correctly answer the item. For example, sickle cell anemia occurs in African American individuals.

When starting to answer each question, carefully look at the stem. The stem is the part of the item that is actually asking the question. It may be stated as a question with a question mark or it may be a statement in which the answer completes the statement. There are other terms that may appear in a stem that also ask for you to prioritize and perform the most important intervention first. If "most appropriate," "most important," "essential," "most likely," "initial," and "best" appear in the stem, the question is asking you to prioritize and decide which intervention should be first because it is more important than all of the other choices.

There are no negative stems in the actual NCLEX examination. You will never find an item that asks for the exception such as: Which of the following would be the exception? The NCLEX examination is not concerned with what the nurse would never do; the NCLEX focuses on what the nurse should do in order to be a safe practitioner.

ALTERNATIVE ITEM FORMAT

In 2003 the NCSBN introduced alternative item format questions that include fill-in-the-blank, multiple response, and "hot spot" questions.

Fill-in-the-Blank Questions

A fill-in-the-blank question may be a short phrase requiring one or two words to complete the sentence or a few descriptive sentences requiring an answer that generally includes one or two words. Additionally, the NCLEX frequently uses this format to write a calculation question. Just enough information is given in a fill-in-the blank question to answer the question. The information is specific so that it leads the test-taker to only one possible answer. Fill-in-the-blank questions may be written at any of the four cognitive levels (knowledge, comprehension, application, or analysis).

The Multiple-Response Question

The multiple-response question may be stated as a complete sentence ending with a question mark or an incomplete sentence requiring one of the options to complete the stem. Instead of having four options, you generally have six options from which to choose the correct keys. Each option will have a little square box to the left of the number. After reading each option, you will choose those options that relate to the stem as true statements and

place an "x" in the boxes. These questions focus heavily on prioritization and critical thinking.

"Hot Spot" Questions

A picture or graph question is the third type of innovative question that NCLEX-RN® has implemented. It asks you to identify something on a picture or graph as asked in the stem. Choosing the location on a picture, supplying some data on a graph, or filling in some information on a graph as asked in the stem is called identifying the hot spot and is considered the key. When you study, think about questions that could ask about anatomy, tables, or graphs.

EXAMINATION APPLICATION PROCESS

Shortly before or following graduation from your school of nursing, you will need to apply for licensure from the board of nursing in the state or territory where you wish to practice. A frequently asked question is, "If I am graduating from nursing school in one state but am moving to another state, where should I take the NCLEX-RN®?" You should always apply for licensure in the state where you want to practice. Although licensure may be transferred from one state to another, taking the NCLEX in the state where you wish to practice saves you the time of applying for licensure in another state and saves you the additional cost of the reciprocity.

After applying to the state board of nursing, you will receive an NCLEX-RN® Examination Candidate Bulletin that contains your application and will give you detailed directions on how to apply for the NCLEX-RN®. It is a good idea to keep the Candidate Bulletin until you take the test and receive your results in case you have questions that the bulletin can answer for you. After completing the application, you should submit it with a certified check, cashier's check, or money to the Pearson VUE group (the National Council's contracted testing service) or register by phone for no additional fee. After receiving your application, Pearson VUE will notify you by mail that they have received your application. Prior to submitting your application you should notify your state board of nursing if you have a disability, so that special accommodations can be provided at the testing center.

Your state board of nursing will let Pearson VUE know of your eligibility to take the NCLEX-RN®. Pearson VUE will send you an Authorization to Test (ATT) and information on how to schedule and take the NCLEX-RN® as well as testing centers for your area generally within 4 weeks of receipt of your Authorization to Test. The NCLEX-RN® is administered at the Sylvan Technology Centers. The Sylvan centers are generally conveniently located in retail areas that have free parking and access to public transportation. It is recommended that you contact the Sylvan center of your choice after receiving your Authorization to Test form as soon as possible to get your desired date and time. You should not wait until you get close to the expiration date on the Authorization to Test form because the Sylvan center may not be able to accommodate your request to test before the expiration date. If you pass the expiration date on the Authorization to Test form, you will have to reapply and pay the fee again. The Sylvan center must schedule an appointment for testing within 30 days of your request if you are a first-time taker of the NCLEX-RN® examination. If you are a repeat taker, the Sylvan center will schedule your test date and time within 45 days of your call.

DAY OF THE TEST

The Sylvan centers are very user friendly and will accommodate the opportunity to test 15 hours a day and 6 days a week. Further testing may occur on Sundays during peak times, such as the summer months when a majority of first-time graduates are taking the NCLEX-RN®. After arranging a testing date and time, you should go to the testing center at least 30 minutes before your scheduled time to ensure you have all your allotted time for the test. If you arrive more than 30 minutes late for your scheduled test, you may have to forfeit your examination and registration fee. The Sylvan center will then notify your board of nursing of your failure to take the test. Family and friends may accompany you to the test center but will not be permitted to wait in the testing center or contact you during any portion of the test.

You will need to take your Authorization to Test form, a current picture identification with your signature such as a driver's license, and a secondary form of identification such as a school ID or Social Security card with you on the day of the test. After displaying your identification, your picture and thumbprint will be taken and you will be asked to sign your name.

You will not be allowed to take personal belongings such as papers, books, scratch paper, school materials, purse, pens, pencils, beepers, cell phones, or handheld calculators into your testing cubicle. There is no eating, drinking, or smoking in the testing area. Taking a nursing textbook or any NCLEX materials into the testing area is strictly prohibited. As a result, you may be asked to leave the testing center, and your examination may be cancelled. You will be given a note board and writing utensil to use during the test; it can be replaced as often as necessary, but at no time is it to be removed from the facility.

You will be escorted to your testing cubicle initially for a brief orientation. Although there is fluorescent lighting used in the testing room, if you wish for a desk light, one will be provided for you.

You will have 5 hours to take the test including a short tutorial before you begin the examination, two scheduled breaks, and unscheduled breaks as necessary. A 10-minute break is mandatory after 2 hours of testing. After 3½ hours there is another 10-minute scheduled break that is optional. You will be notified on the computer screen when it is time for all scheduled breaks, at which point you will be required to leave your testing site. You are also required to show your picture ID and sign your name before leaving and reentering the testing room. During your examination, you must raise your hand if you need anything or want to leave your testing cubicle for any reason.

The pre-examination computer tutorial includes a brief summary of the computer functions needed to answer the items, as well as three sample items. A frequently asked question is, "Do I have to be an expert at operating the computer to take the test?" The answer is no. The tutorial will take you through step by step, how to highlight and record your answer. The tutorial also reviews the use of the on-screen calculator. Its use is optional when you have a calculation item. Even after starting your examination, you may raise your hand if you have a question about any computer function. At the end of your test, you will be given a brief questionnaire asking about your experience with the computerized test. After you have finished the questionnaire, you must raise your hand to be dismissed from the testing area. Your note board and writing utensil will be collected and you will be dismissed.

The actual NCLEX-RN® examination may contain up to 265 items, including 250 real items that will be scored and 15 new "tryout" items. A "tryout" item is a first-time item that is being piloted to evaluate its level of difficulty. It is not scored and does not affect whether your pass or fail the examination. It is very important that you understand that in no way is the test length indicative of passing or failing. You should plan on allowing yourself 1 minute per item, assuming you will need the 5-hour time limit to answer the maximum number of items or 265; you can track your progress by referring to the timer in the upper left corner of the screen and the item number in the upper right corner. The purpose behind displaying the test length and item number is to keep you informed of your progress so you can pace yourself.

TEST SCORING

Using Computer Adaptive Testing (CAT), each candidate begins the examination with an item of the same easy level of difficulty. If a candidate answers this item correctly, the next item will be slightly more difficult. If this item is answered correctly, the following item will be slightly more difficult, and the process will continue with more difficult items until an item is missed. If an item is missed, then the following item will be slightly easier. If that item is also missed, then the next item will be easier than the last one. This process of administering an easier item will continue until an item is correctly answered. Answering an item correctly will result in the subsequent item being more difficult. Putting this into perspective, each item is individualized to fairly and completely evaluate your knowledge, skill, and ability to be a safe registered nurse. After each item, your competency level is computed by the computer and analyzed as to the area of the test plan and level of difficulty of that item.

When you have answered 50% of your items correctly or incorrectly, the margin of error is very small and the indication is clear you have either passed or failed. The goal of your examination and every candidate's examination is to correctly answer 50% of all items. This is why some candidates' examinations are short and may end after 75 items. In this case, 50% or more of the 60 real or scored items were answered either correctly or incorrectly and you either pass or fail. Every candidate's score is computer analyzed after the minimum number of items has been answered. After your items have been analyzed, one of three situations will occur. You will pass, fail, or continue to get more items. A candidate who answers all 265 items has simply taken more time and items to establish the margin of error.

The Sylvan center will transmit your NCLEX test results to Pearson VUE, which in turn transmits the results to your board of nursing. You may have heard a rumor that, at the end of the test, the computer displays the word "pass" or "fail" on the screen. This is not true. Your board of nursing will send you your results. It generally takes 2 to 4 weeks to obtain results. After completing the examination, you will be given information on obtaining quick results after 48 hours of the scheduled exam. There is a small fee to obtain results by the Internet or phone.

RESULTS ANALYSES

A Diagnostic Profile is generated for all candidates who fail the NCLEX-RN®. The Diagnostic Profile, which generally takes 2 to 4 weeks to receive, will come in the mail with the results of your examination. If you opt to obtain your results 48 hours after your examination either by phone or the Internet and you happen to fail, you will have to wait for your mailed results to receive your Diagnostic Profile.

The Diagnostic Profile will provide several pieces of information to help you in preparing for your retake examination. The first piece of information is how close you were to the passage standard. It will also let you know how many total items you answered. Generally candidates who answered all 265 items are either very close to the passing or failing standard.

On the back page of the Diagnostic Profile is an analysis of how well you did on each of the NCLEX-RN® test plan content areas designed to inform you on how to be successful on your future examination. The improvement needed in each of the content areas is outlined on this profile. The amount of improvement needed will range from a "a very small amount of improvement" to "a very large amount of improvement." These descriptions can only be used to identify Client Needs categories and subcategories. For example, you may need "a very large amount of improvement" in the Safety and Infection Control subcategory of the Client Needs of Safe and Effective Care Environment but "a very small amount of improvement" in the Basic Care and Comfort subcategory of the Client Needs of Physiological Integrity. These recommendations can only be used to identify overall weaknesses and strengths and can be used to further guide you in future preparation to retake the examination.

The text's concept, scope, and design represent a commitment to help the graduate RN reach a full professional potential. Good luck on your NCLEX-RN® examination!

Donna Faye Gauwitz, RN, MS

ACKNOWLEDGMENTS

First and foremost, I want to thank Matthew Kane, Director of Learning Solutions at Delmar Cengage Learning, for his belief and support in me and in my ability to write.

A very special thanks goes to Patty Gaworecki, Product Manager, whom I worked with closely over the course of writing this book for her consultations and guidance.

A very special thanks goes to Dave Buddle, Content Project Manager, whom I worked with closely through the copy edit process.

I wish to thank all of the people behind the scenes at Delmar Cengage Learning that contributed in the publication process of this valuable book.

All of the contributors are thanked for their expertise in providing chapter content relevant to a thorough review of the nursing literature. The reviewers are thanked for their valuable comments on the manuscript.

I want to thank all of my nursing students at Methodist Hospital School of Nursing in Peoria, Illinois; Barry University in Miami Shores, Florida; Broward Community College in Pembroke Pines, Florida; and the University of Minnesota in Minneapolis, Minnesota, for their enthusiasm in my NCLEX-style test questions and in my ability to prepare them to take the NCLEX-RN®. I want to thank all of the nursing graduates at Mayo Clinic in Rochester that took my NCLEX-RN® review course in their preparation to take the NCLEX-RN® and their positive feedback.

Lastly and most importantly, I want to thank my husband and best friend, William J. Gauwitz, for his continual support of my commitment to this book over the years of development and when it had to take priority. A very special thanks also goes to him for his computer excellence and skills that were gladly utilized in this book's production.

Donna Faye Gauwitz, RN, MS

ABOUT THE AUTHOR

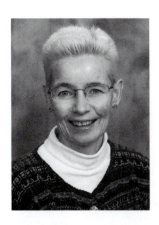

Donna Faye Gauwitz, RN, MS, received her diploma in nursing from St. Francis School of Nursing in Peoria, Illinois. After graduation, she worked on medical-surgical nursing units, specifically neurology, and on the psychiatric unit at St. Francis Hospital, a major acute care facility and trauma center in central Illinois. She immediately began work on her Bachelor of Science degree at Bradley University in Peoria, Illinois. After graduating with a BSN, Donna began her career in nursing education as a staff development coordinator at St. Francis Medical Center, orienting new graduate nurses to a large medical-surgical unit. She was also adjunct faculty at Illinois Central College in East Peoria and at Illinois Wesleyan University in Bloomington, teaching medical-surgical and pediatric nursing. While at Illinois Central College she developed and taught a new college course, "Introduction to Eating Disorders."

Donna further developed her research and publishing interests as a research assistant at the University of Illinois Department of Psychiatry and Behavioral Medicine in Peoria, and at Northwestern University College of Nursing in Chicago, Illinois. She did the research and wrote the proposal for an eating disorder clinic and became the director of the clinic at St. Francis Medical Center in Peoria, Illinois.

Her pursuit of advanced education took her to Northwestern University College of Nursing in Evanston, Illinois, to obtain her master's degree. After graduation from Northwestern University, Donna began her full-time teaching career at Methodist Medical Center in Peoria, Illinois, followed by teaching medical-surgical, orthopedics, rehabilitative, women's health, and neurology nursing at Barry University in Miami Shores, Florida, and Broward Community College in Pembroke Pines, Florida.

After relocating to Minnesota she became a nursing education specialist for an acute care surgical unit at the Mayo Clinic in Rochester, Minnesota. Because of her unique expertise as an NCLEX-RN® item writer, while at the Mayo Clinic she was asked to teach NCLEX review courses for new registered nurse graduates to prepare them to take the NCLEX-RN®. Her love of nursing education then took her to the University of Minnesota as the coordinator of the Nursing Skills Laboratory in Minneapolis, Minnesota.

During her tenure in education she had the opportunity to serve as an item writer eight times for the National Council of State Boards of Nursing in the development of the NCLEX-RN®. She was also asked to publish an article in the *Insight,* a National Council of State Boards of Nursing publication. She further pursued her interest in publishing with three articles in the *Nursing* journal and one article in the *American Journal of Nursing.*

She is also the author of *Administering Medications: Pharmacology for Health Careers.* Donna has also served as a medical expert in several malpractice cases.

Donna is a member of Sigma Theta Tau and has been listed in *Who's Who in American Nursing.*

UNIT I

Medical-Surgical Nursing

Eye, Ear, Nose, and Throat Disorders

1

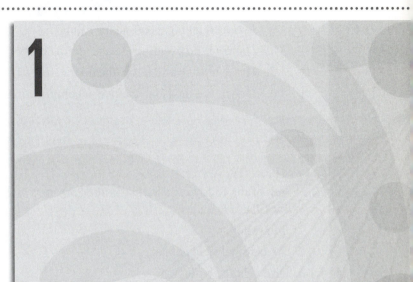

1. Which of the following should the nurse include in the discharge instructions for a client after cataract surgery?

   Select all that apply:

   [   ] 1. Use aseptic technique to apply eye medication

   [   ] 2. Expect an increase in pain after surgery

   [   ] 3. Avoid coughing, bending, or lifting

   [   ] 4. There are no eye drops to use after surgery

   [   ] 5. The eye patch will cover the operative eye for 24 hours

   [   ] 6. A decrease in visual acuity is a complication

2. Which of the following should the nurse include in the assessment of the client's cranial nerves and extraocular eye muscles?

   1. Red reflex

   2. Six cardinal fields of gaze

   3. Disc characteristics

   4. Macular characteristics

3. When completing a measurement of the client's visual acuity, which of the following would be appropriate?

   1. Ophthalmoscope

   2. Penlight

   3. Visual field

   4. Snellen chart

Answer: 1, 3, 5

Rationale: Following cataract surgery, it is appropriate to use aseptic technique to apply eye medications; to instruct the client to avoid coughing, bending, or lifting; and to keep the operative eye patched for 24 hours. Using aseptic technique during the application of eye medications prevents an eye infection. Instructing the client to avoid coughing, bending, or lifting prevents increased intraocular pressure. The client should be instructed that although the eye patch covers the operative eye for only 24 hours, one to two weeks may be necessary to meet visual needs. A decreased visual acuity is not a complication. There should not be an increase in pain after surgery. All pain not relieved by medications should be reported.

Nursing process: Planning

Client need: Health Promotion and Maintenance

Cognitive level: Application

Subject area: Medical-Surgical

Answer: 2

Rationale: When assessing the cranial nerves (III, IV, and VI) and the six extraocular muscles, the six cardinal fields of gaze are utilized. The red reflex, disc characteristics, and macular characteristics are used to inspect the internal eye.

Nursing process: Assessment

Client need: Physiological Adaptation

Cognitive level: Application

Subject area: Medical-Surgical

Answer: 4

Rationale: The measurement of visual acuity includes the Snellen or E chart to test cranial nerve II. The ophthalmoscope and penlight illuminate inner eye structures, while the visual field evaluates cranial nerves and movement in the extraocular eye muscles.

Nursing process: Assessment

Client need: Physiological Adaptation

Cognitive level: Application

Subject area: Medical-Surgical

4. The nurse collects a history from a client suspected of a sensorineural hearing loss. Which of the following findings supports the diagnosis and should be reported?
   1. The ability to hear high-pitched sounds
   2. Frequent ear irrigations for dry, hard cerumen
   3. A history of exposure to excessive noise over a period of time
   4. The client speaks softly

5. Which of the following nursing measures should receive priority in the client's plan of care after eye surgery?
   1. Prevent increased intraocular pressure and infection
   2. Instruct on the importance of follow-up
   3. Instruct on how to perform the Valsalva maneuver
   4. Pain management

6. The nurse should consider which of the following drugs taken by a client with glaucoma? Drugs that
   1. increase intraocular pressure.
   2. decrease intraocular pressure.
   3. decrease vitreous humor.
   4. cause anesthesia.

7. The nurse implements which of the following interventions to reduce intraocular pressure following eye surgery?
   1. Applies hot compresses
   2. Provides bright lighting in the room
   3. Applies gentle pressure on the affected eye
   4. Keeps the head of the bed elevated

Answer: 3

Rationale: Sensorineural hearing loss is a permanent loss that is not correctable. It is a problem with the inner ear caused by excessive noise over a period of time, the aging process, Ménière's disease, ototoxicity, or congenital or other diseases.

Nursing process: Analysis

Client need: Physiological Adaptation

Cognitive level: Application

Subject area: Medical-Surgical

Answer: 1

Rationale: Increased intraocular pressure and infection can cause serious vision complications. Postoperative restrictions on head positioning, bending, coughing, and the Valsalva maneuver will protect the eye from increased intraocular pressure and prevent injury. Follow-up care will be a concern later in the recovery process.

Nursing process: Planning

Client need: Management of Care

Cognitive level: Analysis

Subject area: Medical-Surgical

Answer: 1

Rationale: Glaucoma causes increased intraocular pressure, which can damage the optic nerve. The drugs used to treat glaucoma would decrease intraocular pressure by decreasing aqueous humor in the anterior chamber. An anesthetic would not reduce the intraocular pressure.

Nursing process: Analysis

Client need: Pharmacological and Parenteral Therapies

Cognitive level: Analysis

Subject area: Pharmacologic

Answer: 4

Rationale: Elevating the head of the bed reduces intraocular pressure, as do applying cold compresses and dimming the lights in the room. Applying hot compresses or providing bright lights both would increase intraocular pressure. Pressure on the eye would also increase intraocular pressure.

Nursing process: Implementation

Client need: Physiological Adaptation

Cognitive level: Application

Subject area: Medical-Surgical

8. The nurse assesses which of the following to cause a conductive hearing loss?
Select all that apply:

[   ] **1.** Cerumen

[   ] **2.** Loud noise

[   ] **3.** Otosclerosis

[   ] **4.** Ménière's disease

[   ] **5.** Ototoxicity

[   ] **6.** Middle ear disease

9. The client who just had cataract removal complains of nausea and severe pain in the operative eye. Which of the following nursing actions is the priority in this client's plan of care?

1. Administer drugs for the pain and nausea

2. Notify the physician immediately

3. Assure the client that this is normal after surgery

4. Turn the client to the operative side every two hours

10. The client received instruction following cataract surgery. Which of the following statements by the client indicates the client understood the instruction?

1. "Aspirin is all I need for the soreness."

2. "I will sleep on the operative side."

3. "I will wear an eye shield at night and glasses during the day."

4. "I will not lift anything over 15 pounds."

11. Because a client has glaucoma, plans for nursing interventions should include

1. a decrease in fluid intake.

2. avoiding reading and watching television.

3. a decrease in the salt in the diet.

4. taking eye medications for life.

Answer: 1, 3, 6

Rationale: Conductive hearing loss is a correctable hearing loss that occurs in the middle and outer ear. It affects sound transmitted from the outer to inner ear. Causes include cerumen (earwax), otosclerosis, and middle ear disease. Sustained loud noise, Ménière's disease, and ototoxicity are causes of sensorineural loss.

Nursing process: Assessment

Client need: Physiological Adaptation

Cognitive level: Application

Subject area: Medical-Surgical

Answer: 2

Rationale: Severe pain and pain accompanied by complaints of nausea indicate an increase in intraocular pressure. These complaints need to be reported immediately to prevent damage to the eye. The physician may order drugs or take the client back to surgery. Turning on the operative side is to be avoided because it increases intraocular pressure.

Nursing process: Planning

Client need: Management of Care

Cognitive level: Analysis

Subject area: Medical-Surgical

Answer: 3

Rationale: The client should wear an eye shield or glasses to protect the eye from injury or from rubbing the eye. Tylenol would be ordered for discomfort. Aspirin or drugs containing aspirin would not be used. The client should sleep on the unoperated side. The lifting restriction after surgery is 5 pounds or less. Lifting any more than 5 pounds would increase intraocular pressure.

Nursing process: Evaluation

Client need: Health Promotion and Maintenance

Cognitive level: Analysis

Subject area: Medical-Surgical

Answer: 4

Rationale: Eye medications are critical in the effective treatment of glaucoma. The client needs instruction that these are needed for the rest of his or her life. Decreasing salt and fluids do not decrease intraocular fluids. Normal reading or watching television will not affect glaucoma.

Nursing process: Planning

Client need: Physiological Adaptation

Cognitive level: Application

Subject area: Medical-Surgical

12. Which of the following assessments indicate a client has sustained a retinal detachment? Select all that apply:

[   ] **1.** Floaters

[   ] **2.** A sharp, sudden pain in the eye

[   ] **3.** Photopsia

[   ] **4.** A reddened conjunctiva

[   ] **5.** Glare that is worse at night

[   ] **6.** Ring in the visual field

13. In planning the pre-op care for a client with a retinal detachment, the nurse should include which of the following in the plan of care?

1. Restrict ambulation

2. Maintain flat bed rest

3. Place a patch over the affected eye

4. Have client wear dark glasses for reading and television

14. For a client who sustained a chemical burn from battery acid, the nurse should include which of the following in the emergency procedures?

1. Assess the visual acuity

2. Irrigate the eye with sterile normal saline

3. Swab the eye with antibiotic ointment

4. Cover the affected eye with an eye patch

15. During the initial assessment the nurse observes the presence of bright red drainage on the eye dressing. Which of the following should be the nurse's first action?

1. Report the findings to the physician

2. Continue to monitor the vital signs and pain

3. Note the amount of drainage on the client's record

4. Mark the drainage on the dressing and monitor the amount and color

Answer: 1, 3, 6
Rationale: Retinal detachment is the separation of the retina from the choroid layer, which is the blood supply. Clinical manifestations include photopsia (light flashes), floaters, "cobweb," "hairnet," or ring in the visual field, or loss of peripheral and central vision, all of which are painless.
Nursing process: Assessment
Client need: Physiological Adaptation
Cognitive level: Application
Subject area: Medical-Surgical

Answer: 3
Rationale: Placing an eye patch over the affected eye reduces eye movement. Occasionally bilateral patching may be needed. The size and the location of the retinal break may limit other activities, such as bending, coughing, and the Valsalva maneuver, to prevent further detachment and to promote drainage of fluid. Elevating the head of the bed prevents intraocular pressure.
Nursing process: Planning
Client need: Physiological Adaptation
Cognitive level: Application
Subject area: Medical-Surgical

Answer: 2
Rationale: Emergency care following a chemical burn to the eye includes irrigating the eye immediately with a sterile saline or ocular solution. The irrigation should be continued for at least 10 minutes. After the irrigation, visual acuity will be assessed. Ointment or patching would retain the burn solution on the eye and cause further damage.
Nursing process: Planning
Client need: Safety and Infection Control
Cognitive level: Analysis
Subject area: Medical-Surgical

Answer: 1
Rationale: Bright red drainage on the dressing may indicate hemorrhage and must be reported to the physician immediately. Although monitoring vital signs and the client's pain and recording the amount and color of the drainage are all important interventions, reporting the finding is the priority so emergency measures can be instituted.
Nursing process: Planning
Client need: Management of Care
Cognitive level: Analysis
Subject area: Medical-Surgical

16. How does the nurse correctly straighten the ear canal in preparation to administer eardrops to an adult client? _____

17. The nurse implements which of the following in the plan of care for a client who is hearing impaired?

1. Speaks in a raised voice
2. Speaks slowly
3. Uses exaggerated facial expressions
4. Has the light behind the nurse

18. The nurse is admitting a client in the emergency room with a foreign body in the ear identified as an insect. Which of the following interventions is a priority for the nurse to perform?

1. Irrigate the affected ear
2. Instill diluted alcohol in the affected ear
3. Instill an antibiotic ointment into the affected ear
4. Instill a cortisone ointment into the affected ear

19. The nurse correctly tells a client that the priority goal in the treatment for Ménière's disease is to

1. maintain a sodium-free diet.
2. eliminate environmental noise.
3. preserve the remaining hearing.
4. promote a quiet environment.

Answer: Pull the pinna upward and outward

Rationale: The nurse must pull the pinna upward and outward to straighten the ear canal to administer eardrops in the adult client. The pinna would be pulled down and back in children.

Nursing process: Implementation

Client need: Physiological Adaptation

Cognitive level: Application

Subject area: Medical-Surgical

Answer: 2

Rationale: Speak in a normal tone of voice to the client with impaired hearing. Avoid raising the voice because this does not improve communication. Face the client directly to facilitate lip reading. Moving closer to the better ear may be helpful, but avoid speaking into the impaired ear.

Nursing process: Implementation

Client need: Basic Care and Comfort

Cognitive level: Application

Subject area: Medical-Surgical

Answer: 2

Rationale: Insects are killed before they can be removed unless a flashlight can coax them out. Mineral oil or diluted alcohol will suffocate the insect so that removal by forceps is possible. If the foreign object is vegetable matter it is not irrigated, because this would cause the object to expand and cause a worse impaction. Instilling an antibiotic or cortisone ointment into the affected ear may be done if an infection or inflammation is present.

Nursing process: Planning

Client need: Safety and Infection Control

Cognitive level: Analysis

Subject area: Medical-Surgical

Answer: 3

Rationale: Ménière's disease is an inner ear disease with an unknown etiology that results in vertigo, tinnitus, and a sensorineural hearing loss. The goal of treatment is to preserve the remaining hearing. Nursing interventions include eliminating environmental noise, promoting a quiet environment, and restricting caffeine, nicotine, and alcohol. Prescribing a low-sodium diet has also been proven helpful in some clients.

Nursing process: Implementation

Client need: Management of Care

Cognitive level: Analysis

Subject area: Medical-Surgical

20. The nurse is collecting a history from a client suspected of having Ménière's disease. Which of the following assessment findings support the diagnosis?

Select all that apply:

[   ] **1.** Purulent, foul-smelling drainage

[   ] **2.** Fever

[   ] **3.** Vertigo

[   ] **4.** Tinnitus

[   ] **5.** Increased discrimination in understanding of spoken words

[   ] **6.** Sensorineural hearing loss

21. A client has been receiving streptomycin and develops tinnitus, a disturbance in equilibrium, and hearing loss. The nurse reports this as a result of damage to which cranial nerve? _____

22. A client asks the nurse to explain what glaucoma is. Which of the following is the appropriate response by the nurse?

1. "An opacity of the crystalline lens or its capsule."

2. "A curvature of the cornea that becomes unequal."

3. "A separation of the neural retina from the pigment retina."

4. "An increase in the pressure within the eyeball."

23. Which of the following is the priority for the nurse to include in the teaching plan for a client with acute bacterial conjunctivitis?

1. Instruct the client to avoid rubbing the eyes

2. Apply hot moist compresses to the adherent crust on the eye

3. Stress the importance of hand washing

4. Instruct the client to avoid sharing towels

Answer: 3, 4, 6

Rationale: Clinical manifestations of Ménière's disease include sensorineural hearing loss, vertigo, and tinnitus.

Nursing process: Assessment

Client need: Physiological Adaptation

Cognitive level: Application

Subject area: Medical-Surgical

Answer: Eighth cranial nerve, VIII

Rationale: The eighth cranial nerve is the acoustic nerve that is responsible for hearing. Damage to this cranial nerve results in a hearing loss. Streptomycin is an aminoglycoside anti-infective that may be ototoxic to the eighth cranial nerve.

Nursing process: Analysis

Client need: Pharmacological and Parenteral Therapies

Cognitive level: Application

Subject area: Medical-Surgical

Answer: 4

Rationale: Glaucoma causes an increase in the intraocular pressure inside the eyeball. A cataract is the result of an opacity within the crystalline lens. A curvature of the cornea is an astigmatism. A separation of the retina is a detachment of the retina from its blood supply.

Nursing process: Analysis

Client need: Physiological Adaptation

Cognitive level: Comprehension

Subject area: Medical-Surgical

Answer: 3

Rationale: Acute bacterial conjunctivitis ("pink eye") is very contagious. The priority nursing intervention is strict hand washing to prevent the spread of the infection to others. Then the client would be instructed not to share towels with others and not to rub or touch the eyes. Hot moist compresses may be used to soften adherent eye crusts.

Nursing process: Planning

Client need: Management of Care

Cognitive level: Application

Subject area: Medical-Surgical

24. The nurse caring for a client with presbycusis evaluates the client to be having a problem with _____.

25. A client who has a retinal detachment asks the nurse if a retinal detachment in the good eye is likely to occur. Which of the following responses by the nurse is most appropriate?

   1. "Chances are very high that you will experience another retinal detachment as you get older."

   2. "You should prevent trauma to your good eye because trauma can cause retinal detachment."

   3. "Clinical manifestations of retinal detachment are pain behind the eye, nausea, and dizziness and are to be reported immediately."

   4. "A retinal detachment can be prevented by having yearly ophthalmic examinations."

26. The registered nurse is making out assignments for the day. Which of the following nursing care activities may be delegated to certified assistive personnel?

   1. Instruct a client how to instill artificial tears

   2. Inform the client with cataracts of the post-op care

   3. Assess a client for a hearing loss

   4. Reinforce to a client with bacterial conjunctivitis the importance of hand washing

27. The nurse evaluates which of the following assessment findings to be normal in an older adult client?

   1. Hordeolum

   2. Exophthalmos

   3. Presbyopia

   4. Tinnitus

Answer: hearing high-pitched sounds

Rationale: Presbycusis is a hearing problem that impairs the vibration of the sound through the middle ear due to a bony fixation of the stapes. The result is difficulty hearing high-pitched sounds.

Nursing process: Evaluation

Client need: Physiological Adaptation

Cognitive level: Comprehension

Subject area: Medical-Surgical

Answer: 2

Rationale: There is only a 10% chance of a retinal detachment occurring in the good eye. Risk factors for retinal detachment include high myopia, aphakia, proliferative diabetic retinopathy, retinal lattice degeneration, and ocular trauma.

Nursing process: Analysis

Client need: Physiological Adaptation

Cognitive level: Analysis

Subject area: Medical-Surgical

Answer: 4

Rationale: Only a nurse can instruct, inform, and assess. Certified assistive personnel can reinforce teaching previously taught if it is within the scope of practice, such as hand washing.

Nursing process: Planning

Client need: Management of Care

Cognitive level: Analysis

Subject area: Legal and Ethical Issues

Answer: 3

Rationale: Presbyopia is a condition that causes farsightedness in the older adult client and leads to needing bifocals. A hordeolum is an infection of the sebaceous gland of the eyelid. Exophthalmos is an abnormal protrusion of the globe of the eye frequently seen in hyperthyroidism. Tinnitus is ringing in the ears and can be indicative of various medical conditions.

Nursing process: Evaluation

Client need: Physiological Adaptation

Cognitive level: Application

Subject area: Medical-Surgical

28. The nurse is reviewing the normal limits of a hearing assessment for a client who presents with decreased hearing. Which of the following findings would indicate the need for additional investigation?

1. Sound heard equally in both ears with the Weber test
2. Whispered words are repeated at two feet
3. Bone conduction is heard twice as long as air conduction with the Rinne test
4. Pearly gray tympanic membrane observed with otoscope

29. A client asks the nurse what a hordeolum is. Which of the following is the appropriate response by the nurse?

1. "It is an inflammation of the cornea."
2. "It is a chronic bacterial inflammation of the lid margin."
3. "It is an infection of the conjunctiva."
4. "It is an infection of the sebaceous glands on an eyelid follicle."

30. The registered nurse is preparing to delegate clinical assignments on a medical-surgical nursing unit. Which of the following assignments would be appropriate for the nurse to delegate to a licensed practical nurse?

1. Instruct a client on the postoperative care following surgery for a cataract
2. Develop an activity schedule for a client with glaucoma
3. Perform an assessment of the ears for a client complaining of tinnitus
4. Administer a drug intranasally to a client who has allergic rhinitis

Answer: 3

Rationale: In the Rinne test, the client should hear air conduction twice as long as bone conduction. It is normal for sound to be heard equally in both ears with the Weber test. The tympanic membrane should have a pearly gray appearance with the otoscope. It is also normal to be able to hear whispered words at two feet.

Nursing process: Analysis

Client need: Physiological Adaptation

Cognitive level: Analysis

Subject area: Medical-Surgical

Answer: 4

Rationale: A hordeolum is an infection of the sebaceous glands on an eyelid follicle. A chronic bacterial inflammation of the lid margin is a chalazion. Conjunctivitis is an infection of the conjunctiva.

Nursing process: Analysis

Client need: Physiological Adaptation

Cognitive level: Comprehension

Subject area: Medical-Surgical

Answer: 4

Rationale: A licensed practical nurse may administer a drug intranasally. Assignments involving delegating, developing an activity plan, and performing an ear assessment should all be performed by a registered nurse.

Nursing process: Planning

Client need: Management of Care

Cognitive level: Analysis

Subject area: Legal and Ethical Issues

Respiratory Disorders

2

1. A client is admitted to the intensive care unit 36 hours ago following extensive pulmonary trauma. Which clinical manifestation would first alert the nurse that the client is experiencing adult respiratory distress syndrome (ARDS)?

   1. Blood-tinged, frothy sputum
   2. Dense pulmonary infiltrates with a "whited-out" appearance
   3. An increase in respiratory rate
   4. Increasing hypoxemia

2. A client with a history of asthma presents in the physician's office with complaints of difficulty breathing. While performing the initial assessment, the nurse becomes concerned that the client's respiratory status has worsened based on which of the following?

   1. Wheezing throughout the lung fields
   2. Noticeably diminished breath sounds
   3. Loud wheezing only on expiration
   4. Mild wheezing on inspiration

3. A home health nurse is visiting a client with severe chronic obstructive pulmonary disease (COPD) who is complaining of increased shortness of air. The client is on home oxygen at 2 L/min via an oxygen concentrator with a respiratory rate of 23 breaths/min. The most appropriate nursing action is to

   1. call emergency services to come to the home.
   2. reassure the client of being unnecessarily anxious.
   3. conduct further assessment of the client's respiratory status.
   4. consider increasing the oxygen to 4 L/min during the home visit.

Answer: 3

Rationale: Adult respiratory distress syndrome usually develops within 24 to 48 hours following an acute catastrophic event in clients with no previous pulmonary disease. In most cases, tachypnea and dyspnea are the first clinical manifestations. Blood-tinged, frothy sputum occurs later, after the development of pulmonary edema. The diffuse pulmonary infiltrates, resembling a ground-glass or "whited-out" appearance on a chest x-ray, will appear as ARDS progresses, while early chest x-rays are often normal. Hypoxemia will occur as ARDS progresses and the client becomes refractory to oxygen therapy.

Nursing process: Assessment

Client need: Management of Care

Cognitive level: Analysis

Subject area: Medical-Surgical

Answer: 2

Rationale: The severity of wheezing is not a reliable way to determine severity of an asthma attack. Some clients with minor attacks may have loud wheezing while others may have severe attacks with mild wheezing. The client with severe asthma attacks may have no audible wheezing because of the decrease in airflow. For wheezing to occur, the client must be able to move air to produce sound. Wheezing usually occurs first on exhalation, and as the asthma attack progresses, the client may wheeze during both inspiration and expiration. The significant finding with this assessment is that there are noticeably diminished breath sounds, which means reduced or absence of moving air. This may indicate severe obstruction and respiratory failure.

Nursing process: Assessment

Client need: Physiological Adaptation

Cognitive level: Analysis

Subject area: Medical-Surgical

Answer: 3

Rationale: Further assessment is the most appropriate nursing action. Remember the nursing process; assessment is the first step. Calling for emergency services would be premature. Oxygen is not increased without the approval of the physician, and remember that with COPD the client's drive to breathe is triggered by low oxygen because of the carbon dioxide retention. For clients with COPD, oxygen should not generally be greater than 2 to 3 L/min. Reassurance that the client is unnecessarily anxious is inappropriate.

Nursing process: Implementation

Client need: Physiological Adaptation

Cognitive level: Application

Subject area: Medical-Surgical

4. The nurse is admitting a client with suspected tuberculosis (TB) to the acute care unit. The nurse places the client in airborne precautions until a confirmed diagnosis of active TB can be made. Which of the following tests is a priority to confirm the diagnosis?

   1. Chest x-ray that is positive for lung lesions

   2. Positive purified protein derivative (PPD) test

   3. Sputum positive for blood (hemoptysis)

   4. Sputum culture positive for *Mycobacterium tuberculosis*

5. A student health nurse is conducting tuberculosis (TB) testing. Students who had the purified protein derivative (PPD) test 48 hours ago have returned to have the results read and documented. The nurse determines that the test is positive if which of the following is present?

   1. The client complains of itching at the site

   2. There is a large area of erythema

   3. There is an induration of 10 mm or greater

   4. A bruise is present at the site of injection

6. A client is scheduled for a computerized axial tomography (CAT) scan with contrast as one of several tests to diagnose a respiratory problem. The priority component of the nurse's assessment in preparation for this test would be to ask the client about _____.

Answer: 4

Rationale: The most accurate way to diagnose TB is by sputum culture. Identifying the presence of tubercle bacilli is essential for a definitive diagnosis. Although hemoptysis is associated with more advanced cases of TB, it is not a confirmatory clinical manifestation. A positive PPD indicates exposure to TB, but gives no information about active disease. A chest x-ray with lesions may be present in a number of other diseases, not just TB.

Nursing process: Analysis

Client need: Management of Care

Cognitive level: Analysis

Subject area: Medical-Surgical

Answer: 3

Rationale: An induration of 10 mm or greater is usually considered a positive result. For immunocompromised and HIV-positive clients an induration of 5 mm or greater may be considered a positive result. Erythema is not a positive reaction. Itching or bruising is not indicative of a positive result. Remember, PPD skin tests are read 48 to 72 hours after administration.

Nursing process: Evaluation

Client need: Reduction of Risk Potential

Cognitive level: Analysis

Subject area: Medical-Surgical

Answer: allergy to shellfish or iodine

Rationale: Any client undergoing diagnostic tests should be asked about allergies, in particular to shellfish, seafood, or iodine. Many diagnostic tests, particularly those ordered with contrast, involve the injection of a contrast dye. It is essential to identify the potential risk for allergic reaction.

Nursing process: Assessment

Client need: Reduction of Risk Potential

Cognitive level: Application

Subject area: Medical-Surgical

7. A client with no history of respiratory disease has a sudden onset of dyspnea, chest pain, and tachycardia. A pulmonary embolism is suspected. The nurse anticipates which set of therapeutic orders to be prescribed for this client?

Select all that apply:

[   ] **1.** Semi-Fowler's position

[   ] **2.** Oxygen at 2 L/min

[   ] **3.** High-Fowler's position

[   ] **4.** Morphine sulfate 2 mg intravenously

[   ] **5.** Oxygen at 4 L/min

[   ] **6.** Meperidine hydrochloride (Demerol) 100 mg intramuscular

8. A client with pulmonary edema is currently receiving 6 L/min of oxygen per nasal cannula. The most recent arterial blood gas (ABG) results indicate the following: pH = 7.30, pCO_2 = 50 mm Hg, pO_2 = 56 mm Hg, HCO_3 = 24 mm Hg. The nurse anticipates that the physician will order which of the following?

1. Change nasal cannula to face mask at 6 L/min oxygen

2. Add one ampule of sodium bicarbonate to the client's current intravenous fluids

3. Change nasal cannula to partial rebreather mask at 8 L/min oxygen

4. Intubate the client and place on mechanical ventilation

9. A registered nurse is planning the schedule for the day. Which of the following nursing tasks may the nurse delegate to a licensed practical nurse?

1. Develop instructions for the client on pursed-lip breathing

2. Clarify an order with the physician

3. Instruct a client on a bronchoscopy

4. Administer a purified protein derivative (PPD) to a client

Answer: 1, 4, 5

Rationale: Standard therapeutic interventions for a client with a pulmonary embolism include proper positioning, oxygen, and intravenous analgesics. Semi-Fowler's position is most appropriate because high-Fowler's position creates extreme flexion of the hips and slows venous return from the legs, which increases the risk of new thrombi. This client has no history of respiratory disease and is not limited to 2 to 3 L/min. Therefore, 4 L/min would be appropriate to help relieve dyspnea. Intravenous analgesics are prescribed to relieve chest pain. Morphine sulfate is the drug of choice and 2 mg is the appropriate intravenous dose. Morphine helps reduce pain and anxiety and can diminish congestion of blood in the pulmonary vessels because it causes peripheral venous dilation.

Nursing process: Planning

Client need: Physiological Adaptation

Cognitive level: Application

Subject area: Medical-Surgical

Answer: 4

Rationale: The client is exhibiting respiratory acidosis with severe hypoxemia. Intubation and mechanical ventilation are warranted in this situation. Changing the oxygen delivery system to a mask would not correct the hypoxemia. Changing the oxygen delivery system to partial rebreather mask, even with a slight increase in oxygen, would not correct the significant hypoxia and the rebreather mask would increase the pCO_2 retention. Adding sodium bicarbonate to the IV fluids treats a clinical manifestation, not the underlying condition of respiratory distress, and sodium bicarbonate will not correct the hypoxemia.

Nursing process: Analysis

Client need: Physiological Adaptation

Cognitive level: Analysis

Subject area: Medical-Surgical

Answer: 4

Rationale: It is not appropriate to assign a licensed practical nurse to develop a teaching plan, teach, or clarify an order with the physician. These are tasks reserved for the registered nurse. An LPN may administer a purified protein derivative to a client.

Nursing process: Planning

Client need: Management of Care

Cognitive level: Analysis

Subject area: Legal and Ethical Issues

10. The nurse is assisting the physician with the removal of a chest tube. How should the nurse tell the client to breathe during the procedure? _____

11. The nurse has just received orders to provide chest physiotherapy for a client two times per day. The nurse evaluates which schedule to be most therapeutic?

    1. 7:00 a.m. and 1:00 p.m.

    2. 6:00 a.m. and 4:00 p.m.

    3. 9:00 a.m. and 5:00 p.m.

    4. 8:00 a.m. and 8:00 p.m.

12. The nurse assesses fluctuations in the water seal chamber of a client's closed chest drainage system. The nurse evaluates this finding as indicating

    1. the system is functioning properly.

    2. an air leak is present.

    3. the tubing is kinked.

    4. the lung has reexpanded.

13. The nurse assesses a college-age client complaining of shortness of breath after jogging and tightness in his chest. Upon further questioning, the client denies a sore throat, fever, or productive cough. The nurse notifies the physician that this client's clinical manifestations are most likely related to

    1. pneumonia.

    2. bronchitis.

    3. pneumoconiosis.

    4. asthma.

Answer: Hold his or her breath

Rationale: The client is instructed to hold his or her breath and bear down (Valsalva maneuver) during the chest tube removal to increase intrathoracic pressure and to decrease the potential for air to enter the pleural space.

Nursing process: Implementation

Client need: Reduction of Risk Potential

Cognitive level: Application

Subject area: Medical-Surgical

Answer: 2

Rationale: Chest physiotherapy and postural drainage are most effective upon first awakening and during the day one hour before or two to three hours after meals. This treatment should always be followed by oral hygiene. All of the other options are either at or shortly after meal times.

Nursing process: Evaluation

Client need: Basic Care and Comfort

Cognitive level: Analysis

Subject area: Medical-Surgical

Answer: 1

Rationale: In a closed drainage chest tube system, fluctuations in the water seal chamber during inhalation and exhalation (called tidaling) is a normal finding until the lung reexpands. If the fluctuations are absent, it may mean that there is an air leak, that the tubing is kinked, or that the lung has reexpanded and the client no longer requires chest drainage.

Nursing process: Evaluation

Client need: Physiological Adaptation

Cognitive level: Analysis

Subject area: Medical-Surgical

Answer: 4

Rationale: The exercise may have induced bronchospasms. Lack of fever or productive cough would reduce the possibility of the clinical manifestations representing pneumonia or bronchitis. The occupation as a college student decreases the likelihood of an occupationally related lung disease.

Nursing process: Analysis

Client need: Physiological Adaptation

Cognitive level: Analysis

Subject area: Medical-Surgical

14. Which of the following is a priority to include in the instructions given to a client who has bronchitis?
 1. Avoid cigarette smoking
 2. Decrease overweight status
 3. Increase activity
 4. Avoid malnutrition

15. The nurse is assessing the respiratory status of a client following a thoracentesis. Which finding would indicate further assessment is needed?
 1. Equal bilateral chest expansion
 2. Scattered crackles, unchanged from baseline
 3. Diminished breath sounds on the affected side
 4. Respiratory rate of 22 breaths/minute

16. The nurse is admitting a client who complains of fever, chills, chest pain, and dyspnea. The client has a heart rate of 110, respiratory rate of 28, and a nonproductive hacking cough. A chest x-ray confirms a diagnosis of left lower lobe pneumonia. Upon auscultation of the left lower lobe, the nurse documents which of the following breath sounds?
 1. Bronchial
 2. Bronchovesicular
 3. Vesicular
 4. Absent breath sounds

Answer: 1

Rationale: Cigarette smoking is one of the most significant risk factors for developing bronchitis. Bronchitis involves the major bronchi and is classified as acute or chronic. Acute bronchitis is bronchial airway inflammation related to smoke, irritants, or infection. Chronic bronchitis is a component of chronic obstructive pulmonary disease (COPD). It usually follows an upper respiratory infection such as rhinitis or sore throat. Malnutrition is considered a possible risk factor. Obesity or being active in sports is not correlated with bronchitis.

Nursing process: Planning

Client need: Health Promotion and Maintenance

Cognitive level: Application

Subject area: Medical-Surgical

Answer: 3

Rationale: Following a thoracentesis, the nurse assesses breath sounds and vital signs. The nurse particularly looks for signs that may indicate a pneumothorax as a complication from the procedure. Signs that may indicate a pneumothorax include increased respiratory rate, dyspnea, retractions, diminished breath sounds, or cyanosis. Any of these signs should be reported to the physician immediately. Equal bilateral breath sounds are normal findings and a respiratory rate of 22 is slightly elevated and may be due to pain or anxiety. Scattered crackles, though not normal, have not changed from baseline and would not represent a complication as a result of the procedure.

Nursing process: Evaluation

Client need: Reduction of Risk Potential

Cognitive level: Analysis

Subject area: Medical-Surgical

Answer: 1

Rationale: In the presence of pneumonia there will be bronchial breath sounds over the area of consolidation. The client may also have crackles in the affected side as a result of fluid in the interstitium and alveoli. Absence of breath sounds is not a usual finding and would not likely occur unless there was a serious complication.

Nursing process: Analysis

Client need: Physiological Adaptation

Cognitive level: Application

Subject area: Medical-Surgical

17. The nurse is preparing a client with empyema for a thoracentesis. Which of the following should the nurse have available in the event that the procedure is ineffective?

    1. A ventilator

    2. A chest tube insertion kit

    3. An intubation tray

    4. A crash cart

18. A client is admitted to a burn unit with second and third degree burns over 18% of the body. An inhalation injury is also suspected. The nurse should monitor which of the following to determine the extent of carbon monoxide poisoning?

    1. Pulse oximetry

    2. Urine myoglobin

    3. Arterial blood gases

    4. Serum carboxyhemoglobin levels

19. Which of the following should the nurse include when suctioning a client's tracheostomy?

    1. Instill sterile saline down the trachea to stimulate a cough, then suction with continuous suctioning

    2. Insert the catheter until a cough reflex is obtained or until resistance is felt

    3. Adjust the wall suction to 150 mm Hg for the procedure

    4. Suction the client's mouth before entering the trachea

Answer: 2

Rationale: With empyema, the fluid to be removed from the pleural space is thick and "puslike." The physician may not be able to withdraw the fluid through needle aspiration and the client may require placement of a chest tube to adequately drain the purulent effusion. A ventilator, intubation tray, or crash cart is not likely to be necessary because there was no indication that the client was unstable.

Nursing process: Planning

Client need: Reduction of Risk Potential

Cognitive level: Application

Subject area: Medical-Surgical

Answer: 4

Rationale: Carbon monoxide binds tightly to hemoglobin to form carboxyhemoglobin. Because carbon monoxide binds 200 times greater to hemoglobin than oxygen there is decreased availability of oxygen to the cells. Clients are treated with 100% oxygen. Pulse oximetry will read falsely high, as it is a reading of how well the hemoglobin is bound, but not with oxygen. Urine myoglobin is indicative of byproducts of muscle damage being excreted through the kidneys. Arterial blood gas pCO_2 may falsely represent the client's oxygenation status and is not a measure of carbon monoxide levels.

Nursing process: Assessment

Client need: Reduction of Risk Potential

Cognitive level: Analysis

Subject area: Medical-Surgical

Answer: 2

Rationale: Proper suctioning involves inserting the catheter gently until a cough reflex is stimulated or resistance is felt. It is then withdrawn with intermittent suction and a rotating motion using moderate suction pressure (80 to 120 mm Hg). Nursing research does not support the instillation of saline and the client's risk of aspiration and contamination are increased with this procedure. Airway suctioning is a sterile technique. If the client's mouth is to be suctioned it would be the last thing done, after airway suctioning and before discarding.

Nursing process: Planning

Client need: Physiological Adaptation

Cognitive level: Application

Subject area: Medical-Surgical

20. The nurse is evaluating the respiratory system of a client who admits to smoking a half pack per day for the last 5 years and 1 pack per day for 10 years prior to that. When evaluating the client's risk of developing a respiratory disease, the nurse calculates that the client has a smoking history of how many packs over the years?

 1. 2.5 pack-years

 2. 10 pack-years

 3. 12.5 pack-years

 4. 15 pack-years

21. A client with pneumonia has a poor appetite, is dyspneic and complains of decreased taste sensation, and is receiving chest physiotherapy treatments and breathing treatments. Which of the following actions should the nurse include to improve the client's appetite?

 1. Provide mouth care before meals

 2. Provide juice and fluids at the bedside

 3. Provide three balanced meals each day

 4. Increase fluid intake to 3 L a day

22. A client with left-sided heart failure is progressing to pulmonary edema. The nurse assesses the client and reports which of the following manifestations?

 1. Dry, hacking cough

 2. Bilateral crackles

 3. Fever above 36.8°C or 101.5°F

 4. Peripheral pitting edema

Answer: 3

Rationale: The standard method for determining pack-year smoking history is to take the number of packs per day times the number of years. The number is recorded as the number of pack-years. $(0.50 \times 5) + (1.0 \times 10)$ $= 2.5 + 10 = 12.5$ packs over the years.

Nursing process: Evaluation

Client need: Reduction of Risk Potential

Cognitive level: Application

Subject area: Medical-Surgical

Answer: 1

Rationale: Because of the sputum production and expectoration, particularly during and after treatments, the client will have decreased taste sensation. Providing oral care after pulmonary treatments and before meals will improve taste and appetite. Fatigue from breathing, activity, and treatments will also decrease energy. Providing more frequent small meals (not three large ones), increasing fluid intake, and offering fluids that appeal to the client are appropriate interventions for the client but will not impact appetite.

Nursing process: Planning

Client need: Basic Care and Comfort

Cognitive level: Application

Subject area: Medical-Surgical

Answer: 2

Rationale: A client with left-sided heart failure and pulmonary edema presents primarily with respiratory symptoms. Because of the fluid accumulation in the pulmonary vascular bed there may be a productive cough with pink, frothy sputum. There is no fever associated with pulmonary edema and peripheral pitting edema is more associated with right-sided heart failure.

Nursing process: Assessment

Client need: Physiological Adaptation

Cognitive level: Analysis

Subject area: Medical-Surgical

23. The nurse is performing a respiratory assessment of a client with pleurisy and compares the assessment findings with the previous day's assessment. Currently there is no friction rub, but one was auscultated the previous day. The nurse evaluates this finding as the result of

1. the client taking more shallow breaths.

2. a decreased inflammatory response.

3. the effectiveness of the antibiotics.

4. an accumulation of pleural fluid in the inflamed area.

24. The nurse is caring for a client following a cardiac bypass surgery. The nurse notes that in the first hour the chest tube drainage measured 90 ml. During the second hour the drainage dropped to 5 ml. The nurse suspects that

1. the chest tube may be clotted.

2. the lungs have fully inflated.

3. the client is recovering normally.

4 the physician should be notified.

25. The nurse should monitor a client admitted with a suspected diagnosis of pulmonary emphysema for which of the following clinical manifestations?

Select all that apply:

[   ] **1.** Copious sputum production

[   ] **2.** Bilateral wheezing

[   ] **3.** Marked weight loss

[   ] **4.** Prolonged inspiratory phase

[   ] **5.** Barrel chest appearance

[   ] **6.** Severe dyspnea

Answer: 4

Rationale: Initially a pleural friction rub is auscultated when there is inflammation between the pleural space and visceral pleura. With increasing inflammation, fluid accumulates between the two layers at the inflamed site and reduces the friction. The inflammatory process is still there and would be treated by anti-inflammatory drugs, not necessarily antibiotics (unless there were an infectious process involved). The client should be instructed to take adequately deep breaths for a good assessment of breath sounds and that should be consistent between assessments.

Nursing process: Evaluation

Client need: Physiological Adaptation

Cognitive level: Analysis

Subject area: Medical-Surgical

Answer: 1

Rationale: The first hour after surgery, chest tube draining may be as high as 100 ml/hour but should taper off over the next several hours. There should not be a sudden significant increase or drop in the amount of drainage. In this case, a sudden drop may indicate that a clot has formed in the tube and the nurse will need to gently work the clot out of the tubing to prevent cardiac tamponade. Further assessment would need to be made before notifying the physician. A chest tube is not "milked" but can be gently manipulated. Chest tube drainage is not an indication of lung inflation. Chest drainage may taper off to minimal amounts before the tube is withdrawn, but that is based on the fluctuations in the water seal chamber being minimal and an evaluation by chest x-ray.

Nursing process: Analysis

Client need: Physiological Adaptation

Cognitive level: Analysis

Subject area: Medical-Surgical

Answer: 3, 5, 6

Rationale: Clients with pulmonary emphysema typically manifest symptoms of marked weight loss, barrel chest appearance, prolonged expiratory effort, marked dyspnea, and a cough late in the progression of the disease. There is scant mucus production. Copious sputum production is characteristic of chronic bronchitis. Bilateral wheezing is characteristic of bronchial asthma.

Nursing process: Assessment

Client need: Physiological Adaptation

Cognitive level: Application

Subject area: Medical-Surgical

26. The nurse is preparing to delegate which of the following nursing tasks to a licensed practical nurse?

1. Administer morphine IV to a client experiencing a pulmonary embolism
2. Monitor a client's chest tube for bubbling
3. Assess a client for tactile fremitus
4. Perform a sputum culture for a client

27. The nurse is reviewing the normal limits for a head and neck assessment. Which of the following findings would indicate the need for additional investigation?

1. A small, discrete, movable lymph node
2. The trachea is to the right of the suprasternal notch
3. A thyroid gland that is not visible or palpable
4. The muscles of the neck are symmetrical

28. The nurse is performing an assessment of the thorax and lungs on a 30-year-old client. Which of the following assessments does the nurse evaluate to be a normal adult finding?

1. The thorax is barrel shaped
2. The costal margin is greater than 90°
3. The accessory muscles are used during inspiration and expiration
4. The ribs articulate at a 45° angle with the sternum

29. The nurse correctly documents moist, low-pitched, gurgling breath sounds as

1. sonorous wheezes.
2. coarse crackles.
3. sibilant wheezes.
4. pleural friction rub.

Answer: 4

Rationale: A licensed practical nurse has the knowledge and skill to perform a sputum culture for a client. Administering morphine IV to a client, monitoring a chest tube, or assessing a client for tactile fremitus are nursing tasks reserved for a registered nurse.

Nursing process: Planning

Client need: Management of Care

Cognitive level: Analysis

Subject area: Legal and Ethical Issues

Answer: 2

Rationale: The trachea should be midline in the suprasternal notch. It may be normal to feel a small, discrete, movable lymph node. It is clinically insignificant. The thyroid gland should not be visible or palpable and the muscles of the neck should be symmetrical.

Nursing process: Analysis

Client need: Physiological Adaptation

Cognitive level: Analysis

Subject area: Medical-Surgical

Answer: 4

Rationale: The thorax is generally slightly elliptical in shape although the barrel-shaped chest may be normal in the infant and older adult. The costal angle should be less than 90° during exhalation and at rest. No accessory muscles should be used during normal respirations. The ribs should also articulate at a 45° angle with the sternum.

Nursing process: Evaluation

Client need: Physiological Adaptation

Cognitive level: Analysis

Subject area: Medical-Surgical

Answer: 2

Rationale: Low-pitched gurgling breath sounds are coarse crackles. Sonorous wheezes are low-pitched breath sounds. Sibilant wheezes are high-pitched musical breath sounds. A pleural friction rub is a creaking sound.

Nursing process: Implementation

Client need: Physiological Adaptation

Cognitive level: Comprehension

Subject area: Medical-Surgical

30. When preparing a client to collect a sputum specimen, it would be essential for the nurse to explain which of the following aspects of the procedure?

1. Avoid mouth care prior to collecting the specimen
2. Breathe deeply followed by coughing up sputum
3. Collect the specimen before bedtime
4. Restrict fluids prior to expectorating sputum

Answer: 2

Rationale: Breathing deeply should be followed by coughing up sputum in the collection process of a sputum specimen. Mouth care should be offered prior to collecting a sputum specimen. The specimen should be collected in the morning and fluids encouraged before coughing up the specimen.

Nursing process: Planning

Client need: Reduction of Risk Potential

Cognitive level: Application

Subject area: Medical-Surgical

CHAPTER 3

Cardiovascular Disorders

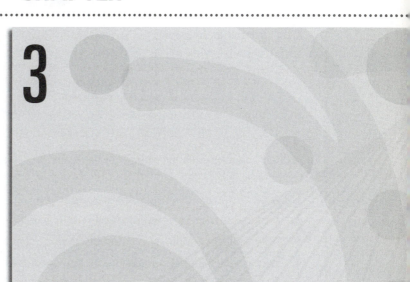

1. During a routine physical examination, a client reports recent occipital headaches, blurred vision, fatigue, and increasing edema. The nurse reports these findings as indicative of
   1. endocarditis.
   2. hypovolemic shock.
   3. hypertension.
   4. ventricular tachycardia.

2. A client's parents ask the nurse, "What is the prognosis of myocarditis?" The most appropriate response by the nurse is
   1. "A heart transplant would be very promising."
   2. "Most often, a person will do well with coronary artery bypass surgery."
   3. "A coronary angioplasty would only involve a one- to three-day hospitalization."
   4. "Recovery usually happens without any special treatment."

3. The nurse is planning the care for a client in the acute stage of bacterial endocarditis. Which of the following interventions should the nurse include?

   Select all that apply:
   [ ] 1. Rest
   [ ] 2. Fluid restriction
   [ ] 3. Vitamin K (Aquamephyton)
   [ ] 4. Analgesics
   [ ] 5. Antibiotics
   [ ] 6. Physical therapy

4. A client who has hypertension asks the nurse why a urine sample is needed. The nurse informs the client it is to check for
   1. protein, which may indicate the kidneys are affected.
   2. illegal drugs, which may have caused the hypertension.
   3. infection, which may cause the blood pressure to rise.
   4. the appropriate drug level of the antihypertensive medication.

Answer: 3

Rationale: Clinical manifestations of hypertension include blurred vision, fatigue, occipital headaches, and increased edema.

Nursing process: Analysis

Client need: Physiological Adaptation

Cognitive level: Application

Subject area: Medical-Surgical

Answer: 4

Rationale: A heart transplant is a late-stage intervention for cardiomyopathy, which rarely results from myocarditis. Coronary artery bypass surgery is indicated for people with > 2 vessel disease not responsive to medical treatment. Coronary angioplasty is indicated for people with coronary artery lesions causing angina-related symptoms. Myocarditis is often asymptomatic and most often resolves spontaneously.

Nursing process: Analysis

Client need: Physiological Adaptation

Cognitive level: Analysis

Subject area: Medical-Surgical

Answer: 1, 4, 5

Rationale: Rest is indicated during the acute stage of bacterial endocarditis, along with acetaminophen (Tylenol) or salicylic acid (aspirin) for aches and antibiotics to fight the infectious organism. Steroids are not indicated and fluids should be encouraged rather than restricted. Vitamin K is used for reversal of warfarin (Coumadin) that would cause the blood to be too thin.

Nursing process: Planning

Client need: Physiological Adaptation

Cognitive level: Application

Subject area: Medical-Surgical

Answer: 1

Rationale: Hypertension is not normally caused by illegal drugs nor by infection. Drug levels are more frequently done by serum analysis rather than urine, and appropriate levels of antihypertensives are judged by the serial blood pressure readings of the client. A urine test that showed high levels of microalbuminuria and proteinuria may indicate that the client's hypertension has caused poor blood supply to the kidneys, resulting in renal dysfunction.

Nursing process: Implementation

Client need: Reduction of Risk Potential

Cognitive level: Analysis

Subject area: Medical-Surgical

5. Which of the following orders should the nurse question in a client who has been admitted with a possible myocardial infarction and active peptic ulcer disease?
   1. Nitroglycerin SL
   2. Oxygen by nasal cannula
   3. Morphine IV
   4. Aspirin PO

6. The nurse's client asks, "How did I get rheumatic heart disease?" The most appropriate response by the nurse is that rheumatic heart disease is frequently a result of
   1. hypertension.
   2. streptococcal infection.
   3. genetic tendency.
   4. pregnancy.

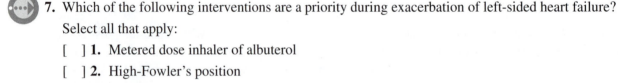

7. Which of the following interventions are a priority during exacerbation of left-sided heart failure? Select all that apply:
   [   ] 1. Metered dose inhaler of albuterol
   [   ] 2. High-Fowler's position
   [   ] 3. Oxygen
   [   ] 4. IV fluids
   [   ] 5. Incentive inspirometer
   [   ] 6. Diuretics

8. The nurse is preparing a client to be discharged after a new diagnosis of heart failure. Which of the following statements by the client shows an appropriate understanding of the nurse's teaching?
   1. "I will do weekly finger-stick monitoring of my sodium levels."
   2. "I will call my doctor if I gain more than two pounds in a day."
   3. "I will take my angiotensin-converting enzyme (ACE) inhibitor as needed for shortness of breath."
   4. "I will not take my diuretic pill on weekends when I am traveling, in order to avoid incontinence."

Answer: 4

Rationale: Nitroglycerin, oxygen, morphine, and aspirin are all appropriate interventions for a client suspected of having a myocardial infarction. However, a client with an active peptic ulcer should not be considered a candidate for aspirin, due to its antiplatelet effects possibly promoting more GI bleeding.

Nursing process: Analysis

Client need: Physiological Adaptation

Cognitive level: Analysis

Subject area: Medical-Surgical

Answer: 2

Rationale: Rheumatic heart disease commonly occurs in children after an infection of group A beta-hemolytic streptococcal pharyngitis.

Nursing process: Analysis

Client need: Physiological Adaptation

Cognitive level: Analysis

Subject area: Medical-Surgical

Answer: 2, 3, 6

Rationale: Nursing interventions that are a priority for a client with an acute exacerbation of left-sided heart failure include having the client assume a high-Fowler's position, oxygen, and diuretics to reduce the fluid volume. Albuterol is used for a client with asthma. IV fluid flush would be harmful for a client experiencing respiratory distress from left-sided heart failure.

Nursing process: Planning

Client need: Management of Care

Cognitive level: Analysis

Subject area: Medical-Surgical

Answer: 2

Rationale: While finger-stick glucose levels are done by clients to monitor their diabetes, sodium finger-stick levels are not done. ACE inhibitors need to be taken daily, as prescribed (not prn). Diuretic pills may be delayed a few hours before a big event, but not skipped or the client may end up with a heart failure exacerbation. A client who calls about a sudden weight gain may receive instructions from the health care provider to come in to be evaluated or may be instructed to take an extra diuretic pill at home.

Nursing process: Planning

Client need: Physiological Adaptation

Cognitive level: Application

Subject area: Medical-Surgical

9. The nurse should monitor a client after a coronary angioplasty for which of the following clinical manifestations indicating cardiac tamponade?

Select all that apply:

[   ] **1.** Muffled heart sounds

[   ] **2.** Headache

[   ] **3.** Hypotension

[   ] **4.** Vision changes

[   ] **5.** Cool, diaphoretic skin

[   ] **6.** Tachycardia

10. The nurse is caring for a client who has an allergy to penicillin. Immediately after receiving cefazolin (Ancef) IV for prophylaxis for a pacemaker insertion, the client becomes restless, tachycardic, and hypotensive. Which of the following interventions should the nurse implement as the priority?

1. Administer epinephrine (adrenaline)

2. Obtain stat blood culture

3. Administer thrombolytic therapy

4. Administer atropine

11. After a myocardial infarction, a client has concerns about when it is safe to resume sexual activity. The most appropriate response by the nurse is

1. "You should really talk to your doctor about that."

2. "Continue with the sexual practice with which you are most comfortable."

3. "You need to first undergo a cardiac stress test."

4. "When you're able to climb two flights of stairs comfortably."

Answer: 1, 3, 5, 6

Rationale: Clinical manifestations of cardiac tamponade include muffled heart sounds, tachycardia, low blood pressure, and cool, diaphoretic skin. These clinical manifestations indicate shock, possibly caused by a dissection (cutting) of a coronary artery, a ventricle, or the septum during the coronary angioplasty.

Nursing process: Assessment

Client need: Physiological Adaptation

Cognitive level: Application

Subject area: Medical-Surgical

Answer: 1

Rationale: Blood cultures and IV antibiotics are appropriate for a client in septic shock. Thrombolytic therapy is indicated for some clients experiencing an acute MI or peripheral clot. Atropine would be appropriate for an individual who has symptomatic bradycardia or heart block. The client has a known allergy to penicillin, and cefazolin (Ancef) is a related cephalosporin, so the client is likely experiencing a severe allergic reaction. The priority intervention for anaphylactic shock would be to monitor the airway and give epinephrine, while infusing rapid IV fluids for hypotension.

Nursing process: Planning

Client need: Management of Care

Cognitive level: Analysis

Subject area: Legal and Ethical Issues

Answer: 4

Rationale: Discussing timing for the client to resume sexual activity should be handled matter-of-factly by the nurse while discussing other activities. The client may not be physically ready to continue with comfortable sexual practices immediately after the myocardial infarction. The client needs an objective indicator. A cardiac stress test is not necessary prior to resuming sexual activity, while the ability to climb two flights of stairs comfortably is a good guideline.

Nursing process: Analysis

Client need: Physiological Adaptation

Cognitive level: Analysis

Subject area: Medical-Surgical

12. In preparing a client for a transesophageal echocardiogram (TEE), the nurse should include which of the following in the client education?

    1. "You will be able to eat only soft foods for the first day after the procedure."

    2. "You will need a designated driver to take you home."

    3. "The procedure involves a series of x-rays that may require you to come back."

    4. "The procedure involves a balloon that will press plaque against the blocked walls of your coronary artery."

13. After receiving a permanent pacemaker, the client asks the nurse if there are any activities to avoid during a vacation scheduled four months after discharge. Which of the following is the most appropriate response by the nurse?

    1. "There are no restrictions on your activity."

    2. "You should avoid working over a running engine."

    3. "Avoid standing in front of microwave ovens."

    4. "Swimming in the ocean should be avoided."

14. After a client with coronary artery disease develops heavy, substernal chest pain, which of the following interventions should the nurse do first?

    1. Administer 2 puffs of albuterol (Proventil) by mouth

    2. Administer 1 tablet of nitroglycerin under the tongue every 5 minutes; call 911 if no relief after 15 minutes

    3. Administer 0.04 mg IV push nitroglycerin slowly over 1 to 2 minutes

    4. Administer immediate synchronized cardioversion

Answer: 2

Rationale: After a transesophageal echocardiogram (TEE), the client should be able to eat lukewarm food as soon as the gag reflex returns, usually just a few hours after receiving anesthetizing spray in the back of the throat. X-rays are not involved, nor is the client undergoing a balloon procedure such as the coronary angioplasty. Having a designated driver will be needed after a transesophageal echocardiogram because the client has received IV sedation.

Nursing process: Analysis

Client need: Health Promotion and Maintenance

Cognitive level: Analysis

Subject area: Medical-Surgical

Answer: 2

Rationale: Early microwave ovens required avoidance by persons with pacemakers, but not current models. Swimming would be contraindicated for the first few weeks due to abduction of the arm while the leads were still adhering to the muscle of the heart. However, four months postoperatively, the client should be able to abduct arms for swimming. Working over a running engine, as well as being near high-frequency power waves, is contraindicated for anyone with a permanent pacemaker.

Nursing process: Analysis

Client need: Reduction of Risk Potential

Cognitive level: Analysis

Subject area: Medical-Surgical

Answer: 2

Rationale: Administering albuterol (Proventil) in a situation where a client had exercise-induced asthma and experienced shortness of breath would be appropriate. However, for a client with known cardiac disease who is experiencing chest pain, the inhaler would not be appropriate. Nitroglycerin is not given IV push. Immediate synchronized cardioversion is appropriate for the client in pulseless ventricular tachycardia or ventricular fibrillation. Correct administration of nitroglycerin for a client who has coronary artery disease involves 1 nitroglycerin tablet every 5 minutes (if blood pressure is above 90 systolic) for up to 3 tablets, then calling 911 if no relief.

Nursing process: Planning

Client need: Physiological Adaptation

Cognitive level: Analysis

Subject area: Medical-Surgical

15. The nurse assists the client with coronary artery disease to select which of the following menu choices? Select all that apply:

[   ] 1. Mozzarella cheese

[   ] 2. Grilled cheddar cheese sandwich

[   ] 3. Tomato juice

[   ] 4. Peanut-butter sandwich

[   ] 5. 2% milk

[   ] 6. Tortilla

16. In caring for a client with a cardiac history, the client has a temperature of 39.4°C or 103°F, and becomes tachycardic, hypotensive, and short of breath while exhibiting cool, clammy skin and a decreased urine output. The client also has positive blood cultures. The nurse should plan to include which of the following in the plan of care for this client?

1. Assistance with pericardiocentesis

2. Administration of antihypertensives

3. Administration of vasopressors

4. Assistance with defibrillation

Subject area: Medical-Surgical

17. Which of the following should the nurse include in the preoperative teaching for a client scheduled for coronary artery bypass graft (CABG) surgery?

1. A liquid diet will be ordered for the first four to five days postoperatively

2. Coughing is to be avoided in order to protect the sternal incision

3. The hospital stay is generally about 10 days

4. High-calorie supplements are encouraged in the first few weeks postoperative

Answer: 1, 6

Rationale: Cheddar cheese has higher fat content than mozzarella cheese, and a canned vegetable drink often has high sodium content. Peanut-butter is a high-fat item. Skim milk is preferred to 2%. Tortilla is a low-fat item.

Nursing process: Implementation

Client need: Basic Care and Comfort

Cognitive level: Analysis

Subject area: Medical-Surgical

Answer: 3

Rationale: A client who is exhibiting a temperature of 39.4°C or 103°F, and becomes tachycardic, hypotensive, and has shortness of breath with cold, clammy skin and a decreased urine output has signs of septic shock (systemic infection) with known positive blood cultures. A pericardiocentesis is an intervention for cardiac tamponade, a condition which may also result in shock, but is also generally accompanied by muffled heart sounds and pulsus paradoxus, neither of which are presented in this client. Antihypertensive drugs would cause the client's blood pressure to drop even further. If the client were in a pulseless ventricular tachycardia or fibrillation, emergency defibrillation would be indicated, but no dysrhythmia is present in the scenario. Vasopressors are indicated to raise the blood pressure. Rapid IV fluid administration and inotropic drugs may be used as well.

Nursing process: Planning

Client need: Physiological Adaptation

Cognitive level: Analysis

Answer: 4

Rationale: The first meal after coronary artery bypass graft surgery may be clear liquids, but the client quickly progresses to low fat and low salt as soon as it can be tolerated. Coughing is important to clear the airways, and is done by splinting the sternum with a pillow. Hospital stays are generally four to five days. A poor appetite may be present for the first few weeks and clients are encouraged to try high-calorie supplements.

Nursing process: Planning

Client need: Physiological Adaptation

Cognitive level: Application

Subject area: Medical-Surgical

18. The nurse observes the ECG rhythm of a client who has received a new permanent pacemaker for third-degree heart block. Several spikes are noted on the rhythm, but are not followed by any other waveforms. The nurse recognizes this as

1. an indication that the pacemaker is adhering to the heart.

2. a normal finding because spikes should never be seen on a pacemaker ECG rhythm strip.

3. the sinoatrial (S-A) node is beating appropriately but may not show up on the rhythm strip.

4. an abnormal finding because every spike on the ECG strip should be followed by a waveform.

19. The nurse assesses the left foot of a client with known coronary artery disease that has become suddenly cold, painful, and pulseless. Which of the following would be the priority intervention for this client?

1. Notify the physician

2. Provide education to the client about probable bypass surgery for the client's leg the following week

3. Instruct the client on importance of daily doses of warfarin (Coumadin)

4. Instruct the client to restrict activity, keeping it warm and elevated until it heals

20. Plans for nursing interventions for a client in the acute stage of bacterial endocarditis should include which of the following interventions?

1. Daily ECGs

2. Administration of analgesics as needed

3. Strict fluid restriction

4. Aggressive physical therapy

Answer: 4

Rationale: While it is true that the pacemaker leads need time to adhere to the heart muscle after implantation, the correct precaution is to keep the affected side's arm near the body for about one to three weeks. It does not mean that the device won't function properly as soon as it is implanted. Spikes are seen on an ECG waveform strip when the pacemaker discharges an electrical stimulus to the heart and should be followed by a P wave (for atrial depolarization) or a QRS wave (ventricular depolarization) as indicated by pacemaker programming.

Nursing process: Analysis

Client need: Physiological Adaptation

Cognitive level: Analysis

Subject area: Medical-Surgical

Answer: 1

Rationale: Scheduling bypass surgery for a week after the left foot of a client has suddenly become cold, painful, and pulseless is not an aggressive enough treatment, as ischemia, tissue necrosis, and gangrene may happen within several hours from an acute arterial occlusion. Warfarin (Coumadin) anticoagulant therapy would be likely after the intervention for this occlusion, but is not the nurse's immediate priority. Keeping the limb elevated may actually cause more pain, and is indicated for someone with venous stasis or venous phlebitis. The nurse needs to notify the physician immediately so this client can be seen and arrangements can be made for immediate transport to a hospital where the client can be evaluated for possible catheter-directed thrombolytic therapy, emergency embolectomy, or bypass surgery.

Nursing process: Planning

Client need: Management of Care

Cognitive level: Analysis

Subject area: Legal and Ethical Issues

Answer: 2

Rationale: Antibiotics to combat the bacterial infection and analgesics for aches that may occur are appropriate interventions for acute-stage bacterial endocarditis. Adequate fluid intake is important also. However, aggressive physical therapy is contraindicated in the acute stage because the client needs to reserve some physical resources for recovery. Daily ECGs are not necessary for acute bacterial endocarditis.

Nursing process: Planning

Client need: Physiological Adaptation

Cognitive level: Application

Subject area: Medical-Surgical

21. Which of the following is a priority for the nurse to report when obtaining a history from a client scheduled for a coronary angiogram?

1. A history of rheumatic heart disease
2. A history of allergy to shellfish
3. A recent diagnosis of hyperlipidemia
4. A previous coronary angioplasty to the right coronary artery

22. Which of the following should the nurse include in the plan of care for a client following a coronary angiogram?

1. Vigorous leg exercises
2. Immediate cardiac stress test
3. Encourage fluids
4. Activity restriction for four to six weeks

23. The nurse is teaching a class to student nurses on rheumatic fever. Which of the following should the nurse include in the class? Rheumatic fever

1. occurs mainly in the elderly.
2. is more likely to develop after a varicella zoster infection.
3. is easy to diagnose with a throat culture and serum antistreptolysin titer.
4. may be diagnosed by a series of two-step blood cultures.

Answer: 2

Rationale: While obtaining a clear record of the client's cardiac history is important prior to a coronary angiogram, it is a priority to notify the physician of an allergy to shellfish. The client with a shellfish allergy is more likely to be allergic to the contrast dye used in the procedure. An order may be given to give diphenhydramine (Benadryl), steroids, or extra IV fluids before the procedure. The chart should be marked for an allergy to shellfish.

Nursing process: Analysis

Client need: Management of Care

Cognitive level: Analysis

Subject area: Medical-Surgical

Answer: 3

Rationale: The client's leg on the side where the cardiologist entered the femoral artery needs to remain still for a period of time after the procedure (usually two to four hours) in order to allow the arterial site to seal. A cardiac stress test would not be indicated because the angiogram provides a more definitive diagnostic work-up. A four to six weeks' activity restriction may be indicated after a large myocardial infarction, but not for a simple coronary angiogram, after which the client can begin walking hours later. The client should be encouraged to drink fluids to protect the kidneys from the contrast dye.

Nursing process: Planning

Client need: Physiological Adaptation

Cognitive level: Application

Subject area: Medical-Surgical

Answer: 3

Rationale: Rheumatic fever occurs primarily in young adults and is mostly likely to develop after a group A beta-hemolytic streptococcal upper respiratory infection. Diagnosis is not done by a series of blood cultures, but rather with a throat culture and serum antistreptolysin titer.

Nursing process: Planning

Client need: Physiological Adaptation

Cognitive level: Application

Subject area: Medical-Surgical

24. Which of the following should the nurse include in the plan of care for the client experiencing pain from a deep vein thrombosis (DVT) of the leg who is receiving heparin and warfarin (Coumadin)? Administration of

    1. aspirin 325 mg p.o. every 4 hours.

    2. patient-controlled analgesic of IV morphine.

    3. meperidine (Demerol) 50 mg IM every 3 hours.

    4. ibuprofen (Motrin) 400 mg p.o. every 6 hours p.r.n.

25. The client with a recent diagnosis of cardiomyopathy asks the nurse, "What contributed to my getting this illness?" The most appropriate response is to say that the majority of clients with cardiomyopathy also have

    1. hypertension.

    2. a viral infection.

    3. a genetic trait.

    4. an unknown cause.

26. The nurse is teaching the client what to expect after coronary artery bypass graft surgery (CABG). Which of the following client statements demonstrates that the client correctly understood the teaching?

    1. "I will be given a pen and paper to communicate, because I will still have a breathing tube in my throat."

    2. "I will be fed with a tube into my stomach until I can eat again."

    3. "Pain medicine is generally not needed after this surgery."

    4. "The nurses will be checking on me every four hours."

Answer: 2

Rationale: A daily dose of aspirin would be ordered for antiplatelet effect, not for pain control. A client with a deep vein thrombosis would be receiving heparin therapy, so intramuscular injections should be avoided (due to possible hematoma formation at injection sites). Ibuprofen (Motrin) is also contraindicated for a client receiving oral anticoagulants due to possible drug interaction. The best solution to this client's pain would be patient-controlled IV analgesic.

Nursing process: Planning

Client need: Pharmacological and Parenteral Therapies

Cognitive level: Application

Subject area: Pharmacologic

Answer: 4

Rationale: Although hypertension, viral infection, or a genetic trait may all be possible reasons for developing cardiomyopathy, the majority of cases are idiopathic (unknown reason).

Nursing process: Analysis

Client need: Physiological Adaptation

Cognitive level: Application

Subject area: Medical-Surgical

Answer: 1

Rationale: A nasogastric tube may be used to decompress the stomach after coronary artery bypass graft surgery, but is not immediately used for feeding unless the client cannot eat in the days following surgery. Pain medication is offered regularly because the client will most likely experience pain in the sternal incision as well as leg, if a graft was taken from there. Immediately after CABG surgery the nurses will be assessing the client every 15 minutes and more frequently as needed until the client becomes stable. It is correct that the client should expect to use hand signals and writing to communicate in the first few hours after surgery while on the ventilator.

Nursing process: Evaluation

Client need: Physiological Adaptation

Cognitive level: Analysis

Subject area: Medical-Surgical

27. Because a client with sinus bradycardia is experiencing hypotension, plans for intervention include administration of what drug? _____

28. The nurse reports the following ECG strip to be indicative of which of the following dysrhythmias?

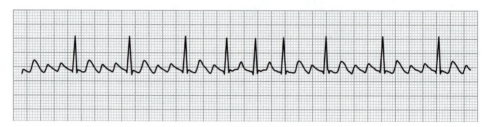

    1. Ventricular fibrillation

    2. Atrial flutter

    3. Atrial fibrillation

    4. Ventricular tachycardia

29. The nurse is evaluating a 28-year-old healthy client admitted to the hospital for abdominal surgery. The client's recovery was uneventful except for some occasional nausea and vomiting. The nurse evaluates the following rhythm on the ECG monitor to be _____.

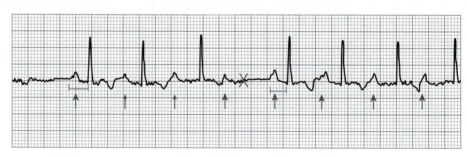

Answer: Atropine

Rationale: Atropine is a cholinergic blocking agent that blocks acetylcholine effects on postganglionic cholinergic receptors in the cardiac muscle and A-V and S-A nodes of the heart. It is used to treat a client with sinus bradycardia who is symptomatic.

Nursing process: Planning

Client need: Pharmacological and Parenteral Therapies

Cognitive level: Analysis

Subject area: Pharmacologic

Answer: 2

Rationale: Atrial flutter is a dysrhythmia characterized by a very irritable atrium. The atria fire at a rate of 250 to 350 beats per minute. The waveforms produced resemble the teeth of a saw. Ventricular fibrillation is a lethal rhythm characterized by a chaotic rhythm that originates in the ventricles. It is an unorganized and uncoordinated series of rapid impulses that cause the heart to fibrillate rather than contract. Atrial fibrillation is an extremely irritable rhythm originating in the atrium. There is a constant generalized quivering with no sign of organized atrial activity. Ventricular tachycardia is a lethal rhythm that exists when three or more premature ventricular contractions (PVCs) occur in a row at a rate greater than 100 beats per minute.

Nursing process: Evaluation

Client need: Physiological Adaptation

Cognitive level: Application

Subject area: Medical-Surgical

Answer: sinus bradycardia

Rationale: Sinus bradycardia is a heart rhythm in which the sinoatrial node (S-A) fires at fewer than 60 beats per minute. It may be an unknown rhythm in a healthy individual. It goes untreated unless the client is symptomatic. Then the drug of choice is atropine. It may be found in athletes, acute myocardial infarction, as an adverse reaction of calcium channel blockers, hyperkalemia, increased intracranial pressure, or manipulation of the abdominal contents during surgery.

Nursing process: Evaluation

Client need: Physiological Adaptation

Cognitive level: Application

Subject area: Medical-Surgical

30. A client is brought to the emergency room with a third-degree heart block after experiencing an acute anterior myocardial infarction. Which of the following interventions is the priority on an emergency basis?

    1. Temporary pacemaker

    2. Administer lidocaine

    3. Cardioversion

    4. Administer atropine

31. The nurse should include which of the following in the plan of care of a client after a pacemaker is inserted?

    1. Instruct the client to avoid lifting the arm on the pacemaker side above shoulder height

    2. Encourage the client to exercise the shoulder and arm on the side of the pacemaker four times a day

    3. Encourage the client to wash the pacemaker incision with warm soapy water twice a day

    4. Instruct the client to avoid the use of microwave ovens

32. Following morning assessments, the registered nurse may delegate which of the following clients with a dysrhythmia to a licensed practical nurse to care for? A client with

    1. ventricular tachycardia.

    2. sinus bradycardia.

    3. ventricular fibrillation.

    4. sinus rhythm with a second-degree A-V block type II (Mobitz II).

Answer: 1

Rationale: A third-degree heart block is a lethal rhythm. It is the complete blockage of the atrial impulses into the ventricles. The block may be at the A-V node, bundle of His, or bundle branches, resulting in the atria and ventricles beating independently of each other. The atrial rate is usually normal while the ventricular rate is very slow and below 55 beats per minute. The causes may be an anterior myocardial infarction, coronary artery disease, surgery, aging, or drug toxicity such as digoxin, procainamide (Procanbid), or verapamil (Calan).

Nursing process: Planning

Client need: Management of Care

Cognitive level: Analysis

Subject area: Medical-Surgical

Answer: 1

Rationale: A client who had a pacemaker inserted should be instructed to stay on bed rest for 12 hours with minimal activity of the affected arm and shoulder to prevent dislodging the leads of the pacemaker. The client should also be instructed to keep the insertion area dry for one week postinsertion. It is not necessary to avoid microwave ovens because they do not threaten the function of the pacemaker.

Nursing process: Planning

Client need: Physiological Adaptation

Cognitive level: Application

Subject area: Medical-Surgical

Answer: 2

Rationale: Ventricular tachycardia and ventricular fibrillation are lethal dysrhythmias that require immediate intervention to maintain life. Sinus rhythm with a second-degree A-V block type II (Mobitz II) requires pacemaker placement. Sinus bradycardia is a dysrhythmia that generally goes unnoticed because the client can compensate for the decreased cardiac output. Treatment is not necessary unless the client becomes symptomatic.

Nursing process: Planning

Client need: Management of Care

Cognitive level: Analysis

Subject area: Legal and Ethical Issues

33. The nurse is monitoring the ECG tracing on the central monitors on a cardiac unit. Which of the following dysrhythmias is a priority for the nurse to report first?

1. Sinus rhythm with a first-degree A-V block

2. Supraventricular tachycardia (SVT)

3. Atrial fibrillation

4. Idioventricular rhythm (ventricular escape rhythm)

34. The nurse prioritizes the following clients with dysrhythmias in order of their care. Prioritize the following clients, from highest to lowest priority, in the order in which care should be performed.

_____ **1.** A client with sinus bradycardia

_____ **2.** A client with atrial flutter

_____ **3.** A client with ventricular fibrillation

_____ **4.** A client with sinus tachycardia

35. In caring for a client with atrial flutter, which of the following goals would have priority?

1. Reduce the ventricular rate to below 100 beats per minute

2. Identify and treat the underlying cause

3. Control the heart rate and maintain cardiac output

4. Increase the heart rate

Answer: 4

Rationale: Idioventricular rhythm (ventricular escape rhythm) is a lethal rhythm in which there is a high pacemaker failure. No impulses are conducted to the ventricles from above the bundle of His. Supraventricular tachycardia (SVT) is a term used to describe tachydysrhythmias that cannot be classified more accurately. Treatment depends on the severity of the client's clinical manifestations. A sinus rhythm with a first-degree A-V block is a consistent delay in the A-V conduction. Generally no intervention is recommended. Atrial fibrillation is a constant quivering of the heart caused by extreme atrial irritability. The atrial rate is controlled with calcium channel blockers and beta blockers. Cardioversion may be necessary and is most successful if performed within three days of treatment.

Nursing process: Implementation

Client need: Management of Care

Cognitive level: Analysis

Subject area: Medical-Surgical

Answer: 3, 2, 4, 1

Rationale: A client with sinus bradycardia is generally symptomatic with treatment not being necessary. A client with sinus tachycardia should be assessed for the cause and treated as needed. The most common drugs used are beta blockers. The ventricular response is controlled in a client with atrial flutter through the administration of calcium channel blockers. Ventricular fibrillation is a lethal rhythm in which the heart fibrillates. A code and CPR must be performed immediately or the client will die.

Nursing process: Analysis

Client need: Management of Care

Cognitive level: Analysis

Subject area: Medical-Surgical

Answer: 3

Rationale: The goal for a client with atrial fibrillation is to reduce the ventricular response rate to below 100 beats per minute. An appropriate goal for a client with sinus tachycardia is to identify and treat the underlying cause. It is a priority to control the heart rate and maintain cardiac output in a client with atrial flutter. A goal of increasing the heart rate would be an appropriate goal for a client with a junctional rhythm.

Nursing process: Planning

Client need: Management of Care

Cognitive level: Analysis

Subject area: Medical-Surgical

36. Which of the following should the nurse include in the plan of care for a client with sinus tachycardia?
  1. Administer lidocaine
  2. Assess the client
  3. Administer atropine
  4. Cardioversion

Answer: 2

Rationale: Sinus tachycardia is a dysrhythmia in which the S-A node discharges at more than 100 beats per minute. The nursing interventions include assessing the client for the cause and treating as needed. The most commonly used drugs are beta blockers.

Nursing process: Planning

Client need: Physiological Adaptation

Cognitive level: Application

Subject area: Medical-Surgical

CHAPTER

Gastrointestinal Disorders

4

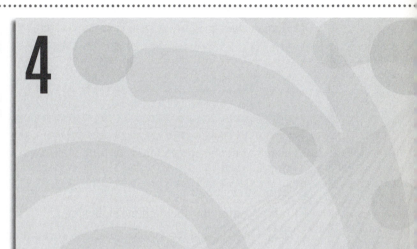

1. The nurse is assessing a client's gastrointestinal tract. Which of the following subjective assessments should be included?

    1. Rebound tenderness

    2. Diarrhea

    3. Generalized red abdominal rash

    4. Hematuria

2. In planning the postprocedure care for a client who has a barium enema, the nurse should include which of the following?

    Select all that apply:

    [   ] **1.** Position the client on the right side

    [   ] **2.** Observe and record the amount of rectal drainage

    [   ] **3.** Encourage fluids

    [   ] **4.** Maintain bed rest for 12 hours

    [   ] **5.** Monitor the client for a rise in body temperature and abdominal pain

    [   ] **6.** Administer a laxative

3. When providing care for a client who has had an upper gastrointestinal endoscopy, the nurse should include which of the following interventions?

    1. Assist the client to maintain a right-side lying position

    2. Provide the client with a fatty test meal

    3. Keep the client NPO until the gag reflex returns

    4. Administer the prescribed bulk-forming laxative

Answer: 1

Rationale: Assessment includes both subjective and objective data. Rebound tenderness is sudden pain when the examiner palpating the abdomen removes the examining fingers and the client complains of pain. Diarrhea, generalized red abdominal rash, and hematuria are all observable and therefore objective, not subjective, data.

Nursing process: Assessment

Client need: Physiological Adaptation

Cognitive level: Application

Subject area: Medical-Surgical

Answer: 3, 6

Rationale: As a result of the barium being administered rectally for a barium enema, increasing fluids and administering a laxative are encouraged to resume normal defecation and prevent an impaction. Positioning the client on the right side and maintaining bed rest for 12 hours is postprocedure care for a liver biopsy. Rectal bleeding would be assessed after a colonoscopy. A rise in body temperature and abdominal pain would indicate a possible perforation following an endoscopy.

Nursing process: Planning

Client need: Reduction of Risk Potential

Cognitive level: Application

Subject area: Medical-Surgical

Answer: 3

Rationale: Because a topical anesthesia spray, usually lidocaine, is administered during an upper gastrointestinal endoscopy to facilitate passage of the endoscopy, assessing the return of the gag reflex is crucial postprocedure prior to administering food and fluids to prevent aspiration. Positioning the client on the right side is postprocedure care following a liver biopsy. Providing the client a fatty test meal may be ordered following an oral cholecystogram to check for gallbladder emptying. Administering a laxative is not necessary because no barium is used during an upper endoscopy to cause constipation.

Nursing process: Planning

Client need: Reduction of Risk Potential

Cognitive level: Application

Subject area: Medical-Surgical

4. The nurse is caring for a client with gastroesophageal reflux disease. Which of the following measures would be essential to include in the client's discharge instructions?

Select all that apply:

[   ] **1.** Small, frequent meals

[   ] **2.** Avoid fluids at mealtime

[   ] **3.** High-calorie and high-protein diet

[   ] **4.** Bulk-forming laxatives

[   ] **5.** Sleep with the head of the bed elevated

[   ] **6.** Avoid caffeine in the diet

5. The nurse is caring for a client with gastroenteritis. Which of the following nursing measures should receive priority in the client's plan of care?

1. Maintain a clean environment free from odors

2. Assist the client to wash hands and face before meals

3. Encourage fluids and monitor intake and output

4. Provide foods the client likes and allow plenty of time for meals

6. The nurse is caring for a client with diverticulitis. Which of the following diets would be essential to include in the client's plan of care?

1. High-fiber diet

2. Low-fat, high-carbohydrate, and high-protein diet, avoiding alcohol

3. High-calorie, high-carbohydrate, and low-fat diet

4. Diet high in protein and calories, low in residue, and milk free

Answer: 1, 5, 6

Rationale: Small, frequent meals, avoiding caffeine, and sleeping with the head of the bed elevated prevent the gastric secretions from going backward through an incompetent lower esophageal sphincter (LES) that occurs in gastroesophageal reflux disease. Avoiding fluids at mealtime and providing for rest after meals is the treatment of dumping syndrome. A high-calorie, high-protein diet with 2000 ml of fluid daily is recommended in malnutrition after certain gastrointestinal diseases or surgery. Low-roughage, high-fiber diet and bulk-forming laxatives are the recommended diet to treat diverticulitis.

Nursing process: Planning

Client need: Physiological Adaptation

Cognitive level: Application

Subject area: Medical-Surgical

Answer: 3

Rationale: Although maintaining a clean environment free from odors, assisting the client to wash the hands and face before meals, and offering foods the client likes are appropriate nursing interventions for a client with gastroenteritis, encouraging fluids and monitoring the intake and output are the priority interventions.

Nursing process: Planning

Client need: Management of Care

Cognitive level: Application

Subject area: Medical-Surgical

Answer: 1

Rationale: Diverticulitis is treated with a high-fiber diet and bulk-forming laxatives. If a diet is low in fiber and with the decreased bulk of the stool, the bowel lumen narrows, leading to high intra-abdominal pressure during defecation. This contributes to the formation of the diverticula. A low-fat, high-carbohydrate, and high-protein diet avoiding alcohol is the diet of choice for pancreatitis. A high-calorie, high-carbohydrate, and low-fat diet is the diet for cirrhosis. A diet high in protein and calories, low in residue, and milk free is the diet for ulcerative colitis.

Nursing process: Planning

Client need: Basic Care and Comfort

Cognitive level: Application

Subject area: Medical-Surgical

7. The registered nurse is making out the clinical assignments for the day. Which of the following nursing tasks is appropriate to delegate to a licensed practical nurse?

   1. Plan an activity schedule for a client following a Billroth I
   2. Develop a plan of care for a client following a total proctocolectomy
   3. Assess the client's understanding of the care following an ileostomy
   4. Assist the client to select a low-fat diet following a cholecystectomy

8. The nurse is collecting a nursing history from a client suspected of having an obstruction of the alimentary canal. Which of the following questions should the nurse ask first to elicit the most accurate assessment?

   1. "Are you frequently awakened during the middle of the night because of pain?"
   2. "Have you recently lost a lot of weight?"
   3. "Do you have difficulty swallowing food or liquids?"
   4. "Have you experienced any bleeding?"

9. The nurse is caring for a client with peptic ulcer disease. Which of the following observations should the nurse report immediately?

   Select all that apply:
   [   ] 1. Hypotension
   [   ] 2. Thirst
   [   ] 3. Headache
   [   ] 4. Tachycardia
   [   ] 5. Restlessness
   [   ] 6. Diarrhea

10. When preparing a client for insertion of a nasogastric tube, it is essential for the nurse to include which of the following aspects of the procedure?

   1. Instruct the client to avoid swallowing when the tube is felt in the back of the throat
   2. Assist the client to assume a left-side lying or recumbent position
   3. Tilt the client's head back when the tube is being inserted
   4. Measure the tube from the tip of the nose to the earlobe to the xiphoid process

Answer: 4

Rationale: A licensed practical nurse may assist a client in selecting the specific foods on a selected diet. Only a registered nurse may develop, assess, and plan interventions.

Nursing process: Planning

Client need: Management of Care

Cognitive level: Analysis

Subject area: Legal and Ethical Issues

Answer: 3

Rationale: Difficulty swallowing food or liquids is the most appropriate assessment to determine the presence of an obstruction of the alimentary canal. Pain and weight loss may also occur with an obstruction but would not be the first clinical manifestation that the client would present with. Bleeding would be diagnostic with cancer, not an obstruction.

Nursing process: Assessment

Client need: Physiological Adaptation

Cognitive level: Analysis

Subject area: Medical-Surgical

Answer: 1, 4, 5

Rationale: Hypotension, tachycardia, and restlessness are all indicative of hemorrhage in a client with a peptic ulcer and must be reported immediately. Thirst, headache, and diarrhea are all clinical manifestations a client may experience with or without peptic ulcer disease but do not indicate an emergency situation.

Nursing process: Analysis

Client need: Reduction of Risk Potential

Cognitive level: Analysis

Subject area: Medical-Surgical

Answer: 4

Rationale: It is correct to measure from the tip of the nose to the tip of the earlobe to the xiphoid process prior to inserting a nasogastric tube to determine correct placement. Instructing the client not to swallow the tube when the tube is felt in the back of the throat is incorrect, because the nurse would encourage a client to swallow as the tube is being passed. The client should be in a high-Fowler's position for insertion of the tube. The head should be tilted forward when the tube is felt in the throat.

Nursing process: Planning

Client need: Reduction of Risk Potential

Cognitive level: Application

Subject area: Medical-Surgical

11. The nurse monitors a client for signs of dumping syndrome. Which of the following does the nurse evaluate as early clinical manifestations?

Select all that apply:

[   ] **1.** Hematemesis

[   ] **2.** Abdominal muscle rigidity

[   ] **3.** Tachycardia

[   ] **4.** Vertigo

[   ] **5.** Sweating

[   ] **6.** Diarrhea

12. A client scheduled for a vagotomy asks the nurse what a vagotomy is. Which of the following statements by the nurse best describes the purpose of the vagotomy?

1. "It decreases food transit time in the stomach."

2. "It regenerates the gastric mucosa."

3. "It reduces the stimulus to acid secretion."

4. "It stops stress-related reactions."

13. The nurse is caring for a client who is jaundiced. The nurse should implement which of the following in the plan for this client's pruritus?

1. Monitor the client's temperature and assess the client's color

2. Instruct the client to scratch with knuckles instead of nails

3. Administer prescribed analgesic and assist the client to bathe frequently

4. Encourage the client to eat a high-protein, low-cholesterol diet

14. A nurse is educating a group of individuals about hepatitis B. The nurse would identify what as the major route of transmission? _____

Answer: 3, 4, 5, 6

Rationale: Vertigo, tachycardia, sweating, and diarrhea are early manifestations that occur in a client with dumping syndrome. Hematemesis, melena, and hypotension occur with a gastrointestinal bleed. Abdominal pain, muscle rigidity, nausea, and vomiting occur in peritonitis. Epigastric distress after meals relieved by vomiting occurs in bile reflux gastritis, another postoperative complication of peptic ulcer surgery.

Nursing process: Assessment

Client need: Physiological Adaptation

Cognitive level: Application

Subject area: Medical-Surgical

Answer: 3

Rationale: A vagotomy severs the vagus nerve and eliminates the hydrochloric acid stimulus.

Nursing process: Analysis

Client need: Physiological Adaptation

Cognitive level: Application

Subject area: Medical-Surgical

Answer: 2

Rationale: Pruritus occurs as a result of an accumulation of bile salts under the skin. Scratching with the knuckles instead of the nails maintains the skin's integrity and prevents tearing.

Nursing process: Implementation

Client need: Physiological Adaptation

Cognitive level: Application

Subject area: Medical-Surgical

Answer: Serum

Rationale: Hepatitis B is transmitted by serum. Poor sanitation plays a role in the transmission of hepatitis A and E. Contaminated shellfish is a source of infection in the spread of hepatitis A. The fecal-oral route is the mode of transmission for hepatitis A and E.

Nursing process: Assessment

Client need: Reduction of Risk Potential

Cognitive level: Comprehension

Subject area: Medical-Surgical

15. The nurse is admitting a client with a diagnosis of preicteric (prodromal phase) hepatitis. Which of the following would the nurse expect to be the priority assessment finding?

    1. Clay-colored stools

    2. Anorexia

    3. Jaundice

    4. Pruritus

16. A client is diagnosed with hepatitis A and asks the nurse how to avoid infecting other family members. The nurse's response would be based on the understanding that the spread of hepatitis A is primarily

    1. sexual contact with an infected person who does not show symptoms of the disease.

    2. by contaminated needles from a person who has some form of hepatitis.

    3. through blood transfusions of improperly prepared blood.

    4. from person to person through fecal contamination or contaminated food and water.

17. The most effective prevention for viral hepatitis the nurse should administer is _____.

18. The nurse is discharging a client with chronic pancreatitis. Which of the following measures would be essential to include in the client's discharge instruction?

    1. Weight reduction and exercise program

    2. Bowel retraining program including daily laxative administration

    3. Diet modifications avoiding high-fat foods, caffeine, and alcohol

    4. Relaxation techniques and stress management

Answer: 2

Rationale: Anorexia is a clinical manifestation that occurs in the preicteric phase of hepatitis. Clay-colored stools, jaundice, and pruritus are all clinical manifestations that occur in the icteric phase of hepatitis.

Nursing process: Assessment

Client need: Physiological Adaptation

Cognitive level: Analysis

Subject area: Medical-Surgical

Answer: 4

Rationale: Hepatitis A is transmitted by the fecal-oral route and by contaminated food and water. Sexual contact with an infected person, contaminated needles, and contaminated blood are modes of transmission for hepatitis B and C.

Nursing process: Analysis

Client need: Physiological Adaptation

Cognitive level: Application

Subject area: Medical-Surgical

Answer: hepatitis B immunization

Rationale: Hepatitis B immunization is the best prevention for a client with viral hepatitis.

Nursing process: Implementation

Client need: Reduction of Risk Potential

Cognitive level: Application

Subject area: Medical-Surgical

Answer: 3

Rationale: A diet low in fat and avoiding caffeine and alcohol are recommended for chronic pancreatitis. Weight reduction, exercise program, bowel retraining program, relaxation techniques, and stress management are not interventions pertinent to pancreatitis.

Nursing process: Planning

Client need: Basic Care and Comfort

Cognitive level: Application

Subject area: Medical-Surgical

19. A client with acute cholelithiasis is experiencing colic pain and is requesting medication. When intervening in this situation, the nurse administers which of the following drugs?

    1. Meperidine (Demerol)

    2. Morphine

    3. Oxycodone and acetaminophen (Percocet)

    4. Propoxyphene hydrochloride (Darvon)

20. In preparing the client for an endoscopic cholecystectomy, the nurse should include which of the following post-op information?

Select all that apply:

    [   ] **1.** "There is a small midline abdominal incision."

    [   ] **2.** "You will be NPO for two days followed by a low-fat diet."

    [   ] **3.** "Your activity will be restricted."

    [   ] **4.** "Generally the pain is minimal."

    [   ] **5.** "There is a low incidence of wound infection."

    [   ] **6.** "The hospital stay is generally one to two days."

21. The nurse performs which part of the gastrointestinal assessment first?

    1. Auscultation

    2. Palpation

    3. Inspection

    4. Percussion

22. When preparing a client for a colonoscopy, it would be essential for the nurse to explain which of the following aspects of the procedure?

    1. Stools will be white until all the barium is expelled

    2. Bowel sounds will be monitored hourly for 12 hours

    3. The client will be positioned on the right side with the legs straight

    4. The client must begin a clear liquid diet beginning at noon the day before

Answer: 1

Rationale: Demerol is the drug of choice for acute cholelithiasis because it causes less spasming of the biliary ducts than morphine. Percocet and Darvocet would not be appropriate drug choices for a client experiencing colic pain in acute cholelithiasis.

Nursing process: Implementation

Client need: Pharmacological and Parenteral Therapies

Cognitive level: Analysis

Subject area: Pharmacologic

Answer: 4, 5, 6

Rationale: The laparoscopic cholecystectomy is a minor procedure with few complications. There is decreased wound infection, minimal pain, and a one to two day hospital stay. An abdominal incision, nasogastric tube, NPO, low-fat diet, pain, Jackson-Pratt drain, and restricted activity would occur in an open cholecystectomy.

Nursing process: Planning

Client need: Physiological Adaptation

Cognitive level: Application

Subject area: Medical-Surgical

Answer: 3

Rationale: Inspection should be the first phase of the gastrointestinal assessment, followed by auscultation, percussion, and palpation. Inspection should be performed first, before there is any stimulation of the intestinal organs and contents.

Nursing process: Implementation

Client need: Physiological Adaptation

Cognitive level: Analysis

Subject area: Medical-Surgical

Answer: 4

Rationale: The client will be on clear liquids beginning at noon and for up to 8 hours before the procedure, then NPO. The client will be placed in the left lateral decubitus position to facilitate the insertion of the colonoscope. There is no barium administered and the vital signs, not the bowel sounds, will be monitored postprocedure for signs of hemorrhage.

Nursing process: Planning

Client need: Reduction of Risk Potential

Cognitive level: Application

Subject area: Medical-Surgical

23. A client experiences regurgitation and dyspepsia. The nurse assists the client to assume an upright position. Which of the following statements by the nurse would best describe the purpose of this measure?

    1. "It prevents the flow of gastric contents into the esophagus."

    2. "It decreases the inflammatory changes in the esophagus."

    3. "It enhances and strengthens esophageal peristalsis."

    4. "It increases the lower esophageal pressure."

24. Because a client has Crohn's disease, plans for nursing intervention should include

    1. weight reduction measures and low-calorie diet.

    2. frequent application of lubricant lotion and discouraging scratching.

    3. teaching the importance of follow-up liver function test after discharge.

    4. perianal care and restoration of fluids and electrolytes.

25. During an acute exacerbation of Crohn's disease, which of the following nursing diagnoses should have priority?

    1. Imbalanced nutrition: less than body requirements related to anorexia and diarrhea

    2. Anxiety related to altered self-concept and health status

    3. Fatigue related to decreased nutrient intake and anemia

    4. Knowledge deficiency related to lack of information about disease process

26. The nurse is evaluating the pain complaints of four clients. Which client does the nurse report to the physician as indicative of peptic ulcer disease?

    1. Low, colicky abdominal pain

    2. A gnawing epigastric pain relieved by food

    3. Left upper-quadrant pain that radiates to the back

    4. Right upper-quadrant pain radiating to the right shoulder

Answer: 1

Rationale: An upright position is the best position for a client experiencing regurgitation and dyspepsia. It prevents the flow of gastric contents into the esophagus.

Nursing process: Evaluation

Client need: Physiological Adaptation

Cognitive level: Application

Subject area: Medical-Surgical

Answer: 4

Rationale: A client with Crohn's disease experiences frequent loose stools. The client may have as many as 20 stools per day so nursing interventions for perianal care and restoration of fluids and electrolytes are important. Weight-reduction measures and a low-calorie diet are appropriate interventions for cholecystitis. Teaching the importance of follow-up liver function tests after discharge would be an intervention for hepatitis. Frequent application of a lubricant lotion and discouraging scratching are appropriate interventions for a client experiencing jaundice.

Nursing process: Planning

Client need: Physiological Adaptation

Cognitive level: Application

Subject area: Medical-Surgical

Answer: 1

Rationale: The priority nursing diagnosis for a client with Crohn's disease is imbalanced nutrition: less than body requirements related to anorexia and diarrhea. Other less important nursing diagnoses include fatigue related to decreased nutrient intake and anemia, knowledge deficiency related to lack of information about the disease process, and anxiety related to altered self-concept and health status.

Nursing process: Evaluation

Client need: Physiological Adaptation

Cognitive level: Analysis

Subject area: Medical-Surgical

Answer: 2

Rationale: A gnawing epigastric pain relieved by food is indicative of peptic ulcer disease. Low, colicky abdominal pain is a clinical manifestation of diverticulitis. Upper left-quadrant pain that radiates to the back is classic in pancreatitis. Right upper-quadrant pain that radiates to the right shoulder is characteristic of cholecystitis.

Nursing process: Analysis

Client need: Physiological Adaptation

Cognitive level: Application

Subject area: Medical-Surgical

27. The nurse observes a staff member caring for a client after a vagotomy and partial gastrectomy. Which of the following indicates that the staff member is irrigating the nasogastric tube correctly?

    1. Inject 10 ml distilled water, clamp tube for 30 minutes, then disconnect suction for 30 minutes
    2. Insert 20 ml of air and clamp off suction for 1 hour
    3. Administer 20 ml of prescribed antibiotic and increase pressure of suction
    4. Fill syringe with 30 ml of normal saline, inject into tube, and withdraw slowly

28. In planning the postoperative care for a client with an ileostomy, the nurse would select which of the following as the priority nursing diagnosis?

    1. Disturbed body image related to the ostomy
    2. Risk for deficient fluid volume related to excess fluid loss
    3. Ineffective sexuality patterns related to loss of sexual desire
    4. Risk for impaired skin integrity related to fecal drainage

29. The nurse is caring for a client receiving continuous nasogastric feedings. The nurse observes the client for aspiration that could be the result of

    1. use of unclean equipment and reflux into the esophagus.
    2. administering tube feedings at either a cold or warm temperature.
    3. too rapid administration and incomplete stomach emptying.
    4. allergic reaction to feeding administered.

30. The nurse is caring for a client receiving medications through a nasogastric tube. Which of the following is the appropriate method for the nurse to administer these medications?

    1. Mix all medications together and administer as a bolus and flush with 20 to 30 ml normal saline or water at the end
    2. Administer those medications which are compatible and flush with 60 ml normal saline or water at the end
    3. Administer each medication individually and flush with 100 ml normal saline or water at the end
    4. Administer each medication individually, flush with 5 to 10 ml normal saline or water between each medication, and flush with 20 ml at the end

Answer: 4

Rationale: The correct procedure for irrigating a nasogastric tube is to fill a syringe with 30 ml normal saline followed by injecting it into the tube and withdrawing slowly.

Nursing process: Evaluation

Client need: Reduction of Risk Potential

Cognitive level: Application

Subject area: Medical-Surgical

Answer: 2

Rationale: The priority nursing diagnosis for a client with an ileostomy is risk for deficient fluid volume related to excess fluid loss. The client with an ileostomy has continuous liquid stools, which can result in a fluid volume deficit unless the client takes in an adequate amount of fluids. Other less important nursing diagnoses include disturbed body image related to the ostomy, ineffective sexuality patterns related to loss of sexual desire, and risk for impaired skin integrity related to fecal drainage.

Nursing process: Planning

Client need: Physiological Adaptation

Cognitive level: Analysis

Subject area: Medical-Surgical

Answer: 3

Rationale: Administering a continuous nasogastric feeding too fast places the client at risk for aspiration. Aspiration could also be the result of incomplete stomach emptying. Use of unclean equipment and reflux into the esophagus places the client at risk for infection manifested by diarrhea. Administering a tube feeding at either too cold or too warm a temperature may result in spasms. An allergic reaction to the feeding administered is the result of an intolerance to the feeding.

Nursing process: Evaluation

Client need: Reduction of Risk Potential

Cognitive level: Analysis

Subject area: Medical-Surgical

Answer: 4

Rationale: The appropriate procedure for administering medications through a nasogastric tube is to administer each medication separately. After each medication is administered individually, 5 to 10 ml of normal saline or water should be administered between medications followed by a 20 ml flush at the end.

Nursing process: Evaluation

Client need: Reduction of Risk Potential

Cognitive level: Application

Subject area: Pharmacologic

31. The nurse is assessing a client postoperatively following a hemorrhoidectomy. Which of the following assessments would be most important for the nurse to include?

1. The client's ability to assume a sitting position
2. The degree of embarrassment the client expresses
3. Inspection of the rectal area for bleeding
4. Presence of nausea and vomiting

32. The nurse is caring for a client two hours after a hemorrhoidectomy. The client asks the nurse, "Should I be having severe pain?" The most appropriate response by the nurse would be

1. "Yes and I'll get you a pain medication."
2. "This is a minor surgery and the pain is also minor."
3. "I'll call your physician because I don't know why you are having so much pain."
4. "Try changing your position and take some deep breaths to relax you."

33. The nurse is caring for a client one week postoperatively following a colostomy. Which of the following assessment findings would be a priority for the nurse to report?

1. The client is experiencing flatulence
2. The color of the stoma is dusky blue
3. The skin under the colostomy bag is red
4. The client appears depressed

34. The nurse is discharging a client with an ileostomy. Which of the following would the nurse include in the discharge instructions?

1. A drainage appliance only needs to be worn in public
2. Bowel regularity will be established within two weeks
3. Report any signs of bleeding from the stoma
4. Increase fluids rich in electrolytes, such as Gatorade

Answer: 3

Rationale: Post-op care following a hemorrhoidectomy includes a high-fiber diet, increased fluid intake, stool softeners, and inspecting the area for bleeding.

Nursing process: Assessment

Client need: Physiological Adaptation

Cognitive level: Application

Subject area: Medical-Surgical

Answer: 1

Rationale: The pain following a hemorrhoidectomy can be persistent and severe. It is important that the nurse understands this and does not disregard the client's complaints.

Nursing process: Analysis

Client need: Physiological Adaptation

Cognitive level: Analysis

Subject area: Medical-Surgical

Answer: 2

Rationale: It is a priority that the nurse reports the stoma of a colostomy that becomes dusky blue. This indicates ischemia. A client who has a colostomy may experience flatulence after eating gas-forming foods. The skin under the colostomy bag that becomes red may be a sign of irritation. A client who is depressed may be having a difficult time adjusting to the colostomy.

Nursing process: Analysis

Client need: Physiological Adaptation

Cognitive level: Analysis

Subject area: Medical-Surgical

Answer: 4

Rationale: Because a client with an ileostomy has continuous liquid stools, the potential for losing electrolytes exists. The client should be encouraged to drink fluids rich in electrolytes, such as Gatorade. Regularity is not established with an ileostomy, so an appliance must be worn at all times.

Nursing process: Planning

Client need: Physiological Adaptation

Cognitive level: Application

Subject area: Medical-Surgical

35. A client with a colostomy is experiencing an increased odor and asks the nurse what is contributing to this. The most appropriate response by the nurse is

  1. "There are no foods that affect odor."

  2. "Food such as eggs, asparagus, fish, and broccoli will increase the odor."

  3. "The odor is normal but a pouch deodorant will help."

  4. "Changing the pouch and washing the stoma daily will eliminate the odor."

36. The nurse evaluates which of the following clients to be at greatest risk for developing alcoholic cirrhosis (Laënnec's)?

  1. A 55-year-old male who has chronic alcoholism

  2. A 28-year-old male who had a recent exposure to a hepatotoxic drug

  3. A 70-year-old male who has a history of right-sided heart failure

  4. A 40-year-old female who has a biliary obstruction

37. The nurse should assess a client suspected of having peritonitis for which of the following clinical manifestations?

  Select all that apply:

  [ ] **1.** Pyrosis

  [ ] **2.** Abdominal tenderness

  [ ] **3.** Diarrhea

  [ ] **4.** Muscle rigidity

  [ ] **5.** Abdominal pain

  [ ] **6.** Tachycardia

Answer: 2

Rationale: Although changing the colostomy pouch and a pouch deodorant may help the odor of a colostomy, the most appropriate intervention is to instruct the client to avoid odor-forming foods such as eggs, asparagus, fish, and broccoli.

Nursing process: Analysis

Client need: Physiological Adaptation

Cognitive level: Analysis

Subject area: Medical-Surgical

Answer: 1

Rationale: Alcoholic (Laënnec's) cirrhosis is associated with alcohol abuse. Postnecrotic cirrhosis is the result of a toxic substance. Chronic biliary obstruction may cause biliary cirrhosis. Cardiac cirrhosis may result from a long-standing right-sided heart failure.

Nursing process: Evaluation

Client need: Physiological Adaptation

Cognitive level: Analysis

Subject area: Medical-Surgical

Answer: 2, 4, 5, 6

Rationale: Clinical manifestations of peritonitis include abdominal pain, tenderness, and distention. Other clinical manifestations include muscle rigidity, fever, nausea, vomiting, tachycardia, and tachypnea. Diarrhea is a characteristic of many gastrointestinal disorders, such as gastroenteritis. Pyrosis may also be included in many other gastrointestinal disorders.

Nursing process: Assessment

Client need: Physiological Adaptation

Cognitive level: Application

Subject area: Medical-Surgical

38. The nurse assesses which of the following clients to most likely develop a problem with constipation?

1. A client who consumes a high-fiber diet

2. A client who is receiving trimethoprim-sulfamethoxazole (Bactrim)

3. A client who is receiving dicyclomine hydrochloride (Bentyl)

4. A client who has a 1500 ml fluid intake per day

39. The nurse assesses a client for the presence of a gastric outlet obstruction. Which of the following findings should be reported?

Select all that apply:

[ ] **1.** Large abdominal peristaltic waves

[ ] **2.** Sudden severe upper abdominal pain

[ ] **3.** Shoulder pain

[ ] **4.** Projectile vomiting

[ ] **5.** Rigid, boardlike abdomen

[ ] **6.** Weight loss

40. The nurse assesses a client with hepatic encephalopathy for asterixis by

1. asking the client to extend an arm, dorsiflex the wrist, and extend the finger.

2. assessing the client for azotemia, oliguria, and intractable ascites.

3. assessing the client for a musty, sweet breath odor.

4. asking the client to draw a cross and noting any deterioration in the figure construction.

Answer: 3

Rationale: Dicyclomine hydrochloride (Bentyl) is a cholinergic blocking drug generally given for hypermotility and spasms of the gastrointestinal tract associated with an irritable colon, spastic colon, or mucous colitis. Constipation is a common adverse reaction to Bentyl. Other gastrointestinal adverse reactions include nausea, vomiting, and dry mouth. A high-fiber diet would be given to prevent constipation. Trimethoprim-sulfamethoxazole (Bactrim) is an antibiotic frequently given for a urinary tract infection. A common adverse reaction is diarrhea. A client with a fluid intake of 1500 ml could develop constipation but Bentyl is a more likely cause of constipation.

Nursing process: Assessment

Client need: Reduction of Risk Potential

Cognitive level: Analysis

Subject area: Medical-Surgical

Answer: 1, 4, 6

Rationale: Clinical manifestations of a gastric outlet obstruction include loud peristalsis, large and visible peristaltic abdominal waves, vomiting that relieves the pain, and accompanying weight loss. Sudden severe upper abdominal pain, shoulder pain, and a rigid, boardlike abdomen are classic in perforation of a peptic ulcer.

Nursing process: Analysis

Client need: Physiological Adaptation

Cognitive level: Analysis

Subject area: Medical-Surgical

Answer: 1

Rationale: Asking the client to extend the arm, dorsiflex the wrist, and extend the finger is asterixis, or liver flap, which is a clinical manifestation that occurs as coma approaches in hepatic encephalopathy. Asking the client to draw a cross and noting any deterioration in the figure construction is also a clinical manifestation of hepatic encephalopathy. A musty, sweet breath odor occurs in some clients with hepatic encephalopathy. Azotemia, oliguria, and intractable ascites are manifestations of hepatorenal syndrome, a serious complication of cirrhosis.

Nursing process: Assessment

Client need: Physiological Adaptation

Cognitive level: Application

Subject area: Medical-Surgical

41. Which of the following should the nurse include when performing a Hematest?

1. Open the front flap on the cover of the slide, and apply a thin smear of stool in the first box only

2. Open the flap on the back of the slide and apply a drop of developing solution

3. Place test tablet on top of the stool specimen on guaiac paper and follow with two drops of water

4. Document results after waiting five minutes to observe color changes

42. The nurse obtains a pH of 8.0 when aspirating for gastric contents when assessing correct tube placement. The nurse evaluates a pH of 8.0 to be

1. alkaline, and indicates respiratory secretions.

2. a neutral pH.

3. acidic, confirming gastric secretions.

4. indicative of intestinal secretions.

43. Based on an understanding of the adverse reactions to drugs, which of the following drugs does the nurse evaluate from the medication history to cause constipation?

1. Fluoxetine (Prozac)

2. Digoxin (Lanoxin)

3. Amoxycillin (Polymox)

4. Amitriptyline (Elavil)

44. When assessing a client with a nasogastric tube, the nurse discovers it is set on continuous high suction. Which of the following nursing actions should the nurse implement?

1. Clamp the tube for 30 minutes, then reconnect it to continuous high suction

2. Call the physician and remove the tube

3. Irrigate the tube with 30 ml of normal saline and record the characteristics of the drainage

4. Change the suction to low intermittent suction

Answer: 3

Rationale: The correct way to perform a Hematest is to place a test tablet on top of the stool on guaiac paper followed by two drops of water. Two minutes should be waited before assessing the results. A Hemoccult slide test is performed by opening the flap of the slide and applying a thin smear of stool in the first box only. The slide cover is then closed and the slide turned over. The flap on the back is open and two drops of Hemoccult developing solution is applied in each box.

Nursing process: Implementation

Client need: Reduction of Risk Potential

Cognitive level: Application

Subject area: Medical-Surgical

Answer: 1

Rationale: When checking for correct nasogastric tube placement, a pH of 8.0 indicates the presence of alkaline and respiratory secretion. Fluid aspirated with a pH higher than 6.0 indicates pleural fluid from the tracheobronchial tree. A range of 1.0 to 4.0 indicates proper tube placement. Fluid aspirated with a pH higher than 6.0 may also indicate the tube is placed in the intestine because the intestinal secretions are less acidic than the stomach.

Nursing process: Evaluation

Client need: Reduction of Risk Potential

Cognitive level: Analysis

Subject area: Medical-Surgical

Answer: 4

Rationale: Fluoxetine (Prozac) is a selective serotonin reuptake inhibitor that causes diarrhea. Digoxin (Lanoxin) is a cardiac glycoside that may cause diarrhea. Amoxycillin (Polymox) is an antibiotic that causes diarrhea. Amitriptyline (Elavil) is a tricyclic antidepressant that may cause constipation.

Nursing process: Evaluation

Client need: Pharmacological and Parenteral Therapies

Cognitive level: Analysis

Subject area: Pharmacologic

Answer: 4

Rationale: A nasogastric tube should be set on low intermittent suction to prevent trauma to the stomach. A tube set on continuous high suction may cause trauma to the gastric tissue and may actually suck out the stomach wall.

Nursing process: Implementation

Client need: Reduction of Risk Potential

Cognitive level: Application

Subject area: Medical-Surgical

45. During an inspection of the abdomen, which of the abdominal findings should the nurse report as abnormal?
1. Bilateral symmetrical abdomen
2. Flat abdominal contour
3. Strong abdominal pulsations
4. Depressed umbilicus beneath the abdominal surface

Answer: 3

Rationale: A strong abdominal pulsation may indicate a widened pulse pressure and an aortic aneurysm. A bilateral symmetrical abdomen, flat abdominal contour, and a depressed umbilicus beneath the abdominal surface are all normal findings.

Nursing process: Analysis

Client need: Physiological Adaptation

Cognitive level: Application

Subject area: Medical-Surgical

Endocrine Disorders

5

1. The nurse assesses which of the following assessments in a client with severe anterior pituitary deficiency caused by the growth of a tumor?

Select all that apply:

[   ] **1.** Intolerance to heat

[   ] **2.** Hyperglycemia

[   ] **3.** Polyuria

[   ] **4.** Bradycardia

[   ] **5.** Hypoglycemia

[   ] **6.** Dehydration

2. The nurse should include which of the following in preoperative instructions for a client with an anterior pituitary tumor who is scheduled for a total hypophysectomy using the transsphenoid approach?

1. Avoid sneezing or blowing the nose after surgery

2. Drink 10 glasses of fluids the day before surgery

3. Do not rinse the mouth with any solutions until the packing is removed

4. Support the neck when getting out of bed

3. The nurse is collecting a nursing history from a client admitted with diabetes insipidus. Which of the following questions should the nurse ask?

1. "Have you experienced a change in temperature where you feel very hot or very cold?"

2. "Have you noticed a change in how you react to people or situations?"

3. "Have you experienced a change in urinary frequency or amount?"

4. "Have you noticed a change in how you function sexually?"

Answer: 4, 5

Rationale: The anterior pituitary gland secretes several hormones, primarily ACTH, TSH, FSH, LH, and prolactin. A tumor in the anterior pituitary gland results in hyposecretion of one or more of the hormones secreted. Bradycardia would indicate a deficiency in thyroid hormones and hypoglycemia would indicate a deficiency in adrenocorticotrophic hormones. Intolerance to heat would be characteristic of hyperthyroidism and hyperglycemia would indicate an increase in ACTH. Polyuria would be characteristic of excessive secretion of ADH from the posterior pituitary or excessive secretion of ACTH. Dehydration and polyuria are characteristics of diabetes insipidus, a posterior pituitary disorder.

Nursing process: Assessment

Client need: Physiological Adaptation

Cognitive level: Application

Subject area: Medical-Surgical

Answer: 1

Rationale: A transsphenoid hypophysectomy is a surgical approach through the oral-nasal cavity. Any stress on the nasal cavity, such as sneezing or blowing one's nose, may precipitate the leakage of cerebrospinal fluid. These clients are not dehydrated prior to surgery, so they don't need increased fluids. Postoperatively, clients may rinse their mouths with warm saline. Since the surgery involves the upper lip and nose, supporting the neck is not necessary.

Nursing process: Planning

Client need: Health Promotion and Maintenance

Cognitive level: Application

Subject area: Medical-Surgical

Answer: 3

Rationale: The client with diabetes insipidus has a deficiency in ADH (antidiuretic hormone) secreted from the posterior pituitary gland. The client will experience voiding frequent large volumes of dilute urine. Questions regarding changes in heat and cold tolerance and mental status would be appropriate for thyroid disorders. Changes in sexual function are appropriate for anterior pituitary disorders and disorders with the sexual organs.

Nursing process: Assessment

Client need: Physiological Adaptation

Cognitive level: Application

Subject area: Medical-Surgical

4. The nurse should include which of the following in the discharge instructions of a client with diabetes insipidus?

  1. Follow-up appointments are not necessary with the physician unless there is an acute illness

  2. The prescribed hormone drugs will need to be taken for a lifetime

  3. Extra fluids should be taken cautiously when experiencing a major stressor

  4. Changes in diet and exercise may require changes in medication dosages

5. The nurse should report which of the following client assessments as consistent with a diagnosis of Graves' disease?

Select all that apply:

  [   ] **1.** Lethargy

  [   ] **2.** Exophthalmus

  [   ] **3.** Heat intolerance

  [   ] **4.** Weight loss

  [   ] **5.** Cold, clammy skin

  [   ] **6.** Bradycardia

6. Which of the following client statements should the nurse report to the physician prior to scheduling a radioactive iodine uptake and excretion test?

  1. "I've been taking over-the-counter cough medicine for the past two weeks."

  2. "My husband and I are vegetarians."

  3. "We like to drink a glass of wine with our meals."

  4. "I take a baby aspirin every day since my heart attack last year."

Answer: 2

Rationale: Clients with disorders involving a deficiency in hormone production will need to take replacement hormones for the rest of their lives. The client with diabetes insipidus is deficient in ADH so he or she will need to take the replacement vasopressin for a lifetime. These clients need periodic follow-up to monitor response to medication dose and route. Major stressors, such as illness or surgery, will affect hormone requirements so a client with diabetes insipidus will need increased fluids for fluid replacement until vasopressin dosages can be regulated. Diet and exercise do not have an effect on medication dosages for diabetes insipidus but do have an effect on diabetes mellitus.

Nursing process: Planning

Client need: Health Promotion and Maintenance

Cognitive level: Application

Subject area: Medical-Surgical

Answer: 2, 3, 4

Rationale: Hyperthyroidism, also known as Graves' disease (an increase in the production of thyroid hormones), is characterized by an increase in the metabolic rate, protruding eyeballs (exophthalmus), and an accumulation of fluid in the fat pads behind the eyes. The client also experiences hyperexcitability, nervousness, heat intolerance, and weight loss despite increased appetite. Lethargy and bradycardia are characteristics of decreased metabolism. An increased metabolic rate results in increased body warmth.

Nursing process: Assessment

Client need: Physiological Adaptation

Cognitive level: Application

Subject area: Medical-Surgical

Answer: 1

Rationale: Medications and foods containing iodine alter the results of radioactive iodine tests. Over-the-counter cough medicines may contain iodine. A vegetarian diet and wine are not food sources of iodine. Aspirin is not a medicinal source of iodine.

Nursing process: Analysis

Client need: Physiological Adaptation

Cognitive level: Application

Subject area: Medical-Surgical

7. Which of the following should the nurse include in the teaching plan for a client who has hyperthyroidism and is treated with ^{123}I?

   1. A single dose of the radioactive iodine is sufficient
   2. Body excretions are considered radioactive for one week
   3. An increase in temperature and pulse rate should be reported
   4. Symptoms of hyperthyroidism should subside in one to two weeks

8. The nurse develops a plan of care for the immediate postoperative period for a client who had a thyroidectomy. The plan should include measures to

   1. correct fluid and electrolyte balance.
   2. administer medications to decrease vascularity of the thyroid glands.
   3. promote range-of-motion exercises to the neck.
   4. prevent complications of respiratory obstruction.

9. The nurse implements which of the following interventions in the plan of care for a client with hypothyroidism?

   1. Applying lotion for skin care
   2. Providing a cool temperature in the room
   3. Scheduling periods of rest
   4. Administering p.r.n. medications for diarrhea

Answer: 3

Rationale: Hyperthyroid clients treated with ^{123}I need to be observed closely for signs of hyperthyroidism indicating treatment was not successful. Hypothyroidism results indicate overresponse. Some clients need a second dose. Clients have a fear about radioactive substances but they are not considered to be radioactive and no radiation precautions are necessary. It takes approximately three to four weeks before the symptoms of hyperthyroidism subside.

Nursing process: Planning

Client need: Health Promotion and Maintenance

Cognitive level: Analysis

Subject area: Medical-Surgical

Answer: 4

Rationale: A thyroidectomy is removal of the thyroid gland through a neck incision. Immediately postoperatively there is the potential complication of airway obstruction by edema formation. Fluid and electrolyte balance would be monitored during the operative period and would not be imbalanced immediately post-op. Medications to decrease the vascularity of the thyroid glands would be done preoperatively. Range-of-motion exercises to the neck are not started until several days postoperatively.

Nursing process: Planning

Client need: Physiological Adaptation

Cognitive level: Application

Subject area: Medical-Surgical

Answer: 1

Rationale: The client with hypothyroidism has decreased metabolism, which results in a slowing down of all body processes. Characteristically, the skin is very dry and thickened and requires lubrication. With a decrease in metabolic rate, the client will be cold and will be prone to constipation. These clients are very lethargic and sleep much of the time and therefore need to be encouraged to participate in activities to the greatest extent possible.

Nursing process: Implementation

Client need: Physiological Adaptation

Cognitive level: Application

Subject area: Medical-Surgical

10. The nurse is caring for a client with myxedema. Which of the following would indicate to the nurse that the client's condition is deteriorating?

    1. An increase in pulse rate and respirations

    2. Cold skin and episodes of chills

    3. Difficulty in arousing the client for medications

    4. Client complaints of palpitations

11. The nurse should include which of the following in the preoperative teaching plan for a client with hyperparathyroidism who is scheduled to have a portion of his parathyroid gland removed?

    1. Force fluids to at least 3000 ml per day

    2. Take over-the-counter supplements of vitamin D daily

    3. Maintain bed rest as much as possible

    4. Adhere strictly to the high-calcium diet

12. The postoperative orders for a client who has had the parathyroid gland removed include using Chvostek's sign to assess for signs of tetany. Which of the following is the appropriate assessment technique the nurse should implement?

    1. Occlude the blood flow in the wrist

    2. Observe respiratory rate and depth

    3. Listen for a crowing sound with inspirations

    4. Tap sharply over the facial nerves

Answer: 3

Rationale: The most life-threatening complication for the client with myxedema is myxedema coma. This client already has decreased metabolism and as the condition worsens, cardiac, respiratory, and neurological systems slow down even more. The client then goes into a coma and may die from circulatory and respiratory collapse. If a client with myxedema becomes unable to be aroused, the client may be progressing into a coma. In myxedema the client experiences a decrease in pulse rate and respirations, has cold skin, and often has complaints of being chilled due to the decreased metabolic rate. Clients with increased metabolism complain of palpitations.

Nursing process: Evaluation

Client need: Reduction of Risk Potential

Cognitive level: Analysis

Subject area: Medical-Surgical

Answer: 1

Rationale: Hyperparathyroidism is caused by an overproduction of the parathyroid hormone, parathormone, from the parathyroid glands. Parathormone takes calcium from the bone and concentrates it in the blood. As a result, these clients are prone to renal stones. Forcing fluids dilutes the urine and prevents precipitation of kidney stones. Remaining in bed contributes to stone formation. With an increased level of calcium in the blood, the client should be on a diet low in calcium. Vitamin D would not be necessary to enhance the absorption of calcium.

Nursing process: Planning

Client need: Health Promotion and Maintenance

Cognitive level: Application

Subject area: Medical-Surgical

Answer: 4

Rationale: Tetany is neuromuscular irritability characterized by tremors and spasms. Chvostek's sign is performed by tapping sharply over the facial nerves and is positive if that causes twitching or spasms in the region of the eyes, nose, and mouth. Occluding the blood flow in the wrist is Trousseau's sign. Assessing for respiratory obstruction and laryngeal spasm are important measures to detect impending tetany but are not Chvostek's sign.

Nursing process: Assessment

Client need: Physiological Adaptation

Cognitive level: Application

Subject area: Medical-Surgical

13. The diet prescribed for a client with hypoparathyroidism should be high in calcium and low in phosphorus. The nurse instructs the client to eat which of the following foods?

1. Milk

2. Green leafy vegetables

3. Cauliflower

4. Cheese

14. The nurse is admitting a client suspected of having Cushing's syndrome. Which of the following assessments supports the diagnosis of Cushing's syndrome?

Select all that apply:

[ ] 1. Slender trunk with enlarged arms and legs

[ ] 2. Hypertension

[ ] 3. Hyperglycemia

[ ] 4. Decreased body and facial hair

[ ] 5. Hyperpigmentation of the skin on the breasts and abdomen

[ ] 6. Fat pad accumulations above the clavicles

15. The nurse evaluates which of the following nursing diagnoses to be most important for a client with Cushing's syndrome?

1. Ineffective breathing patterns related to depressed respirations

2. Risk for infection related to altered protein metabolism and inflammatory response

3. Pain related to tissue and nerve injury and anxiety

4. Ineffective therapeutic regimen management related to lack of knowledge about the need for lifelong replacement therapy

16. The nurse would report which of the following laboratory results as consistent with a diagnosis of primary aldosteronism?

1. Serum potassium of 3 mEq/L

2. Serum phosphorus of 3 mg/dL

3. Serum sodium of 130 mEq/L

4. Serum calcium of 12 mg/dL

Answer: 2

Rationale: Milk and cheese products are high in calcium but also high in phosphorus. Green leafy vegetables have a higher calcium, lower phosphorus ratio but spinach should be avoided as it contains oxalate, which forms insoluble calcium substances. Cauliflower has a high phosphorus content in relation to calcium.

Nursing process: Implementation

Client need: Basic Care and Comfort

Cognitive level: Application

Subject area: Medical-Surgical

Answer: 2, 3, 6

Rationale: Cushing's syndrome is an overproduction of glucocorticoids and androgens from the adrenal cortex. These hormones produce fat pad accumulations, a "buffalo hump" in the neck and supraclavicular areas. Hypertension and hyperglycemia are also clinical manifestations. The client has fat pad accumulations in the trunk. Protein wasting results in slender arms and legs. The excessive androgens cause virilization with increased body and facial hair. Hyperpigmentation of the skin is a result of insufficient adrenal cortex hormones.

Nursing process: Assessment

Client need: Physiological Adaptation

Cognitive level: Application

Subject area: Medical-Surgical

Answer: 2

Rationale: The anti-inflammatory effects of increased corticosteroids may mask the signs of inflammation and infection. These clients do not have changes in respiratory status or pain. Lifelong replacement therapy is not necessary unless the client had an adrenalectomy.

Nursing process: Evaluation

Client need: Physiological Adaptation

Cognitive level: Analysis

Subject area: Medical-Surgical

Answer: 1

Rationale: Excessive production of aldosterone from the adrenal cortex (primary aldosteronism) is characterized by a severe decline in serum potassium levels causing muscle weakness and fatigue and decline in serum hydrogen ions leading to alkalosis. Hypertension is the major sign of primary aldosteronism with serum sodium levels that are normal or elevated. Serum calcium levels are low, as the hypokalemic alkalosis may decrease the ionized serum calcium levels leading to tetany. A serum phosphorus level of 3 mg/dL is within the normal range.

Nursing process: Analysis

Client need: Physiological Adaptation

Cognitive level: Analysis

Subject area: Medical-Surgical

17. Which of the following nursing interventions should be included in a plan of care for a client with Addison's disease?

   1. Administer the prescribed diuretics

   2. Give diet instructions for a low-carbohydrate, low-protein diet

   3. Monitor for signs of Na^+ and K^+ imbalances

   4. Encourage self-care activities

18. Which of the following questions should the nurse ask during an admission interview for a client admitted with a diagnosis of pheochromocytoma?

   1. "Do you ever notice or feel an increase in your heart beating?"

   2. "Do you suddenly feel warm and flushed when you get out of bed?"

   3. "Do your symptoms subside when you eat simple sugars?"

   4. "Do the attacks make you feel like you want to rest awhile and sleep?"

19. The nurse conducts a health history for a client with type 1 diabetes mellitus. Which of the following client statements best describes the onset characteristics of this type of diabetes?

   1. "I was diagnosed during the fifth month of my pregnancy."

   2. "One day I passed out after I had terrible nausea, vomiting, and abdominal pain."

   3. "When I hit 40, I began to notice I was picking up weight and urinating more frequently."

   4. "My fasting blood sugars are always between 110 mg/dL and 126 mg/dL."

20. Which of the following should be included in the assessment of a client with diabetes mellitus who is experiencing a hypoglycemic reaction?

   Select all that apply:

   [ ] **1.** Tremors

   [ ] **2.** Nervousness

   [ ] **3.** Extreme thirst

   [ ] **4.** Flushed skin

   [ ] **5.** Profuse perspiration

   [ ] **6.** Constricted pupils

Answer: 3

Rationale: Addison's disease is a deficiency of adrenal glucocorticoids and mineralocorticoids resulting in major disturbances in sodium (hyponatremia) and potassium (hyperkalemia). These clients need lifelong replacement therapy of glucocorticoids and mineralocorticoids. A high-carbohydrate, high-protein diet is ordered. With insufficient glucocorticoids and mineralocorticoids, the client is at risk for developing Addisonian crisis when under any stress, including self-care activities.

Nursing process: Planning

Client need: Physiological Adaptation

Cognitive level: Application

Subject area: Medical-Surgical

Answer: 1

Rationale: Pheochromocytoma is a tumor in the adrenal medulla that secretes excessive amounts of epinephrine and norepinephrine. Palpitations are a major clinical manifestation. Postural hypotension occurs frequently and would be noted with dizziness and cold and clammy skin. Hyperglycemia is another classic manifestation. Clinical manifestations that subside when simple sugars are eaten are characteristic of hypoglycemia. The "attacks" that occur are a result of the release of the catecholamines and cause the client to be extremely anxious, tremulous, and weak.

Nursing process: Assessment

Client need: Physiological Adaptation

Cognitive level: Application

Subject area: Medical-Surgical

Answer: 2

Rationale: Type 1 diabetes mellitus usually has an acute onset with nausea, vomiting, and abdominal pain and is often diagnosed after the client becomes comatose with ketoacidosis. Diabetes mellitus diagnosed during pregnancy is classified as gestational diabetes. Type 2 diabetes mellitus has a gradual onset and usually occurs in clients over 30. Clients with consistent fasting blood sugar levels that are slightly over normal are classified as borderline diabetics with impaired glucose intolerance.

Nursing process: Evaluation

Client need: Physiological Adaptation

Cognitive level: Application

Subject area: Medical-Surgical

Answer: 1, 2, 5

Rationale: In hypoglycemia, the blood glucose levels fall, resulting in sympathetic nervous system responses such as sweating, tremors, and nervousness. Extreme thirst and flushed skin are clinical manifestations present in hyperglycemia. Dilated pupils are a sympathetic response.

Nursing process: Assessment

Client need: Physiological Adaptation

Cognitive level: Application

Subject area: Medical-Surgical

21. The client with diabetes mellitus asks the nurse which blood sugar test is most significant in determining that one is diabetic. The best response of the nurse would be

    1. "When you have two consecutive fasting blood sugars of 126 or more in a short period of time."

    2. "Whenever you have a blood sugar taken and it is 150 or more."

    3. "When your blood sugar is in the range of 150 and 190 a couple of hours after you drink a special glucose solution."

    4. "When your blood sugar is 175 or more an hour after you have eaten a meal."

22. Which of the following nutritional goals would be most important in the teaching plan for a client with diabetes mellitus?

    1. Limit saturated fats to 20% of total calories

    2. Maintain body weight at 10 to 15 lbs above ideal body weight

    3. Avoid eating snacks between meals

    4. Include all essential food components in the diet plan

23. The nurse should instruct a client with diabetes mellitus and the client's family about the clinical manifestations of diabetic ketoacidosis before discharge. Which of the following should be included? Select all that apply:

    [ ] **1.** Dehydration

    [ ] **2.** Shallow, labored respirations

    [ ] **3.** Acetone breath

    [ ] **4.** Tremors

    [ ] **5.** Cold, clammy skin

    [ ] **6.** Abdominal pain

24. Which of the following should the nurse include in the instructions given to a client with diabetes mellitus on how to prevent hypoglycemia?

    1. Eat a meal or snack every four to five hours while awake

    2. Have a family member learn to inject insulin if symptoms appear

    3. Increase insulin if moderate exercise is planned

    4. Ingest complex carbohydrates if symptoms appear

Answer: 1

Rationale: Fasting plasma glucose levels are abnormal if they are 126 mg/dL or more and two consecutive fasting blood sugars of 126 mg/dL or more is indicative of diabetes mellitus. Random plasma glucose levels and two-hour postload glucose are not abnormal until they are more than 200 mg/dL. A one-hour postmeal plasma glucose level of 175 mg/dL is within the normal range.

Nursing process: Analysis

Client need: Physiological Adaptation

Cognitive level: Analysis

Subject area: Medical-Surgical

Answer: 4

Rationale: The diabetic diet should be a well-balanced meal including all the essential food elements. Saturated fats should be limited to 10% of total calories. Achieving and maintaining ideal weight is necessary to gain control of blood sugar levels. Spacing meals throughout the day is less taxing on the pancreas.

Nursing process: Evaluation

Client need: Health Promotion and Maintenance

Cognitive level: Application

Subject area: Medical-Surgical

Answer: 1, 3, 6

Rationale: In diabetic ketoacidosis (DKA), the body burns fats, which increases the amount of ketone bodies. An increase in ketone bodies causes acetone breath, which has a fruity odor. In DKA the respirations are deep but not labored. Other clinical manifestations of DKA include hydration, abdominal pain, orthostatic hypotension, and tachycardia. DKA is a state of hyperglycemia. Tremulousness and cold, clammy skin are signs of hypoglycemia.

Nursing process: Planning

Client need: Physiological Adaptation

Cognitive level: Application

Subject area: Medical-Surgical

Answer: 1

Rationale: Meals or snacks every four to five hours while awake will maintain consistent blood sugar levels and should help to prevent hypoglycemia. Hypoglycemia is treated with injections of glucagon to raise the blood sugar level. Exercise burns calories so that less insulin is needed. Hypoglycemia is treated by ingesting simple carbohydrates.

Nursing process: Planning

Client need: Reduction of Risk Potential

Cognitive level: Application

Subject area: Medical-Surgical

25. The nurse instructs a client with diabetes mellitus that the priority self-care activity for preventing the complication of diabetes is
    1. Learn to administer insulin properly and know the signs of hyperglycemia and hypoglycemia
    2. Follow the prescribed diabetic diet closely unless medical condition changes
    3. Keep the blood glucose levels controlled at or near normal levels
    4. Report to the physician immediately any kidney, vascular, or neurological changes

26. The nurse is observing a staff member preparing to give a client in diabetic ketoacidosis 40 units of NPH insulin IV bolus. Which of the following interventions by the nurse is appropriate?
    1. Assist the staff member preparing the injection by rotating the vial of NPH insulin prior to drawing up the insulin
    2. Instruct the staff member to follow the NPH IV bolus with 5 to 10 units per hour in normal saline
    3. Ask the staff member to give the client the NPH insulin IV bolus for the experience
    4. Tell the staff member that only regular insulin may be administered intravenously

27. The registered nurse is delegating tasks to be performed to a nursing unit. Which of the following tasks may be delegated to a licensed practical nurse?
    1. Develop the nutritional plan for a client with diabetes mellitus
    2. Assess ECG changes in a client with pheochromocytoma who had an adrenalectomy
    3. Implement the teaching plan for a client with Addison's disease
    4. Monitor the blood pressure in a client with primary aldosteronism

28. The nurse is caring for a client with diabetes mellitus who received six units of regular insulin at 0730. The nurse should monitor the client for clinical manifestations of hypoglycemia at which of the following times?
    1. 0930 to 1030
    2. 0800 to 0830
    3. 1200 to 1400
    4. 1500 to 1700

Answer: 3

Rationale: The main goal in the management of the diabetic is to prevent the vascular and neuropathic complications from occurring by keeping the blood glucose levels at normal or near normal levels through an interrelated mix of insulin, diet, and exercise. Proper administration of insulin and adherence to diet will not prevent complications. The renal, vascular, and neurological changes have already begun by the time the client notices changes.

Nursing process: Implementation

Client need: Management of Care

Cognitive level: Application

Subject area: Medical-Surgical

Answer: 4

Rationale: Only regular insulin, which is clear, may be administered intravenously.

Nursing process: Evaluation

Client need: Physiological Adaptation

Cognitive level: Analysis

Subject area: Medical-Surgical

Answer: 4

Rationale: A licensed practical nurse cannot perform tasks that involve developing, assessing, or implementing. Those are tasks that only the registered nurse can perform. A licensed practical nurse may monitor the blood pressure in a client with aldosteronism.

Nursing process: Analysis

Client need: Management of Care

Cognitive level: Analysis

Subject area: Legal and Ethical Issues

Answer: 1

Rationale: Regular insulin is a short-acting insulin that has an onset of 30 minutes to one hour. The peak is between two to three hours and the duration is between four to six hours. A hypoglycemia reaction is most likely to occur during the peak, so if regular insulin was given at 0730, a hypoglycemic reaction would occur between 0930 and 1030.

Nursing process: Assessment

Client need: Physiological Adaptation

Cognitive level: Application

Subject area: Medical-Surgical

29. Which of the following is a priority for the nurse to monitor in a client with pheochromocytoma?
    1. Weight
    2. Serum glucose level
    3. Blood pressure
    4. Temperature

30. The nurse identifies which of the following clients to be at greatest risk for developing primary hyperaldosterism?
    1. A client with untreated lung cancer
    2. A client with a lesion of the hypothalamus
    3. A client with a history of meningitis and peripheral neuropathy
    4. A client with hypertension and hypokalemia not treated with diuretics

Answer: 3

Rationale: Pheochromocytoma is a disorder caused by a tumor of the adrenal medulla characterized by intermittent or persistent hypertension. It is a priority to stabilize the blood pressure so surgery may be performed to remove the tumor.

Nursing process: Assessment

Client need: Management of Care

Cognitive level: Analysis

Subject area: Legal and Ethical Issues

Answer: 4

Rationale: Primary hyperaldosterism should be suspected in a client with hypertension and hypokalemia not treated with diuretics.

Nursing process: Evaluation

Client need: Physiological Adaptation

Cognitive level: Analysis

Subject area: Medical-Surgical

Neurological Disorders

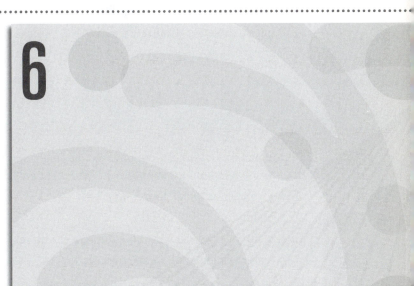

6

1. Which of the following would the nurse assess in a client who has a degeneration of the neurons that synthesize and release dopamine?

   1. Bradycardia and hypotension

   2. Insomnia and mania

   3. Hand tremors and muscle rigidity

   4. Pupil dilation and dysuria

2. As the nurse assesses a client undergoing diagnostic testing for myasthenia gravis, which of the following findings would be most supportive of the diagnosis of myasthenia gravis?

   1. A history of a spinal cord injury

   2. A history of a viral infection

   3. A history of muscle weakness improved with rest

   4. A history of an autoimmune disease

3. Which of the following clinical manifestations would the nurse expect to find in a client with meningitis? Select all that apply:

   [   ] **1.** Headache

   [   ] **2.** Dysphagia

   [   ] **3.** Nuchal rigidity

   [   ] **4.** Fever

   [   ] **5.** Dysarthria

   [   ] **6.** Vomiting

4. The nurse correctly explains to a client's family that the reason a stroke on the right side of the brain results in paralysis on the left side of the body is because the pyramidal pathways cross over at the end of which of the following?

   1. Medulla

   2. Thalamus

   3. Pons

   4. Midbrain

Answer: 3

Rationale: Dopamine is a neurotransmitter that inhibits the excitatory functions of acetylcholine-producing neurons. It is through dopamine's ability to inhibit and balance the excitatory functions that coordinated, refined movement can occur. Without the inhibiting effects of dopamine, the client experiences difficulty initiating voluntary movement and muscle rigidity. A "pill-rolling" tremor is present. Bradycardia, hypotension, insomnia, mania, pupil dilation, and dysuria are not signs of the lack of dopamine.

Nursing process: Assessment

Client need: Physiological Adaptation

Cognitive level: Application

Subject area: Medical-Surgical

Answer: 4

Rationale: Myasthenia gravis is an autoimmune disease of the neuromuscular junction that is manifested by a fluctuating skeletal muscle weakness. Antibodies attack the acetylcholine at the neuromuscular junction, preventing muscle contraction. There is no correlation to a spinal cord injury. Although there is no known cause of multiple sclerosis, there is research indicating a correlation to a viral infection. Muscle strength is generally increased after rest.

Nursing process: Assessment

Client need: Physiological Adaptation

Cognitive level: Analysis

Subject area: Medical-Surgical

Answer: 1, 3, 4, 6

Rationale: Headache, nuchal rigidity or resistance to flexion of the neck, fever, nausea, and vomiting are the classic clinical manifestations of meningitis.

Nursing process: Assessment

Client need: Physiological Adaptation

Cognitive level: Application

Subject area: Medical-Surgical

Answer: 1

Rationale: The crossover of the pyramidal pathways at the end of the medulla results in the opposite side of the body being affected when the cerebrovascular accident (CVA) occurs in the other side. For example, when the CVA is on the right side, the paralysis is on the left side of the body. The pons and midbrain, like the medulla, are parts of the midbrain. The thalamus is located in the cerebrum and lies above the brainstem.

Nursing process: Analysis

Client need: Physiological Adaptation

Cognitive level: Analysis

Subject area: Medical-Surgical

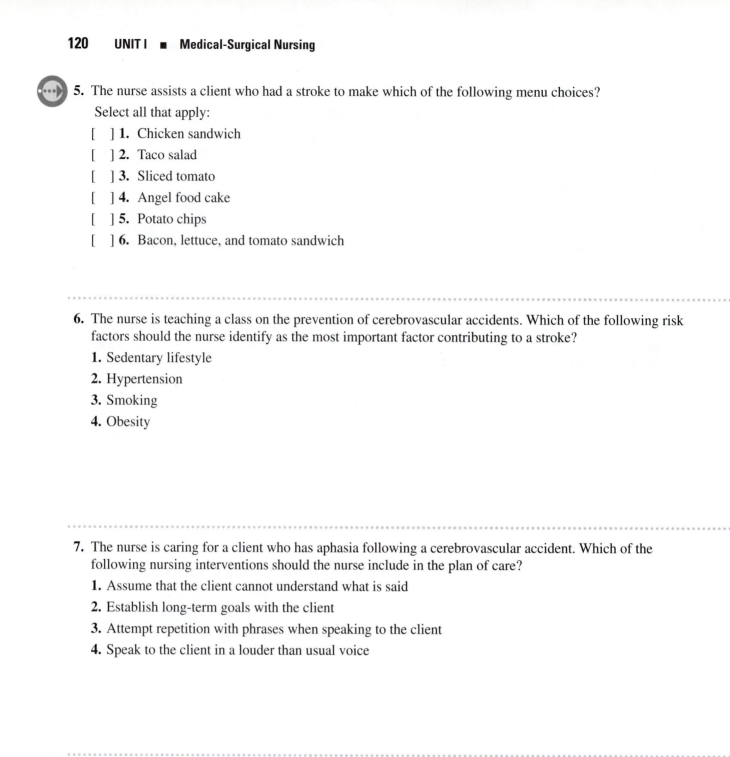

5. The nurse assists a client who had a stroke to make which of the following menu choices?
   Select all that apply:
   [   ] 1. Chicken sandwich
   [   ] 2. Taco salad
   [   ] 3. Sliced tomato
   [   ] 4. Angel food cake
   [   ] 5. Potato chips
   [   ] 6. Bacon, lettuce, and tomato sandwich

6. The nurse is teaching a class on the prevention of cerebrovascular accidents. Which of the following risk factors should the nurse identify as the most important factor contributing to a stroke?
   1. Sedentary lifestyle
   2. Hypertension
   3. Smoking
   4. Obesity

7. The nurse is caring for a client who has aphasia following a cerebrovascular accident. Which of the following nursing interventions should the nurse include in the plan of care?
   1. Assume that the client cannot understand what is said
   2. Establish long-term goals with the client
   3. Attempt repetition with phrases when speaking to the client
   4. Speak to the client in a louder than usual voice

8. The nurse assesses that neither the client's sounds of speech or the meanings can be distinguished, and comprehension of both written and spoken language is impaired. The nurse documents this as _____.

Answer: 1, 3, 4

Rationale: A high-fat diet is a modifiable risk factor in clients at risk for a cerebrovascular accident. Chicken sandwich, sliced tomato, and angel food cake is the menu with the lowest fat content. Bacon, potato chips, and taco salad are not only high in fat but also high in sodium, which would predispose a client to hypertension and risk for another stroke.

Nursing process: Implementation

Client need: Basic Care and Comfort

Cognitive level: Application

Subject area: Medical-Surgical

Answer: 2

Rationale: A sedentary lifestyle predisposes a client to obesity and cardiovascular disease, which increases the risk of a cerebrovascular accident. Smoking and obesity are modifiable risk factors that do increase the risk of a stroke, but hypertension is supported by research to put the client at the greatest risk for a stroke. Successful treatment of hypertension is the best prevention of a CVA.

Nursing process: Evaluation

Client need: Reduction of Risk Potential

Cognitive level: Application

Subject area: Medical-Surgical

Answer: 3

Rationale: When aphasia occurs with a cerebrovascular accident, repetition proves beneficial in enhancing the client's understanding of what is said. An assumption should never be made that the client understood what was said. The client may be experiencing expressive, receptive, or global aphasia. The client cannot focus to plan a long-term goal. Speaking louder to the client serves no purpose because the client is not hard of hearing. The client benefits most from presenting only one idea at a time, simple yes and no questions, repetition, and never rushing the client.

Nursing process: Planning

Client need: Physiological Adaptation

Cognitive level: Application

Subject area: Medical-Surgical

Answer: receptive aphasia

Rationale: Receptive aphasia is the inability to distinguish between sounds, meaning, and the comprehension of those words whether written or spoken. Expressive aphasia is the inability to express oneself in either spoken or written words. Dysarthria is the impairment in the muscular control of speech. It does not mean that the client cannot understand or express him- or herself correctly, but does mean that there is an impairment in the ability to phonate, articulate, or pronounce the words.

Nursing process: Assessment

Client need: Physiological Adaptation

Cognitive level: Application

Subject area: Medical-Surgical

9. During an initial interview with a client who has had an anterior cord syndrome spinal cord injury, the nurse would expect to find which of the following assessment findings?

Select all that apply:

[   ] **1.** Motor weakness that is greater in the upper extremities than in the lower ones

[   ] **2.** Impairment in the sensations of touch, position, vibration, and motion

[   ] **3.** Hypoesthesia

[   ] **4.** Flaccid bowel and bladder function

[   ] **5.** Decreased pain

[   ] **6.** Loss of temperature below the level of the injury

10. Which of the following actions is a priority for the nurse to perform first in a client with a spinal cord injury who complains of a headache?

1. Administer a beta adrenergic blocker

2. Take the blood pressure

3. Assess the pupillary reaction

4. Insert a Foley catheter

11. The nurse is caring for a client suspected of botulism. The nurse should assess the client for which of the following?

Select all that apply:

[   ] **1.** Headache

[   ] **2.** Muscle weakness

[   ] **3.** Drowsiness

[   ] **4.** Stiff jaw and neck

[   ] **5.** Respiratory and eye problems

[   ] **6.** Opisthotonos

Answer: 3, 5, 6

Rationale: Motor weakness that is greater in the upper extremities than the lower ones is present in a central cord syndrome. Impairment in the sense of touch, position, vibration, and motion is present in Brown-Sequard's syndrome in which a disruption in one half of the spinal cord has occurred, either from a lesion or a transection. Flaccid bowel and bladder function and paralysis of the lower extremities represent damage to the lowest portion of the spinal cord. Hypoesthesia, decreased pain, and loss of temperature below the level of injury represent the anterior cord syndrome because the posterior cord is still intact and, therefore, the sensations of touch, vibration, motion, and position are unaffected.

Nursing process: Assessment

Client need: Physiological Adaptation

Cognitive level: Analysis

Subject area: Medical-Surgical

Answer: 2

Rationale: The priority action in a client who has sustained a spinal cord injury and is complaining of a severe headache is to take the blood pressure. A severe headache and a systolic blood pressure of 300 mm Hg are suggestive of autonomic dysreflexia or hyperreflexia, which are life threatening if left untreated.

Nursing process: Planning

Client need: Management of Care

Cognitive level: Application

Subject area: Medical-Surgical

Answer: 2, 5

Rationale: General gastrointestinal symptoms (nausea, vomiting, and abdominal pain) occur 6 to 48 hours after ingestion of food suspected to be contaminated. However, involvement of the nervous system progresses very quickly over two to four days with symptoms of eye problems, muscle weakness, and respiratory problems that can be life threatening. Headache, fever, nausea, and vomiting occur with meningitis. Drowsiness, confusion, and seizures are all findings that may occur with a head injury or brain abscess. Opisthotonos, stiff jaw, and stiff neck are clinical manifestations that are classic in tetanus.

Nursing process: Assessment

Client need: Physiological Adaptation

Cognitive level: Application

Subject area: Medical-Surgical

12. Because a client with a spinal cord injury is at risk for pneumonia, atelectasis, and respiratory arrest, the nurse should plan to

1. position the client in a prone position.

2. monitor the hemoglobin and hematocrit levels.

3. administer propoxyphene (Darvon) 65 mg p.o. every four hours.

4. have the client count to 10 out loud without taking a breath.

13. The nurse is caring for a client with Parkinson's disease. Which of the following nursing interventions should the nurse include in the plan of care?

1. Elevate the client's legs

2. Offer the client the bedpan every two hours

3. Encourage the client to sit in a reclining, soft chair without arms

4. Instruct the client to eat a high-calcium diet

14. The physician tells a client with multiple sclerosis that it is a chronic progressive neurologic condition. The client asks the nurse, "Will I experience pain?" The most appropriate response by the nurse is

1. "Tell me about your fears regarding pain."

2. "Analgesics will be ordered to control the pain."

3. "Pain is not a characteristic symptom of this disease process."

4. "Let's make a list of the things you need to ask your physician."

Answer: 4

Rationale: A prone position is not desirable for a client who has sustained a spinal cord injury because it would further decrease the vital capacity and could even predispose the client to a cardiac arrest. Monitoring the hemoglobin and hematocrit levels would be important interventions when there is blood loss from other injuries. Administering Darvon is not an appropriate intervention for a client with a spinal cord injury.

Nursing process: Planning

Client need: Physiological Adaptation

Cognitive level: Application

Subject area: Medical-Surgical

Answer: 1

Rationale: Elevating the legs is an important intervention in the client with Parkinson's disease because ankle edema occurs. Offering the bedpan every two hours is an intervention for multiple sclerosis. Reclining in a soft chair without arms is incorrect because a client with Parkinson's disease needs an upright, firm chair with arms to facilitate getting out of the chair because of the decrease in mobility. A high-calcium diet is incorrect because a diet with foods that are easily chewed and high in roughage is recommended for the difficulties with chewing and also to prevent constipation.

Nursing process: Planning

Client need: Physiological Adaptation

Cognitive level: Application

Subject area: Medical-Surgical

Answer: 3

Rationale: The clinical manifestations of multiple sclerosis include weakness or paralysis of the extremities, numbness or tingling, visual disturbances, bowel or bladder disturbances, and gait and balance difficulties. Pain is not a clinical manifestation of multiple sclerosis. By providing this information, the nurse educates and reassures the client. Telling the client to make a list for the physician shifts responsibility from the nurse to the physician. Reflecting the client's fears about pain is not the most appropriate response. Providing accurate information is most appropriate.

Nursing process: Analysis

Client need: Physiological Adaptation

Cognitive level: Analysis

Subject area: Medical-Surgical

15. The nurse is caring for a client with amyotrophic lateral sclerosis. Which of the following nursing diagnoses should have priority?

1. Impaired skin integrity related to disuse

2. Anticipatory grieving related to inevitable death

3. Acute pain related to inflammation

4. Self-care deficit related to paralysis

16. The nurse is caring for a client with Guillain-Barré syndrome. Which of the following would indicate the client's condition is deteriorating?

1. Weakness and paresthesia

2. Pain and muscle aches

3. Urinary retention

4. Respiratory infection

17. A client's family asks the nurse what meningitis is. The nurse's response should be based on an understanding that meningitis is.

1. a fatal form of polyneuritis.

2. a cerebrospinal infection.

3. a collection of pus in the brain tissue.

4. a rare progressive loss of motor neurons.

18. The nurse is admitting a client diagnosed to have a cerebrovascular accident involving left-brain damage. The nurse evaluates which of the following to be clinical manifestations of a cerebrovascular accident involving left-brain damage?

Select all that apply:

[   ] **1.** Paralyzed right side

[   ] **2.** Aphasia

[   ] **3.** Left-sided neglect

[   ] **4.** Paralyzed left side

[   ] **5.** Depression

[   ] **6.** Denial of deficits

Answer: 2

Rationale: The priority nursing diagnosis for a client with amyotrophic lateral sclerosis is anticipatory grieving related to inevitable death. ALS is a fatal neurological disease in which there is a loss of motor neurons. Death generally results when the respiratory muscles are affected and respiratory function is compromised.

Nursing process: Analysis

Client need: Physiological Adaptation

Cognitive level: Application

Subject area: Medical-Surgical

Answer: 4

Rationale: Guillain-Barré syndrome is a fatal disease that is characterized by an ascending paralysis affecting the peripheral nervous system. Respiratory infection and failure are the most common complications.

Nursing process: Analysis

Client need: Physiological Adaptation

Cognitive level: Analysis

Subject area: Medical-Surgical

Answer: 2

Rationale: Meningitis is a cerebrospinal infection. Purulent exudate forms in bacterial meningitis, but does not form in viral meningitis. Meningitis is not associated with polyneuritis or a progressive loss of motor neurons.

Nursing process: Analysis

Client need: Physiological Adaptation

Cognitive level: Analysis

Subject area: Medical-Surgical

Answer: 1, 2, 5

Rationale: Clients who have left-sided brain damage are aware of their deficits and often experience anxiety or depression. Aphasia and paralysis on the right side are also common clinical manifestations of left-side brain damage. Paralysis or neglect of the left side and a denial of any deficits are common in right-sided brain damage.

Nursing process: Evaluation

Client need: Physiological Adaptation

Cognitive level: Application

Subject area: Medical-Surgical

19. Which of the following is a priority when suctioning a client with increased intracranial pressure?

    1. Limit the suction passes to 30 seconds

    2. Suction the client as needed

    3. Suction the client at least every hour

    4. Schedule the suctioning with other nursing tasks

20. The nurse is caring for a client with an arterioventricular malformation who is scheduled for surgery. Which of the following should be the priority in the care provided to this client?

    1. Offer psychologic support

    2. Encourage a high-protein and high-calorie diet

    3. Avoid activities that will increase the blood pressure

    4. Administer intravenous fluids to prevent dehydration

21. The nurse is caring for a client in the first 48 hours following a spinal cord trauma. Which of the following nursing interventions should the nurse include in the plan of care?

    1. Encourage a high-protein and high-roughage diet

    2. Insert a nasogastric tube

    3. Position the client in a prone position

    4. Administer a daily tap water enema

22. Immediately following a spinal cord injury, a client's family asks the nurse, "Is the damage the client presents with in the emergency room as bad as it seems?" The most appropriate response by the nurse is

    1. "Because of edema around the spinal cord, it is difficult to evaluate the extent of the injury for up to one week."

    2. "Unfortunately yes, the injury is exactly as it appears."

    3. "Probably not, because the client will probably regain a lot of function."

    4. "The injury is so severe that death is imminent within days."

Answer: 1

Rationale: Suctioning can cause an increase in intracranial pressure and should be used cautiously. The client must be closely assessed during suctioning and suction passes should be limited to 30 seconds. The client should be allowed to rest for several minutes between suction passes, manually hyperventilated, and preoxgenated with 100% oxygen prior to suctioning.

Nursing process: Implementation

Client need: Physiological Adaptation

Cognitive level: Application

Subject area: Medical-Surgical

Answer: 3

Rationale: Arterioventricular malformation is a congenital malformation that results in a tangled web of dilated and thin-walled vessels. The abnormality in the capillary network of these vessels develops an impaired communication between the arterial and venous systems. Any increase in the pressure within the vessels may cause them to rupture. As a result, all activities should be avoided that increase the blood pressure.

Nursing process: Planning

Client need: Physiological Adaptation

Cognitive level: Application

Subject area: Medical-Surgical

Answer: 2

Rationale: A nasogastric tube connected to low intermittent suction may be inserted following a spinal cord trauma to relieve gastric distention. This is particularly necessary if the injury is above the T5 level. Hypomotility results with the possibility of a paralytic ileus or gastric distention.

Nursing process: Planning

Client need: Physiological Adaptation

Cognitive level: Application

Subject area: Medical-Surgical

Answer: 1

Rationale: It is difficult to ascertain the client's permanent level of disability until after the resolution of edema surrounding the spinal cord. It is edema that can cause compression of the spinal cord and increase ischemic damage to the spinal cord. The spinal cord damage caused by edema is typically evident within a week. Telling the family not to worry about the extent of the injury, as the injury is lethal, may be inaccurate and robs the family of any hope.

Nursing process: Analysis

Client need: Physiological Adaptation

Cognitive level: Analysis

Subject area: Medical-Surgical

23. The nurse is admitting a client suspected of Parkinson's disease. Which of the following does the nurse observe that supports the diagnosis?

Select all that apply:

[ ] **1.** Chorea movements

[ ] **2.** Tremor noticeable at rest

[ ] **3.** Paresthesia

[ ] **4.** Rigidity

[ ] **5.** Bradykinesia

[ ] **6.** Muscle wasting

24. The nurse is admitting a client with severe involuntary twisting movements of the face, limbs, and body and a deterioration of the intellect and emotions. The nurse suspects what disease? _____

25. The nurse is preparing a client with myasthenia gravis for a plasmapheresis. Which of the following laboratory tests must be obtained and assessed prior to this procedure?

Select all that apply:

[ ] **1.** Creatine phosphokinase (CPK)

[ ] **2.** Complete blood count (CBC)

[ ] **3.** Blood urea nitrogen (BUN)

[ ] **4.** Platelets

[ ] **5.** Clotting studies

[ ] **6.** Urine for protein

26. The nurse is assessing a client with myasthenia gravis at 1600. Which of the following assessment findings should the nurse anticipate the client to report?

1. Double vision and a muffled nasal quality speech

2. Tremors of the hands when attempting to lift objects

3. Improvement of muscle strength with mild exercise

4. Numbness and tingling of the extremities

Answer: 2, 4, 5

Rationale: Parkinson's disease is a neurological disorder with three classic features: tremor, rigidity, and bradykinesia.

Nursing process: Assessment

Client need: Physiological Adaptation

Cognitive level: Application

Subject area: Medical-Surgical

Answer: Huntington's disease

Rationale: Huntington's disease, also known as Huntington's chorea, is characterized by "chorea," writhing movements of the limbs and body. Eventually, the client shows a severe decline in cognitive functions. Parkinson's disease is associated with tremor, rigidity, and bradykinesia. Guillain-Barré syndrome is associated with spreading weakness and paralysis. Amyotrophic lateral sclerosis is associated with progressive weakness of the upper extremities, muscle wasting, and fasciculations.

Nursing process: Assessment

Client need: Physiological Adaptation

Cognitive level: Application

Subject area: Medical-Surgical

Answer: 2, 4, 5

Rationale: Plasmapheresis is a procedure that removes anti-Ach receptor antibodies by way of a machine called a cell separator. This machine separates the plasma from the blood. Plasmapheresis may be useful in clients in crisis being prepared for surgery or when corticosteroids are to be avoided.

Nursing process: Assessment

Client need: Reduction of Risk Potential

Cognitive level: Analysis

Subject area: Medical-Surgical

Answer: 1

Rationale: Myasthenia gravis is an autoimmune disease resulting in alterations of the skeletal muscles. The clinical manifestations are more prominent late in the day because the skeletal muscles are weakest then and strongest early in the day. The eye, breathing, speaking, chewing, and swallowing muscles are predominantly involved.

Nursing process: Assessment

Client need: Physiological Adaptation

Cognitive level: Analysis

Subject area: Medical-Surgical

27. The nurse's plan of care for a client with Guillain-Barré syndrome is based on an understanding of which of the following disease processes?

1. Decreased secretion of acetylcholine and an increase of cholinesterase at the myoneural junction

2. Segmental demyelination of the ventral and dorsal nerve roots in the spinal cord and medulla

3. Chronic inflammation, demyelination, and scarring of the CNS

4. Decreased secretion of the neurotransmitter dopamine with an anticholinergic effect

28. Which of the following should the nurse assess to provide the most accurate information regarding a client suspected of having a C4 injury?

1. Ask the client to shrug the shoulders while applying downward pressure

2. Ask the client to straighten the flexed arms while applying resistance

3. Ask the client to grasp an object and make a fist

4. Ask the client to lift the arms while applying resistance

29. A client has difficulty communicating because of expressive aphasia following a cerebrovascular accident. When the nurse asks how the client is feeling, the spouse answers for the client. The nurse should

1. ask how the spouse knows how the client is feeling.

2. acknowledge the spouse but look at the client for a response.

3. instruct the spouse to let the client answer.

4. return later to speak to the client after the spouse has gone home.

30. Which statement made by the spouse of a client with multiple sclerosis indicates to the nurse an understanding of the home-care needs for this client?

1. "I'm going to feed my spouse from now on."

2. "I've learned how to take care of a Foley catheter."

3. "I will put up handrails in the shower."

4. "I will make my spouse stay in bed as much as possible."

Answer: 2

Rationale: Guillain-Barré syndrome, often referred to as postinfectious polyneuropathy, is a segmental demyelination of the ventral and dorsal nerve roots in the spinal cord and medulla. A decrease in acetylcholine at the neuromuscular junction is myasthenia gravis. Parkinson's disease is a decrease in the secretion of dopamine. A chronic inflammation, demyelination, and scarring of the CNS is characteristic of multiple sclerosis.

Nursing process: Analysis

Client need: Physiological Adaptation

Cognitive level: Analysis

Subject area: Medical-Surgical

Answer: 1

Rationale: Asking a client to shrug the shoulders while applying resistance will provide the most accurate information in a client suspected of a C4 injury. Asking a client to straighten the flexed arms while applying resistance would assess for a C7 injury. Asking the client to grasp an object and make a fist would assess for a C8 injury. Asking the client to lift the arms while applying resistance would assess for a C5 injury.

Nursing process: Assessment

Client need: Physiological Adaptation

Cognitive level: Application

Subject area: Medical-Surgical

Answer: 3

Rationale: Expressive aphasia is a difficulty in both writing and speech. It is important to allow a client with expressive aphasia sufficient time to speak. No one should speak for the client because this serves only to increase the client's frustration.

Nursing process: Implementation

Client need: Physiological Adaptation

Cognitive level: Analysis

Subject area: Medical-Surgical

Answer: 3

Rationale: A goal in the nursing management of multiple sclerosis is to promote the client's independence while ensuring the client's comfort and safety. Assistive devices like handrails in the shower encourage independence and safety. It is also essential to promote mobility and prevent complications.

Nursing process: Evaluation

Client need: Physiological Adaptation

Cognitive level: Analysis

Subject area: Medical-Surgical

31. The nurse should consider which of the following when planning the care of a client with Lou Gehrig disease?

    1. Death frequently occurs from decreased respiratory function

    2. Successful treatment consists of IV methylprednisolone (Solu-Medrol)

    3. Life expectancy after diagnosis is 25 years

    4. Higher incidence in females between the ages of 15 and 50

32. The nurse is caring for a client with a spinal cord trauma following a motorcycle accident. It is a priority for the nurse to monitor for and immediately report which of the following findings?

    Select all that apply:

    [   ] **1.** Hypotension

    [   ] **2.** Bradycardia

    [   ] **3.** Pain

    [   ] **4.** Inflammation at the site of the injury

    [   ] **5.** Ecchymosis

    [   ] **6.** Warm, dry extremities

33. Passive range of motion exercises have been prescribed for a recent cerebral vascular (CVA) client with left hemiplegia. Which of the following would be most important for the nurse to include in the exercise treatment plan?

    1. Begin the exercises on the first day of hospitalization during the acute phase

    2. Perform each movement slowly and smoothly repeating five times during the exercise period

    3. Position each joint higher than the joint proximal to it

    4. Schedule the exercises once a shift along with another nursing activity

34. A new nurse caring for a client with glioblastoma asks a nurse the prognosis for this client. Based on an understanding of a glioblastoma, the nurse informs the new nurse that the prognosis is

    1. successful with chemotherapy.

    2. dependent on the client's overall condition.

    3. curable with surgery.

    4. extremely grave.

Answer: 1

Rationale: Death from amyotrophic lateral sclerosis (ALS), also known as Lou Gehrig disease, typically comes from a respiratory infection related to decreased respiratory function. There is no cure for ALS. Riluzole (Rilutek) may be given to retard the progression of the disease. Clients typically live for only two to six years after learning of their diagnosis. The disease affects twice as many men as women.

Nursing process: Planning

Client need: Physiological Adaptation

Cognitive level: Analysis

Subject area: Medical-Surgical

Answer: 1, 2, 6

Rationale: Hypotension, bradycardia, and warm, dry extremities indicate the presence of neurogenic shock and occur as the result of a loss of vasomotor tone. Neurogenic shock most commonly occurs with a cervical or high-thoracic injury.

Pain would indicate the preservation of sensation. Ecchymosis and inflammation at the site of the injury would be expected with the injury.

Nursing process: Analysis

Client need: Reduction of Risk Potential

Cognitive level: Analysis

Subject area: Medical-Surgical

Answer: 1

Rationale: Although positioning each joint of a CVA client higher than the joint proximal to it is worthy, the nursing goal is to maintain musculoskeletal function. This is accomplished by initiating passive range of motion exercises during the acute phase and on the first day of hospitalization. Muscle atrophy secondary to lack of innervation and to inactivity can develop in as little as a month.

Nursing process: Planning

Client need: Physiological Adaptation

Cognitive level: Application

Subject area: Medical-Surgical

Answer: 4

Rationale: A glioblastoma is a highly malignant brain tumor with a very poor prognosis.

Nursing process: Implementation

Client need: Physiological Adaptation

Cognitive level: Analysis

Subject area: Medical-Surgical

35. The nurse should implement which of the following methods of assisting during a seizure?
Select all that apply:

[   ] **1.** Turn the client on the side

[   ] **2.** Restrain the client

[   ] **3.** Turn on the lights

[   ] **4.** Observe the seizure activity

[   ] **5.** Open the airway with a padded tongue blade

[   ] **6.** Provide for client privacy

36. The nurse should inform a client with a seizure disorder to avoid which of the following?
Select all that apply:

[   ] **1.** Excess noise

[   ] **2.** Stress

[   ] **3.** Infections

[   ] **4.** A high chocolate intake

[   ] **5.** Alcohol

[   ] **6.** Fatigue

37. In planning the post-op care after cranial surgery, the nurse should place the client in which of the following positions?

1. Flat bed rest

2. Side-lying position

3. Elevate the head of bed 30°

4. Trendelenburg

38. The nurse is preparing a plan of a care for a client post-op following a craniotomy. The nurse formulates which of the following goals as the priority goal when caring for this client?

1. Prevent increased intracranial pressure

2. Maintain a safe environment

3. Prevent infection

4. Maintain skin integrity

Answer: 1, 4, 6

Rationale: When a client is having a seizure, it is a priority for the nurse to place the client on the side, observe all seizure activity, and protect the client from harm.

The purpose of placing the client on the side is to prevent aspiration. Nothing should be given by mouth nor should the client be restrained.

Privacy should be provided for the client.

Nursing process: Implementation

Client need: Basic Care and Comfort

Cognitive level: Analysis

Subject area: Medical-Surgical

Answer: 2, 5, 6

Rationale: It is important for the nurse to instruct a client who has had a seizure to avoid stress, fatigue, and alcohol. The nurse should instruct the client on stress control techniques and methods to promote sleep. A well-balanced diet is also recommended.

Nursing process: Implementation

Client need: Basic Care and Comfort

Cognitive level: Application

Subject area: Medical-Surgical

Answer: 3

Rationale: Following a craniotomy, the best position to place the client in is to have the head of the bed elevated 30° to prevent increased intracranial pressure.

Nursing process: Planning

Client need: Basic Care and Comfort

Cognitive level: Analysis

Subject area: Medical-Surgical

Answer: 1

Rationale: The primary goal following a craniotomy is to prevent increased intracranial pressure. Fluid and electrolytes and body position are crucial to prevent an increased intracranial pressure. An elevated head position should be maintained and extreme neck flexion avoided. Maintaining a head elevated position decreases sagittal sinus pressure, promotes venous drainage, and decreases vascular congestion.

Nursing process: Planning

Client need: Reduction of Risk Potential

Cognitive level: Analysis

Subject area: Medical-Surgical

39. The nurse reviews the report of a client's cerebrospinal fluid analysis. Which of the following findings should the nurse report?

  1. Glucose 60 mg/dl

  2. Total protein 30 mg/dl

  3. Clear, colorless appearance

  4. White blood cells 100/μl

40. When assessing cranial nerve X, the nurse will need which of the following?

  1. A tongue blade

  2. A tuning fork

  3. An ophthalmoscope

  4. Cotton and a safety pin

41. The nurse assesses the Achilles tendon reflex by striking the Achilles tendon with a reflex hammer. The reflex the nurse is assessing is the _____.

42. A mother asks the nurse if the seizures her child is experiencing will last a lifetime. The appropriate response by the nurse would be

  1. "The tonic-clonic seizures your child is experiencing will last a lifetime but can be successfully controlled with an antiepileptic drug."

  2. "Your child is experiencing a type of seizure called typical absence seizure and it may or may not go away. Each child is different."

  3. "The type of seizure your child has is called akinetic seizure and it may or may not go away. Each child is different."

  4. "Psychomotor seizures are hard to predict and you should ask your doctor."

Answer: 4

Rationale: Normal cerebrospinal fluid should have a clear and colorless appearance. Protein should be 15 to 45 mg/dl. Higher protein levels may indicate a tumor or an infection. Normal glucose ranges between 45 to 75 mg/ml. Glucose levels higher than 75 mg/ml indicate the presence of an infection, leukemia, or cancer. The white blood cells range is 0.8/µl. Higher levels indicate an infection or a tumor.

Nursing process: Analysis

Client need: Reduction of Risk Potential

Cognitive level: Analysis

Subject area: Medical-Surgical

Answer: 1

Rationale: Cranial nerve X is the vagus nerve and is responsible for the gag reflex. Assessment of the gag reflex is done with a tongue blade inserted in the mouth and gently touched to the posterior pharynx or soft palate. It is essential to assess CN X in a client suspected of a decreased level of consciousness or after certain procedures where an anesthetic or an anesthetic spray was used.

Nursing process: Assessment

Client need: Reduction of Risk Potential

Cognitive level: Application

Subject area: Medical-Surgical

Answer: plantar reflex

Rationale: The Achilles tendon is assessed by asking the client to flex the leg at the knee while the examiner dorsiflexes the foot at the ankle and strikes the Achilles tendon with a reflex hammer. The normal response is plantar flexion at the ankle.

Nursing process: Assessment

Client need: Reduction of Risk Potential

Cognitive level: Application

Subject area: Medical-Surgical

Answer: 2

Rationale: Typical absence (petit mal) seizures occur in children but rarely extend into adolescence. These seizures may completely cease or develop into another type of seizure.

Nursing process: Analysis

Client need: Physiological Adaptation

Cognitive level: Analysis

Subject area: Medical-Surgical

43. The nurse is caring for a client with increased intracranial pressure. Which of the following assessment findings should the nurse immediately report?

1. Nausea

2. Fever

3. Headache

4. Absence of papillary response

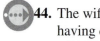**44.** The wife of a client who is experiencing blurred vision and having difficulty focusing on objects asks the nurse what area of the brain is affected. Using a diagram for illustration, the nurse points to which lobe of the brain that is responsible for vision and visual perception? _____

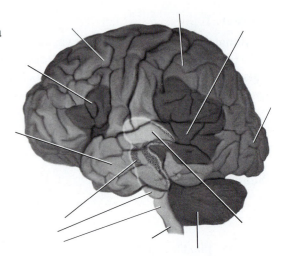

45. The registered nurse is delegating nursing tasks for the day. Which of the following tasks may be appropriately delegated to unlicensed assistive personnel?

1. Instruct a client with headaches to keep a diary of the characteristics of the headaches

2. Plan sample menu selections for a client who had a stroke

3. Monitor the temperature in a client who had a spinal cord injury

4. Assess cranial nerve VII in a client suspected of having trigeminal neuralgia

Answer: 4

Rationale: Absence of papillary response is an ominous sign and may indicate impending herniation and should be reported immediately to the physician. Fever is a common complication following an injury to the brain and should also be reported, but absence of papillary response is a priority. Headache and nausea are all clinical manifestations a client may experience but do not indicate an emergency.

Nursing process: Analysis

Client need: Reduction of Risk Potential

Cognitive level: Analysis

Subject area: Medical-Surgical

Answer: Occipital lobe

Rationale: The occipital lobe is the lobe of the brain that is responsible for vision and visual perception.

Nursing process: Analysis

Client need: Physiological Adaptation

Cognitive level: Comprehension

Subject area: Medical-Surgical

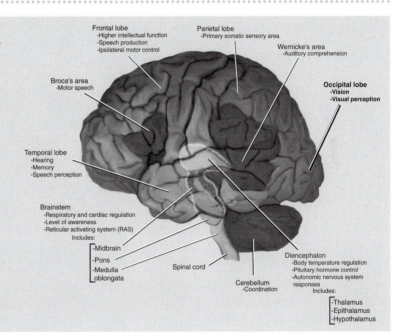

Answer: 3

Rationale: Unlicensed assistive personnel cannot instruct or plan nursing activities. Performing assessment techniques are also not a function of the unlicensed assistive personnel.

Nursing process: Planning

Client need: Management of Care

Cognitive level: Analysis

Subject area: Medical-Surgical

CHAPTER

Integumentary Disorders

7

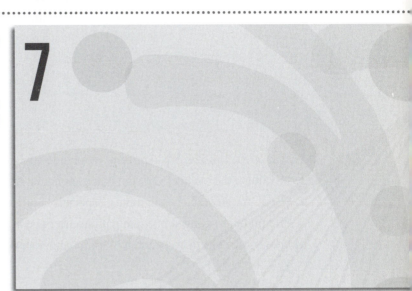

1. Which of the following nursing activities should the registered nurse delegate to a licensed practical nurse?
   1. Instruct a client with acne vulgaris on the use of tretinoin (Retin-A)
   2. Develop a plan of care on the irrigation of a skin ulcer with normal saline
   3. Obtain a health history from a client admitted with a pressure sore on the coccyx
   4. Monitor the vital signs of a client with cellulitis for evidence of sepsis

2. Which of the following is a priority to include when instructing a client to perform a skin assessment?
   1. "Evaluate the evenness of skin color, moisture, and temperature."
   2. "Look for any changes in moles, especially color and size."
   3. "Begin performing skin examinations after age 40."
   4. "Assess the entire body and look for changes in skin or moles."

3. The nurse assesses a client's skin and finds an elevated, solid lesion on the client's great toe. It is pink, nontender, and 0.5 cm in size. Which of the following is the most appropriate action by the nurse?
   1. Notify the physician immediately
   2. Gather more information about the lesion from the client
   3. Instruct the client to cover the lesion with an adhesive bandage
   4. Determine what the client has been doing to treat the lesion

Answer: 4

Rationale: A licensed practical nurse may not instruct, develop a teaching plan, or obtain a health history. Those are activities reserved for the registered nurse. A licensed practical nurse may monitor the vital signs of a client with cellulitis for evidence of sepsis. A licensed practical nurse is trained to monitor vital signs for deviations from normal and then report those changes to a registered nurse.

Nursing process: Planning

Client need: Management of Care

Cognitive level: Analysis

Subject area: Legal and Ethical Issues

Answer: 4

Rationale: Skin self-examination includes the entire body, looking for any changes in skin color as well as changes in moles. Although evaluating the evenness of skin color, moisture, and temperature is an appropriate intervention, it is limited in its focus to two insignificant characteristics of skin moisture and temperature. These do not change with development of skin cancer. Inspecting moles is also an important part of a skin examination, but limits the skin assessment to moles only and negates the rest of the assessment. Performing a skin examination is an ongoing assessment and not just something that begins after age 40.

Nursing process: Planning

Client need: Physiological Adaptation

Cognitive level: Application

Subject area: Medical-Surgical

Answer: 2

Rationale: More information is needed about the lesion to help determine an appropriate course of action. The findings do not require immediate attention from the physician. It is inappropriate to determine a plan of action without completing a thorough assessment. Determining what the client has been doing to treat the lesion only gathers part of the data needed to determine a plan of action.

Nursing process: Implementation

Client need: Physiological Adaptation

Cognitive level: Analysis

Subject area: Medical-Surgical

4. The nurse instructs a client with pruritis to apply an emollient immediately after bathing. The nurse understands that the rationale for this intervention is

   1. to prevent evaporation of water from the epidermis.

   2. to cause vasodilation that will reduce the symptoms of pruritis.

   3. to provide extra fat to the subcutaneous tissue.

   4. to protect the skin from further irritation.

5. The nurse is discharging a client who developed a skin tear while hospitalized for surgery. The nurse instructs the client in wound care for the skin tear. Which of the following would be essential to include in the wound care instructions for this client?

   1. Cover the skin tear with a transparent dressing

   2. Use a nonadherent dressing over the wound

   3. Eat a high-fat diet to help the wound heal more quickly

   4. Drink 3000 ml of water every day to keep the skin hydrated

6. The nurse is teaching a mother about caring for her 4-year-old with atopic dermatitis. Which of the following statements by the mother indicates that the teaching has been successful?

   1. "I prevent the spread of dermatitis by using separate towels for the children."

   2. "We will all switch to soy milk."

   3. "I will keep my child out of the sun."

   4. "I will avoid using fabric softeners in the laundry."

7. The nurse is teaching a class on the treatment of psoriasis with methotrexate. Which of the following should the nurse include in her teaching?

   1. Methotrexate is recommended only for those over the age of 50

   2. It is important to monitor serum albumin, total protein, and blood glucose

   3. An effective birth control for both men and women must be taken

   4. Topical steroids used with methotrexate provide the most effective therapy

Answer: 1

Rationale: Emollients seal in water and hydrate the skin. Emollients do not affect the blood vessels. The emollient is not in contact with the subcutaneous tissue. The primary function of an emollient is to rehydrate the skin. Intact skin is the best defense against irritation.

Nursing process: Analysis

Client need: Basic Care and Comfort

Cognitive level: Application

Subject area: Medical-Surgical

Answer: 2

Rationale: Use of a nonadherent dressing is the most helpful in treatment of skin tears. A transparent dressing causes maceration of the skin and may cause further skin trauma with removal. A diet high in fat does not help with healing. A diet high in protein and vitamin C is more likely to help healing. The primary treatment of skin tears is protecting them from further trauma so they can heal.

Nursing process: Planning

Client need: Physiological Adaptation

Cognitive level: Application

Subject area: Medical-Surgical

Answer: 4

Rationale: Fabric softeners often contain chemicals or components that are irritants for those with atopic dermatitis. Dermatitis is not a contagious condition, so using separate towels is not necessary. Avoidance of certain foods in treating atopic dermatitis is controversial. It is recommended that only known allergens be avoided. The sun is not a trigger for atopic dermatitis.

Nursing process: Evaluation

Client need: Physiological Adaptation

Cognitive level: Analysis

Subject area: Medical-Surgical

Answer: 3

Rationale: Because methotrexate is associated with chromosomal abnormalities, both men and women must use highly effective birth control during therapy. Methotrexate may be used in clients with very severe disease who have been unresponsive to other therapies regardless of age. The appropriate lab work to monitor when a client is taking methotrexate includes blood chemistry and liver and renal function studies. Methotrexate is only used when all other treatment options fail.

Nursing process: Planning

Client need: Physiological Adaptation

Cognitive level: Application

Subject area: Medical-Surgical

8. The nurse is providing diet instructions for a client with acne rosacea. Which of the following describes the most appropriate dietary restrictions?

Select all that apply:

[   ] **1.** Avoid spicy foods

[   ] **2.** Limit the intake of foods rich in omega-3 fatty acids

[   ] **3.** Avoid chocolate

[   ] **4.** Avoid caffeine

[   ] **5.** Restrict the use of products containing phenylalanine

[   ] **6.** Avoid fried foods

9. The nurse is evaluating the following four clients for the development of a pressure ulcer. Which of the following clients is at greatest risk for the development of a pressure ulcer?

1. A 52-year-old obese female, two days post-op for a knee replacement, who has an indwelling urinary catheter

2. A 74-year-old thin male, who is awaiting surgery for a fractured left hip

3. A 91-year-old emaciated female with a blood sugar of 160 mg/dl, who is sitting in a wheelchair

4. A 67-year-old obese male, who has cellulitis of his right lower leg

10. The nurse is instructing a client with herpes zoster on self-care. Which of the following statements by the client indicates the teaching has been successful?

1. "I will stay away from my young grandchildren."

2. "Frequent cool baths will help my herpes heal more quickly."

3. "I will use topical diphenhydramine to dry up the lesions."

4. "I will avoid using fabric softener in the laundry."

11. When assessing for changes in skin color in an African-American client, the nurse should assess which of the following first?

1. Soles of the feet

2. Palms of the hand

3. Conjunctiva or sclera

4. Nail beds or oral mucosa

Answer: 1, 4

Rationale: Spicy foods, hot and cold caffeine, and alcohol are all foods that worsen acne rosacea. Foods rich in omega-3 fatty acids, chocolate, fried foods, and products containing phenylalanine are unrelated to controlling rosacea.

Nursing process: Evaluation

Client need: Basic Care and Comfort

Cognitive level: Application

Subject area: Medical-Surgical

Answer: 2

Rationale: Risk factors for the development of pressure sores include bony prominences, inability to change position independently, and a bed rest status. These factors pose the highest risk for the client.

Nursing process: Evaluation

Client need: Physiological Adaptation

Cognitive level: Analysis

Subject area: Medical-Surgical

Answer: 1

Rationale: People who have not had chickenpox may get it from exposure to those with herpes zoster. Cool baths, although soothing, do not speed up the healing process. Topical diphenhydramine is useful for itching but will not accelerate the healing process. The use of fabric softener is unrelated to herpes zoster.

Nursing process: Evaluation

Client need: Physiological Adaptation

Cognitive level: Analysis

Subject area: Medical-Surgical

Answer: 4

Rationale: Assessment of the skin of those with naturally darker pigmentation should be done in an area where the epidermis is thin or in areas of least pigmentation, such as the nail beds or oral mucosa. The soles of the feet and palms of the hands are the second best options. It would not be appropriate to inspect the conjunctiva or sclera of an African-American client for skin color because of the possibility of yellowing.

Nursing process: Assessment

Client need: Physiological Adaptation

Cognitive level: Application

Subject area: Medical-Surgical

12. The nurse is preparing to teach a class on the prevention of skin problems. Which of the following is a priority for the nurse to instruct clients to avoid?

1. Sunlight
2. Radiation
3. Alkaline soaps
4. Vitamin E

13. The nurse is caring for a client during the emergent phase of a burn injury. Which of the following assessments would provide the nurse with the most accurate information regarding this client's full-thickness burns?

1. Leathery, dry, hard skin
2. Red, fluid-filled vesicles
3. Massive edema at the injury site
4. Serous exudates from a shiny, dark-brown wound

14. Prioritize the emergency management of a burn, from highest to lowest priority, with 1 as the highest priority.

_____ **1.** Establish and maintain an airway
_____ **2.** Assess for associated injuries
_____ **3.** Establish an IV line with a large-gauge needle
_____ **4.** Remove the client from the burning source

15. Using an open method of skin care, which of the following should the nurse include when caring for a client with deep partial-thickness burns of both legs?

1. Ensure that sterile water is used in the debridement tank
2. Apply topical silver sulfadiazine (Silvadene) with clean gloves
3. Use clean gloves to remove the dressings and wash the wounds
4. Wear a cap, mask, gown, and gloves when caring for the client

Answer: 1

Rationale: Limiting exposure to the sun is the most important preventive measure in reducing the risk of developing skin cancer and premature aging. Radiation and alkaline soaps are less common causes of skin problems. Overexposure to vitamin E does not cause skin problems.

Nursing process: Planning

Client need: Management of Care

Cognitive level: Application

Subject area: Medical-Surgical

Answer: 1

Rationale: A burn that has leathery, dry, and hard skin describes a full-thickness burn in the emergent phase. A burn that is a red, fluid-filled vesicle with massive edema at the injury site describes a deep, partial-thickness burn during the emergent phase. Serous exudate from a shiny, dark-brown wound describes a partial-thickness burn in the acute phase.

Nursing process: Assessment

Client need: Physiological Adaptation

Cognitive level: Application

Subject area: Medical-Surgical

Answer: 4, 1, 3, 2

Rationale: It is a priority to remove a client from the burning source, followed by establishing and maintaining an airway. Establishing an IV line with a large-gauge needle and assessing for associated injuries would follow in priority.

Nursing process: Implementation

Client need: Reduction of Risk Potential

Cognitive level: Analysis

Subject area: Medical-Surgical

Answer: 2

Rationale: The open method requires cleansing the wounds, applying a topical antimicrobial, and leaving the wounds open to air. Either saline or an electrolyte solution is best to use in the debridement tank. It would be inappropriate to use the open method with a partial-thickness burn because there are no dressings in place.

Nursing process: Planning

Client need: Physiological Adaptation

Cognitive level: Application

Subject area: Medical-Surgical

16. The nurse notifies the physician that a client who is 12 hours postburn has abdominal distention and faint, intermittent bowel sounds. Which of the following should the nurse perform?

    1. Withhold oral intake except water

    2. Insert a nasogastric tube

    3. Administer a histamine-blocking medication

    4. Reposition the client in preparation for an enema

17. The nurse is caring for a client with a burn injury who has a nursing diagnosis of impaired physical mobility related to limited range of motion secondary to pain. Which of the following is the priority nursing intervention for this client?

    1. Encourage the client to perform range of motion exercises in the absence of pain

    2. Instruct the client on the importance of exercise to prevent contractures

    3. Provide an analgesic medication before physical activity and exercise

    4. Arrange for the physical therapist to increase activity during hydrotherapy

18. Which of the following statements by a client who received instructions on pain control prior to a dressing change indicates the instructions were understood?

    1. "I will ask for my midazolam (Versed) one hour before the dressing change."

    2. "I will ask for acetaminophen (Tylenol) two hours before my dressing change."

    3. "I will put on my favorite music to take my mind off my pain."

    4. "I will ask the nurse for IV morphine five minutes before my dressing change."

19. The client who has burns on the face, neck, and chest asks why a pressure garment must be worn so many hours a day prior to dressing changes. Which of the following statements by the nurse provides the most accurate explanation?

    1. "The pressure garment protects your skin from sunlight and further damage."

    2. "It provides support and splinting to keep your body in alignment."

    3. "It reduces the thickness of the scar tissue."

    4. "The pressure garment helps trap the oils in your skin."

Answer: 2

Rationale: Paralytic ileus is common in the postburn phase and is best treated with a nasogastric tube to suction for decompression. All oral intake should be withheld. Administering a histamine-blocking medication will not improve peristalsis, although it may be given to reduce the possibility of aspirating acidic stomach contents. It would not be appropriate to prepare the client at this time for administration of an enema. Once there is evidence of peristalsis (bowel sounds are present, the client passes flatus), an enema may be administered.

Nursing process: Implementation

Client need: Physiological Adaptation

Cognitive level: Application

Subject area: Medical-Surgical

Answer: 3

Rationale: Control of pain is crucial before clients will participate in their prescribed exercise routine. This is best facilitated by administering an analgesic medication before physical activity. Controlling the pain should be followed by encouraging range of motion and instructing the client on the importance of exercise to prevent contractures. Arranging for a client to see a physical therapist does not address pain control. In fact, most burn patients find hydrotherapy to be very painful because of the debridement that must occur at that time.

Nursing process: Implementation

Client need: Management of Care

Cognitive level: Analysis

Subject area: Medical-Surgical

Answer: 4

Rationale: Pain control in a burn injury includes administering IV morphine just prior to the dressing change. Midazolam (Versed) is a good drug for pain control but it must be administered too far in advance to be of maximal benefit. Acetaminophen (Tylenol) is not an adequate analgesic for pain associated with full-thickness burns. Listening to music may be a good adjunct therapy to medication to control pain prior to a dressing change for a burn, but it is usually not enough by itself to control a client's pain.

Nursing process: Evaluation

Client need: Physiological Adaptation

Cognitive level: Analysis

Subject area: Legal and Ethical Issues

Answer: 3

Rationale: Pressure garments flatten scar tissue, giving the client more mobility and better cosmetic appearance. Wearing a pressure dressing does protect the site from further injury, but this is not the major reason for wearing a pressure garment. Wearing a pressure dressing does not support or splint the body part, nor does it trap the oils in the skin.

Nursing process: Evaluation

Client need: Reduction of Risk Potential

Cognitive level: Analysis

Subject area: Medical-Surgical

20. The nurse is planning to debride and remove scales and crusts of skin lesions to the left leg of a client. Which of the following is a priority intervention for this client?

1. Cool oatmeal bath

2. Warm saline dressings

3. Cool sodium bicarbonate bath

4. Warm magnesium sulfate dressings

21. A client with chronic skin lesions on the face and arms admits to the nurse of being unable to look in the mirror. Based on this information, which of the following nursing diagnoses would the nurse identify?

1. Anxiety related to personal appearance

2. Disturbed body image related to perception of unsightly lesions

3. Social isolation related to poor self-image

4. Deficient knowledge related to lack of understanding of use of cover-up techniques

22. The nurse is caring for a client with full-thickness burns who is receiving fluid replacement. Which of the following would indicate to the nurse that the client's condition is deteriorating?

1. Systolic BP of 86

2. 30 to 50 ml/hr urine output

3. Respiratory rate of 18/minute

4. Pulse rate of 85

23. During the acute phase of a burn injury, the nurse assists a client with deep partial-thickness burns of the left arm to make which of the following menu choices that are most appropriate?

Select all that apply:

[ ] **1.** Fried chicken

[ ] **2.** Turkey sandwich with lettuce and tomato

[ ] **3.** Barbecued pork on a roll

[ ] **4.** Mashed potatoes

[ ] **5.** Milkshake

[ ] **6.** Cola beverage

Answer: 2

Rationale: Debridement is best accomplished using a warm solution. Saline is the best choice. A cool oatmeal or sodium bicarbonate bath is best used for pruritis. Magnesium sulfate will not be helpful for the person with scaly and crusty skin.

Nursing process: Implementation

Client need: Physiological Adaptation

Cognitive level: Application

Subject area: Medical-Surgical

Answer: 2

Rationale: Defining characteristics for disturbed body image include verbalization of self-disgust and inability to look at oneself in the mirror. Anxiety would be an appropriate nursing diagnosis only if the client verbalizes or demonstrates anxiety related to the appearance. Social isolation or deficient knowledge would be an appropriate diagnosis only if the client verbalizes these as problems.

Nursing process: Evaluation

Client need: Management of Care

Cognitive level: Application

Subject area: Medical-Surgical

Answer: 1

Rationale: A decrease in the systolic blood pressure to less than 90 mm Hg indicates evaporation, plasma loss, and a fluid shift into the interstitium secondary to the burn injury. A urinary output of between 30 and 50 ml per hour, respiration rate of 18, and a pulse rate of 85 are all considered normal.

Nursing process: Analysis

Client need: Reduction of Risk Potential

Cognitive level: Analysis

Subject area: Medical-Surgical

Answer: 2, 4, 5

Rationale: A turkey sandwich with lettuce and tomato, mashed potatoes, and a milkshake provide the highest quality protein with the best representation of food groups for a client who has a partial-thickness burn of one arm. It is also manageable by a client who has only one hand that is usable. Fried chicken is high in fat and barbecued pork is spicy and may not be tolerated well. A cola beverage, although high in calories, is void of nutrients.

Nursing process: Implementation

Client need: Basic Care and Comfort

Cognitive level: Application

Subject area: Medical-Surgical

24. A client with psoriasis is being treated with psoralen plus UVA light phototherapy. During the course of therapy, the client is instructed to wear protective eyewear to block all UV rays. Which of the following statements by the client indicates a correct understanding of the teaching?

1. "I should wear sunglasses continuously for 6 hours after taking the medication."

2. "I should wear sunglasses until my pupils can constrict when exposed to light."

3. "I will wear sunglasses for 12 hours after treatment to prevent retinal damage."

4. "I should wear sunglasses for 24 hours following treatment when indoors near a bright window."

25. Which of the following assessments would provide the nurse with the most accurate information regarding a client in the emergent phase of burn care?

Select all that apply:

[   ] **1.** Extreme thirst

[   ] **2.** Decreased pulse

[   ] **3.** Warm and flushed feeling

[   ] **4.** Decreased bowel sounds

[   ] **5.** Dehydration

[   ] **6.** Decreased blood pressure

26. A client with burns over the face, arms, and trunk is requesting pain medication. When intervening in this situation, the nurse should administer which of the following drugs of choice for pain control in burn management?

1. Meperidine (Demerol)

2. Morphine

3. Oxycodone/aspirin (Percodan)

4. Propoxyphene/acetaminophen (Darvocet)

Answer: 4

Rationale: Psoralen is absorbed by the lens of the eye, so protective eyewear must be used for 24 hours after taking the medication. Since UVA penetrates glass, the sunglasses must also be worn inside.

Nursing process: Evaluation

Client need: Physiological Adaptation

Cognitive level: Analysis

Subject area: Medical-Surgical

Answer: 1, 4, 6

Rationale: The emergent phase of a burn injury is also called the resuscitative phase. It begins with the onset of the burn and generally lasts one to two days but may continue for approximately five days. Initially there is fluid loss and the presence of edema. It continues until diuresis begins. The client will exhibit thirst and chilling due to fluid and heat loss. Decreased bowel sounds or even absent bowel sounds may be present from an adynamic ileus resulting from trauma or a potassium shift. Signs of hypovolemic shock would include decreased blood pressure and increased pulse.

Nursing process: Assessment

Client need: Physiological Adaptation

Cognitive level: Application

Subject area: Medical-Surgical

Answer: 2

Rationale: Morphine sulfate is the drug of choice in the treatment of burns. Meperidine (Demerol) may also be used but is not the drug of choice. Oxycodone/aspirin (Percodan) and propoxyphene/acetaminophen (Darvocet) are not strong enough drugs to provide adequate pain relief.

Nursing process: Implementation

Client need: Pharmacological and Parenteral Therapies

Cognitive level: Analysis

Subject area: Pharmacologic

27. In planning the care for a severely burned client, the nurse should select which of the following as the priority nursing diagnosis?

 1. Pain related to burn injury and treatments

 2. Impaired physical mobility related to contractures

 3. Risk for deficient fluid volume related to a fluid shift, evaporation, and plasma loss

 4. Imbalanced nutrition: less than body requirements related to the body's need for an increased calorie intake

28. The nurse implements which of the following nursing measures as preventing dilutional hyponatremia in a client with burns?

 1. Instruct the client on the sodium content in foods

 2. Administer a diuretic

 3. Encourage the client to drink fluids other than water

 4. Encourage the client to exercise vigorously

29. Which of the following nursing interventions should the nurse include in the rehabilitative phase of burn care?

 1. Establish and maintain a patent airway

 2. Insert two large-bore catheters percutaneously

 3. Administer range of motion exercises

 4. Use Parkland formula to calculate fluid requirement

30. Which of the following nursing tasks should the nurse delegate to unlicensed assistive personnel?

 1. Remove a dressing to a skin tear of a client's leg

 2. Advise a client with acne to use water-based cosmetics

 3. Assist with bathing of a client with a burn

 4. Encourage a client with acne rosacea to verbalize feelings

Answer: 3

Rationale: The priority nursing diagnosis for a client with burns is risk for deficient fluid volume related to a fluid shift, evaporation, and plasma loss.

Nursing process: Planning

Client need: Management of Care

Cognitive level: Analysis

Subject area: Medical-Surgical

Answer: 3

Rationale: The client is encouraged to drink fluids other than water as a means of preventing dilutional hyponatremia, also known as water intoxication. Fluids rich in electrolytes and calories are offered.

Nursing process: Implementation

Client need: Physiological Adaptation

Cognitive level: Application

Subject area: Medical-Surgical

Answer: 3

Rationale: Administering range of motion exercises is an appropriate intervention for the rehabilitative phase of burn care. Establishing and maintaining a patent airway, inserting two large-bore catheters percutaneously, and using the Parkland formula to calculate fluid requirement are interventions reserved for the emergent and acute phase of burn management.

Nursing process: Planning

Client need: Physiological Adaptation

Cognitive level: Application

Subject area: Medical-Surgical

Answer: 3

Rationale: Removing a dressing, providing a client instructions, or encouraging a client to verbalize feelings are all activities that require the skills of a qualified nurse. Although socialization is a skill that unlicensed assistive personnel may perform, encouraging a client to verbalize feelings is a skill that requires the expertise of the nurse in assisting the client to deal with the expressed feelings. Unlicensed assistive personnel may assist with the bathing of a client who sustained a burn.

Nursing process: Planning

Client need: Management of Care

Cognitive level: Analysis

Subject area: Medical-Surgical

CHAPTER

Musculoskeletal Disorders

8

1. The nurse is caring for a client who just returned from surgery with a long leg cast. Which of the following interventions is the priority in the first 24 hours?

   1. Position the client supine to facilitate drying of the cast
   2. Dangle the client on the side of the bed in the evening
   3. Elevate the leg on a pillow above heart level
   4. Assess the cast for rough edges and smoothness

2. Immediately after application of a plaster of paris cast, the client asks the nurse when weight bearing may begin. The most appropriate response by the nurse is

   1. "I do not know. I will ask your physician."
   2. "It is all individualized based on how you feel."
   3. "Within 8 hours, you will be standing next to the bed."
   4. "Generally after 24 to 48 hours."

3. The client asks the nurse after a total hip replacement with a cemented prosthesis when ambulation and weight bearing may begin. The nurse bases the answer on the knowledge that weight bearing and ambulation

   1. are permitted after four weeks.
   2. are individualized and difficult to predict.
   3. may begin with a walker the first postoperative day.
   4. occur within three to five months.

4. The nurse is caring for a client who has a compression dressing in place after an amputation. The nurse appropriately removes the dressing

   1. for bathing and physical therapy.
   2. when getting the client in a chair.
   3. for two hours once a shift.
   4. when the pain has stopped.

Answer: 3
Rationale: The priority nursing intervention for a client with a long leg cast in the first 24 hours is to elevate the extremity above the level of the heart by placing the leg on several pillows to prevent edema. The edges of the cast may be checked for smoothness or roughness.
Nursing process: Implementation
Client need: Management of Care
Cognitive level: Application
Subject area: Medical-Surgical

Answer: 4
Rationale: Generally for 24 to 48 hours after direct cast application, direct weight bearing is contraindicated. After the 24 to 48 hour time frame, a walking heel will be applied to the cast.
Nursing process: Analysis
Client need: Physiological Adaptation
Cognitive level: Application
Subject area: Medical-Surgical

Answer: 3
Rationale: Weight bearing and ambulation following a total hip replacement with a cemented prosthesis may begin with a walker the first postoperative day.
Nursing process: Analysis
Client need: Physiological Adaptation
Cognitive level: Application
Subject area: Medical-Surgical

Answer: 1
Rationale: The compression dressing that is applied immediately following surgery is only removed for bathing and physical therapy. The purpose of the compression dressing is to support the soft tissues while reducing edema and promoting limb shrinkage to ensure a good prosthetic fit at a later date.
Nursing process: Implementation
Client need: Physiological Adaptation
Cognitive level: Application
Subject area: Medical-Surgical

5. The nurse is discharging a client with rheumatoid arthritis who complains of morning stiffness. Which of the following measures should the nurse include in the discharge instructions?

   1. Encourage the client to sleep with pillows under the knees

   2. Instruct the client to apply ice packs to the joints before getting out of bed

   3. Instruct the client to take a warm shower in the morning when getting up

   4. Teach the client to perform all of the household chores at one time

6. Before a client has skin traction applied, which of the following should the nurse include in the instructions given to the client?

   1. Skin traction may be used for long periods of time

   2. Skin traction is applied until surgery can be performed

   3. A pin will be put in the bone

   4. Weights up to 45 pounds will be applied

7. In planning the post-op care for a client with a hip spica cast, the nurse should know the best method of positioning this client would be

   1. maintain the client in a prone position.

   2. use the support bar between the thighs to turn the client.

   3. turn the client side to side and support with pillows.

   4. allow the client to turn into any position that offers comfort.

8. Which of the following dietary guidelines should the nurse provide to a client with a fracture?

   1. Three large, high-calorie meals

   2. High-fiber foods and 2000 to 3000 ml of fluids daily

   3. Low-protein and low-fat foods

   4. Limit milk and milk products to two servings daily

Answer: 3

Rationale: Morning stiffness is a common complaint of clients with rheumatoid arthritis because of the limited joint movements. A warm shower upon arising is recommended to increase mobility and decrease discomfort associated with the limited mobility. Cold packs may be used during exacerbations of the disease, but heat is most effective to relieve stiffness. The work of cleaning the house should be spread out throughout the week and not done at one time.

Nursing process: Planning

Client need: Health Promotion and Maintenance

Cognitive level: Application

Subject area: Medical-Surgical

Answer: 2

Rationale: The purpose of skin traction such as Buck's, Bryant's, Russell, a pelvic belt, or a sling is simply to stabilize the affected part and maintain alignment until surgery or skeletal traction can be performed. Skin traction is only a short-term treatment and generally for no longer than 48 to 72 hours. Generally the weight for skin traction does not exceed 7 to 10 pounds.

Nursing process: Planning

Client need: Health Promotion and Maintenance

Cognitive level: Application

Subject area: Medical-Surgical

Answer: 3

Rationale: A client with a hip spica cast should be turned from side to side and supported with pillows. The prone position and turning the client by using the support bar is contraindicated because they can cause the cast to break.

Nursing process: Planning

Client need: Basic Care and Comfort

Cognitive level: Application

Subject area: Medical-Surgical

Answer: 2

Rationale: Although three well-balanced meals are encouraged following a fracture, an excessive calorie intake is to be avoided because of the limited mobility that predisposes the client to weight gain. A high-fiber diet and increased fluid intake are necessary to prevent constipation. Adequate protein and calcium intake must be maintained to ensure adequate healing.

Nursing process: Implementation

Client need: Basic Care and Comfort

Cognitive level: Analysis

Subject area: Medical-Surgical

9. Which of the following changes in a client's neurovascular assessment should be reported as a critical sign of arterial insufficiency?

1. Pale extremity that is cool to touch

2. Hypersensation below the injury

3. Pain unrelieved by analgesic

4. Reduced motion in affected extremity

10. In planning the postoperative care for a client with a cast, the nurse would select which of the following as an appropriate nursing diagnosis?

1. Risk for deficient fluid volume related to excess fluid loss

2. Total urinary incontinence: related to aging process

3. Constipation related to decreased mobility

4. Imbalanced nutrition: less than body requirements related to lack of knowledge of appropriate food choices

11. A client's x-ray reveals a fracture in which one bone fragment is forced into or onto another fragment. The nurse interprets this finding as indicative of what type of fracture? _____

Answer: 1

Rationale: A pale and cool extremity following a musculoskeletal injury is the classic indication of arterial insufficiency and must be immediately reported. Hypersensation below the injury as well as other abnormal sensations may be experienced, but they are not the priority finding. An evaluation of a potential problem including a comparison of the affected and unaffected extremity will prove beneficial. Pain unrelieved by analgesics is indicative of compartment syndrome. Reduced movement in the affected extremity should be investigated as potential damage to the motor component of the affected nerves.

Nursing process: Analysis

Client need: Reduction of Risk Potential

Cognitive level: Analysis

Subject area: Medical-Surgical

Answer: 3

Rationale: Constipation related to decreased mobility is an appropriate nursing diagnosis for a client with a cast.

Nursing process: Analysis

Client need: Physiological Adaptation

Cognitive level: Analysis

Subject area: Medical-Surgical

Answer: Impacted

Rationale: An impacted bone fracture occurs as a result of a comminuted fracture (fracture in which the bone is broken into several pieces or shattered). As a result of the bone being broken into several pieces, two or more fragments are forced into each other.

Nursing process: Implementation

Client need: Physiological Adaptation

Cognitive level: Comprehension

Subject area: Medical-Surgical

12. Which of the following interventions would be appropriate for the nurse to include in the treatment plan of a client with a stump?

1. Expose the stump to air for 20 minutes
2. Generously apply lotion to the stump
3. Administer skin care by rubbing with alcohol
4. Scrub the stump daily to prevent infection

13. The nurse is assisting a client to walk with a crutch for the first time after an amputation. Which of the following indicates the nurse correctly understands the principles of crutch walking after an amputation?

1. Instruct the client to remove the compression dressing before crutch walking
2. Encourage the client to place the weight of the body on the axilla
3. Administer an analgesic 30 minutes prior to crutch walking
4. Assist the client to crutch walk for no more than five minutes

14. Because a client has bursitis, plans for nursing interventions should include

1. aggressive antibiotic therapy.
2. rest.
3. range of motion activities.
4. high-protein diet.

15. The nurse is admitting a client with rheumatoid arthritis. Which of the following laboratory test results would the nurse evaluate as being elevated and used to monitor disease activity?

1. Serum uric acid
2. Erythrocyte sedimentation rate
3. Bence Jones protein
4. White blood cell count

Answer: 1

Rationale: Following an amputation, the stump is exposed to air for 20 minutes daily after washing to promote adequate drying. Lotion and alcohol are contraindicated unless specifically prescribed by the physician. Scrubbing a stump is strictly contraindicated. The stump should be gently cleansed.

Nursing process: Planning

Client need: Physiological Adaptation

Cognitive level: Application

Subject area: Medical-Surgical

Answer: 4

Rationale: Initially following an amputation, crutch walking is limited to five minutes to avoid dependent edema. A client should never place weight on the axilla. This can compromise the nerve passing through the axilla. A compression dressing would not be removed prior to ambulation. Administration of an analgesic 30 minutes prior to ambulation could cause sedation and predispose a client to a fall.

Nursing process: Analysis

Client need: Physiological Adaptation

Cognitive level: Application

Subject area: Medical-Surgical

Answer: 2

Rationale: Bursitis is inflammation of the bursa (small sacs of the connective tissues lined with synovial fluid). Bursitis is generally the result of some kind of mechanical injury and is most successfully treated by rest.

Nursing process: Planning

Client need: Basic Care and Comfort

Cognitive level: Application

Subject area: Medical-Surgical

Answer: 2

Rationale: Although no single laboratory test is used for rheumatoid arthritis, the erythrocyte sedimentation rate (ERS) is elevated in over 80% of clients and is used to monitor disease activity and the response to treatment.

Nursing process: Evaluation

Client need: Reduction of Risk Potential

Cognitive level: Analysis

Subject area: Medical-Surgical

16. The nurse is caring for a client with gout. Which of the following dietary selections should the nurse include in the dietary instructions?

Select all that apply:

[   ] 1. Salmon

[   ] 2. Macaroni

[   ] 3. Sardines

[   ] 4. Cheese

[   ] 5. Spinach

[   ] 6. Venison

17. The nurse assesses which of the following clinical manifestations in a client with osteomyelitis?

Select all that apply:

[   ] 1. Night sweats

[   ] 2. Cool extremities

[   ] 3. Petechiae

[   ] 4. Fever

[   ] 5. Nausea

[   ] 6. Restlessness

18. The nurse assists a client with osteoporosis to make which of the following menu selections?

1. Scrambled eggs and a banana

2. Bagel with cream cheese and half a grapefruit

3. 3 oz grilled chicken and a baked potato

4. Sardines and cooked broccoli

19. The nurse expects to find which of the characteristic clinical manifestations in a client with osteoarthritis?

1. Loss of function from Bouchard's and Heberden's nodes

2. Joint pain that is relieved by rest

3. Joint stiffness that is worse with activity

4. Pain and stiffness that improve with humidity and low barometric pressure

Answer: 2, 4

Rationale: Foods high in purine are limited for a client with gout. Gout is repeated arthritic episodes associated with high levels of serum uric acid. Uric acid is the end product of purine catabolism. Liver, salmon, sardines, venison, and sweetbreads are high in purine content. Macaroni and cheese are lower purine food choices.

Nursing process: Planning

Client need: Basic Care and Comfort

Cognitive level: Application

Subject area: Medical-Surgical

Answer: 1, 4, 5, 6

Rationale: Osteomyelitis is an infection of the bone characterized by both local and systemic manifestations. Systemic manifestations include fever, chills, night sweats, nausea, malaise, and restlessness.

Nursing process: Assessment

Client need: Physiological Adaptation

Cognitive level: Application

Subject area: Medical-Surgical

Answer: 4

Rationale: Osteoporosis is characterized by a deterioration of bone and increased bone fragility. An adequate intake of calcium is essential in both the prevention and treatment of osteoporosis. Foods high in calcium include milk and milk products, sardines, salmon, and certain green leafy vegetables such as broccoli. Eggs, fruits, poultry, and potatoes are poor calcium food choices.

Nursing process: Implementation

Client need: Basic Care and Comfort

Cognitive level: Application

Subject area: Medical-Surgical

Answer: 2

Rationale: Joint pain that is relieved by rest is characteristic of osteoarthritis. Pain and stiffness are made worse with increased humidity and a low barometric pressure. Heberden's nodes are bony overgrowths at the distal interphalangeal joints. Bouchard's nodes involve the proximal interphalangeal joints. Although these nodes are generally red, swollen, and tender, they do not cause a significant loss of function.

Nursing process: Assessment

Client need: Physiological Adaptation

Cognitive level: Application

Subject area: Medical-Surgical

20. The nurse is admitting a client for possible systemic lupus erythematosus (SLE). When assessing this client, the nurse understands that the most significant clinical manifestation present in SLE is

    1. petechiae on the abdomen.

    2. low-grade afternoon fever.

    3. discoid rash over the face and upper chest.

    4. multiple ecchymoses over the body.

21. The nurse is admitting a client after falling from a ladder and recognizes that the grating sound when the ends of a broken bone are moved is known as _____.

22. The nurse is caring for a client with an open fracture. Which of the following would be the priority to include in this client's treatment plan?

    1. A high-protein diet

    2. Insertion of a Foley catheter

    3. Tetanus toxoid

    4. Passive range of motion exercises

23. Because a client is at risk for back pain and falls, the nurse should instruct a client that the three concepts necessary to achieve good body mechanics and prevent pain and injury are _____.

Answer: 3

Rationale: A discoid (coinlike) rash is the classic dermatologic manifestation of systemic lupus erythematosus. It characteristically takes on a butterfly appearance.

Nursing process: Assessment

Client need: Physiological Adaptation

Cognitive level: Analysis

Subject area: Medical-Surgical

Answer: crepitation

Rationale: Crepitation is a grating sound heard on movement after a bone fracture.

Nursing process: Assessment

Client need: Physiological Adaptation

Cognitive level: Comprehension

Subject area: Medical-Surgical

Answer: 3

Rationale: The priority nursing intervention for an open fracture in which the skin integrity is broken is to administer a tetanus toxoid. A high-protein diet would be important but not the priority.

Nursing process: Planning

Client need: Management of Care

Cognitive level: Analysis

Subject area: Medical-Surgical

Answer: body alignment, balance, and coordinated movement

Rationale: Sensors in muscles and joints tell the cerebellum and other parts of the brain where and how the arm or leg is moving and what position it is in (feedback results in balance with smooth, coordinated motion).

Nursing process: Implementation

Client need: Reduction of Risk Potential

Cognitive level: Analysis

Subject area: Medical-Surgical

24. A client is scheduled for an open reduction internal fixation (ORIF) of a fracture. The nurse is explaining to the client why this procedure is necessary. Which of the following is the primary reason for the nurse to give a client that best describes the purpose of the ORIF?

1. "It is used when the client is in too much pain to do a closed reduction."

2. "It is completed whenever a client cannot maintain long-term immobility."

3. "It is necessary when no other realignment method can be completed."

4. "It is necessary when a cast would be too large to provide adequate mobility."

25. Which of the following neurovascular complications should the nurse assess for after a fracture?

Select all that apply:

[   ] **1.** Petechiae over all extremities

[   ] **2.** Pallor

[   ] **3.** Exaggerated extremity movement

[   ] **4.** Decreased sensation distal to the fracture site

[   ] **5.** Purulent drainage at the site of an open fracture

[   ] **6.** Pulselessness

26. A client with a fractured pelvis has a nursing diagnosis of impaired mobility related to bed rest, weakness, and traction. The nurse should inform the client that the rationale for maintaining good body alignment in the bed is to

1. decrease protein catabolism.

2. minimize the workload on the heart.

3. increase body strength and muscle mass.

4. reduce musculoskeletal strain and enhance lung expansion.

27. A nurse is developing a care plan for a client with an open fracture of the femur. Which of the following nursing diagnoses would the nurse choose as the priority nursing diagnosis?

1. Risk for constipation related to immobilization

2. Activity intolerance related to prolonged immobility

3. Risk for impaired skin integrity related to immobility

4. Impaired neurovascular status related to compression of nerves

Answer: 3

Rationale: When no other method, such as long-term immobility, can accomplish realignment for a fracture, open reduction internal fixation (ORIF) will be completed. Pain is evident in a fracture; however, with the medications available today, pain can usually be controlled enough to complete a closed reduction either under IV conscious sedation or with general anesthesia.

Nursing process: Evaluation

Client need: Physiological Adaptation

Cognitive level: Application

Subject area: Medical-Surgical

Answer: 2, 4, 6

Rationale: Neurovascular complications are assessed by a neurovascular check. Clinical manifestations of a possible neurovascular problem include pain with passive motion, pallor, pulselessness, parethesia, pressure, and paralysis. Loss of sensation is an indication of parethesia.

Nursing process: Assessment

Client need: Physiological Adaptation

Cognitive level: Application

Subject area: Medical-Surgical

Answer: 4

Rationale: Fractures cause damage to the affected bone, placing additional strain on the surrounding tissues, ligaments, and joints. Traction places the affected bone in proper alignment to reduce the strain on the surrounding parts. A client who has bed rest ordered may have a rapid deconditioning resulting in decreased lung capacity and orthostatic hypotension. Proper body alignment reduces the strain and increases lung expansion.

Nursing process: Implementation

Client need: Physiological Adaptation

Cognitive level: Analysis

Subject area: Medical-Surgical

Answer: 4

Rationale: Compression of the nerves is the most serious complication from an open fracture and is caused by edema or bone displacement. Compression of nerves can cause cell death. Risk for constipation, activity intolerance, and risk for impaired skin integrity are all important nursing diagnoses, but they are not the priority.

Nursing process: Implementation

Client need: Management of Care

Cognitive level: Analysis

Subject area: Medical-Surgical

28. The nurse has given discharge instructions to a client with an above-the-knee amputation who will be fitted with a prosthesis when healing is complete. Which of the following statements by the client would indicate that the client has understood the instructions?

1. "I should lie on my abdomen for 30 minutes three or four times a day."

2. "I should change the limb sock when it becomes soiled or stretched out."

3. "I should use lotion on the stump to prevent drying and cracking of the skin."

4. "I should elevate the residual limb on a pillow several times a day to decrease edema."

29. The nurse assesses that a client has lower-extremity weakness on the left. What should the nurse observe the client doing to evaluate the client's ability to use a walker?

1. Moving both the walker and the left leg forward 6 inches, then moving the right leg while the body weight is supported by the arms and the left leg

2. Moving both the walker and the right leg forward 6 inches, then moving the left leg while the body weight is supported by the arms and the right leg

3. Moving the walker forward 12 inches, bearing the body weight on the arms and extremities, then walking up to the walker

4. Moving both the walker and the left leg forward 12 inches, then moving the right leg while the body weight is supported by the arms and the left leg

30. A client has been admitted to the hospital with a diagnosis of osteoporosis resulting in a compression fracture of the spine. The physician has ordered complete bed rest and has ordered a dietary consultation. Which of the following is the priority for the nurse to include in the nutritional counseling?

1. Protein intake should be increased to 50% of the calorie intake daily

2. Vitamin D should be taken in the diet as food, not as an oral medication

3. Calcium intake should be 1500 mg daily

4. Calorie and fat intake should not exceed 1500 calories daily

31. Two days postoperatively a client who had a right lower-leg amputation is complaining of pain in the right toe. The nurse should report this as which kind of pain? _____

Answer: 1

Rationale: Lying on the abdomen will help to make a well-rounded stump and prevent hip contractures. The limb sock should always be changed daily. Lotion is never used on a stump. Elevation is not a treatment of amputation. Pressure on the stump and hip contractures are to be avoided.

Nursing process: Evaluation

Client need: Physiological Adaptation

Cognitive level: Analysis

Subject area: Medical-Surgical

Answer: 1

Rationale: A walker is a mechanical aid used for walking assistance by clients who need more support than a cane. Instructions for use of a walker are to move the walker and affected leg ahead 6 inches, then move the stronger leg ahead, and repeat. Arms bear the weight in the second step after the affected leg is moved forward 6 inches.

Nursing process: Evaluation

Client need: Physiological Adaptation

Cognitive level: Analysis

Subject area: Medical-Surgical

Answer: 3

Rationale: Calorie, protein, and fat intake if adequate for sustaining health are not a concern in osteoporosis. It is true that getting vitamins in the food is best; however, if additional vitamin D is required, a supplement is good if the client gets at least 15 minutes of sunlight per day. Calcium intake for women before menopause should be at least 1000 mg/day and after menopause should increase to at least 1500 mg/day. In a client with osteoporosis at any age, adequate calcium intake is at least 1500 mg/day.

Nursing process: Planning

Client need: Basic Care and Comfort

Cognitive level: Analysis

Subject area: Medical-Surgical

Answer: Phantom

Rationale: Phantom pain occurs in 80% of clients with an amputation. This pain is real to the client and the client should be medicated for the pain. Some clients have phantom pain for years after the amputation.

Nursing process: Analysis

Client need: Physiological Adaptation

Cognitive level: Application

Subject area: Medical-Surgical

32. Which of the following is a priority for the nurse to include in the preoperative teaching plan for a client scheduled for a total hip arthroplasty?

1. Signs of prosthetic dislocation

2. Methods to prevent dehydration

3. Exercises to promote hip flexion

4. Measures to prevent malnutrition

33. Which of the following would be the priority nursing action after being unable to palpate the client's pedal pulse after an open reduction of a tibia fracture?

1. Notify the physician of the inability to detect the pedal pulse

2. Check the lower extremity for pallor

3. Use a Doppler to check for the pedal pulse

4. Measure both extremities for comparison

34. A client has received teaching on the use of a cane to assist with ambulation. Which of the following statements by the client would indicate to the nurse that further teaching is needed?

1. "My elbows should be slightly bent when I use the cane."

2. "I should hold the cane on my unaffected side."

3. "A walker would be more difficult to use than a cane."

4. "While walking, I should have shoes and socks on at all times."

35. During an exercise session, the nurse assists the client to dorsiflex and plantarflex the foot. The client asks what kind of exercise this is. Which of the following is the appropriate response by the nurse?

1. Active range of motion

2. Passive range of motion

3. Isometric

4. Isotonic

Answer: 1

Rationale: When a hip is replaced, dislocation is a real problem; it is very important to teach the signs of dislocation to the client both preoperatively and postoperatively. Dehydration and malnutrition are not usual manifestations of hip arthroplasty and hip flexion is not a desired outcome. Hip flexion can cause dislocation of the arthroplasty.

Nursing process: Planning

Client need: Management of Care

Cognitive level: Analysis

Subject area: Medical-Surgical

Answer: 3

Rationale: To ensure that the circulation is intact when the pulse is not palpable, the nurse should use a Doppler. It is inappropriate to notify the physician without collecting all the appropriate data. Although checking the lower extremity pallor and measuring circumference will provide data of circulation, it does not ensure that a pedal pulse is present.

Nursing process: Implementation

Client need: Management of Care

Cognitive level: Analysis

Subject area: Medical-Surgical

Answer: 3

Rationale: The client should use the cane on the unaffected side. The elbow is held slightly flexed. There are different reasons to use a walker versus a cane; however, neither one is "better." Shoes must be worn. Never use socks alone. Socks may be optional to wear with the shoes.

Nursing process: Evaluation

Client need: Physiological Adaptation

Cognitive level: Analysis

Subject area: Medical-Surgical

Answer: 2

Rationale: Passive range of motion is exercise conducted with the assistance of another individual. Active range of motion is done by the client alone. Isometric exercise involves resistance and isotonic exercise does not use resistance.

Nursing process: Analysis

Client need: Physiological Adaptation

Cognitive level: Application

Subject area: Medical-Surgical

36. A client with systemic lupus erythematosus (SLE) is admitted to a nursing unit. Which of the following would indicate to the nurse that the client's condition is deteriorating?

   1. A serum sodium of 145 mEq/L

   2. A serum potassium of 5.5 mEq/L

   3. Large amounts of glucose in the urine

   4. Large amounts of protein in the urine

37. The registered nurse delegates which of the following nursing tasks to unlicensed assistive personnel?

   1. Perform active range of motion activities on a client who had a hip arthroplasty

   2. Reinforce the instruction given on how to perform a two-point crutch walk

   3. Instruct a client on how to use a walker

   4. Walk a client who has an ankle sprain to the bathroom

38. Which of the following crutch gaits should the nurse instruct the client to use who has bilateral paralysis of the hips and legs?

   1. Swing-to gait

   2. Four-point gait

   3. Three-point gait

   4. Two-point gait

Answer: 4

Rationale: Protein in the urine indicates renal failure and lupus nephritis is the number one cause of death in SLE. Serum sodium and potassium and glucose in the urine are not indicative of complications resulting from SLE. A serum sodium level of 145 mEq/L and a serum potassium level of 5.5 mEq/L are normal.

Nursing process: Analysis

Client need: Reduction of Risk Potential

Cognitive level: Analysis

Subject area: Medical-Surgical

Answer: 4

Rationale: Unlicensed assistive personnel cannot reinforce instruction or provide instruction. Performing active range of motion exercises on a client who had a hip arthroplasty is not an appropriate job assignment for unlicensed assistive personnel and active range of motion is likely to dislocate the hip (particularly adduction). Unlicensed assistive personnel may walk a client who has an ankle sprain to the bathroom.

Nursing process: Planning

Client need: Management of Care

Cognitive level: Analysis

Subject area: Medical-Surgical

Answer: 1

Rationale: A swing-to gait is a crutch gait that is used by clients who have paralysis of the hips and legs or wear bilateral braces on the legs. A four-point gait may be used by arthritic clients. A three-point gait may be used by a client with a broken leg or sprained ankle. A two-point gait requires more weight bearing on each foot. It is a faster crutch gait than a four-point gait.

Nursing process: Planning

Client need: Health Promotion and Maintenance

Cognitive level: Analysis

Subject area: Medical-Surgical

39. Which of the following should the nurse include when instructing a client with crutches on the two-point gait?

   1. Move the right crutch followed by the left foot, then move the left crutch forward followed by the right foot

   2. Move both crutches forward together and bring the legs through beyond the crutches

   3. Move the left crutch and right foot forward together, followed by moving the right crutch and the left foot forward together

   4. Move both crutches and the weaker leg forward, followed by moving the stronger leg forward

40. The nurse should include which of the following in the teaching plan for a client who has a cane prescribed?

   1. Move the cane forward two feet to ensure that the body weight is supported on both legs

   2. Hold the cane with the hand on the weaker side of the body

   3. Position the arm holding the cane so the elbow is completely straight to ensure maximum support

   4. Position the cane six inches to the side and six inches to the front of the foot of the strongest leg

Answer: 3

Rationale: When using the two-point gait, the left crutch and right foot are moved forward together, followed by moving the right crutch and left foot forward together. The crutch walk requires some weight bearing on each foot. During the four-point gait, the right crutch is moved forward followed by the left foot, then the left crutch is moved forward followed by the right foot. This is the most stable of all crutch walks. It provides the most support while requiring weight bearing on both legs. This gait may be used for some types of paralysis such as in children with cerebral palsy. In the three-point gait, both crutches are moved forward with the weaker leg, followed by moving the stronger leg forward. In this gait, the client is required to bear all weight on the unaffected leg. In the swing-to gait, both crutches are moved forward together followed by bringing the legs through beyond the crutches. This gait is used by clients who have a paralysis of their lower extremities.

Nursing process: Planning

Client need: Health Promotion and Maintenance

Cognitive level: Analysis

Subject area: Medical-Surgical

Answer: 4

Rationale: To provide a wide base of support, the cane should be positioned both six inches to the side and six inches to the front of the foot of the strongest leg. The cane should be held on the stronger side of the body. The elbow is bent to correctly use a cane. A cane is not an appropriate assistive device for someone with bilateral leg weakness.

Nursing process: Planning

Client need: Health Promotion and Maintenance

Cognitive level: Analysis

Subject area: Medical-Surgical

CHAPTER

Genitourinary Disorders

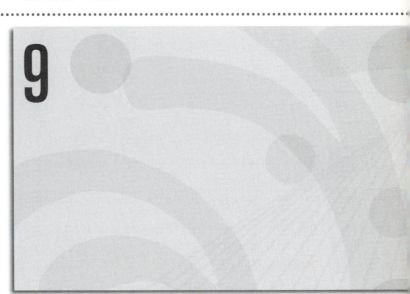

9

1. The nurse is teaching a class on urinary infections. Which of the following should the nurse include?
   1. The urinary tract below the urethra is sterile
   2. Pyelonephritis is a common infection of the lower urinary tract
   3. *E. coli* is the most common cause of urinary infections
   4. Males are more prone to urinary tract infections than females

2. The nurse tells a student nurse that the normal constituents of urine are the following.
   Select all that apply:
   [ ] 1. Protein
   [ ] 2. Sodium chloride
   [ ] 3. Ketones
   [ ] 4. Urea
   [ ] 5. Epithelial cells
   [ ] 6. Water

3. The nurse assesses a client's hourly output of urine to be 70 ml. Which of the following is the most appropriate action by the nurse?
   1. Notify the physician immediately
   2. Encourage the client to drink more fluids
   3. Instruct the client on the importance of ambulation
   4. Recognize this as a normal hourly output

4. The nurse instructs a client with pyelonephritis to drink 3000 ml of fluids per day. The nurse understands that the rationale for this intervention is
   1. to prevent reflux of urine.
   2. to prevent stasis of urine.
   3. to decrease urine output.
   4. to decrease residual urine.

Answer: 3

Rationale: *E. coli* is the most common organism causing urinary infections. The urinary tract above the urethra is sterile. Pyelonephritis is an infection of the kidneys or upper urinary tract. The incidence of urinary tract infections is greater in the female because the urethra is shorter than that of the male and also is closer to the vagina and rectum.

Nursing process: Planning

Client need: Physiological Adaptation

Cognitive level: Application

Subject area: Medical-Surgical

Answer: 2, 4, 6

Rationale: Urine is normally made up of sodium chloride, urea, and water. Protein is an abnormal constituent of urine indicating renal disease. Ketones may be found in a client who is in diabetic ketoacidosis. The presence of epithelial cells is found in a urinary tract infection.

Nursing process: Implementation

Client need: Physiological Adaptation

Cognitive level: Comprehension

Subject area: Medical-Surgical

Answer: 4

Rationale: The average 24 hour daily output for an adult is approximately 1500 ml or 62.5 ml per hour, so 70 ml is considered normal and no further action is necessary.

Nursing process: Planning

Client need: Physiological Adaptation

Cognitive level: Application

Subject area: Medical-Surgical

Answer: 2

Rationale: Increasing the fluid intake promotes the flushing out of the urinary tract and prevents stasis of urine. Preventing reflux of urine and decreasing urinary output or residual urine do not provide rationales for increasing fluid intake in pyelonephritis.

Nursing process: Analysis

Client need: Reduction of Risk Potential

Cognitive level: Analysis

Subject area: Medical-Surgical

5. A nurse is discharging a client who was hospitalized with calcium oxalate calculi. The nurse instructs the client regarding which of the following food selections contribute to the development of calcium oxalate calculi?

Select all that apply:

[   ] **1.** Celery

[   ] **2.** Salmon

[   ] **3.** Beets

[   ] **4.** Bacon

[   ] **5.** Whole wheat bread

[   ] **6.** Asparagus

6. The nurse is teaching a class on renal disease. Which of the following should the nurse include?

1. 90% of the nephrons are involved in acute renal failure

2. There is a direct correlation between the amount of urine produced and the severity of renal failure

3. Acute renal failure follows prolonged hypotension

4. The most diagnostic lab test for renal failure is the blood urea nitrogen

7. The nurse administers which of the following prescribed medications to a client with recurrent urinary tract infections caused by *Escherichia coli?*

1. Hyoscyamine sulfate (Levsin)

2. Bethanechol chloride (Urecholine)

3. Sulfamethoxazole and trimethoprim (Bactrim DS)

4. Phenazopyridine hydrochloride (Pyridium)

8. The nurse is caring for a client experiencing renal colic associated with nephrolithiasis. Which of the following nursing measures should receive priority in the client's plan of care?

1. Strain urine

2. Administer morphine sulfate

3. Monitor intake and output

4. Encourage ambulation

Answer: 1, 3, 6

Rationale: The goal of dietary management in calcium oxalate calculi is to encourage an acid-ash diet and reduce dietary oxalate. Celery, beets, and asparagus are all high in dietary oxalate. Salmon, bacon, and whole wheat bread are all meats or whole grains that are permitted on an acid-ash diet.

Nursing process: Planning

Client need: Basic Care and Comfort

Cognitive level: Application

Subject area: Medical-Surgical

Answer: 3

Rationale: Acute renal failure does occur after prolonged hypovolemia or hypotension. Involvement of 95% of the nephrons is found in end-stage renal disease. There is no direct correlation between the amount of urine produced and the severity of renal failure. Even though acute renal failure is often associated with a urinary output of less than 400 ml per day, it is possible to have a normal or even an increased urinary output. Creatinine is the most diagnostic test for renal failure.

Nursing process: Planning

Client need: Physiological Adaptation

Cognitive level: Application

Subject area: Medical-Surgical

Answer: 3

Rationale: Sulfamethoxazole and trimethoprim (Bactrim DS) is an antibiotic and a drug of choice in the treatment of urinary tract infections. Hyoscyamine sulfate (Levsin) is an anticholinergic used in specific spastic disorders. Bethanechol chloride (Urecholine) is a cholinergic agonist used in urinary retention. Phenazopyridine hydrochloride (Pyridium) is a urinary analgesic given to produce an analgesic effect on the urinary mucosa.

Nursing process: Implementation

Client need: Pharmacological and Parenteral Therapies

Cognitive level: Application

Subject area: Pharmacologic

Answer: 2

Rationale: Straining the urine, monitoring intake and output, and encouraging ambulation are all appropriate interventions in the management of renal calculi, but administering an analgesic is the priority intervention for a client experiencing renal colic. Renal colic is an excruciating pain that occurs when a stone passes into the ureter.

Nursing process: Planning

Client need: Management of Care

Cognitive level: Analysis

Subject area: Medical-Surgical

9. The nurse is caring for a client suspected of sustaining renal trauma following an automobile accident. It is a priority that the nurse monitor and report which of the following findings?
   1. Lethargy
   2. Hypertension
   3. Hematuria
   4. Bradycardia

10. The nurse is caring for a client in acute renal failure. Which of the following clinical manifestations is a priority for the nurse to monitor in this client?
    1. Infection
    2. Pain
    3. Oliguria
    4. Anemia

11. The nurse is caring for a client in acute renal failure. Which of the following would indicate to the nurse that the client is uremic?
    1. BUN of 32 mg/dl
    2. Serum calcium of 10.5 mg/dl
    3. Serum potassium of 2.8 mg/dl
    4. Urine specific gravity of 1.030

12. The nurse is preparing a client for an intravenous pyelogram (IVP). Which of the following would be essential for the nurse to include?
    1. Instruct the client that no fasting is required
    2. Inform the client that a ureteral catheter will be inserted during the procedure
    3. Administer a laxative the night before the procedure
    4. Monitor for bladder spasms after the procedure

Answer: 3

Rationale: When monitoring a client for hematuria who has sustained a renal trauma, it is important to detect hemorrhage, which can be a life-threatening complication.

Nursing process: Analysis

Client need: Management of Care

Cognitive level: Analysis

Subject area: Medical-Surgical

Answer: 1

Rationale: The nurse should closely monitor a client in acute renal failure for the presence of an infection, which constitutes the greatest mortality. The incidence may be as high as 70% in clients who developed acute renal failure resulting from an infection following trauma or surgery. Pain is generally not a clinical manifestation in acute renal failure. Although a client may die from oliguria, it is generally reversible and the mortality rate is approximately 50%. Anemia occurs in chronic, not acute, renal failure.

Nursing process: Assessment

Client need: Management of Care

Cognitive level: Analysis

Subject area: Medical-Surgical

Answer: 1

Rationale: An elevated BUN, or increased nitrogenous wastes in the blood, is classic uremia in a client in acute renal failure. A normal BUN is 10 to 20 mg/dl. A serum calcium of 10.5 mg/dl and a urine specific gravity of 1.030 are at the upper range for normal calcium (9 to 10.5 mg/dl) and specific gravity (1.010 to 1.030). A serum potassium of 2.8 mg/dl is low (3.5 to 5.5 mEq/L) and is not indicative of acute renal failure.

Nursing process: Evaluation

Client need: Reduction of Risk Potential

Cognitive level: Application

Subject area: Medical-Surgical

Answer: 3

Rationale: Administering a laxative the evening before an IVP is correct. Fasting for 8 hours is required. There is no fasting before a KUB (kidneys, ureters, bladder) x-ray. Inserting a ureteral catheter occurs during a retrograde pyelogram, not an IVP. Bladder spasms occur after a retrograde pyelogram, not an IVP.

Nursing process: Planning

Client need: Reduction of Risk Potential

Cognitive level: Application

Subject area: Medical–Surgical

13. The nurse identifies which of the following hospitalized clients to be at greatest risk for the development of a nosocomial urinary tract infection?

   1. A 48-year-old male suspected of Parkinson's disease who had been jogging prior to admission

   2. A 75-year-old male who has pancreatic cancer

   3. A 34-year-old male who drinks 2500 ml of fluids daily, following a fracture of the fibula

   4. A 60-year-old obese female with cholecystitis

14. The nurse correctly collects urine by which of the following methods to establish the diagnosis of urethritis?

   1. Obtain a specimen in the beginning and in the middle of the urine flow

   2. Obtain the first voided specimen in the morning

   3. Collect all urine for 24 hours

   4. Collect any voided specimen during the day

15. The nurse identifies which of the following diagnostic laboratory tests as the one the nurse should assess first to establish a diagnosis for renal disease?

   1. Blood urea nitrogen (BUN)

   2. Serum creatinine

   3. Serum uric acid

   4. Serum potassium

16. The nurse is collecting a nursing history from a client admitted with acute pyelonephritis. Which of the following questions should the nurse ask?

   1. "Have you noticed any blood in your urine?"

   2. "Have you experienced a decrease in your urinary output?"

   3. "Do you have pain when urinating?"

   4. "Do you find you are experiencing dribbling at the end of urinating?"

Answer: 2
Rationale: Although nosocomial urinary infections may occur in any hospitalized client, the incidence is significantly impacted by the client's overall state of health. A client who is male, older, and has a terminal cancer receiving chemotherapy is immunosuppressed and at the greatest risk.
Nursing process: Analysis
Client need: Reduction of Risk Potential
Cognitive level: Analysis
Subject area: Medical-Surgical

Answer: 1
Rationale: Obtaining a urine specimen in the beginning and again in the middle of the urine flow (split urine collections) for the purpose of performing a culture is the correct procedure for diagnosing urethritis.
Nursing process: Implementation
Client need: Reduction of Risk Potential
Cognitive level: Application
Subject area: Medical-Surgical

Answer: 2
Rationale: Although serum potassium, uric acid, and blood urea nitrogen are all useful diagnostic tests in the diagnosis of renal disease, the serum creatinine is the most diagnostic.
Nursing process: Assessment
Client need: Reduction of Risk Potential
Cognitive level: Analysis
Subject area: Medical-Surgical

Answer: 3
Rationale: Dysuria, or painful urination, does occur in acute pyelonephritis. Blood in the urine and dribbling at the end of urinating are not clinical manifestations. An increased urinary output, and not a decreased output, occurs in pyelonephritis.
Nursing process: Assessment
Client need: Physiological Adaptation
Cognitive level: Application
Subject area: Medical-Surgical

17. The nurse identifies which of the following clients to be at greatest risk for the development of struvite calculi?

   1. A Jewish male with a history of gout
   2. A male with idiopathic hypercalcuria
   3. A female with an autosomal recessive defect
   4. A female with a urinary tract infection

18. The nurse monitors a client who has chronic renal failure and a potassium level of 5.8 mEq/L for which of the following clinical manifestations?

   Select all that apply:
   [   ] 1. Dry skin
   [   ] 2. Lethargy
   [   ] 3. Weakness
   [   ] 4. Muscle irritability
   [   ] 5. Loss of deep tendon reflexes
   [   ] 6. Diarrhea

19. When preparing a client for a renal biopsy, it would be essential for the nurse to explain which of the following aspects of the procedure?

   1. Inform the client that the procedure involves insertion of a catheter and installation of saline solution into the bladder
   2. Explain to the client that burning on urination following the procedure is expected
   3. Inform the client that prior to the procedure typing and cross-matching blood will be done
   4. Explain to the client that before the procedure a cathartic or enema will be administered

20. The nurse monitors an increased incidence of stress incontinence in a client during which of the following activities?

   1. Eating
   2. Sleeping
   3. Walking
   4. Laughing

Answer: 4

Rationale: Women who experience frequent urinary tract infections are more likely to develop struvite calculi that take on a staghorn appearance from repeated *Proteus* urinary tract infections. A Jewish male with a history of gout is at risk for uric acid calculi. A male with idiopathic hypercalcuria is at risk for calcium oxalate. A female with an autosomal recessive defect is at risk for cystine calculi.

Nursing process: Analysis

Client need: Reduction of Risk Potential

Cognitive level: Analysis

Subject area: Medical-Surgical

Answer: 3, 4, 6

Rationale: Weakness, muscle irritability, and diarrhea are all indications of hyperkalemia. Confusion, lethargy, and depression occur in hyponatremia. Hypotension, drowsiness, and loss of deep tendon reflexes occur in hypermagnesemia. Dry skin, nausea, and vomiting occur in hypernatremia.

Nursing process: Assessment

Client need: Physiological Adaptation

Cognitive level: Application

Subject area: Medical-Surgical

Answer: 3

Rationale: A client scheduled for a renal biopsy will routinely be typed and cross-matched for blood because of the risk of bleeding. The insertion of a catheter and installation of saline solution into the bladder occur with a cystometrogram. Burning on urination is an anticipated outcome following a cystoscopy. Administering an enema or cathartic before the procedure may occur with several procedures, such as intravenous pyelography, retrograde pyelogram, or a cystoscopy.

Nursing process: Planning

Client need: Reduction of Risk Potential

Cognitive level: Application

Subject area: Medical-Surgical

Answer: 4

Rationale: Stress incontinence occurs during periods of increased abdominal pressure such as that which occurs with laughing. Eating, sleeping, and walking do not alter the abdominal pressure.

Nursing process: Assessment

Client need: Physiological Adaptation

Cognitive level: Application

Subject area: Medical-Surgical

21. After inserting an indwelling Foley catheter, the nurse begins to inflate the balloon and the client complains of pain. Which of the following would be the priority action for the nurse to implement?

   1. Aspirate back solution from the balloon and remove the catheter

   2. Insert the remainder of the solution in the balloon and pull back gently until resistance is felt

   3. Aspirate back solution from the balloon and advance the catheter further

   4. Withdraw the catheter slightly and insert an additional 1 ml into the balloon

22. Which of the following principles of catheter care should the nurse consider before catheterizing a client?

   1. Place a urinary catheter in a client who is geriatric to prevent urinary incontinence

   2. Use catheterization as a last resort

   3. Keep the catheter bag on the bed and at the level of the bladder

   4. Sprinkle powder in the perineal area and around the catheter insertion site

23. The nurse should include which of the following in the procedure for female urinary catheterization?

   1. Expose the urinary meatus with the dominant hand

   2. Lubricate two inches of the catheter

   3. Insert the catheter 8 inches with the sterile gloved hand

   4. Allow the labia to relax after the meatus is cleansed

24. Before calculating the urinary output of a client suspected of decreased renal perfusion and possible renal failure, the nurse understands that the minimum hourly urinary output must not fall below how many milliliters per hour? _____

Answer: 3

Rationale: When a client complains of pain during inflation of the balloon after inserting an indwelling catheter, the nurse should aspirate back the inserted solution and advance the catheter further to ensure the catheter is in the bladder and not lodged in the urethra.

Nursing process: Implementation

Client need: Reduction of Risk Potential

Cognitive level: Analysis

Subject area: Medical-Surgical

Answer: 2

Rationale: Catheterization may be used as a last resort after all noninvasive measures to promote urination, such as encouraging ambulation and fluids, have failed. Catheterization should never be used for clients who are geriatric to prevent urinary incontinence. The catheter bag should always be kept below the level of the bladder. Applying powder to the perineal area and around the catheter insertion site should never be used, because this practice promotes infection.

Nursing process: Analysis

Client need: Reduction of Risk Potential

Cognitive level: Analysis

Subject area: Medical-Surgical

Answer: 2

Rationale: For the female client, the urinary catheter should be lubricated two inches to facilitate easy insertion. The urinary meatus is exposed with the gloved nondominant hand. The catheter is inserted until urine begins to flow, which is generally two to three inches. Allowing the labia to relax after the meatus is cleansed results in contamination and increases the risk of infection.

Nursing process: Planning

Client need: Reduction of Risk Potential

Cognitive level: Analysis

Subject area: Medical-Surgical

Answer: 30

Rationale: An hourly urinary output less than 30 ml per hour is indicative of decreased blood flow to the kidneys and should be reported.

Nursing process: Analysis

Client need: Reduction of Risk Potential

Cognitive level: Analysis

Subject area: Medical-Surgical

25. When preparing a client for an intravenous pyelography (IVP), the nurse should explain which of the following aspects of the procedure?

Select all that apply:

[   ] **1.** Fasting is not required

[   ] **2.** A laxative will be given the evening before the procedure

[   ] **3.** A contrast dye will be given intravenously

[   ] **4.** A ureteral catheter will be inserted during the procedure

[   ] **5.** A sedative will be given

[   ] **6.** Mild discomfort may be experienced during the procedure

26. The registered nurse may delegate which of the following nursing tasks to unlicensed assistive personnel (UAP)?

Select all that apply:

[   ] **1.** Perform a glucose test on a urine specimen for a client who has diabetes mellitus

[   ] **2.** Monitor a client's intravenous line for patency

[   ] **3.** Provide teaching to a client on how to prevent urinary tract infections

[   ] **4.** Assist a client who has calcium oxalate calculi in making appropriate menu selections

[   ] **5.** Take the vital signs of a client in renal failure

[   ] **6.** Record the intake and output of a client experiencing urinary incontinence

27. The nurse evaluates a client with a diagnosis of dehydration to have which of the following specific gravity readings?

1. 1.000

2. 1.017

3. 1.023

4. 1.035

28. The nurse is reviewing the normal limits for a urinalysis. Which of the following findings would indicate to the nurse the need for additional investigation?

1. Dark amber-colored urine

2. Faint, aromatic odor

3. Specific gravity of 1.015

4. pH of 6.0

Answer: 2, 3

Rationale: A laxative is given the evening before an IVP and a contrast dye is administered intravenously. The client should be NPO for eight hours. No fasting is required for a renal scan, a nephrotomogram, an MRI, an ultrasound, and a kidney, ureters, bladder x-ray. A ureteral catheter is inserted by cystoscopy during a retrograde pyelogram. Sedation medication may be administered before an MRI if a client is claustrophobic. Discomfort may be associated with a retrograde pyelogram, renal angiogram, renal biopsy, and cystoscopy.

Nursing process: Planning

Client need: Reduction of Risk Potential

Cognitive level: Application

Subject area: Medical-Surgical

Answers: 1, 5, 6

Rationale: It is the responsibility of the registered nurse to know or reasonably believe that unlicensed assistive personnel have the appropriate training, orientation, and documented competencies. The UAP cannot do assessments or evaluate responses.

Nursing process: Implementation

Client need: Management of Care

Cognitive level: Application

Subject area: Medical-Surgical

Answer: 4

Rationale: Normal specific gravity is 1.003 to 1.030. An elevated specific gravity occurs with albuminuria, glycosuria, and dehydration. A decreased specific gravity occurs with diabetes insipidus.

Nursing process: Evaluation

Client need: Reduction of Risk Potential

Cognitive level: Analysis

Subject area: Medical-Surgical

Answer: 1

Rationale: Normal urine specific gravity is 1.003 to 1.030. Normal urine pH is 4.0 to 8.0. Urine is normally yellow in color and faint in odor. Dark amber urine may indicate dehydration, infection, or blood in the urine.

Nursing process: Analysis

Client need: Reduction of Risk Potential

Cognitive level: Application

Subject area: Medical-Surgical

29. Which of the following should the nurse include to correctly collect a timed urine specimen?

   1. Instruct the client to save the first voided specimen when the urine collection time starts

   2. Instruct the client on the importance of continuing to save all urine even if one specimen is missed

   3. Place the collection container in a location that is room temperature and away from accidental spillage

   4. Encourage the client to empty the bladder and save this specimen at the end of the collection time

Answer: 4

Rationale: The first voided specimen for a timed urinary test should be discarded. The collection container should be kept in the refrigerator or on ice in the bathroom. If a urine specimen is missed, the whole timed test must start again. It is helpful to have a sign on the bathroom door and above the toilet to save all urine. At the conclusion of the test, the client should be encouraged to empty the bladder and save this specimen.

Nursing process: Planning

Client need: Reduction of Risk Potential

Cognitive level: Application

Subject area: Medical-Surgical

Oncology Disorders

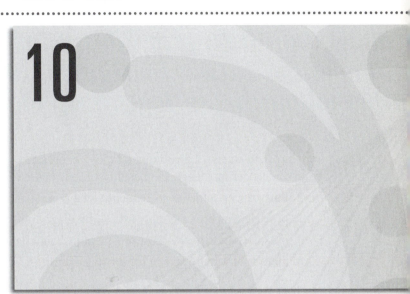

10

1. A client asks the nurse, "Does everyone who gets cancer die of it?" The nurse's best response is based on the understanding that
    1. about five million people in the U.S. survive cancer for five or more years.
    2. all one million people diagnosed in the U.S. annually will eventually die of their disease.
    3. cancer is the leading cause of adult death in the U.S.
    4. it destroys hope to discuss dying with a client with cancer.

2. The client states, "I heard that all men get prostate cancer sometime in their lives." In teaching the client about cancer incidence, the best response is based on the understanding that
    1. lung cancer is the most frequently diagnosed cancer in men.
    2. prostate cancer is the most frequently diagnosed cancer in men.
    3. prostate cancer is the most prevalent in Caucasian men.
    4. there is no way to screen for prostate cancer, so it is the most common cause of cancer death in men.

3. When planning the discharge of a client with cancer, which of the following should the nurse include as a priority?
    1. Encouragement to drink no alcoholic beverages
    2. Information on all local hospices
    3. Plans for a visiting nurse
    4. Information on stress reduction techniques

4. While assessing a client's skin, the nurse should report which of the following findings as a possible skin cancer?
    1. Red, swollen plaques
    2. A bull's-eye rash
    3. A blue-black appearing mole
    4. Spider angiomas

Answer: 1

Rationale: Over one million Americans are diagnosed with cancer each year. However, only 500,000 die annually and approximately five million are cancer free for five or more years. Heart disease, not cancer, is the leading cause of adult death in the U.S.

Nursing process: Analysis

Client need: Physiological Adaptation

Cognitive level: Application

Subject area: Medical-Surgical

Answer: 2

Rationale: Prostate cancer is the most common cancer in men in the U.S., with lung cancer being second. The incidence of prostate cancer is significantly higher in black men worldwide. Screening is available for prostate cancer.

Nursing process: Analysis

Client need: Physiological Adaptation

Cognitive level: Application

Subject area: Medical-Surgical

Answer: 4

Rationale: Reducing stress in a person's life is one of the recommended methods of cancer risk reduction. Clients with cancer are at a higher risk of a new cancer or recurrence, and therefore should be instructed in risk-reduction methods. Limiting alcoholic beverages is encouraged to reduce cancer risk, but it is not required that the client abstain completely unless there are other medical reasons to do so. Not all clients will require home or hospice care after discharge, as many clients with cancer lead long, productive lives.

Nursing process: Planning

Client need: Management of Care

Cognitive level: Analysis

Subject area: Medical-Surgical

Answer: 3

Rationale: A blue-black appearing mole is one of the cardinal signs of melanoma skin cancer. Red swollen plaques, bull's-eye rash, and spider angiomas are not indicative of skin cancer, but other dermatologic abnormalities.

Nursing process: Analysis

Client need: Reduction of Risk Potential

Cognitive level: Application

Subject area: Medical-Surgical

5. The nurse is collecting a health history on a client admitted for colon cancer. Which of the following questions would be a priority to ask this client?

   1. "Have you noticed any blood in the stool?"
   2. "Have you been experiencing nausea?"
   3. "Do you have any back pain?"
   4. "Have you noticed your abdomen has swollen?"

6. A nurse is educating a group of clients on cancer screening practices. Which of the following instructions should the nurse include as a recommended screening pattern?

   1. Annual Pap and pelvic examination should begin at age 40
   2. Annual cancer check-ups for all persons over age 40
   3. Annual mammography should begin at age 30
   4. Annual fecal occult blood test and colonoscopy at age 40

7. The client with cancer states, "My pain is a 10!" on a 0 to 10 scale (10 being worst possible pain). Which of the following is the appropriate nursing intervention?

   1. Instruct the client that no more narcotic analgesia can be given at this time in order to prevent addiction
   2. Ask the client if the pain is really that bad, since narcotic analgesia will be given as a last resort for severe pain
   3. Assure that a strong opioid, nonopioid, and adjuvant are ordered and administer per order
   4. Administer another dose of meperidine (Demerol) as prescribed

Answer: 1

Rationale: Although early colon cancer is asymptomatic, occult or frank blood in the stool is often an assessment finding in a client diagnosed with colon cancer. If pain is present, it is usually lower abdominal cramping. Constipation and diarrhea are more frequent findings than nausea, and ascites is more likely to be present in very advanced disease of ovarian and liver cancers.

Nursing process: Assessment

Client need: Management of Care

Cognitive level: Analysis

Subject area: Medical-Surgical

Answer: 2

Rationale: Nationally recognized cancer screening guidelines recommend everyone over age 40 visit the doctor annually for cancer assessment. Pap and pelvic examinations, screening for cervical and uterine cancer, should begin at age 18. Mammographic screening for breast cancer is not recommended on an annual basis until at least age 40, and colorectal screening is recommended beginning at age 50, with colonoscopy only every 5 to 10 years.

Nursing process: Planning

Client need: Health Promotion and Maintenance

Cognitive level: Application

Subject area: Medical-Surgical

Answer: 3

Rationale: Fewer than 1% of clients become addicted to narcotic analgesics when used appropriately for pain management; therefore, in this case, addiction should not be a concern. Narcotic doses can be increased as pain increases, and therefore do not need to be reserved for fear of using them too early. Meperidine (Demerol) is seldom used to treat cancer pain because of metabolites that accumulate with continued use. If this is ordered, the nurse should consult with the physician regarding a change. According to the World Health Organization analgesic ladder for pain management, severe pain should be treated with a strong opioid (e.g., morphine), with a nonopioid analgesic (e.g., acetaminophen), and an adjuvant (e.g., nonsteroidal anti-inflammatory).

Nursing process: Evaluation

Client need: Physiological Adaptation

Cognitive level: Analysis

Subject area: Medical-Surgical

8. In planning the care of a client experiencing fatigue related to chemotherapy, which of the following is the most appropriate nursing intervention?

   1. Prioritize and administer nursing care throughout the day

   2. Accomplish all the nursing care early in the day so the client can rest the remainder of the day

   3. Perform all nursing care during the evening shift when the client is the most rested

   4. Limit the number of visitors, promoting a maximum opportunity for sleep

9. The nurse is caring for a client who underwent a bone marrow transplant 10 days ago. The nurse should monitor the client for which of the following clinical manifestations that indicates a potentially life-threatening situation?

   1. Mucositis

   2. Confusion

   3. Depression

   4. Mild temperature elevation

10. Six days after receiving chemotherapy, the client reports that, "My mouth feels like it's on fire!" Which of the following is the priority nursing action?

    1. Encourage rinsing the mouth several times per day with an over-the-counter mouthwash

    2. Administer analgesics as ordered

    3. Assess the oral mucosa for signs of infection and tissue breakdown

    4. Instruct the client to eat small, frequent meals of soft food such as applesauce

Answer: 1

Rationale: Clients should be taught to pace their activities throughout the day in order to conserve energy; therefore, nursing care should be paced as well. Fatigue is the most common side effect of cancer and its treatment; therefore, it needs to be appropriately managed. While adequate sleep is important, maximal sleep will not completely resolve clinical manifestations. Completely restricting visitors does not promote healthy coping and may result in isolation.

Nursing process: Planning

Client need: Physiological Adaptation

Cognitive level: Application

Subject area: Medical-Surgical

Answer: 4

Rationale: During the first 100 days post-transplant, clients are at high risk for life-threatening infections. This is especially true prior to marrow engraftment, which occurs at approximately two to three weeks post-transplant. The earliest sign of infection in an immunocompromised client may be a mild fever. Mucositis, confusion, and depression are possible clinical manifestations but represent less life-threatening complications.

Nursing process: Assessment

Client need: Reduction of Risk Potential

Cognitive level: Analysis

Subject area: Medical-Surgical

Answer: 3

Rationale: Adverse reactions of chemotherapy include stomatitis and mucositis in some clients. The nurse should always first assess the client's oral mucosa for signs of breakdown and infection. Pain medication may be necessary to administer, but this is not the first action the nurse should take. Rinsing the oral mucosa is encouraged, but with salt or soda solution, not over-the-counter mouthwashes, which can be drying. Clients should eat small, frequent meals of soothing foods after chemotherapy, but usually this is not required after the first week, and again, the nurse should perform an assessment before implementing a plan of care.

Nursing process: Planning

Client need: Physiological Adaptation

Cognitive level: Analysis

Subject area: Medical-Surgical

11. The nurse finds the client vomiting on the second day after chemotherapy. Antiemetics and IV fluids have been administered as ordered. The nurse should include which of the following as an appropriate intervention for this client?

    1. Offer music therapy to decrease nausea

    2. Encourage the client to remain in an upright position for two hours after eating

    3. Obtain an order for a tube feeding to assure adequate nutrition

    4. Discuss decreasing the next dose of chemotherapy with the physician

12. In preparing a client on oral narcotic analgesics for discharge after a mastectomy, the nurse should include the following in postoperative teaching.

    1. Use oral narcotics sparingly to avoid constipation

    2. Bowel-training program

    3. High-protein, low-carbohydrate diet plan

    4. Upper extremity weight-training program

13. While caring for the client with superior vena cava syndrome, the nurse should include which of the following interventions?

    1. Restrict visitors, since the client will be anxious

    2. Withhold chemotherapy until the syndrome resolves

    3. Instruct the client in Valsalva's maneuver

    4. Elevate the head of the bed

Answer: 1

Rationale: The addition of complementary therapies, such as music therapy, relaxation techniques, distraction, and imagery, have been shown to provide additional relief from nausea and vomiting. The client should remain in an upright position after eating, but 30 minutes is usually sufficient. A tube feeding would be inappropriate since nausea and vomiting after chemotherapy are usually a short-term problem, after which the client will be able to return to normal eating patterns. Unless extremely severe and unmanageable, it would not be appropriate to decrease the dose of chemotherapy at the next administration.

Nursing process: Planning

Client need: Physiological Adaptation

Cognitive level: Application

Subject area: Medical-Surgical

Answer: 2

Rationale: Surgery, narcotic analgesics, and client immobility promote constipation postoperatively. Therefore, clients should be instructed in a bowel-training program that includes use of suppositories or oral stool softener as needed, physical activity such as walking, and intake of fruits, fiber, and fluid. Oral narcotics should be used as needed for pain while managing the adverse reaction of constipation. The diet should be high in fiber, not necessarily protein. A weight-training program would not be appropriate until surgical drains are removed, although use of the affected side with gentle arm motion is advocated.

Nursing process: Planning

Client need: Health Promotion and Maintenance

Cognitive level: Application

Subject area: Medical-Surgical

Answer: 4

Rationale: Superior vena cava syndrome is compression of the superior vena cava by enlarged lymph nodes, clot, or tumor, thus restricting the flow of blood out of the head, neck, and upper extremities. This results in swelling of these areas and shortness of breath. Elevating the head of the bed decreases the pressure in the head and upper body by allowing gravity to assist in blood flow. The client should not perform Valsalva's maneuver, as this increases that pressure. The client will be anxious about this, so providing resources to decrease anxiety, including supportive friends and family, would be advocated. Chemotherapy or radiation to decrease the size of a tumor or lymph node is one of the treatments for superior vena cava syndrome, so chemotherapy should be administered as ordered, and not withheld.

Nursing process: Implementation

Client need: Physiological Adaptation

Cognitive level: Application

Subject area: Medical-Surgical

14. The nurse is caring for a client with small cell lung cancer. Which of the following observations would be a priority that the nurse should report immediately?

    1. Weight loss

    2. Serum sodium less than 130 mEq/L

    3. Headache

    4. Urinary output greater than 60 ml/hour

15. The nurse is caring for a client who received chemotherapy for leukemia 24 hours ago and is now complaining of flank pain. The client's urinary output has decreased to less than 30 ml/hour. The nurse evaluates which of the following conditions as the most likely cause of the client's clinical manifestations?

    1. Syndrome of inappropriate antidiuretic hormone (SIADH)

    2. Tumor lysis syndrome

    3. Superior vena cava syndrome

    4. Hypercalcium

16. The nurse should instruct a client that which of the following is the most effective prevention against bladder cancer?

    1. Drink 8 to 10 glasses of fluid per day

    2. Void at least five times per day

    3. Stop smoking

    4. Take herbal supplements

Answer: 2

Rationale: Clients most at risk for syndrome of inappropriate antidiuretic hormone (SIADH) are those with small cell lung cancer, as well as several other cancers. Therefore, the nurse should be alert for clinical manifestations of this, such as weight gain, decreased urinary output, and dilutional hyponatremia. Headache may occur, but this is not a common clinical manifestation of SIADH.

Nursing process: Analysis

Client need: Management of Care

Cognitive level: Analysis

Subject area: Medical-Surgical

Answer: 2

Rationale: Tumor lysis is most common in clients who have received chemotherapy for leukemia lymphoma, or small cell lung cancer, within 24 to 48 hours of administration. Flank pain is a clinical manifestation of renal failure associated with tumor lysis syndrome. Flank pain is not a typical clinical manifestation of syndrome of inappropriate antidiuretic hormone (SIADH), superior vena cava syndrome, or hypercalcium.

Nursing process: Evaluation

Client need: Reduction of Risk Potential

Cognitive level: Analysis

Subject area: Medical-Surgical

Answer: 3

Rationale: Persons at greatest risk for bladder cancer are Caucasian men over 50 years of age who have had occupational exposures to dyes, rubber, and leather industries, and who smoke. Since age, race, and occupation are not alterable, the best alternative is to stop smoking. Clients should be provided with smoking-cessation information and support to reduce their risk of several cancers and other health problems.

Nursing process: Planning

Client need: Reduction of Risk Potential

Cognitive level: Analysis

Subject area: Medical-Surgical

17. Which of the following should the nurse include in the preoperative care plan of a client with head and neck cancer?

    1. Instruct the client and family in communicating with a picture board

    2. Assess the client's favorite foods to assure these are provided postoperatively

    3. Plan for a volunteer to take the client outside for cigarette breaks

    4. Provide frequent oral care, including rinsing with mouthwash

18. A client who has been treated for lung cancer returns to the clinic and during the nursing assessment reports recent problems with balance and memory. Based on the nurse's understanding of lung cancer, the appropriate action would be

    1. reassure the client that these are just common signs of aging.

    2. recommend that the client obtain gingko from the health food store.

    3. perform a more thorough assessment.

    4. call for an ambulance, since this is an oncology emergency.

19. The nurse is caring for a client following lobectomy lung cancer. Which of the following should the nurse include in the plan of care for this client?

    1. Position the client on the operative side only

    2. Avoid administering narcotic pain medication

    3. Maintain strict bed rest

    4. Instruct the client on the importance of coughing and deep breathing

Answer: 1

Rationale: Surgery is the primary treatment for head and neck cancer and may involve removal of part of the tongue, larynx, and other structures. This surgery is often disfiguring and often makes eating and communicating with staff and family very difficult. Losses can lead to difficulties in coping, so nursing interventions to lessen losses and promote coping (such as communicating with a picture board) have a major role for the nurse in this setting. Mouthwash should not be used because it is drying to the oral mucosa. Smoking should be highly discouraged; it is one of the leading risk factors for this cancer and it dries the oral mucosa. The diet for this client should be developed in collaboration with physician and therapists and often includes tube feeding, followed by soft mechanical diet, due to swallowing difficulties. Unfortunately, the client will not be able to have favorite foods for a while.

Nursing process: Planning

Client need: Physiological Adaptation

Cognitive level: Application

Subject area: Medical-Surgical

Answer: 3

Rationale: Lung cancer often metastasizes to the brain, causing the neurologic symptoms the client is describing. Providing reassurance is minimizing the client's concerns, and making recommendations for herbal supplements without a thorough assessment is not an appropriate nursing intervention. The client is not in immediate danger, so calling an ambulance is not appropriate either.

Nursing process: Analysis

Client need: Physiological Adaptation

Cognitive level: Analysis

Subject area: Medical-Surgical

Answer: 4

Rationale: Postoperatively, deep breathing is important to promote oxygenation and clear secretions, so strict bed rest is discouraged and ambulation is encouraged. Additionally, administration of pain medication to lessen pain and promote deep breathing is essential and should not be avoided. After a lobectomy, prolonged lying on the operative side is to be avoided.

Nursing process: Planning

Client need: Physiological Adaptation

Cognitive level: Application

Subject area: Medical-Surgical

20. The spouse of a client with early stage prostate cancer asks the nurse, "Why isn't the physician treating my husband's cancer?" The nurse's best response should be based on which of the following?

1. Watchful waiting is often appropriate for men over age 70

2. The client must really have Stage IV cancer, which is not curable

3. All prostate cancer should be treated, and this client should get another opinion

4. The client is being treated with hormonal manipulation, which isn't perceived as treatment by clients

21. While performing a nursing assessment, a female client informs the nurse of vague abdominal discomfort, bloating, and unexplained indigestion and flatulence for the last few months. What should the nurse ask in order to elicit the most important information for completing the assessment?

1. "Do you often eat spicy food?"

2. "Tell me about your family's medical history."

3. "Have you had weight loss recently?"

4. "Are you experiencing unusual menstrual bleeding?"

22. The nurse should instruct a client following a colostomy from the ascending colon that the stool will be characteristically _____.

Answer: 1

Rationale: Prostate cancer is very slow growing in older men, and therefore no intervention is recommended. "Watchful waiting" is appropriate for men over age 70 with small, early stage cancers. Transurethral resection of the prostate and external beam radiation are used to treat advanced disease. The client may be receiving hormonal therapy, but it is primarily used for advanced disease.

Nursing process: Analysis

Client need: Physiological Adaptation

Cognitive level: Analysis

Subject area: Medical-Surgical

Answer: 2

Rationale: Vague abdominal discomfort, bloating, and unexplained indigestion and flatulence are unfortunately the only clinical manifestations of ovarian cancer, and the reason it is often overlooked. Therefore, to more thoroughly complete the assessment, the nurse should take a complete family cancer history to aid in determining the client's risk of ovarian cancer. Women with a family history of ovarian cancer are at higher risk. If anything, the client would probably be gaining weight, not losing, from abdominal ascites. Unusual menstrual bleeding is an important clinical manifestation related to uterine, rather than ovarian, cancer.

Nursing process: Analysis

Client need: Physiological Adaptation

Cognitive level: Analysis

Subject area: Medical-Surgical

Answer: loose and liquid

Rationale: A colostomy formed from the ascending colon produces liquid stool, since it contains the fluid that would normally be removed while traveling through the remainder of the colon.

Nursing process: Planning

Client need: Health Promotion and Maintenance

Cognitive level: Application

Subject area: Medical-Surgical

23. The nurse is teaching a class on breast self-examination. Which of the following should the nurse include in the class?

   1. Use only deep pressure when palpating the breast

   2. Include both inspection and palpation of the breast in the exam

   3. Use fingertips while palpating the breast

   4. Perform breast palpation exam in front of a mirror

24. A client states, "I'm worried about being burned by radiation therapy." The most appropriate response is based on the nurse's understanding that

   1. applying hand lotion to the area being radiated will reduce the chance of burns.

   2. darker-skinned persons burn more easily during radiation therapy.

   3. burns are very rare with today's technology.

   4. washing the radiated area with strong soap will reduce the chance of burns.

25. When planning care for a client being treated for cervical cancer, it would be a priority for the nurse to include which of the following in the plan of care?

   1. Instruction on birth control methods

   2. Vigorous fluid hydration

   3. Assessment of sexual function

   4. Daily weights

Answer: 2

Rationale: Breast self-exam should include inspection of the breasts in front of a mirror. According to national authorities, it should also include palpation using light, medium, and deep pressure with the pads of the first three fingers (not the fingertips) while in the shower and while lying down. It is not necessary to perform the palpation exam in front of a mirror.

Nursing process: Planning

Client need: Health Promotion and Maintenance

Cognitive level: Application

Subject area: Medical-Surgical

Answer: 3

Rationale: The equipment and techniques used to deliver radiation therapy today very rarely result in skin burns. Local skin reaction such as redness, dryness, desquamation, and irritation may occur. These reactions occur most often in fair-skinned persons, and are potentially worse if there are oils on the skin from hand lotion, soap, or deodorant; therefore, application of these is discouraged. Washing the area receiving radiation with plain water and patting dry is preferred to strong soap.

Nursing process: Analysis

Client need: Physiological Adaptation

Cognitive level: Application

Subject area: Medical-Surgical

Answer: 3

Rationale: Surgery and radiation therapy for cervical cancer often result in shortening of the vagina, vaginal dryness, and loss of libido due to emotional issues related to sexuality and femininity. Therefore, the client's feelings about sexuality and the partner's feelings should be assessed. If a client is not sexually active, instructions should be given in the use of a vaginal dilator and lubricant to prevent adhesion of the vaginal walls. While instruction about birth control methods may be needed for some clients, treatment for cervical cancer may include total abdominal hysterectomy, so that this would not be appropriate for all clients. Encouraging fluids and daily weights are not priorities in cervical cancer care.

Nursing process: Planning

Client need: Management of Care

Cognitive level: Application

Subject area: Medical-Surgical

26. The registered nurse is making out the nursing tasks for the day. Which of the following nursing tasks may be delegated to a licensed practical nurse?

   1. Administer 3% saline solution IV to a client with severe syndrome of inappropriate antidiuretic hormone (SIADH)

   2. Assess for an electrolyte imbalance in a client with tumor lysis syndrome

   3. Administer prescribed anticonvulsant to prevent seizure in a client who has a central nervous system tumor

   4. Monitor the serum calcium level in a client who has hypercalcemia

27. The nurse is teaching a class on breast cancer. Which of the following should the nurse include as risk factors?

   1. Menopause at an early age and excessive caffeine use

   2. Slender build and first birth before the age of 20 years

   3. Menarche at an early age and nulliparous

   4. Asian descent and lower socioeconomic status

28. Which of the following findings on a female breast exam should the nurse report as suspicious of breast cancer?

   1. Multiple, bilateral, round, lumpy tissue that is tender

   2. A soft, mobile, single lobular nodule that is nontender

   3. A poorly defined, firm lump that is nontender and fixed to the skin

   4. A single soft lump that is well defined and tender

Answer: 3

Rationale: Syndrome of inappropriate antidiuretic hormone (SIADH), tumor lysis syndrome, and hypercalcemia are all oncology medical emergencies, requiring the attention of a registered nurse. Administering an IV solution, assessing for an electrolyte imbalance, and monitoring the serum calcium are all nursing tasks reserved for the registered nurse. Hypercalcemia is also an oncology medical emergency, so monitoring the serum calcium is a nursing task reserved for the registered nurse. A licensed practical nurse may administer an anticonvulsant to a client who has a central nervous system tumor.

Nursing process: Planning

Client need: Management of Care

Cognitive level: Analysis

Subject area: Legal and Ethical Issues

Answer: 3

Rationale: Risk factors for breast cancer include being white over being nonwhite. The incident of breast cancer is higher in obese females. Additional risk factors include menarche at an early age and being nulliparous.

Nursing process: Planning

Client need: Reduction of Risk Potential

Cognitive level: Analysis

Subject area: Medical-Surgical

Answer: 3

Rationale: A poorly defined, firm lump that is nontender and fixed to the skin is characteristic of breast cancer.

Nursing process: Analysis

Client need: Reduction of Risk Potential

Cognitive level: Analysis

Subject area: Medical-Surgical

29. The nurse is admitting a client with vaginal cancer. Which of the following questions should the nurse ask to elicit the most likely causative factor?

    1. "Did you experience your first menses before the age of 11 years?"

    2. "Did your mother take diethylstilbestrol (DES) during pregnancy?"

    3. "Have you ever taken tamoxifen?"

    4. "Do you have a history of a sexually transmitted disease?"

30. The nurse should instruct a female client that the best time to perform a breast self-examination is which of the following?

    1. At the onset of menstruation

    2. The last day of the menstrual period

    3. Every month during ovulation

    4. Weekly at the same time of day

31. Which of the following instructions should the nurse give a male client on how to perform a testicular self-examination (TSE)?

    1. Examine the testicle while lying down

    2. Gently feel the testicle with one finger to feel for a growth

    3. The best time to examine the testicle is after a shower

    4. A testicular exam should be done once every six months

Answer: 2

Rationale: A client whose mother had taken diethylstilbestrol (DES) during pregnancy is more likely to develop vaginal cancer. There is no correlation with the age of the first menses, having taken tamoxifen, or having had a history of a sexually transmitted disease.

Nursing process: Analysis

Client need: Reduction of Risk Potential

Cognitive level: Analysis

Subject area: Medical-Surgical

Answer: 2

Rationale: The best time to perform a breast self-examination is the last day of the menstrual period.

Nursing process: Planning

Client need: Health Promotion and Maintenance

Cognitive level: Analysis

Subject area: Medical-Surgical

Answer: 3

Rationale: The best time to perform a testicular self-examination is after a shower. The warmth of the shower causes the testes to position themselves lower in the scrotum. The testes should be examined by both hands by rolling each testis between the thumb and first three fingers until the surface has been covered. The examination should be performed each month at a consistent time such as the first of the month.

Nursing process: Planning

Client need: Health Promotion and Maintenance

Cognitive level: Application

Subject area: Medical-Surgical

Hematological Disorders

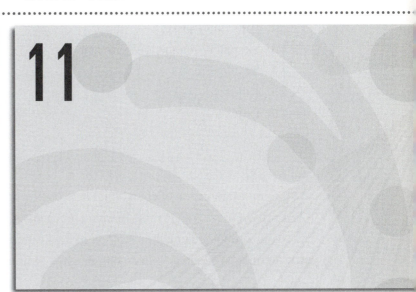

11

1. The nurse is admitting a client suspected of having sickle cell anemia. The client has a fever of 38.9°C or 102°F, faint yellow-tinged sclera, and is complaining of abdominal pain. Which of the following clinical manifestations further support this diagnosis?

   Select all that apply:

   [   ] 1. Rapid but regular breathing

   [   ] 2. Pale, dilute urine

   [   ] 3. Skin ulcers on the lower extremities

   [   ] 4. Swollen fingers

   [   ] 5. Pallor

   [   ] 6. Fatigue

2. The nurse making a care plan for a client with severe thrombocytopenia should include which of the following?

   1. Careful examination of spinal fluid obtained by lumbar puncture

   2. A private room with reverse isolation precautions

   3. Avoid intramuscular administration of medications

   4. Careful monitoring of urinary output while titrating the dosage of furosemide (Lasix)

3. A client with lung cancer is admitted with a new diagnosis of acute disseminated intravascular coagulation (DIC). Which of the following actions is a priority?

   1. Obtain a diet history from the client for the last three days

   2. Assess the client for any indications of internal or external bleeding

   3. Take the family to the family lounge and discuss home care for a client with DIC

   4. Call the dialysis unit to determine when the client may be transferred

4. The nurse has instructed a client with a hematological disorder about the functions of the hematologic system. The client indicates a need for further teaching by describing the function of the hematologic system as

   1. "The coagulation and clotting of blood."

   2. "The exchange of oxygen and carbon dioxide at the alveoli."

   3. "The transportation of oxygen and carbon dioxide to cells of the body."

   4. "To fight infection."

Answer: 3, 4, 5, 6

Rationale: The client with sickle cell anemia develops skin ulcers on the lower extremities from the vaso-occlusive aspects of the disease. The client would have shortness of breath and be fatigued and pale. The client may have swollen fingers. The hemolysis of red blood cells results in bilirubinuria. The client's urine is dark colored.

Nursing process: Analysis

Client need: Physiological Adaptation

Cognitive level: Application

Subject area: Medical-Surgical

Answer: 3

Rationale: Severe thrombocytopenia is a platelet count of <10,000 to 20,000/mm^3. The client with this low number of platelets is at great risk of bleeding from any invasive procedure. Intramuscular injections can cause a hematoma in the muscle and should be avoided if possible. A lumbar puncture would put the client at an unnecessary risk of bleeding. A private room is not indicated unless there are other reasons for isolation (infection, neutropenia). Furosemide is a diuretic and not used as therapy for thrombocytopenia.

Nursing process: Planning

Client need: Physiological Adaptation

Cognitive level: Application

Subject area: Medical-Surgical

Answer: 2

Rationale: Acute disseminated intravascular coagulation (DIC) is a serious disorder resulting in bleeding and clotting. It is a priority that the client must be assessed frequently by the nurse for bleeding. After ensuring that there is no active bleeding, the nurse may obtain a detailed diet history or implement family teaching. A delay to do family teaching away from the client or to dwell on diet history would not be appropriate. Some clients with chronic DIC may eventually require dialysis.

Nursing process: Analysis

Client need: Management of Care

Cognitive level: Analysis

Subject area: Medical-Surgical

Answer: 2

Rationale: Oxygen and carbon dioxide are transported in the blood. Air exchange occurs in the lungs, which are a part of the respiratory system. The blood also contains substances that help to form clots and mount immune responses to infectious agents.

Nursing process: Evaluation

Client need: Physiological Adaptation

Cognitive level: Comprehension

Subject area: Medical-Surgical

5. The nurse is admitting a client with severe shortness of breath. The nurse assesses which of the following clinical manifestations to be present in the client with pernicious anemia?

Select all that apply:

[   ] 1. Oral temperature greater than 38°C or 100.5°F

[   ] 2. Dark-brown urine

[   ] 3. Paresthesia

[   ] 4. White and yellow patches on the tongue

[   ] 5. Mental confusion

[   ] 6. Muscle weakness

6. The nurse is discharging a client with aplastic anemia. Which of the following statements made by the client would demonstrate the need for additional teaching by the nurse?

1. "I'm a little nervous about the side effects of my medicines and will call if I have questions."

2. "I have a lot of sisters and brothers. I hope one of them will match for my bone marrow transplant."

3. "I'm going back to my job in the toddler room at a day care center tomorrow."

4. "Diabetes runs in my family so we will be checking my glucose levels while I am on the prednisone."

7. A client with a chronic bleeding duodenal ulcer is admitted to the hospital. What clinical manifestations should the nurse assess for in a client with a 30% blood volume loss?

Select all that apply:

[   ] 1. Postural hypotension

[   ] 2. Dizziness

[   ] 3. Tachycardia with activity

[   ] 4. Swelling

[   ] 5. Blood pressure below normal at rest

[   ] 6. Pain

8. Which of the following should the nurse include in the instructions provided to a client with sickle cell anemia?

Select all that apply:

[   ] 1. Administer pain medications

[   ] 2. Encourage fluids

[   ] 3. Treat the presence of infection

[   ] 4. Avoid informing others of the condition

[   ] 5. Vigorous exercise is permitted

[   ] 6. Inform the client that the disorder is not hereditary

Answer: 3, 5, 6

Pernicious anemia results from a deficiency of the vitamin cobalamin. The client may be short of breath and have muscle weakness. Neurology changes, such as paresthesia and mental confusion, can also occur in severe cases. Elevated temperature and dark-colored urine may be present in sickle cell anemia. A client with pernicious anemia may have a sore tongue but not white patches, which is characteristic of candidiasis.

Nursing process: Assessment

Client need: Physiological Adaptation

Cognitive level: Application

Subject area: Medical-Surgical

Answer: 3

Rationale: A client newly treated for aplastic anemia may be immunocompromised for weeks, at risk of bleeding, and fatigued. Returning to work in a day care center may be unrealistic and risky to the client. The nurse should be sure the client and family understand the risks before discharge.

Nursing process: Evaluation

Client need: Physiological Adaptation

Cognitive level: Analysis

Subject area: Medical-Surgical

Answer: 1, 3

Rationale: An acute blood loss of 30% may appear more severe than a slower rate of blood loss. The client would not be showing signs of shock (clammy skin) nor would the vital signs be completely normal. It is important for the nurse to assess the client in various positions and states of activity in order to elicit the signs of significant blood loss. Pain, dizziness, and swelling occur with a 50% blood loss.

Nursing process: Assessment

Client need: Physiological Adaptation

Cognitive level: Analysis

Subject area: Medical-Surgical

Answer: 1, 2, 3

Rationale: Recognition of the signs of a vaso-occlusive crisis and the measures to prevent it are very important in keeping the health of a client with sickle cell anemia in control. It is essential to administer pain medications, encourage fluids, and treat infections. Individuals may fear the disease but educating friends of the client is a healthy approach to the disease. Dehydration from excessive exercise or heat can precipitate a cycle of pain. Sickle cell anemia is a genetic disorder and counseling of couples before they have offspring is recommended.

Nursing process: Planning

Client need: Physiological Adaptation

Cognitive level: Application

Subject area: Medical-Surgical

9. The nurse is evaluating a client with an enlarged spleen. Which of the following diagnostic tests would confirm the diagnosis?

1. Urinalysis

2. CAT scan of the chest

3. Blood cultures

4. CAT scan of the abdomen

10. The nurse has started a transfusion of packed red blood cells. The nurse should immediately stop the transfusion when which of the following occurs?

1. Fever and back pain

2. Dry mouth

3. Hypothermia and pallor

4. Heart rate of 74 beats per minute

11. The nurse is caring for a client with neutropenia. Which of the following blood tests would indicate to the nurse the desired response to treatment?

1. Increased granulocytes

2. Decrease in platelet count

3. Normal hemoglobin

4. Liver functions above normal

12. The nurse is preparing to administer a red blood cell transfusion to a client. The client tells the nurse of being terrified of contracting HIV from the transfusion. Which of the following statements is the most appropriate by the nurse?

1. "Don't worry. I've given a lot of transfusions and I've never had a client get HIV, yet."

2. "I understand your concerns. The blood supply is not 100% safe. Why don't you get someone in your family to donate blood for you?"

3. "This blood was given by screened donors and tested for HIV. The chances of getting HIV from a blood transfusion are very small."

4. "You are much more likely to die if you don't get this transfusion than if you do."

Answer: 4

Rationale: Complications from an enlarged spleen can be reflected in the complete blood count. Cell morphology may be abnormal in certain conditions that are associated with splenomegaly. The spleen is located in the abdomen and visualization of the spleen and surrounding structures with a CAT scanner may be helpful in finding an etiology.

Nursing process: Evaluation

Client need: Reduction of Risk Potential

Cognitive level: Application

Subject area: Medical-Surgical

Answer: 1

Rationale: Fever and back pain can occur in hemolytic blood transfusion reaction caused by the mismatch of blood types. If the transfusion is not stopped immediately, the client could go into shock and die. Dry mouth could be caused by an antihistamine given as a premedication or from dehydration, but it is not a reason to stop the transfusion. Blood products expire in a few hours and interruptions should be minimized. A heart beat of 74 beats per minute is not too high or too low. The client may also spike a temperature and have flushed skin.

Nursing process: Implementation

Client need: Physiological Adaptation

Cognitive level: Analysis

Subject area: Medical-Surgical

Answer: 1

Rationale: Neutropenia is an abnormally low white blood or granulocyte count. The goal of treatment would be an increase in the granulocyte count. Platelets, hemoglobin level, and liver function test changes may indicate response to some treatments, but are not measures of neutrophil count.

Nursing process: Evaluation

Client need: Reduction of Risk Potential

Cognitive level: Analysis

Subject area: Medical-Surgical

Answer: 3

Rationale: Informing the client of the blood donation process is an objective way to allay the fear of transfusion. Blood from related donors is not safer because of a family member's motivation to hide a possible health history.

Nursing process: Analysis

Client need: Reduction of Risk Potential

Cognitive level: Analysis

Subject area: Medical-Surgical

13. Which of the following is essential for the nurse to assess in the health history of a client with a hematologic disorder?

   1. The client's occupation

   2. The client's recreational activities

   3. The client's menstrual history

   4. The client's recent trip to Canada

14. A student nurse is reviewing the chart of a client with a long-standing anemia. The student asks the nurse what the term koilonychias means. The nurse should inform the student that koilonychias means the

   1. fingernails are spoon shaped.

   2. skin is flushed.

   3. mucous membranes are pink and moist.

   4. white count is elevated.

15. A client returns to the clinic after a procedure complaining of pain in the left lower back. The nurse suspects the client most likely is experiencing

   1. a hematoma from a bone marrow biopsy and aspiration performed two days ago.

   2. splenomegaly following a Schilling test.

   3. viral hepatitis B infection from a blood transfusion.

   4. folic acid deficiency.

16. A client with an enlarged lymph node in the neck is scheduled to have an open biopsy of the node. Which of the following client statements would alert the nurse to an inadequate understanding of the procedure?

   1. "I have to go to the hospital really early in the morning and I can't drink or eat anything after midnight."

   2. "My husband will have to drive me home after the biopsy."

   3. "They are going to find cancer and I have to stay in the hospital overnight."

   4. "I will know the results of my biopsy within a couple of days."

Answer: 3

Rationale: A woman's reproductive history can help explain if the client is anemic from an abnormal menstrual flow. Transfusion reactions (alloimmunization from multiple pregnancies) may also occur. Occupation, recreational activities, and travel to Canada would have little relevance to the hematologic health history.

Nursing process: Assessment

Client need: Reduction of Risk Potential

Cognitive level: Analysis

Subject area: Medical-Surgical

Answer: 1

Rationale: Spoon-shaped fingernails, or koilonychias, are a sign of long-standing chronic anemia.

Nursing process: Planning

Client need: Physiological Adaptation

Cognitive level: Comprehension

Subject area: Medical-Surgical

Answer: 1

Rationale: The most common site for biopsy and aspiration of the bone marrow is the posterior iliac crest bone. A hematoma from inadequate pressure applied to the site postprocedure could cause pain. Splenomegaly does not cause pain in this area and does not result from a Schilling test for pernicious anemia. Hepatitis from a blood transfusion would typically take weeks to cause symptoms, and pain in this specific site is unlikely. Folic acid deficiency is not painful and usually is the result of poor dietary intake and not of a procedure.

Nursing process: Analysis

Client need: Reduction of Risk Potential

Cognitive level: Analysis

Subject area: Medical-Surgical

Answer: 3

Rationale: Open biopsies of lymph nodes may be done in the operating room under local anesthesia. The client may be told to be NPO as a precaution. The client should be able to go home that same day if someone else drives. The biopsy is being done to determine why the lymph node is swollen. Cancer could be found on a lymph node biopsy, but there may be other causes of an enlarged node. Usually the pathological results are available within two days.

Nursing process: Evaluation

Client need: Physiological Adaptation

Cognitive level: Analysis

Subject area: Medical-Surgical

17. The nurse is admitting a client with a hematologic disorder. During the dietary history, the client states eating clay regularly. The nurse reports this client as exhibiting what clinical manifestation of anemia? _____

18. The admitting nurse is making room assignments for a client admitted with aplastic anemia. The nurse appropriately selects which of the following room assignments for this client?

1. Semiprivate room with strict hand washing

2. Private room, protective isolation, and HEPA filtration

3. Semiprivate room with no special precautions

4. Private room with ECG monitoring on a cardiac care unit

19. During an IV antibiotic administration, the nurse inspects a 2-day-old IV site on a client who is neutropenic and observes redness without swelling. The client complains of tenderness. Which of the following interventions is the priority for the nurse to implement?

1. Check the client's vital signs before going to care for another client

2. Inform the client that the IV will need to be changed to a new site

3. Administer prescribed pain medications

4. Inform the client that medication is causing a rash

20. A client with iron deficiency anemia is very pale, has shortness of breath, and records a hemoglobin level of 7.5 grams. Which of the following is a priority for the nurse to implement?

1. Administer an iron supplement

2. Instruct the client on a diet high in iron

3. Administer packed red cells

4. Instruct the client to conserve energy

Answer: Pica

Rationale: Pica is the compulsive ingestion of clay and can occur in persons with iron deficiency anemia.

Nursing process: Analysis

Client need: Physiological Adaptation

Cognitive level: Comprehension

Subject area: Medical-Surgical

Answer: 2

Rationale: The aplastic anemia client has neutropenia and needs protection from other clients and staff. A private room with protective isolation and special air filtration is ideal.

Nursing process: Implementation

Client need: Reduction of Risk Potential

Cognitive level: Analysis

Subject area: Medical-Surgical

Answer: 2

Rationale: A client who is neutropenic is susceptible to infection. In the absence of white blood cells, the inflammatory response to infection and the ability to produce pus is suppressed. Redness and pain may be the only clinical manifestations. Changing the 2-day-old IV site is appropriate. Vital signs may further indicate infection if abnormal, but not always. Administering pain medications will ease the pain but not the infection, which could become rapidly severe. Notifying the physician is not a priority.

Nursing process: Implementation

Client need: Management of Care

Cognitive level: Analysis

Subject area: Medical-Surgical

Answer: 3

Rationale: A client with a hemoglobin of 7.5 grams classifies as severe anemia. The client is symptomatic and the administration of packed red cells is the priority. Administering an iron supplement, instructing the client on a diet high in iron, and conserving energy are all important interventions but not the priority.

Nursing process: Analysis

Client need: Management of Care

Cognitive level: Analysis

Subject area: Medical-Surgical

21. During a therapeutic phlebotomy of a client with hemochromatosis, the nurse explains the rationale for the procedure by telling the client

    1. "You may need several phlebotomies during your lifetime to keep the iron from damaging your pancreas and heart."

    2. "The blood is being removed so your blood is available for future transfusions."

    3. "If you hadn't been a vegetarian you wouldn't have gotten this disease."

    4. "You have too much blood and some of it has to be removed to make you less prone to infections."

22. Which of the following should the nurse include in the plan of care for a client scheduled for a bone marrow biopsy?

    1. Assist the client on the abdomen with arms toward the head preprocedure

    2. Place the client NPO preprocedure

    3. Position the client on the abdomen for one hour postprocedure

    4. Place a light gauze dressing on the insertion site

23. A nurse caring for a client with acute disseminated intravascular coagulation (DIC) should monitor the client for which of the following clinical manifestations?

    Select all that apply:

    [   ] **1.** Bleeding from the nose and mouth

    [   ] **2.** Hypertension

    [   ] **3.** Jaundiced sclera

    [   ] **4.** Elevated platelet count

    [   ] **5.** Oliguria

    [   ] **6.** Dizziness

24. The nurse should monitor a client with a blood type A who received a transfusion from a type O donor for which of the following?

    1. A febrile reaction because of the blood type mismatch

    2. An expected rise in hemoglobin and hematocrit

    3. A conversion from Rh negative to Rh positive because of the mismatched blood type

    4. Fluid overload symptoms

Answer: 1

Rationale: Hemochromatosis is a genetic disorder that may require a periodic series of phlebotomies to remove iron from the body. The purpose is not to save the blood for later transfusion back to the client. Diet cannot cause the disease. Having too much blood does not cause infections.

Nursing process: Analysis

Client need: Reduction of Risk Potential

Cognitive level: Analysis

Subject area: Medical-Surgical

Answer: 1

Rationale: The bone marrow biopsy is an aspiration of bone marrow performed with a needle and syringe. The posterior iliac crest is the best bone site for this test. The client does not have to be NPO. The client should lie on the back for 20 to 30 minutes postprocedure. A pressure dressing should be applied to the area.

Nursing process: Planning

Client need: Reduction of Risk Potential

Cognitive level: Application

Subject area: Medical-Surgical

Answer: 1, 5, 6

Rationale: Disseminated intravascular coagulation is a serious bleeding disorder which results in both thrombosis and bleeding. Bleeding occurs due to a very low platelet count. The client would be most likely to have hypotension rather than hypertension. Jaundiced sclera indicates hemolysis or liver disease.

Nursing process: Assessment

Client need: Physiological Adaptation

Cognitive level: Application

Subject area: Medical-Surgical

Answer: 2

Rationale: The type O blood would not cause a febrile transfusion reaction because it contains neither A nor B antigens to which the recipient's antibodies react. Type O is a universal donor for this reason. Nothing in the case was mentioned about the Rh status of the donor or recipient, thus no conclusion about this can be made. A fluid overload reaction is caused by volume and rate of transfusion, not by the blood type.

Nursing process: Assessment

Client need: Pharmacological and Parenteral Therapies

Cognitive level: Analysis

Subject area: Medical-Surgical

25. The nurse is caring for a client with a severe anemia. A transfusion of two units of packed red blood cells has been ordered. The nurse should start an infusion of which solution prior to hanging the blood? _____

Answer: Normal saline

Rationale: Normal saline is the only solution compatible to run in an IV with red blood cells.

Nursing process: Implementation

Client need: Pharmacological and Parenteral Therapies

Cognitive level: Application

Subject area: Medical-Surgical

Fluid, Electrolyte, and Acid–Base Disorders

12

1. A client with hypoparathyroidism complains of numbness and tingling in his fingers and around the mouth. The nurse would assess for what electrolyte imbalance? _____

2. The nurse evaluates which of the following clients to be at risk for developing hypernatremia?
   1. 50-year-old with pneumonia, diaphoresis, and high fevers
   2. 62-year-old with congestive heart failure taking loop diuretics
   3. 39-year-old with diarrhea and vomiting
   4. 60-year-old with lung cancer and syndrome of inappropriate antidiuretic hormone (SIADH)

3. A client is admitted with diabetic ketoacidosis who, with treatment, has a normal blood glucose, pH, and serum osmolality. During assessment, the client complains of weakness in the legs. Which of the following is a priority nursing intervention?
   1. Request a physical therapy consult from the physician
   2. Ensure the client is safe from falls and check the most recent potassium level
   3. Allow uninterrupted rest periods throughout the day
   4. Encourage the client to increase intake of dairy products and green leafy vegetables

4. A client with a potassium level of 5.5 mEq/L is to receive sodium polystyrene sulfonate (Kayexalate) orally. After administering the drug, the priority nursing action is to monitor
   1. urine output.
   2. blood pressure.
   3. bowel movements.
   4. ECG for tall, peaked T waves.

Answer: Hypocalcemia

Rationale: Hypoparathyroidism can cause low serum calcium levels. Numbness and tingling in extremities and in the circumoral area around the mouth are the hallmark signs of hypocalcemia. Normal calcium level is 9 to 11 mg/dl.

Nursing process: Assessment

Client need: Physiological Adaptation

Cognitive level: Application

Subject area: Medical-Surgical

Answer: 1

Rationale: Diaphoresis and a high fever can lead to free water loss through the skin, resulting in hypernatremia. Loop diuretics are more likely to result in a hypovolemic hyponatremia. Diarrhea and vomiting cause both sodium and water losses. Clients with syndrome of inappropriate antidiuretic hormone (SIADH) have hyponatremia, due to increased water reabsorption in the renal tubules.

Nursing process: Evaluation

Client need: Reduction of Risk Potential

Cognitive level: Analysis

Subject area: Medical-Surgical

Answer: 2

Rationale: In the treatment of diabetic ketoacidosis, the blood sugar is lowered, the pH is corrected, and potassium moves back into the cells, resulting in low serum potassium. Client safety and the correction of low potassium levels are a priority. The weakness in the legs is a clinical manifestation of the hypokalemia. Dairy products and green, leafy vegetables are a source of calcium.

Nursing process: Implementation

Client need: Management of Care

Cognitive level: Analysis

Subject area: Medical-Surgical

Answer: 3

Rationale: Kayexalate causes potassium to be exchanged for sodium in the intestines and excreted through bowel movements. If client does not have stools, the drug cannot work properly. Blood pressure and urine output are not of primary importance. The nurse would already expect changes in T waves with hyperkalemia. Normal serum potassium is 3.5 to 5.5 mEq/L.

Nursing process: Implementation

Client need: Management of Care

Cognitive level: Analysis

Subject area: Medical-Surgical

5. The nurse is caring for a client who has been in good health up to the present and is admitted with cellulitis of the hand. The client's serum potassium level was 4.5 mEq/L yesterday. Today the level is 7 mEq/L. Which of the following is the next appropriate nursing action?

   1. Call the physician and report results

   2. Question the results and redraw the specimen

   3. Encourage the client to increase the intake of bananas

   4. Initiate seizure precautions

6. A client is receiving an intravenous magnesium infusion to correct a serum level of 1.4 mEq/L. Which of the following assessments would alert the nurse to immediately stop the infusion?

   1. Absent patellar reflex

   2. Diarrhea

   3. Premature ventricular contractions

   4. Increase in blood pressure

7. A client with chronic renal failure reports a 10 pound weight loss over 3 months and has had difficulty taking calcium supplements. The total calcium is 6.9 mg/dl. Which of the following would be the first nursing action?

   1. Assess for depressed deep tendon reflexes

   2. Call the physician to report calcium level

   3. Place an intravenous catheter in anticipation of administering calcium gluconate

   4. Check to see if a serum albumin level is available

 8. A client with heart failure is complaining of nausea. The client has received IV furosemide (Lasix), and the urine output has been 2500 ml over the past 12 hours. The client's home drugs include metoprolol (Lopressor), digoxin (Lanoxin), furosemide, and multivitamins. Which of the following are the appropriate nursing actions before administering the digoxin?

   Select all that apply:

   [ ] **1.** Administer an antiemetic prior to giving the digoxin

   [ ] **2.** Encourage the client to increase fluid intake

   [ ] **3.** Call the physician

   [ ] **4.** Report the urine output

   [ ] **5.** Report indications of nausea

   [ ] **6.** Monitor continuous ECG for peaked T waves and widened QRS

Answer: 2

Rationale: A client who has been in good health up to the present is admitted for cellulitis of the hands. When the serum potassium goes from 4.5 mEq/L to 7.0 mEq/L with no risk factors for hyperkalemia, false high results should be suspected because of hemolysis of the specimen. The physician would likely question results as well. Bananas are a food high in potassium. Seizures are not a clinical manifestation of hyperkalemia.

Nursing process: Implementation

Client need: Management of Care

Cognitive level: Analysis

Subject area: Medical-Surgical

Answer: 1

Rationale: An intravenous magnesium infusion may be used to treat a low serum magnesium level. Normal serum magnesium is 1.5 to 2.5 mEq/L. Clinical manifestations of hypermagnesemia are the result of depressed neuromuscular transmission. Absent reflexes indicate a magnesium level around 7 mEq/L. Diarrhea and PVCs are not clinical manifestations of high magnesium levels. Hypermagnesemia causes hypotension.

Nursing process: Evaluation

Client need: Management of Care

Cognitive level: Analysis

Subject area: Legal and Ethical Issues

Answer: 4

Rationale: A client with chronic renal failure who reports a 10 pound weight loss over 3 months and has difficulty taking calcium supplements is poorly nourished and likely to have hypoalbuminemia. A drop in serum albumin will result in a false low total calcium level. Placing an IV is not a priority action. Depressed reflexes are a sign of hypercalcemia. Normal serum calcium is 9 to 11 mg/dl.

Nursing process: Implementation

Client need: Management of Care

Cognitive level: Analysis

Subject area: Medical-Surgical

Answer: 3, 4, 5

Rationale: Potassium is lost during diuresis with a loop diuretic such as furosemide (Lasix). Hypokalemia can cause digitalis toxicity, which often results in nausea. The physician should be notified, and digoxin should be held until potassium levels and digoxin levels are checked. Peaked T waves and widened QRS are manifestations of hyperkalemia.

Nursing process: Evaluation

Client need: Pharmacological and Parenteral Therapies

Cognitive level: Analysis

Subject area: Medical-Surgical

9. The nurse is caring for a bedridden client admitted with multiple myeloma and a serum calcium level of 13 mg/dl. Which of the following is the most appropriate nursing action?

1. Provide passive ROM exercises and encourage fluid intake

2. Teach the client to increase intake of whole grains and nuts

3. Place a tracheostomy tray at the bedside

4. Administer calcium gluconate IM as ordered

10. An older adult client admitted with heart failure and a sodium level of 113 mEq/L is behaving aggressively toward staff and does not recognize family members. When the family expresses concern about the client's behavior, the nurse would respond most appropriately by stating

1. "The client may be suffering from dementia, and the hospitalization has worsened the confusion."

2. "Most older adults get confused in the hospital."

3. "The sodium level is low, and the confusion will resolve as the levels normalize."

4. "The sodium level is high and the behavior is a result of dehydration."

11. A client with a serum sodium of 115 mEq/L has been receiving 3% NS at 50 ml/hr for 16 hours. This morning the client feels tired and short of breath. Which of the following interventions is a priority?

1. Turn down the infusion

2. Check the latest sodium level

3. Assess for signs of fluid overload

4. Place a call to the physician

12. A client with chronic renal failure receiving dialysis complains of frequent constipation. When performing discharge teaching, which over-the-counter products should the nurse instruct the client to avoid at home?

1. Bisacodyl (Dulcolax) suppository

2. Fiber supplements

3. Docusate sodium

4. Milk of magnesia

Answer: 1

Rationale: A client who has a serum calcium of 13 mg/dl has hypercalcemia. Normal serum calcium is 9 to 11 mg/dl. Fluid intake promotes renal excretion of excess calcium. ROM exercises promote reabsorption of calcium into bone. Placing a tracheostomy at the bedside is a nursing intervention for hypocalcemia. Although calcium gluconate may be administered in hypocalcemia, it is never administered IM.

Nursing process: Planning

Client need: Physiological Adaptation

Cognitive level: Application

Subject area: Medical-Surgical

Answer: 3

Rationale: Normal serum level is 135 to 145 mEq/L. Neurological symptoms occur when sodium levels fall below 120 mEq/L. The confusion is an acute condition that will go away as the sodium levels normalize. Dementia is an irreversible condition.

Nursing process: Analysis

Client need: Physiological Adaptation

Cognitive level: Analysis

Subject area: Medical-Surgical

Answer: 3

Rationale: A complication of hypertonic sodium solution administration is fluid overload. While turning down the infusion, checking the latest sodium level, and notifying the physician may all be reasonable, the priority intervention is to assess for manifestations of fluid overload. Assessment is always the priority to determine what action to take next.

Nursing process: Evaluation

Client need: Management of Care

Cognitive level: Analysis

Subject area: Medical-Surgical

Answer: 4

Rationale: Milk of magnesia contains magnesium, an electrolyte that is excreted by kidneys. Clients with renal failure are at risk for hypermagnesemia, since their bodies cannot excrete the excess magnesium. The client should avoid magnesium-containing laxatives.

Nursing process: Planning

Client need: Health Promotion and Maintenance

Cognitive level: Application

Subject area: Medical-Surgical

13. A client is receiving intravenous potassium supplementation in addition to maintenance fluids. The urine output has been 120 ml every 8 hours for the past 16 hours and the next dose is due. Before administering the next potassium dose, which of the following is the priority nursing action?

1. Encourage the client to increase fluid intake

2. Administer the dose as ordered

3. Draw a potassium level and administer the dose if the level is low or normal

4. Notify the physician of the urine output and hold the dose

14. The nurse should monitor for clinical manifestations of hypophosphatemia in which of the following clients?

1. A client with osteoporosis taking vitamin D and calcium supplements

2. A client who is alcoholic receiving total parenteral nutrition

3. A client with chronic renal failure awaiting the first dialysis run

4. A client with hypoparathyroidism secondary to thyroid surgery

15. A client admitted with squamous cell carcinoma of the lung has a serum calcium level of 14 mg/dl. The nurse should instruct the client to avoid which of the following foods upon discharge?

Select all that apply:

[   ] **1.** Fish

[   ] **2.** Eggs

[   ] **3.** Broccoli

[   ] **4.** Organ meats

[   ] **5.** Nuts

[   ] **6.** Canned salmon

16. A client with pancreatitis has been receiving potassium supplementation for four days since being admitted with a serum potassium of 3.0 mEq/L. Today the potassium level is 3.1 mEq/L. Which of the following laboratory values should the nurse check before notifying the physician of the client's failure to respond to treatment?

1. Sodium

2. Phosphorus

3. Calcium

4. Magnesium

Answer: 4

Rationale: Urine output is an indication of renal function. Normal urine output is at least 30 ml/hour. Clients with impaired renal function are at risk for hyperkalemia. Initiating a lab draw requires a physician order.

Nursing process: Planning

Client need: Management of Care

Cognitive level: Analysis

Subject area: Medical-Surgical

Answer: 2

Rationale: A client with osteoporosis taking vitamin and calcium supplements, a client with chronic renal failure awaiting dialysis, and a client with hypoparathyroidism secondary to thyroid surgery are at risk for hyperphosphatemia. Alcoholics and clients receiving TPN are at risk for low phosphorus levels, due to poor intestinal absorption and shifting of phosphorus into cells along with insulin and glucose.

Nursing process: Assessment

Client need: Reduction of Risk Potential

Cognitive level: Analysis

Subject area: Medical-Surgical

Answer: 3, 5, 6

Rationale: Fish, eggs, and organ meats are high in phosphorus. Broccoli, nuts, and canned salmon are high in calcium. Clients with lung or breast cancer often have elevated calcium levels due to tumor-induced hyperparathyroidism.

Nursing process: Implementation

Client need: Basic Care and Comfort

Cognitive level: Application

Subject area: Medical-Surgical

Answer: 4

Rationale: Low serum magnesium levels can inhibit potassium ions from crossing cell membranes, resulting in potassium loss through the urine. Generally, low magnesium levels must be corrected before potassium replacement is effective.

Nursing process: Evaluation

Client need: Reduction of Risk Potential

Cognitive level: Analysis

Subject area: Medical-Surgical

17. The nurse should include which of the following instructions to assist in controlling phosphorus levels for a client in renal failure?

    1. Increase intake of dairy products and nuts

    2. Take aluminum-based antacids such as aluminum hydroxide (Amphojel) with or after meals

    3. Reduce intake of chocolate, meats, and whole grains

    4. Avoid calcium supplements

18. A client with pneumonia presents with the following arterial blood gases: pH of 7.28, $PaCO_2$ of 74, HCO_3 of 28 mEq/L, and PO_2 of 45. Which of the following is the most appropriate nursing intervention?

    1. Administer a sedative

    2. Place client in left lateral position

    3. Place client in high-Fowler's position

    4. Assist the client to breathe into a paper bag

19. A client with COPD feels short of breath after walking to the bathroom on 2 liters of oxygen nasal cannula. The morning's ABGs were pH of 7.36, $PaCO_2$ of 62, HCO_3 of 35 mEq/L, O_2 at 88% on 2 liters. Which of the following should be the nurse's first intervention?

    1. Call the physician and report the change in client's condition

    2. Turn the client's O_2 up to 4 liters nasal cannula

    3. Encourage the client to sit down and to take deep breaths

    4. Encourage the client to rest and to use pursed-lip breathing technique

20. A client who had a recent surgery has been vomiting and becomes dizzy while standing up to go to the bathroom. After assisting the client back to bed, the nurse notes that the blood pressure is 55/30 and the pulse is 140. The nurse hangs which of the following IV fluids to correct this condition?

    1. D5.45 NS at 50 ml/hr

    2. 0.9 NS at an open rate

    3. D5W at 125 ml/hr

    4. 0.45 NS at open rate

Answer: 2

Rationale: Aluminum-based antacids are often prescribed in the treatment of renal failure to bind with phosphate and increase elimination through the GI tract. Dairy products and nuts are foods high in phosphorus. Chocolate, meats, and whole grains are foods high in magnesium. Clients with renal failure often require calcium supplements as a result of poor vitamin D metabolism and in order to prevent hyperphosphatemia.

Nursing process: Planning

Client need: Health Promotion and Maintenance

Cognitive level: Analysis

Subject area: Medical-Surgical

Answer: 3

Rationale: The client with a pH of 7.28, $PaCO_2$ of 74, HCO_3 of 28 mEq/L, and PO_2 of 45 is in a state of respiratory acidosis. Placing the client in high-Fowler's position will facilitate the expansion of the lungs and help the client blow off the excess CO_2. Sedatives would impede respirations. The question does not indicate which is the affected lung, so left lateral position would not be a first choice. Breathing into a paper bag will cause the PCO_2 to rise higher.

Nursing process: Planning

Client need: Physiological Adaptation

Cognitive level: Application

Subject area: Medical-Surgical

Answer: 4

Rationale: Clients with COPD, especially those who are in a chronic compensated respiratory acidosis, are very sensitive to changes in O_2 flow, because hypoxemia rather than high CO_2 levels stimulates respirations. Deep breaths are not helpful, because clients with COPD have difficulty with air trapping in alveoli. There is no need to call the physician, since this client is presently most likely at baseline.

Nursing process: Planning

Client need: Management of Care

Cognitive level: Analysis

Subject area: Medical-Surgical

Answer: 2

Rationale: A client who recently had surgery, is vomiting, becomes dizzy when standing up, has a blood pressure of 55/30, and has a pulse of 140 is hypovolemic and requires plasma volume expansion. Isotonic fluids such as 0.9 NS will expand volume. Hypotonic fluids such as 0.45 NS will leave the intravascular space. D5W will metabolize into free water and leave the intravascular space. D5.45 NS is a good maintenance fluid but a rate of 50 ml per hour is not sufficient to expand the vascular volume quickly.

Nursing process: Implementation

Client need: Pharmacological and Parenteral Therapies

Cognitive level: Analysis

Subject area: Pharmacologic

21. A client with renal failure enters the emergency room after skipping three dialysis treatments to visit family out of town. Which set of ABGs would indicate to the nurse that the client is in a state of metabolic acidosis?

    1. pH of 7.43, PCO_2 of 36, HCO_3 of 26
    2. pH of 7.41, PCO_2 of 49, HCO_3 of 30
    3. pH of 7.33, PCO_2 of 35, HCO_3 of 17
    4. pH of 7.25, PCO_2 of 56, HCO_3 of 28

22. A client with a small bowel obstruction has had an NG tube connected to low intermittent suction for two days. The nurse should monitor for clinical manifestations of which acid-base disorder?

    1. Respiratory alkalosis
    2. Respiratory acidosis
    3. Metabolic alkalosis
    4. Metabolic acidosis

23. A client who suffers from an anxiety disorder is very upset, has a respiratory rate of 32, and is complaining of lightheadedness and tingling in the fingers. ABG values are pH of 7.48, $PaCO_2$ of 29, HCO_3 of 24, and O_2 is at 93% on room air. The nurse performs which of the following as a priority nursing intervention?

    1. Monitor intake and output
    2. Encourage client to increase activity
    3. Institute deep breathing exercises every hour
    4. Provide reassurance to the client and administer sedatives

Answer: 3

Rationale: A pH of 7.33, PCO_2 of 35, and HCO_3 of 17 and a pH of 7.25, PCO_2 of 56, and HCO_3 of 28 both indicate acidosis. The pH of 7.25 is a respiratory acidosis. A pH of 7.41, PCO_2 of 49, and HCO_3 of 30 is a compensated metabolic alkalosis. A pH of 7.43, PCO_2 of 36, and HCO_3 of 26 is normal.

Nursing process: Analysis

Client need: Reduction of Risk Potential

Cognitive level: Analysis

Subject area: Medical-Surgical

Answer: 3

Rationale: Clients with gastric suctioning can lose hydrogen ions resulting in a metabolic alkalosis.

Nursing process: Assessment

Client need: Physiological Adaptation

Cognitive level: Analysis

Subject area: Medical-Surgical

Answer: 4

Rationale: A client who is anxious and upset, gets lightheaded, and has tingling in the fingers is in respiratory alkalosis. The arterial blood gases include a pH of 7.48, $PaCO_2$ of 29, and HCO_3 of 24. Administering sedatives will assist the client to slow breathe and retain more CO_2, thus bringing the pH back into normal range. Deep breathing exercises may worsen the client's condition. Encouraging the client to increase activity is contraindicated because clients are often exhausted and require rest after expending so much energy breathing. Monitoring intake and output is not a priority.

Nursing process: Implementation

Client need: Management of Care

Cognitive level: Analysis

Subject area: Medical-Surgical

24. Which of the following assessment findings would indicate to the nurse that a client's diabetic ketoacidosis is deteriorating?

    1. Deep tendon reflexes decreasing from +2 to +1

    2. Bicarbonate rising from 20 mEq/L to 22 mEq/L

    3. Urine pH less than 6

    4. Serum potassium decreasing from 6.0 mEq/L to 4.5 mEq/L

25. A client who is admitted with malnutrition and anorexia secondary to chemotherapy is also exhibiting generalized edema. The client asks the nurse for an explanation for the edema. Which of the following is the most appropriate response by the nurse?

    1. "The fluid is an adverse reaction to the chemotherapy."

    2. "A decrease in activity has allowed extra fluid to accumulate in the tissues."

    3. "Poor nutrition has caused decreased blood protein levels, and fluid has moved from the blood vessels into the tissues."

    4. "Chemotherapy has increased your blood pressure, and fluid was forced out into the tissues."

26. A client with a recent thyroidectomy complains of numbness and tingling around the mouth. Which of the following findings indicates the serum calcium is low?

    1. Bone pain

    2. Depressed deep tendon reflexes

    3. Positive Chvostek's sign

    4. Nausea

27. A client recently diagnosed with syndrome of inappropriate antidiuretic hormone (SIADH) complains of headache, weight gain, and nausea. Which of the following is an appropriate nursing diagnosis for this client?

    1. Deficient fluid volume related to decreased fluid intake

    2. Excess fluid volume related to increased water retention

    3. Deficient fluid volume related to excessive fluid loss

    4. Risk for injury related to fluid volume loss

Answer: 1

Rationale: A decrease in deep tendon reflexes is a sign that pH is dropping and that metabolic acidosis is worsening in diabetic ketoacidosis. An increase in bicarbonate would indicate that the acidosis is being corrected. A urine pH less than 6 indicates the kidneys are excreting acid. Serum potassium levels are expected to fall because acidosis is corrected and potassium moves back into the intracellular space.

Nursing process: Analysis

Client need: Reduction of Risk Potential

Cognitive level: Analysis

Subject area: Medical-Surgical

Answer: 3

Rationale: Generalized edema, or anasarca, is often seen in clients with low albumin levels secondary to poor nutrition. Decreased oncotic pressure within the blood vessels allows fluid to move from the intravascular space to the interstitial space.

Nursing process: Analysis

Client need: Physiological Adaptation

Cognitive level: Analysis

Subject area: Medical-Surgical

Answer: 3

Rationale: Numbness and tingling around the mouth indicate hypocalcemia, which results in neuromuscular irritability. A positive Chvostek's sign is the contraction of facial muscles when the facial nerve in front of the ear is tapped. Bone pain, nausea, and depressed deep tendon reflexes are signs of hypercalcemia.

Nursing process: Analysis

Client need: Reduction of Risk Potential

Cognitive level: Analysis

Subject area: Medical-Surgical

Answer: 2

Rationale: The client exhibits signs of excess fluid volume. Syndrome of inappropriate antidiuretic hormone (SIADH) is the release of excess ADH by the pituitary gland, which results in hypervolemic hyponatremia and clinical manifestations of headache, weight gain, and nausea.

Nursing process: Analysis

Client need: Management of Care

Cognitive level: Analysis

Subject area: Medical-Surgical

28. The registered nurse is delegating nursing tasks for the day. Which of the following tasks may the nurse delegate to a licensed practical nurse?

   1. Assess a client for metabolic acidosis
   2. Evaluate the blood gases of a client with respiratory alkalosis
   3. Obtain a glucose level on a client admitted with diabetes mellitus
   4. Perform a neurological assessment on a client suspected of having hypocalcemia

29. A client who is post-gallbladder surgery has a nasogastric tube, decreased reflexes, pulse of 110 weak and irregular, and blood pressure of 80/50 and is weak, mildly confused, and has a serum of potassium of 3.0 mEq/L. Based on the assessment data, which of the following is the priority intervention?

   1. Withhold furosemide (Lasix)
   2. Notify the physician
   3. Administer the prescribed potassium supplement
   4. Instruct the client on foods high in potassium

30. The nurse is admitting a client with a potassium level of 6.0 mEq/L. The nurse reports this finding as a result of

   1. acute renal failure.
   2. malabsorption syndrome.
   3. nasogastric drainage.
   4. laxative abuse.

Answer: 3

Rationale: A licensed practical nurse may obtain a finger-stick glucose on a client with diabetes mellitus. A licensed practical nurse may not assess a client for metabolic acidosis, evaluate blood gases on a client with respiratory alkalosis, or perform a neurological assessment on a client suspected of hypocalcemia.

Nursing process: Planning

Client need: Management of Care

Cognitive level: Analysis

Subject area: Medical-Surgical

Answer: 2

Rationale: The priority intervention for a client who had gallbladder surgery, has a nasogastric tube, decreased reflexes, pulse of 110 weak and irregular, and blood pressure of 80/50 and is weak, mildly confused, and has a serum potassium of 3.0 mEq/L would be to notify the physician that the potassium level is low. After notifying the physician, the furosemide (Lasix) may be withheld and potassium supplement should be administered as prescribed and may even be increased after talking with the physician. The client may also be instructed on foods high in potassium. These are all appropriate interventions but not the priority.

Nursing process: Planning

Client need: Management of Care

Cognitive level: Analysis

Subject area: Medical-Surgical

Answer: 2

Rationale: A serum potassium level of 6.0 mEq/L is indicative of acute renal failure. Malabsorption syndrome, nasogastric drainage, and laxative abuse may result in a low serum potassium level, because output may be greater than input. Diarrhea results in malabsorption syndrome and can come from laxative abuse. Fluids and electrolytes may be lost in the nasogastric drainage. Normal serum potassium is 3.5 to 5.5 mEq/L.

Nursing process: Analysis

Client need: Physiological Adaptation

Cognitive level: Application

Subject area: Medical-Surgical

31. Which of the following should the nurse include in the diet teaching for a client with a sodium level of 158 mEq/L?

    Select all that apply:

    [   ] 1. Peanut butter sandwich

    [   ] 2. Pretzels

    [   ] 3. Baked chicken

    [   ] 4. Chicken bouillon

    [   ] 5. Baked potato

    [   ] 6. Baked ham

32. The nurse assesses a client to be experiencing muscle cramps, numbness, and tingling of the extremities, and twitching of the facial muscle and eyelid when the facial nerve is tapped. The nurse reports this assessment as consistent with which of the following?

    1. Hypokalemia

    2. Hypernatremia

    3. Hypermagnesemia

    4. Hypocalcemia

33. Which of the following should the nurse include when preparing to teach a class on the regulation and functions of electrolytes?

    1. Sodium is essential to maintain intracellular fluid water balance

    2. Magnesium is essential to the function of muscle, red blood cells, and nervous system

    3. Less calcium is excreted with aging

    4. Chloride is lost in hydrochloride acid

34. The nurse assists a client with a serum potassium of 3.2 mEq/L to make which of the following menu selections?

    Select all that apply:

    [   ] 1. Baked cod

    [   ] 2. Ham and cheese omelet

    [   ] 3. Fried eggs

    [   ] 4. Baked potato

    [   ] 5. Whole grain muffin

    [   ] 6. Spinach

Answer: 3, 5

Rationale: Normal serum sodium is between 135 and 145 mEq/L. A sodium level of 158 mEq/L is elevated and a low sodium diet should be prescribed. A peanut butter sandwich, pretzels, chicken bouillon, and baked ham are all foods high in sodium content. Baked chicken and baked potato are low-sodium food choices.

Nursing process: Planning

Client need: Basic Care and Comfort

Cognitive level: Application

Subject area: Medical-Surgical

Answer: 4

Rationale: Normal serum calcium is 9 to 11 mg/dl. A client who has hypocalcemia would experience muscle cramps, numbness, and twitching of the facial muscles and eyelid when the facial nerve is tapped. Hypocalcemia may result from renal failure, hypoparathyroidism, acute pancreatitis, liver disease, malabsorption syndrome, and vitamin D deficiency. Normal serum potassium level is 3.5 to 5.5 mEq/L. Normal serum sodium is 135 to 145 mEq/L. Normal serum magnesium is 1.5 to 2.5 mEq/L.

Nursing process: Analysis

Client need: Physiological Adaptation

Cognitive level: Analysis

Subject area: Medical-Surgical

Answer: 4

Rationale: Sodium is essential to maintain extracellular fluid water balance. Phosphate is the major anion in intracellular fluid water balance that is essential in the function of muscle, red blood cells, and nervous system. A person tends to excrete more calcium with age. Chloride is lost through hydrochloride acid.

Nursing process: Planning

Client need: Physiological Adaptation

Cognitive level: Analysis

Subject area: Medical-Surgical

Answer: 1, 4, 6

Rationale: Normal serum potassium is 3.5 to 5.5 mEq/L. A client who has a potassium of 3.2 mEq/L would benefit from a diet high in potassium. Baked cod, baked potato, and spinach are all food selections high in potassium. A ham and cheese omelet is high in sodium. Fried eggs are high in cholesterol. A whole grain muffin is high in grains.

Nursing process: Implementation

Client need: Basic Care and Comfort

Cognitive level: Application

Subject area: Medical-Surgical

35. The nurse evaluates which of the following clients to have hypermagnesemia?

   1. A client who has chronic alcoholism and a magnesium level of 1.3 mEq/L

   2. A client who has hyperthyroidism and a magnesium level of 1.6 mEq/L

   3. A client who has renal failure, takes antacids, and has a magnesium level of 2.9 mEq/L

   4. A client who has congestive heart disease, takes a diuretic, and has a magnesium level of 2.3 mEq/L

36. The nurse is evaluating the serum laboratory results on the following four clients. Which of the following laboratory results is a priority for the nurse to report first?

   1. A client with osteoporosis and a calcium level of 10.6 mg/dl

   2. A client with renal failure and a magnesium level of 2.5 mEq/L

   3. A client with bulimia and a potassium level of 3.6 mEq/L

   4. A client with dehydration and a sodium level of 149 mEq/L

37. The registered nurse is delegating client assignments to unlicensed assistive personnel. Which of the following clients does not require additional monitoring and assessment and may be delegated to unlicensed assistive personnel?

   1. A client who has been experiencing diarrhea and has a serum chloride level of 100 mEq/L

   2. A client with renal failure who has a serum magnesium level of 3.0 mEq/L

   3. A client who has experienced a fracture of the femur and has a serum phosphate of 5.0 mg/dl

   4. A client with dehydration who has a serum sodium level of 128 mEq/L

Answer: 3

Rationale: Normal serum magnesium is 1.5 to 2.5 mEq/L. Clients who have chronic alcoholism and hyperthyroidism are prone to hypomagnesemia. A client who has congestive heart failure, takes a diuretic, and has a magnesium level of 2.3 mEq/L falls within the normal magnesium range.

Nursing process: Evaluation

Client need: Reduction of Risk Potential

Cognitive level: Application

Subject area: Medical-Surgical

Answer: 4

Rationale: Although a client with acute osteoporosis may have a high serum calcium, a level of 10.6 mg/dl is normal. Normal serum calcium is 9 to 11 mg/dl. Normal serum magnesium is 1.5 to 2.5 mEq/L. A client who has renal failure is prone to hypermagnesemia, but a level of 2.5 mEq/L is at the upper limit of normal. A client who has bulimia generally vomits enough to result in a low potassium level, but a potassium level of 3.6 mEq/L is low normal. Normal serum potassium is 3.5 to 5.5 mEq/L. Normal serum sodium is 135 to 145 mEq/L. The sodium level generally goes up with dehydration. A sodium level of 149 mEq/L is elevated.

Nursing process: Evaluation

Client need: Management of Care

Cognitive level: Analysis

Subject area: Medical-Surgical

Answer: 1

Rationale: Normal serum chloride is 95 to 105 mEq/L. A client with diarrhea may experience a low chloride level, but 100 mEq/L is within the normal range and may be delegated to unlicensed assistive personnel. Normal serum magnesium is 1.5 to 2.5 mEq/L. A magnesium level of 3.0 mEq/L is elevated and may occur in renal failure. Phosphate levels may be elevated with healing fractures. A phosphate level of 5.0 mg/dl is elevated. Normal serum phosphate is 2.8 to 4.5 mg/dl. A sodium level of 128 mEq/L is decreased and may be found with dehydration. Normal serum sodium is 135 to 145 mEq/L.

Nursing process: Planning

Client need: Management of Care

Cognitive level: Analysis

Subject area: Legal and Ethical Issues

Perioperative Nursing

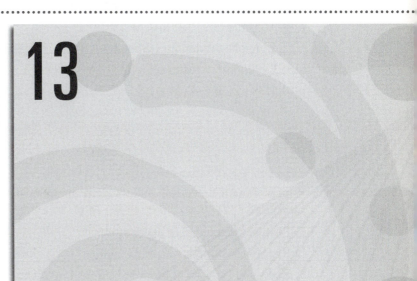

13

1. The nurse evaluates which of the following drugs to place the surgical client at risk for perioperative complications?

Select all that apply:

[   ] 1. Acetaminophen (Tylenol)

[   ] 2. Acetylsalicylic acid (aspirin)

[   ] 3. Omeprazole (Prilosec)

[   ] 4. Diphenhydramine (Sominex)

[   ] 5. Ibuprofen (Motrin)

[   ] 6. Sertraline (Zoloft)

2. Which of the following should the nurse include when teaching a client about an upcoming outpatient surgery?

1. Postoperative nursing interventions

2. Risk for postoperative complications

3. Risks and benefits of proposed surgical procedure

4. Risks and benefits of anesthetic choices

3. In reviewing the chart of a client about to undergo general anesthesia, which of the following is the greatest risk factor? The client who

1. expresses anxiety about the upcoming procedure.

2. ate a snack within the last three hours.

3. smokes and states his last cigarette was 24 hours ago.

4. has a history of hypertension controlled by diet and exercise.

Answer: 2, 4, 5, 6

Rationale: Drugs that place clients at risk during the perioperative period include aspirin, antidepressants, anticholinergics, steroids, nonsteroidal anti-inflammatory, antihypertensives, tranquilizers, diuretics, and drugs containing bromide. Acetylsalicylic acid (aspirin) may increase bleeding during surgery. Diphenhydramine (Sominex) contains bromide, which can accumulate in the body and produce manifestations of dementia. Nonsteroidal anti-inflammatory drugs such as ibuprofen (Motrin) may increase the risk of stress ulcers and displace other drugs from blood proteins. Antidepressants such as sertraline (Zoloft) may lower blood pressure during anesthesia. Acetaminophen (Tylenol) and omeprazole (Prilosec) have no effect on the surgical process.

Nursing process: Evaluation

Client need: Pharmacological and Parenteral Therapies

Cognitive level: Analysis

Subject area: Pharmacologic

Answer: 1

Rationale: Preoperative teaching involves educating the client about anticipated postoperative nursing interventions including turning, coughing, deep breathing, and leg exercises. Risks of complications, proposed surgical procedures, and anesthetic choices are primarily discussed with the client by the surgical and anesthetic team.

Nursing process: Planning

Client need: Physiological Adaptation

Cognitive level: Application

Subject area: Medical-Surgical

Answer: 2

Rationale: Aspiration poses a risk during general anesthesia. Clients are instructed not to eat or drink anything prior to general anesthesia in order to reduce the risk of aspiration. While cigarette smoking and controlled hypertension may increase risks of complications postoperatively, aspiration poses a more significant risk in this situation. Anxiety does not pose a risk factor for general anesthesia.

Nursing process: Assessment

Client need: Reduction of Risk Potential

Cognitive level: Analysis

Subject area: Medical-Surgical

4. Which of the following is a priority in the nursing assessment of a client preoperatively?

1. Question the client about any known allergies

2. Verification of client identification

3. Determination of client's nutritional status

4. Verification of client's neurological status

5. The nurse is obtaining a nursing history from a client suspected to be at risk for malignant hyperthermia. Which of the following should the nurse assess first to elicit the most accurate risk assessment?

1. Previous history of complications associated with surgery

2. Drug allergies

3. Over-the-counter medication usage

4. History of unexplained fevers

6. The nurse is concerned about a client's risk for impaired gas exchange related to ineffective airway clearance. Which of the following would be a priority assessment?

1. Number of respirations per minute

2. Number of liters of oxygen per minute inspired

3. Decreased air movement

4. Capillary refill

7. The nurse is caring for a postoperative client who has received a general anesthetic. Which of the following observations is the priority to be immediately reported?

1. Complaints of nausea

2. Mild hypertension

3. Decreased urine output

4. Rising body temperature

Answer: 2

Rationale: Prior to completing any assessment of a client preoperatively, it is imperative to correctly verify the client's identity. After verification of client identity, the nursing assessment can continue; this would include assessing the client's allergies, as well as, nutritional and neurological status.

Nursing process: Evaluation

Client need: Management of Care

Cognitive level: Analysis

Subject area: Medical-Surgical

Answer: 1

Rationale: An integral part of the preoperative nursing assessment is the determination of previous complications associated with surgery. Drug allergies, over-the-counter medication usage, and a history of unexplained fevers are not associated with malignant hyperthermia. Malignant hyperthermia is a potentially life-threatening syndrome characterized by a hypermetabolic state caused by certain anesthetic agents, such as succinylcholine.

Nursing process: Assessment

Client need: Reduction of Risk Potential

Cognitive level: Application

Subject area: Medical-Surgical

Answer: 3

Rationale: Decreased air movement may indicate a significant respiratory compromise. Assessing the client's ability to move air is a priority nursing assessment. The number of respirations per minute, number of liters of oxygen inspired, and capillary refill are important assessment data, but are not priority assessments.

Nursing process: Assessment

Client need: Management of Care

Cognitive level: Analysis

Subject area: Medical-Surgical

Answer: 4

Rationale: A rising body temperature can indicate malignant hyperthermia, a rare but life-threatening complication to general anesthesia. Complaints of nausea, mild hypertension, and decreased urine output would need to be conveyed to the anesthesia or surgical team, but are not the emergent complaints.

Nursing process: Analysis

Client need: Management of Care

Cognitive level: Analysis

Subject area: Medical-Surgical

8. The nurse is caring for a client who is perioperative. Which of the following is a priority nursing intervention utilized to prevent infection in this client?

    1. Preparation of the skin overlying the surgical site

    2. Maintenance of hemodynamic status

    3. Maintenance of client's temperature

    4. Determination of estimated blood loss

9. When caring for a client receiving conscious sedation, which of the following should the perioperative nurse routinely monitor?

    1. Temperature

    2. Level of consciousness

    3. Dermatome level

    4. Urine output

10. Which of the following should the perioperative nurse monitor when evaluating the presence of ineffective thermoregulation in a client?

    1. Cardiac rhythm

    2. Blood pressure

    3. Oxygen saturation level

    4. Temperature

11. Which of the following is the priority nursing intervention that the nurse should perform for a client in the postoperative period after surgery?

    1. Establish a patent airway

    2. Maintain adequate blood pressure

    3. Establish level of consciousness

    4. Assess level of pain

Answer: 1

Rationale: Preparation of the skin is a priority nursing intervention utilized to prevent infection. Maintenance of hemodynamic status, temperature, and estimated blood loss do not impact on a client's risk for infection.

Nursing process: Planning

Client need: Management of Care

Cognitive level: Analysis

Subject area: Medical-Surgical

Answer: 2

Rationale: Level of consciousness is routinely monitored in the provision of conscious sedation. Temperature and urine output are monitored in the postoperative phase. Dermatome level is monitored postoperatively after the provision of regional anesthesia.

Nursing process: Assessment

Client need: Reduction of Risk Potential

Cognitive level: Analysis

Subject area: Medical-Surgical

Answer: 4

Rationale: Body temperature is the primary method of assessment utilized by nurses to determine the client's thermoregulation. Cardiac rhythm, blood pressure, and oxygen saturation levels are all monitored, but give little indication of the client's risk for altered body temperature.

Nursing process: Assessment

Client need: Reduction of Risk Potential

Cognitive level: Application

Subject area: Medical-Surgical

Answer: 1

Rationale: The first priority in caring for a client in the postoperative period is the establishment of a patent airway. Maintenance of hemodynamic stability, determination of level of consciousness, and assessment of pain are all important aspects in postoperative care, but are not the priorities.

Nursing process: Implementation

Client need: Management of Care

Cognitive level: Analysis

Subject area: Medical-Surgical

12. The nurse is caring for a client postoperatively. Which of the following would indicate that the client has a compromised airway? The client
    1. complains of anxiety.
    2. complains of pain.
    3. has a pulse oximetry reading of 90%.
    4. is slightly cool and clammy.

13. The nurse is caring for a client who developed a compromised airway. Which of the following interventions is the priority to perform first?
    1. Reposition the client in a supine position
    2. Open the airway with a chin lift or jaw thrust
    3. Prepare for reintubation of the client
    4. Notify the surgeon

14. Which of the following nursing measures should the nurse include in the plan of care to help reduce the clinical manifestations of laryngospasm?
    1. Administer atropine
    2. Reposition the client in a supine position
    3. Administer high-flow oxygen via face mask
    4. Administer succinylcholine (Anectine)

15. The nurse is caring for a client in the immediate postoperative period. Which of the following would indicate that the client is becoming hypovolemic?
    1. A diastolic blood pressure of 100 mm Hg
    2. The client complains of excruciating pain
    3. The client complains of anxiety
    4. Blood loss of 500 ml

Answer: 1

Rationale: Hypoxemia is often associated with complaints of anxiety. A complaint of pain is a common postoperative complaint but is not associated with airway compromise. Normal pulse oximetry levels are above 90%. The assessment finding of coolness and clamminess is a nonspecific assessment finding that may indicate a wide variety of problems.

Nursing process: Evaluation

Client need: Physiological Adaptation

Cognitive level: Application

Subject area: Medical-Surgical

Answer: 2

Rationale: The initial priority nursing intervention for a client experiencing a compromised airway is the reestablishment of the airway. The client may need to be repositioned but often to a Fowler's or lateral position. The client may need to be reintubated and the surgeon should be notified, but these are not the priority interventions.

Nursing process: Implementation

Client need: Management of Care

Cognitive level: Analysis

Subject area: Medical-Surgical

Answer: 4

Rationale: With severe laryngospasm, a client may require the administration of a muscle relaxant like succinylcholine (Anectine) to relax the muscles of the larynx. Clients experiencing laryngospasm are often repositioned into a semi-Fowler's position. The administration of high-flow oxygen is based upon client's oxygen saturation levels and may be used to treat hypoxia, but will not directly reduce the clinical manifestations of laryngospasm.

Nursing process: Planning

Client need: Physiological Adaptation

Cognitive level: Analysis

Subject area: Medical-Surgical

Answer: 4

Rationale: Blood loss and resulting low fluid volume may result in hypovolemia in the postoperative period. Anxiety and pain may cause hypertension in the perioperative client, but would not cause hypovolemia. An elevated diastolic blood pressure is not indicative of hypovolemia.

Nursing process: Analysis

Client need: Physiological Adaptation

Cognitive level: Application

Subject area: Medical-Surgical

16. The nurse is caring for a client postoperatively who develops sinus tachycardia. Which of the following interventions should the nurse perform?

   1. Apply warmed blankets

   2. Administer atropine sulfate

   3. Position the client in a left lateral position

   4. Manage the client's anxiety

17. The nurse is caring for a client postoperatively who has become hypothermic. The nurse's best action would be to

   1. position the client in a left lateral position.

   2. administer an analgesic.

   3. remove clothing saturated with blood.

   4. monitor the intake and output.

18. A client is experiencing confusion in the immediate postoperative period. Which of the following assessments is essential to determine the reason for the confusion?

   1. Airway status

   2. Cardiac rhythm

   3. Level of consciousness

   4. Level of anxiety

19. The nurse admits a client scheduled for surgery. Which of the following findings should the nurse report as a risk factor for aspiration?

   1. Obesity

   2. Cigarette smoking

   3. An elevated serum sodium level

   4. A history of sleep apnea

Answer: 4

Rationale: Treatment of sinus tachycardia involves treating the underlying cause. Sinus tachycardia is a common dysrhythmia often caused by anxiety. Atropine is a drug commonly used to treat sinus bradycardia. Applying warmed blankets and positioning a client in the left lateral position would not be performed for sinus tachycardia.

Nursing process: Implementation

Client need: Physiological Adaptation

Cognitive level: Application

Subject area: Medical-Surgical

Answer: 3

Rationale: The nurse removes clothing saturated with blood and reapplies clean and dry clothing in order to maintain a client's body temperature. Repositioning a client, medicating a client for pain, or monitoring intake and output do not treat a client's low body temperature.

Nursing process: Planning

Client need: Physiological Adaptation

Cognitive level: Application

Subject area: Medical-Surgical

Answer: 1

Rationale: The nurse must first rule out hypoxemia as being the cause of a client's confusion. A client with an impaired airway may be experiencing confusion due to hypoxemia. Cardiac rhythm, level of consciousness, and anxiety are all important assessments in the postoperative period, but are not the initial assessment in a client presenting with confusion.

Nursing process: Assessment

Client need: Physiological Adaptation

Cognitive level: Application

Subject area: Medical-Surgical

Answer: 1

Rationale: Obesity increases a client's risk for aspiration due to increased pressure of abdominal contents on the lower esophageal sphincter. Cigarette smoking, an elevated serum sodium level, or a history of sleep apnea do not increase the risk of aspiration.

Nursing process: Analysis

Client need: Reduction of Risk Potential

Cognitive level: Analysis

Subject area: Medical-Surgical

20. Which of the following is a priority in the plan of care for a client who has had abdominal surgery and complains of pain in the immediate postoperative period?

    1. Monitor the client's blood pressure

    2. Teach the client to splint the abdomen

    3. Reposition the client for comfort

    4. Ask the client to describe the pain

21. A 16-year-old client has a medical history of anorexia nervosa. The nurse is preparing the client for abdominal surgery. The nurse is most concerned about the client's risk for

    1. aspiration.

    2. infection.

    3. hypovolemia.

    4. tissue perfusion.

22. A client is scheduled for an operative procedure to rule out cancer. When the nurse assesses the client, the nurse observes tears in the client's eyes. Which of the following would be the most therapeutic nursing intervention?

    1. Contact the surgeon to alleviate the client's concerns

    2. Ask the client to describe his or her feelings

    3. Medicate the client with a preoperative analgesic

    4. Reassure the client that there is nothing to be concerned about

23. A client is admitted for emergency surgery for a bowel obstruction. The perioperative nurse understands that the client is at greatest risk during the perioperative period for

    1. infection.

    2. electrolyte imbalances.

    3. aspiration.

    4. airway obstruction.

Answer: 4

Rationale: A priority assessment for a client's pain includes a description of the severity and nature of the pain as experienced by the client. Monitoring blood pressure, repositioning of the client, and teaching the client to splint the abdomen are all important postoperative nursing interventions, but are not priority interventions in the management of the client's postoperative pain.

Nursing process: Planning

Client need: Management of Care

Cognitive level: Analysis

Subject area: Medical-Surgical

Answer: 2

Rationale: Clients who have experienced anorexia nervosa are at risk for malnutrition and lowered immune function, and may experience an increased risk of infection and tissue healing. A history of anorexia nervosa does not pose a greater than average risk for aspiration, hypovolemia, or altered tissue perfusion.

Nursing process: Analysis

Client need: Reduction of Risk Potential

Cognitive level: Analysis

Subject area: Medical-Surgical

Answer: 2

Rationale: Assessing what the client is actually experiencing will assist the nurse in selecting the most appropriate nursing intervention. Supporting and advocating for the client are nursing responsibilities. The surgeon may be contacted if the client has specific concerns, but would not be contacted prior to an initial assessment. Medicating the client with a preoperative analgesic would be inappropriate without first addressing the client's concerns or questions.

Nursing process: Planning

Client need: Physiological Adaptation

Cognitive level: Application

Subject area: Medical-Surgical

Answer: 3

Rationale: Clients who have bowel obstructions are at increased risk of aspiration because the intestinal contents can be vomited and aspirated during induction of anesthesia. Clients who have bowel obstructions are not at an increased risk during the perioperative period for infection or airway obstruction. Fluid shifts may occur in the client with a bowel obstruction, but aspiration presents a greater risk for the client.

Nursing process: Analysis

Client need: Reduction of Risk Potential

Cognitive level: Analysis

Subject area: Medical-Surgical

24. A client admitted to the postanesthesia care unit (PACU) after abdominal surgery complains of "feeling a pop" and a gush of warm fluid at the incision site. The nurse concludes that the client has experienced a wound dehiscence. The priority nursing interventions would be which of the following?

Select all that apply:

[   ] **1.** Position the client in a supine position

[   ] **2.** Obtain a complete set of vital signs

[   ] **3.** Cover the incision with a sterile dressing

[   ] **4.** Apply oxygen via nasal cannula at 8 L per minute

[   ] **5.** Contact the surgical team

[   ] **6.** Increase the IV fluid rate

25. A client has a PCA (patient-controlled analgesia) machine ordered to manage postoperative pain. The PACU (postanesthesia care unit) nurse determines that the best time to initiate the PCA machine is

1. when the client complains of pain.

2. when the client arrives at the PACU.

3. just prior to transfer of the client to the floor.

4. when the client shows evidence of nonverbal signs of pain.

26. The registered nurse is preparing the clinical assignments for the day. Which of the following may the nurse delegate to a licensed practical nurse?

1. Inform a client scheduled for surgery on the surgical procedure

2. Instruct a client scheduled for surgery on the preoperative preparation

3. Obtain an informed consent from a client

4. Administer the preoperative intramuscular medication

Answer: 1, 3, 5

Rationale: The priority nursing interventions include repositioning the client in a supine position to prevent evisceration of abdominal contents, covering the wound with a sterile dressing, and notifying the surgical team immediately. Administering oxygen may be applied if the client's oxygen saturation is low. The IV rate may be increased if there is an indication to do so, but is not a priority intervention.

Nursing process: Implementation

Client need: Management of Care

Cognitive level: Analysis

Subject area: Medical-Surgical

Answer: 2

Rationale: PCA (patient-controlled analgesia) is an effective mechanism for the management of client pain. It is initiated upon arrival to the postanesthesia care unit (PACU) and client education is reinforced during the client's stay in the PACU. A delay in initiation of the PCA device may cause an increase in client pain.

Nursing process: Implementation

Client need: Pharmacological and Parenteral Therapies

Cognitive level: Application

Subject area: Medical-Surgical

Answer: 4

Rationale: A licensed practical nurse may administer a preoperative intramuscular medication to a client scheduled for surgery. Informing a client scheduled for surgery on the surgical procedure and instructing a client scheduled for surgery on the preoperative preparation are job tasks reserved for the registered nurse. A licensed practical nurse may not obtain an informed consent because the surgeon must inform the client about the surgical procedure and obtain the informed consent.

Nursing process: Planning

Client need: Management of Care

Cognitive level: Analysis

Subject area: Legal and Ethical Issues

UNIT II

Pharmacologic Nursing

Medication Therapy

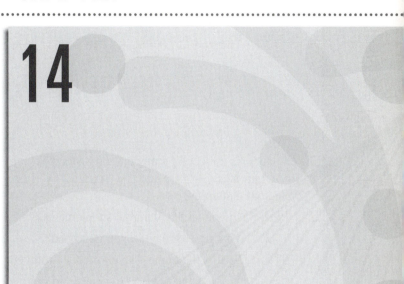

14

1. The nurse is preparing to administer insulin to a client with diabetes mellitus for which of the following purposes?

    1. Relief of disease manifestations

    2. Preventive

    3. Health maintenance

    4. Curative

2. The nurse is collecting a medication history. Which of the following questions would elicit the most accurate information?

    Select all that apply:

    [　] **1.** "Do you take any herbal supplements?"

    [　] **2.** "What time of day do you go to bed?"

    [　] **3.** "What is the highest level of education you completed?"

    [　] **4.** "Do you have a vision or hearing impairment?"

    [　] **5.** "Where do you eat most of your meals?"

    [　] **6.** "Do you have drug insurance coverage?"

3. Which of the following should the nurse include in the oral drug administration procedure? Administer

    1. a drug to a 3-year-old child as a capsule.

    2. two drugs at a time to an older adult client.

    3. a carbonated beverage over ice following a drug.

    4. a sustained action buccal drug under the tongue.

4. When documenting, the nurse correctly abbreviates a drug administered by mouth as _____.

Answer: 3

Rationale: Health maintenance drugs, such as insulin, vitamins, and minerals, are used to keep the body healthy. Relief of disease manifestations, such as antihistamines, is the most common use of drugs used in treatment. Preventive drugs, such as a hepatitis vaccine, are used to prevent disease. Curative drugs, such as antibiotics, are used to cure disease.

Nursing process: Planning

Client need: Pharmacological and Parenteral Therapies

Cognitive level: Analysis

Subject area: Pharmacologic

Answer: 1, 3, 4, 6

Rationale: When obtaining a medication history, it is important to assess if herbal supplements are taken, because of drug and herb interactions. Assessing an impairment of vision or hearing would evaluate the client's inability to correctly administer the drugs. Drug insurance coverage assures that the client is more likely to obtain the drug and comply with the treatment plan. It is important to assess the client's level of education to facilitate appropriate teaching.

Nursing process: Assessment

Client need: Pharmacological and Parenteral Therapies

Cognitive level: Analysis

Subject area: Pharmacologic

Answer: 3

Rationale: Pouring a carbonated beverage over ice and administering it after a drug will decrease nausea. Drugs should be administered in liquid form to children under the age of 5 years. Administering one drug at a time is recommended for an older adult client because of a possibility of impaired swallowing. A buccal drug is a drug to be placed inside the mouth or cheek.

Nursing process: Planning

Client need: Pharmacological and Parenteral Therapies

Cognitive level: Application

Subject area: Pharmacologic

Answer: PO

Rationale: The correct abbreviation for by mouth is PO or po.

Nursing process: Implementation

Client need: Pharmacological and Parenteral Therapies

Cognitive level: Comprehension

Subject area: Pharmacologic

5. Which of the following should the nurse include when administering drugs by a nasogastric tube?
    1. Crush the drug before administering through a feeding tube
    2. Flush between drugs with 10 ml of sterile water
    3. Administer one drug with 30 ml of water
    4. Maintain the client in an upright position for 15 minutes following drug administration

6. Which of the following principles of parenteral drug administration is a priority for the nurse to consider before administering a parenteral injection to a 2-year-old child?
    1. Apply EMLA (lidocaine 2.5% and prilocaine 2.5%) to the injection site one hour before administering the injection
    2. Lightly tap the injection site before administering the injection
    3. Administer up to 1 ml of the prescribed drug to the injection site
    4. Select the vastus lateralis for the administration of the drug

7. The nurse selects which of the following isotonic intravenous solutions for the primary purpose of promoting rehydration and elimination, while providing a good vehicle for potassium replacement?
    1. Sodium chloride 0.45%
    2. Dextrose 5% in water
    3. Dextrose 5% in 0.45% saline
    4. Ringer's lactate

Answer: 3

Rationale: One drug should be administered at a time through a nasogastric tube, but it is better to avoid administering drugs through a feeding tube because the lumen is much smaller than a nasogastric tube. Administer each drug with 5 to 30 ml of water and flush with 5 to 30 ml of water between drugs. The client should be placed in an upright position for at least 30 minutes following drug administration.

Nursing process: Planning

Client need: Pharmacological and Parenteral Therapies

Cognitive level: Application

Subject area: Pharmacologic

Answer: 4

Rationale: The priority of any intramuscular injection is the selection of the appropriate site. The vastus lateralis is the preferred site of drug administration in children under the age of 3. EMLA (lidocaine 2.5% and prilocaine 2.5%) may be applied to an intramuscular injection site one to two hours before administering an injection to a child, but the priority is site selection. Tapping the injection site before administering an injection to a child is helpful because it distracts the child (who then focuses on the tap and not the injection). No more than 1 ml should be administered to a child.

Nursing process: Planning

Client need: Management of Care

Cognitive level: Application

Subject area: Pharmacologic

Answer: 2

Rationale: Dextrose 5% in water is an isotonic intravenous solution with the primary purpose of promoting rehydration and elimination, while providing a good vehicle for potassium replacement. Sodium chloride 0.45% is a hypotonic solution that moves fluids into the cells. It is used to provide daily maintenance of body fluid and establishment of renal function. The client should be monitored for water intoxication. Dextrose 5% in 0.45% saline is a hypertonic solution that draws fluids from the cells. The client should be monitored for dehydration. Ringer's lactate is an isotonic solution that resembles the normal composition of blood serum and plasma. It contains sodium, potassium, calcium, chloride, lactate, but no dextrose.

Nursing process: Implementation

Client need: Pharmacological and Parenteral Therapies

Cognitive level: Analysis

Subject area: Pharmacologic

8. The nurse selects which of the following IV site locations when starting an IV in the medial antebrachial vein? (Label the medial antebrachial vein on the accompanying figure.)

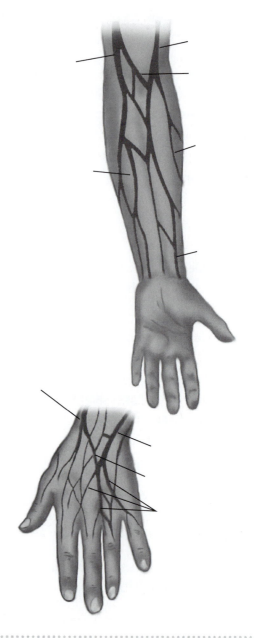

9. The nurse is preparing the client assignments for the day. Which of the following assignments would be appropriate for the registered nurse (RN) to assign to a licensed practical nurse (LPN)?

   1. Administer a drug to a client who has an implantable intravenous infusion port

   2. Insert an angiocath into the medial antebrachial vein of a client going to surgery

   3. Instruct a client on the advantages of an autologous blood transfusion

   4. Discontinue a client's peripheral IV site

Answer:

> **Rationale:** None
>
> **Nursing process:** Implementation
>
> **Client need:** Pharmacological and Parenteral Therapies
>
> **Cognitive level:** Application
>
> **Subject area:** Pharmacologic

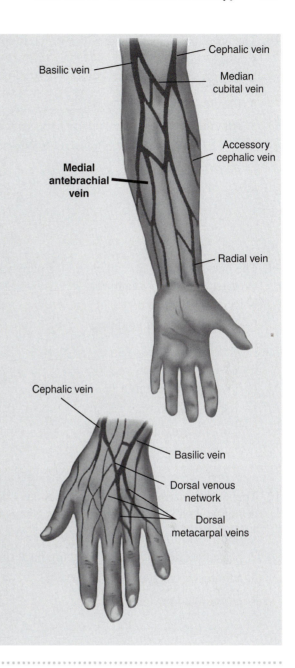

Cephalic vein

Basilic vein

Median cubital vein

Accessory cephalic vein

Medial antebrachial vein

Radial vein

Cephalic vein

Basilic vein

Dorsal venous network

Dorsal metacarpal veins

Answer: 4

Rationale: A licensed practical nurse may discontinue an uncomplicated peripheral IV site. An LPN or any RN who has not been specially trained may not access an implantable intravenous infusion port, because of the risk of infection. Only an RN may insert an IV line such as an angiocath. An LPN may not instruct a client on the various types of blood transfusions. That is a task for an RN.

Nursing process: Planning

Client need: Management of Care

Cognitive level: Analysis

Subject area: Legal and Ethical Issues

10. The nurse prepares to hang which of the following for a client with thrombocytopenia?

   1. Whole blood

   2. Packed red blood cells

   3. Platelets

   4. Albumin

11. The nurse is caring for a client with a peripheral IV. Which of the following would indicate the client is experiencing hypervolemia?
Select all that apply:

   [   ] **1.** Nausea and vomiting

   [   ] **2.** Headache

   [   ] **3.** Dyspnea

   [   ] **4.** Hypertension

   [   ] **5.** Fever

   [   ] **6.** Tachycardia

12. The nurse is caring for a client with an IV who is experiencing dyspnea, hypotension, a weak, rapid pulse, a decreased level of consciousness, and who is becoming cyanotic. The priority nursing intervention is to

   1. notify the physician.

   2. place the client in a Trendelenburg position.

   3. administer oxygen.

   4. discontinue the IV.

Answer: 3

Rationale: Platelets are administered in the treatment of bleeding disorders, such as thrombocytopenia. Whole blood is not used as much as packed red blood cells but may be used in cases of hemorrhage. Red blood cells are used to replace erythrocytes in conditions such as anemia or blood loss. Albumin is used to restore intravascular volume in the treatment of shock and hypoproteinemia.

Nursing process: Implementation

Client need: Pharmacological and Parenteral Therapies

Cognitive level: Analysis

Subject area: Pharmacologic

Answer: 3, 4, 6

Rationale: Clinical manifestations of hypervolemia with intravenous therapy include dyspnea, hypertension, tachycardia, coughing, pulmonary edema, cyanosis, rales, and increased venous pressure. Nausea, vomiting, and fever are clinical manifestations of a pyrogenic reaction.

Nursing process: Evaluation

Client need: Pharmacological and Parenteral Therapies

Cognitive level: Application

Subject area: Pharmacologic

Answer: 4

Rationale: A client who is dyspneic, has hypotension and a weak, rapid pulse, a decreased level of consciousness, and is cyanotic is experiencing an air embolism. Administering oxygen, notifying the physician, and placing the client in a Trendelenburg position are all appropriate interventions, but the priority intervention is to immediately stop the entrance of air into the vein. As little as 10 ml of air may be fatal. An air embolism may result from a loose connection, tubing change, or inappropriately primed tubing. To assure that the entrance of air is stopped from entering the vein, it is safest and quickest to discontinue the IV instead of risking further air to enter the vein.

Nursing process: Implementation

Client need: Management of Care

Cognitive level: Application

Subject area: Pharmacologic

13. Because a client is receiving fresh plasma, the nurse should evaluate which of the following laboratory results for the effectiveness of therapy?

    1. Hemoglobin and hematocrit

    2. Platelets

    3. Prothrombin (PT) and partial thromboplastin (PTT)

    4. White blood cells

14. The nurse is teaching a class on controlled substances. Which of the following should the nurse include in the class?

    1. There is no accepted medical use for schedule I controlled substances

    2. Examples of schedule II drugs include glutethimide (Doriden), secobarbital (Seconal), and hydrocodone with acetaminophen (Vicodin)

    3. Schedule III controlled substances have a high potential for abuse

    4. Schedule IV controlled substances are over-the-counter narcotics that must be sold by a registered pharmacist

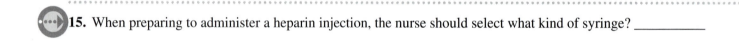

15. When preparing to administer a heparin injection, the nurse should select what kind of syringe? _____

16. The nurse prepares to administer meperidine (Demerol) intramuscularly to an adult client by selecting which of the following gauge needles?

    1. 16 gauge

    2. 18 gauge

    3. 23 gauge

    4. 26 gauge

Answer: 3

Rationale: The prothrombin (PT) and partial thromboplastin (PTT) laboratory tests should be evaluated to determine the effectiveness of receiving fresh plasma. The hematocrit and hemoglobin are evaluated to indicate successful red blood cell therapy. The platelets should be monitored to evaluate successful platelet therapy. The white blood cell count would be evaluated to determine effective granulocyte therapy.

Nursing process: Evaluation

Client need: Pharmacological and Parenteral Therapies

Cognitive level: Analysis

Subject area: Pharmacologic

Answer: 1

Rationale: Schedule I controlled substances have no acceptable medical use and are used for research purposes only. Glutethimide (Doriden), secobarbital (Seconal), and hydrocodone with acetaminophen (Vicodin) are examples of schedule III drugs. Schedule II controlled substances have a high potential for abuse and schedule III drugs have a moderate potential for abuse. Schedule V controlled substances are over-the-counter narcotics that must be sold by a registered pharmacist.

Nursing process: Planning

Client need: Pharmacological and Parenteral Therapies

Cognitive level: Analysis

Subject area: Pharmacologic

Answer: Tuberculin

Rationale: A tuberculin syringe has a volume of 1 ml with a scale of 0.01 ml and is used for heparin injections.

Nursing process: Planning

Client need: Pharmacological and Parenteral Therapies

Cognitive level: Comprehension

Subject area: Pharmacologic

Answer: 3

Rationale: The appropriate gauge needle to administer an intramuscular injection to an adult client is 21 to 23 gauge.

Nursing process: Implementation

Client need: Pharmacological and Parenteral Therapies

Cognitive level: Comprehension

Subject area: Pharmacologic

17. The client is receiving a unit of packed red blood cells. Which of the following observations indicate to the nurse that the client is having an acute hemolytic reaction?
Select all that apply:

[   ] **1.** Tachycardia

[   ] **2.** Headache

[   ] **3.** Fever

[   ] **4.** Hypertension

[   ] **5.** Dyspnea

[   ] **6.** Back pain

18. The nurse should select what gauge needle to administer blood? _____

19. The nurse should instruct a client receiving a blood transfusion to notify the nurse if itching, urticaria, wheezing, or a rash appears for how many hours after completion of the transfusion? _____

20. When administering intravenous therapy to a client, it would be essential for the nurse to include which of the following aspects of the procedure?

1. Make a time strip on the bag with a felt-tip marker

2. Change the tubing every 24 hours

3. Replace the intravenous solution with the same solution when the current solution runs out

4. Avoid letting the intravenous solution hang more than 24 hours

Answer: 1, 2, 5, 6

Rationale: Clinical manifestations of an acute hemolytic reaction include tachycardia, headache, hypotension, dyspnea, back pain, chest pain, and cyanosis.

Nursing process: Evaluation

Client need: Pharmacological and Parenteral Therapies

Cognitive level: Application

Subject area: Pharmacologic

Answer: 16

Rationale: Blood is administered with a 16-gauge needle.

Nursing process: Implementation

Client need: Pharmacological and Parenteral Therapies

Cognitive level: Comprehension

Subject area: Pharmacologic

Answer: One

Rationale: Itching, urticaria, wheezing, or a rash are all clinical manifestations of a mild allergic reaction to a blood transfusion and may occur immediately or up to one hour after the transfusion.

Nursing process: Implementation

Client need: Pharmacological and Parenteral Therapies

Cognitive level: Application

Subject area: Pharmacologic

Answer: 4

Rationale: An intravenous solution should not hang more than 24 to 72 hours. Intravenous tubing should be changed every 48 to 72 hours. The IV solution to be hung should always be checked against the current doctor's order. It is unsafe practice to just hang the solution running out, because the order may have been changed. A time strip should never be made with a felt-tip marker because the ink from the marker may leech through the plastic bag and contaminate the solution.

Nursing process: Planning

Client need: Pharmacological and Parenteral Therapies

Cognitive level: Application

Subject area: Pharmacologic

21. The nurse should include which of the following in the administration of an intravenous solution?

    1. Select a microdrip chamber for medications administered to a pediatric client
    2. Set the end time of an infusion on a controller to initiate the alarm 20 minutes before the scheduled end time
    3. Select a macrodrip chamber for medications administered to a geriatric client
    4. Choose a volume-control administration set to deliver a large amount of an intravenous solution

22. After initiating intravenous therapy, a client experiences chills, headaches, backache, and a temperature of 38.3°C, or 101°F. The nurse should report this as which of the following types of intravenous reactions?

    1. Phlebitis
    2. Pyrogenic reaction
    3. Thrombophlebitis
    4. Air embolism

23. Which of the following is a priority for the nurse to perform on a client who has a thrombophlebitis?

    1. Apply warm moist compresses to the area
    2. Document the appearance of the IV site
    3. Discontinue the IV
    4. Notify the physician

24. The nurse is observing another nurse start an intravenous infusion. Which of the following would indicate the nurse starting the IV does not understand the procedure?

    1. Select a butterfly needle for an endoscopy procedure
    2. Select the scalp vein for an infant
    3. Cleanse the selected IV site with Betadine followed by alcohol
    4. Use a venoscope to find a difficult vein

Answer: 1

Rationale: A microdrip chamber should be selected when administering medications to both pediatric and geriatric clients. As a safety feature, the infusion controller alarm should be set to go off 50 ml before the volume is infused. A volume-control administration set delivers a small amount of IV fluid to a pediatric client or in a critical care situation.

Nursing process: Planning

Client need: Pharmacological and Parenteral Therapies

Cognitive level: Application

Subject area: Pharmacologic

Answer: 2

Rationale: Clinical manifestations of a pyrogenic reaction include a sudden increased temperature, chills, backache, headache, general malaise, and nausea and vomiting.

Nursing process: Analysis

Client need: Pharmacological and Parenteral Therapies

Cognitive level: Application

Subject area: Pharmacologic

Answer: 3

Rationale: Discontinuing the IV is the priority nursing intervention when a thrombophlebitis is present. After discontinuing an intravenous solution, warm moist compresses are applied to the area, the physician is notified, the incident is documented, and the IV is restarted at another site.

Nursing process: Implementation

Client need: Pharmacological and Parenteral Therapies

Cognitive level: Application

Subject area: Pharmacologic

Answer: 3

Rationale: Cleansing the selected IV with Betadine followed by alcohol may form a toxic material that may be absorbed through the skin. It is appropriate to select a butterfly needle for an endoscopy procedure, use the scalp vein for an infant, or find a difficult vein with a venoscope.

Nursing process: Evaluation

Client need: Pharmacological and Parenteral Therapies

Cognitive level: Application

Subject area: Pharmacologic

25. The nurse should monitor a client with a central venous catheter for which of the following manifestations of a pneumothorax?
Select all that apply:

[   ] **1.** Hypertension

[   ] **2.** Shortness of breath

[   ] **3.** Flushing

[   ] **4.** Lethargy

[   ] **5.** Chest pain

[   ] **6.** Weak, rapid pulse

26. A client receiving a blood transfusion complains of chills, headache, backache, and suddenly spikes in temperature. The priority nursing action is to

1. flush the tubing with normal saline.

2. slow the transfusion.

3. discontinue the transfusion.

4. continue to monitor the client.

27. The nurse identifies which of the following orders as an intermittent intravenous infusion?

1. Diazepam (Valium) 5 mg IV push

2. 500 ml intralipids IV in 6 hours

3. Potassium chloride 20 mEq in 1000 ml every 8 hours

4. Ranitidine (Zantac) 0.5 mg in 50 ml 0.9% NaCl over 20 minutes every 6 hours

28. Which of the following principles of intravenous push does the nurse consider before administering a drug by this route?

1. There is less of a risk of adverse reactions with the IV push route

2. The rate of IV push administration must be verified in a drug book

3. All IV push drugs must be diluted in 50 ml of NaCl before administration

4. All IV push drugs should be administered within one minute or less

Answer: 2, 5, 6

Rationale: Clinical manifestations of a pneumothorax include sudden shortness of breath, sharp chest pain, hypotension, pallor, cyanosis, and a weak, rapid pulse, which may indicate the pleural membrane has been punctured.

Nursing process: Assessment

Client need: Pharmacological and Parenteral Therapies

Cognitive level: Application

Subject area: Pharmacologic

Answer: 3

Rationale: Blood administration reactions generally occur within the first 15 minutes. Chills, headache, backache, and a sudden spike in temperature indicate a reaction. The priority nursing action is to discontinue the transfusion and notify the physician immediately.

Nursing process: Implementation

Client need: Pharmacological and Parenteral Therapies

Cognitive level: Application

Subject area: Pharmacologic

Answer: 4

Rationale: An intermittent intravenous infusion is the administration of an IV drug without the infusion of solution. These infusions are administered at regularly scheduled times. An example of an intermittent intravenous infusion is ranitidine (Zantac) 0.5 mg in 50 ml 0.9% NaCl over 20 minutes every 6 hours.

Nursing process: Analysis

Client need: Pharmacological and Parenteral Therapies

Cognitive level: Application

Subject area: Pharmacologic

Answer: 2

Rationale: Administering a drug by the IV push rate is a way to administer a small amount of a drug in a short period of time. The rate of any IV drug must be verified in a drug book before administration. Because this is a rapid way of administering drugs to a client, there is a high risk of adverse reactions possible. If the drug is given too quickly, such as in one minute or less, there is no opportunity to discontinue the drug should a reaction occur.

Nursing process: Implementation

Client need: Pharmacological and Parenteral Therapies

Cognitive level: Application

Subject area: Pharmacologic

29. What type of IV solution should the nurse use to prime blood tubing? _____

- -

30. The nurse is observing another nurse administer blood. Which of the following indicates to the observing nurse that the administering nurse does not understand blood administration?

1. Run the blood slowly for the first 15 minutes at 20 drops per minute

2. Establish the required flow rate after 15 minutes if no signs of a reaction

3. Infuse the transfusion slowly over 6 hours

4. Assess the vital signs every 30 minutes until one hour post-transfusion

- -

31. The nurse assesses which of the following clients to be most appropriate for the selection of the central venous catheter?

1. A client who is dehydrated with hypokalemia requiring fluid and electrolyte replacement

2. A client who has cancer of the esophagus and is receiving chemotherapy

3. A client who has an infection and needs short-term antibiotics

4. A client who had gallbladder surgery and is experiencing post-op nausea

- -

32. Which of the following should the nurse include when caring for a client with a peripherally inserted central venous catheter (PICC)?

1. Weigh the client daily

2. Avoid taking the blood pressure in the arm on the side of the PICC

3. Take the temperature every four hours

4. Monitor the client's response to fluid and electrolyte therapy

- -

Answer: 0.9% NaCl

Rationale: Only 0.9% NaCl should be used to prime blood tubing. Any IV solution with dextrose in it causes coagulation of the blood cells.

Nursing process: Implementation

Client need: Pharmacological and Parenteral Therapies

Cognitive level: Comprehension

Subject area: Pharmacologic

Answer: 3

Rationale: Blood should not hang for more than four hours. If it hangs for more than four hours, there is a risk of bacterial growth. Blood should be run slowly for the first 15 minutes at 20 drops per minute. If no reaction occurs after 15 minutes, the flow rate may be established. The vital signs should be assessed every 30 minutes until one hour after transfusion to make sure that no reaction is occurring.

Nursing process: Evaluation

Client need: Pharmacological and Parenteral Therapies

Cognitive level: Analysis

Subject area: Pharmacologic

Answer: 2

Rationale: A central venous catheter is generally inserted into the internal jugular and subclavian veins with the distal tip located in the superior vena cava to minimize vessel irritation and sclerosis. It is used for long-term therapy, such as for a client who has cancer of the esophagus and is receiving chemotherapy.

Nursing process: Assessment

Client need: Pharmacological and Parenteral Therapies

Cognitive level: Analysis

Subject area: Pharmacologic

Answer: 2

Rationale: The taking of blood pressure should be avoided in the arm on the side of a peripherally inserted central catheter (PICC).

Nursing process: Planning

Client need: Pharmacological and Parenteral Therapies

Cognitive level: Application

Subject area: Pharmacologic

33. The nurse is caring for a client with a central venous access device. Which of the following clinical manifestations does the nurse interpret as indicative of a dislodged catheter?
Select all that apply:

[   ] **1.** Pain in the neck

[   ] **2.** Bleeding from the site

[   ] **3.** Gurgling sounds

[   ] **4.** Skin that is pale and cool to touch

[   ] **5.** Palpitations

[   ] **6.** Chills

34. The nurse is caring for a client with a central venous catheter who is experiencing chest pain, dyspnea, coughing, and apprehension. The nurse reports this as indicative of

1. an infection.

2. a thrombus.

3. a phlebitis.

4. an air embolism.

35. A student nurse asks the nurse where a peripherally inserted central catheter is inserted. Which of the following is the appropriate response by the nurse?

1. Subclavian vein

2. Jugular vein

3. Antecubital area of the basilic vein

4. Directly into the superior vena cava

Answer: 1, 3, 5

Rationale: Clinical manifestations of a dislodged catheter in a client with a central venous access device include pain in the neck, gurgling sounds, and palpitations.

Nursing process: Analysis

Client need: Pharmacological and Parenteral Therapies

Cognitive level: Analysis

Subject area: Pharmacologic

Answer: 4

Rationale: Clinical manifestations of an air embolism in a client with a central venous catheter include chest pain, dyspnea, coughing, and apprehension.

Nursing process: Analysis

Client need: Pharmacological and Parenteral Therapies

Cognitive level: Analysis

Subject area: Pharmacologic

Answer: 3

Rationale: A peripherally inserted central catheter is inserted into the antecubital area of the basilic vein.

Nursing process: Analysis

Client need: Pharmacological and Parenteral Therapies

Cognitive level: Analysis

Subject area: Pharmacologic

36. The nurse selects which of the following intravenous fluids to administer to a client who is very dehydrated with a serum potassium of 2.2 mEq/L, sodium of 129 mEq/L, and calcium of 7.5 mg/dl?

    1. Sodium chloride 0.45%
    2. Ringer's lactate
    3. Dextrose 5% in water
    4. Dextrose 10% in water

37. Which of the following evaluations does the nurse make when the venipuncture site has an observable swelling and is tender and cool to touch?

    1. An infection has developed
    2. Bleeding into the surrounding tissue has occurred
    3. The IV site has infiltrated
    4. A phlebitis is developing

38. A client receiving continuous intravenous therapy is complaining of dyspnea, cough, and tachycardia. The nurse auscultates crackles bilaterally. In determining what action to take next, which of the following factors should the nurse consider?

    1. The client is apprehensive about receiving continuous IV fluids
    2. The client has developed a respiratory infection or pneumonia
    3. The client is exhibiting signs of hypervolemia
    4. The client is experiencing internal bleeding

Answer: 2

Rationale: A client who has a serum potassium of 2.2 mEq/L, sodium of 129 mEq/L, and a calcium of 7.5 mg/dl would benefit from an intravenous solution that resembles the normal composition of the blood serum and plasma with a potassium level below the daily requirement. Ringer's lactate is an isotonic solution that provides sodium, potassium, calcium, chloride, and lactate. Sodium chloride 0.45% is an isotonic solution that may be used for a daily maintenance of body fluid and establishment of renal function. Dextrose 5% in water is an isotonic solution that promotes rehydration and elimination. Administering D_5W may cause a sodium loss but does provide a good medium for administration of potassium. Dextrose 10% in water also contains a higher percentage of dextrose.

Nursing process: Implementation

Client need: Pharmacological and Parenteral Therapies

Cognitive level: Analysis

Subject area: Pharmacologic

Answer: 3

Rationale: An intravenous solution that has infiltrated develops a noticeable swelling and is tender and cool to touch. Infiltration may be caused by using the wrong gauge catheter, the wrong type of device, or by dislodgement of the device from the vein. A phlebitis results from a mechanical or chemical trauma. Tenderness is the first indication. Other clinical manifestations include a reddened area or pink or red stripe along the vein, warmth, and swelling. If the IV site develops an infection, the area becomes red, warm to touch, and may have an observable drainage. Bleeding into the surrounding tissue around an IV site may become swollen and red.

Nursing process: Evaluation

Client need: Pharmacological and Parenteral Therapies

Cognitive level: Application

Subject area: Pharmacologic

Answer: 3

Rationale: A client receiving a continuous intravenous solution who is complaining of dyspnea, cough, tachycardia, and who has crackles auscultated bilaterally is exhibiting clinical manifestations of hypervolemia, or an increased circulating volume. This may cause cardiac overload that can lead to pulmonary edema and cardiac failure. Hypervolemia may be caused by an intravenous solution running at too rapid a rate. Upon detection, the IV should be slowed to a keep-open rate and the physician should be notified.

Nursing process: Analysis

Client need: Reduction of Risk Potential

Cognitive level: Analysis

Subject area: Pharmacologic

39. Which of the following solutions should the nurse administer to correct an excessive fluid loss and provide sodium chloride to a client?

    1. Dextrose 5% in water
    2. Sodium chloride 0.45%
    3. Ringer's lactate
    4. Dextrose 5% in 0.45% normal saline

40. The nurse should perform which of the following CDC guidelines to decrease intravascular infection to intravenous therapy in adult clients?

    1. Routinely apply topical antimicrobial ointment to the insertion site of peripheral venous catheter
    2. Replace the IV tubing, including secondary tubing, and stopcocks every 24 hours
    3. Cleanse the skin site before the venipuncture with warm soapy water
    4. Replace short peripheral venous catheter and rotate sites every 48 to 72 hours

41. Which of the following should the nurse consider when selecting a site for venipuncture?

    1. Shave the insertion site and surrounding area
    2. Select a vein distal to a previously used venipuncture site
    3. Use the same finger to palpate a vein by pressing downward
    4. Apply the tourniquet two inches above the selected venipuncture site

Answer: 4

Rationale: Dextrose 5% in 0.45% normal saline promotes renal function and urinary output while providing calories and sodium to a client. It also corrects an excessive fluid loss. Although sodium chloride 0.45% establishes renal function while providing a daily maintenance of body fluids, it does not provide a source of calories. Ringer's lactate resembles the normal composition of blood and serum while replacing potassium in a client who is hypokalemic. Ringer's lactate contains sodium, potassium, calcium, chloride, and lactate. Dextrose 5% in water promotes rehydration and elimination, and serves as a good medium for the administration of potassium. It may also cause a loss of urinary sodium. D₅W is a source of calories, but does not provide a source of sodium.

Nursing process: Planning

Client need: Pharmacological and Parenteral Therapies

Cognitive level: Analysis

Subject area: Pharmacologic

Answer: 4

Rationale: In an adult client, short peripheral venous catheters should be replaced and the site rotated every 48 to 72 hours. Topical antimicrobial ointment should not be applied to the insertion site of a peripheral or central venous catheter. Prior to insertion, the insertion site should be cleansed with 70% alcohol or 10% povidone-iodine. IV tubing, including secondary tubing, and stopcocks should not be changed more frequently than every 72 hours.

Nursing process: Implementation

Client need: Reduction of Risk Potential

Cognitive level: Analysis

Subject area: Pharmacologic

Answer: 3

Rationale: The nurse should use the same finger to palpate the vein by pressing downward to determine resilience of the vein. The insertion site should not be shaved, because shaving may cause abrasions that predispose the site to infection. The tourniquet should be applied four to five inches above the proposed insertion site. An insertion site should not be selected if it is distal to a previous insertion site. This may cause the new IV to infiltrate.

Nursing process: Analysis

Client need: Pharmacological and Parenteral Therapies

Cognitive level: Analysis

Subject area: Pharmacologic

42. Which of the following gerontological considerations should the nurse include when selecting a venipuncture site and initiating intravenous therapy on an older adult client?

   1. Use a 22- to 24-gauge needle for the venipuncture

   2. Apply the tourniquet tightly and vigorously massage the selected vein

   3. Select a vein on the back of the dominant hand

   4. Secure the needle after the venipuncture with an adhesive tape and avoid covering the site

Answer: 1

Rationale: When initiating an intravenous solution in an older adult client, a 22- to 24-gauge needle is the best. A 22- to 24-gauge needle is used for the delivery of fluid and drugs. The dorsal metacarpal veins are the best veins. Because the veins of an older adult client are fragile, a loosely applied tourniquet or no tourniquet should be used. Adhesive tape should be avoided because the older adult client has fragile skin that can be easily torn. Paper tape is recommended.

Nursing process: Planning

Client need: Pharmacological and Parenteral Therapies

Cognitive level: Analysis

Subject area: Pharmacologic

Measurement and Drug Calculations

15

1. A physician has ordered acetylsalicylic acid (aspirin) 10 gr every 4 hours p.r.n. The available dose for aspirin is 325 mg per tablet. What will the nurse administer?

   1. 2 tabs

   2. 1 tab

   3. 6.6 tabs

   4. 1.5 tabs

2. The physician has ordered guaifenesin (Robitussin) expectorant syrup 1½ ounces p.o. every 4 hours. One 90 ml bottle of guaifenesin (Robitussin) syrup is available. What will the nurse administer?

   1. 30 ml

   2. 45 ml

   3. 15 ml

   4. 10 ml

Answer: 1

Rationale: Find the number of tablets to be administered.

1 gr = 60 mg and 1 tablet = 325 mg

First convert grains to milligrams.

1 gr = 60 mg, 10 gr = 600 mg

660 mg is the desired dose

Set up the ratio:

$$\frac{325 \text{ mg}}{1 \text{ tab}} = \frac{600 \text{ mg}}{x}$$

$$x = \frac{660}{325}$$

$$x = 2.03$$

Because conversions between apothecary and metric systems are not exact, two 325 mg tablets may be administered for the 600 mg (10 grains). The nurse will administer two tablets.

Nursing process: Implementation

Client need: Pharmacological and Parenteral Therapies

Cognitive level: Application

Subject area: Pharmacologic

Answer: 2

Rationale: Find the amount of expectorant that should be administered.

1 ounce = 30 ml

Convert ounces to milliliters.

1 ounce = 30 ml, 1½ ounces = 45 ml, x = 45 ml

The nurse will administer 45 ml.

Nursing process: Implementation

Client need: Pharmacological and Parenteral Therapies

Cognitive level: Application

Subject area: Pharmacologic

3. The physician's order reads phenytoin sodium (Dilantin) 0.1 g p.o. now. On hand are phenytoin sodium (Dilantin) capsules, 100 mg per capsule. The nurse will give

   1. 1 capsule.

   2. 3 capsules.

   3. 2 capsules.

   4. 1½ capsules.

4. The order reads levodopa (Dopar) 1.5 g p.o. b.i.d. On hand are levodopa (Dopar) tablets in a 500 mg strength. The nurse will give

   1. 1.5 tablets.

   2. 3 tablets.

   3. ½ tablet.

   4. 2 tablets.

Answer: 1

Rationale: Find the number of capsules to be administered.

The order is for 0.1 g and each capsule = 100 mg

Convert grams to milligrams.

1 gram = 1000 mg, 0.1 g = 100 mg,

x = 1 capsule

The nurse will administer one capsule.

Nursing process: Implementation

Client need: Pharmacological and Parenteral Therapies

Cognitive level: Application

Subject area: Pharmacologic

Answer: 2

Rationale: Find the number of tablets to be administered.

The order is for 1.5 g, and the tablets on hand are 500 mg.

First convert 1.5 g to milligrams.

1 gram = 1000 mg, 1.5 g = 1500 mg

Determine the number of tablets to be administered.

$$\frac{500 \text{ mg}}{1 \text{ tablet}} = \frac{1500 \text{ mg}}{x}$$

$$x = \frac{1500 \text{ mg}}{500 \text{ mg}} \text{ tablets,}$$

x = 3 tablets

The nurse will administer three tablets of levodopa (Dopar).

Nursing process: Implementation

Client need: Pharmacological and Parenteral Therapies

Cognitive level: Application

Subject area: Pharmacologic

5. The doctor's order states glipizide (Glucotrol) 5000 mcg daily. On hand the nurse has glipizide (Glucotrol) 2.5 mg tablets. How many tablets will the nurse administer?

   1. 1 tablet

   2. 2.5 tablets

   3. 0.2 tablets

   4. 2 tablets

6. The nurse reads a physician's order, which states atropine sulfate 0.5 mg IM stat. The nurse has atropine sulfate 0.3 mg/0.5 ml for injection available. What volume of the atropine solution should the nurse administer IM?

   1. 0.1 ml

   2. 0.5 ml

   3. 0.8 ml

   4. 1.0 ml

Answer: 4

Rationale: Find the number of tablets to be administered.

The order is for 5000 mcg, and the tablets on hand are 2.5 mg.

Convert 5000 mcg to milligrams.

1000 mcg = 1 mg, then 5000 mcg = 5 mg

Set up the ratio to determine the number of tablets to deliver.

$$\frac{2.5 \text{ mg}}{1 \text{ tab}} = \frac{5 \text{ mg}}{x}$$

$$x = \frac{5 \text{ mg}}{2.5 \text{ mg}} \text{ tablets}$$

x = 2 tablets

The nurse will administer two tablets of glipizide (Glucotrol).

Nursing process: Implementation

Client need: Pharmacological and Parenteral Therapies

Cognitive level: Application

Subject area: Pharmacologic

Answer: 3

Rationale: Find the volume for this injection.

Set up a ratio:

$$\frac{0.3 \text{ mg}}{5 \text{ ml}} = \frac{0.5 \text{ mg}}{x}$$

$$x = 5 \text{ ml} \times \frac{0.5 \text{ mg}}{0.3 \text{ mg}}$$

$$x = \frac{2.5}{0.3} \text{ ml}$$

x = 0.80 ml

The nurse will administer 0.8 ml of the injectable solution intramuscularly.

Nursing process: Implementation

Client need: Pharmacological and Parenteral Therapies

Cognitive level: Application

Subject area: Pharmacologic

7. The order reads hydromorphone HCl (Dilaudid) 1.5 mg s.q. every 4 to 6 hours p.r.n. The nurse has injectable hydromorphone HCl (Dilaudid) ampules gr 1/30 per ml. What volume will the nurse administer?

   1. 0.9 ml
   2. 7.5 ml
   3. 0.5 ml
   4. 0.75 ml

8. The doctor's order reads vitamin B_{12} injection 1000 mcg once a month. The nurse has injectable vitamin B_{12} available in a concentration of 0.5 mg/ml. What volume should the nurse administer?

   1. 2.5 ml
   2. 2 ml
   3. 0.5 ml
   4. 1 ml

Answer: 4

Rationale: Find the volume to inject.

Conversion: 1 gr = 60 mg, and the drug has 1/30 grain per ml

Convert 1/30 grain and 1.5 mg to the same units.

Note: It is generally easier to convert grains to milligrams.

$$1 \text{ gr} = 60 \text{ mg}, 1/30 \text{ gr} = \frac{60}{30} \text{ mg}$$

The medicine has a strength of 2 mg/ml.

Then set up the ratio:

$$2 \text{ mg/ml} = \frac{1.5 \text{ mg}}{x}$$

$$x = \frac{1.5 \text{ mg}}{2 \text{ mg}} \text{ ml} = .75 \text{ ml}$$

The nurse will administer 0.75 ml of the injectable solution.

Nursing process: Implementation

Client need: Pharmacological and Parenteral Therapies

Cognitive level: Application

Subject area: Pharmacologic

Answer: 2

Rationale: Find the volume for this injection.

The concentration available is 0.5 mg/ml.

Convert mcg to mg:

1 mg = 1000 mcg

Then set up the ratio:

$$\frac{0.5 \text{ mg}}{1 \text{ ml}} = \frac{1 \text{ mg}}{x}$$

$$x = \frac{1 \text{ mg}}{0.5 \text{ mg}} \text{ ml}$$

$$x = 2 \text{ ml}$$

The nurse will administer 2 ml injectable vitamin B_{12}.

Nursing process: Implementation

Client need: Pharmacological and Parenteral Therapies

Cognitive level: Application

Subject area: Pharmacologic

9. The doctor has ordered furosemide (Lasix) 40 mg IV push. The nurse has injectable furosemide (Lasix) 20 mg in 2 ml available. What should the nurse administer?

   1. 4 ml

   2. 0.4 ml

   3. 2 ml

   4. 3 ml

10. The doctor has ordered diazepam (Valium) 2.5 mg IV push stat. Available is injectable furosemide (Valium) 5 mg/ml. How much will the nurse administer?

   1. 0.75 ml

   2. 1 ml

   3. 0.5 ml

   4. 5 ml

Answer: 1

Rationale: Find the volume to inject.

The order is for 40 mg; available is 20 mg/2 ml

Set up the ratio:

$$\frac{20 \text{ mg}}{2 \text{ ml}} = \frac{40 \text{ mg}}{x}$$

$$x = \frac{40 \times 2}{20 \text{ ml}}$$

$$x = 4 \text{ ml}$$

The nurse will administer 4 ml of injectable furosemide (Lasix) IV push.

Nursing process: Implementation

Client need: Pharmacological and Parenteral Therapies

Cognitive level: Application

Subject area: Pharmacologic

Answer: 3

Rationale: Find the volume to be injected.

The order is for 2.5 mg; the available solution is 5 mg/ml.

Set up a ratio:

$$\frac{5 \text{ mg}}{1 \text{ ml}} = \frac{2.5 \text{ mg}}{x}$$

$$x = \frac{2.5 \text{ mg}}{5 \text{ mg}} \text{ ml}$$

$$x = 0.5 \text{ ml}$$

The nurse will administer 0.5 ml of the injectable furosemide (Valium) solution.

Nursing process: Implementation

Client need: Pharmacological and Parenteral Therapies

Cognitive level: Application

Subject area: Pharmacologic

11. The order reads ceftriaxone (Rocephin) 1.4 g IM b.i.d. Available is a ceftriaxone (Rocephin) 1 g vial; when reconstituted with 2.1 ml, it results in a concentration of 350 mg per ml. What volume will the nurse administer?

1. 3 ml/1 vial

2. 4 ml/2 vials

3. Add more diluent to yield 4 ml in 1 vial

4. 5 ml total/2 vials

12. Amoxicillin with clavulanic acid (Augmentin) powder reconstituted with 69 ml water results in a 75 ml suspension with a 200 mg/5 ml concentration. The doctor's order reads Augmentin 600 mg oral suspension p.o. every 12 hours. What volume of the suspension will the nurse administer?

1. 30 ml

2. 10 ml

3. 15 ml

4. 20 ml

Answer: 2

Rationale: Find the volume to be administered.

The order is for 1.4 g; the available solution is 350 mg/ml.

Convert the grams to mg:

1 g = 1000 mg, 1.4 g = 1400 mg

Convert 1.4 g to milligrams (move the decimal point three places) to equal 1400 mg.

Set up a ratio:

$$350 \text{ mg/ml} = \frac{1400 \text{ mg}}{x}$$

$$x = \frac{1400 \text{ mg}}{350 \text{ mg}} \text{ ml}$$

$$x = 4 \text{ ml}$$

The nurse will need to administer 4 ml of the ceftriaxone (Rocephin). There is not enough medication in one vial to administer 4 ml. Therefore the nurse will need to reconstitute two vials for the prescribed dose.

Nursing process: Implementation

Client need: Pharmacological and Parenteral Therapies

Cognitive level: Application

Subject area: Pharmacologic

Answer: 3

Rationale: Determine the volume to be administered.

The order is for 600 mg; available is 200 mg/5 ml.

Set up a ratio:

$$\frac{200 \text{ mg}}{5 \text{ ml}} = \frac{600 \text{ mg}}{x}$$

$$x = \frac{5 \times 600 \text{ mg}}{200 \text{ mg}} \text{ ml}$$

$$x = 15 \text{ ml}$$

The nurse will administer 15 ml of the reconstituted Augmentin suspension.

Nursing process: Implementation

Client need: Pharmacological and Parenteral Therapies

Cognitive level: Application

Subject area: Pharmacologic

13. Administer 800 ml IV D$_5$W at 75 ml/hour. The drop factor is 10 gtt/ml. How many drops per minute will the nurse administer?

    1. 13

    2. 10

    3. 17

    4. 21

14. Infuse heparin 40,000 units in 1000 ml of normal saline IV over 24 hours. The administration set has a drop factor of 10 gtt/ml. The nurse will set the gtt per minute at what rate?

    1. 14 gtt

    2. 42 gtt

    3. 17 gtt

    4. 7 gtt

Answer: 1

Rationale: Determine the drip rate per minute in gtt.

The order is for a rate of 75 ml/hr; the drop factor is 10 gtt/ml.

Convert the order to ml/minute:

1 hour = 60 minutes, $1/60 \times 75$ ml/hr = 1.25 ml/minute

Determine the drip rate:

x = order × drop factor

x = 1.25 ml/min × 10 gtt/ml

x = 12.5 gtt/min, rounded to 13

The nurse will administer 13 gtt/minute.

Nursing process: Implementation

Client need: Pharmacological and Parenteral Therapies

Cognitive level: Application

Subject area: Pharmacologic

Answer: 4

Rationale: Determine the gtt/minute rate.

The order is for a rate of 1000 ml/day; the drop factor is 10 gtt/ml.

Convert the order to ml/minute:

1 day= 24 hours/day × 60 minutes/hour

$$1000 \text{ ml/day} = \frac{1000}{24 \times 60 \text{ minutes/day}} = 0.69 \text{ ml/minute}$$

Determine the drip rate:

x = order × drop factor

x = 0.69 ml/minute × 10 gtt/ml

x = 6.9 gtt/minute, rounded to 7

The nurse will administer 7 gtt/minute.

Nursing process: Implementation

Client need: Pharmacological and Parenteral Therapies

Cognitive level: Application

Subject area: Pharmacologic

15. The order reads heparin 2000 units s.q. The nurse has on hand heparin 2500 units/ml. How much will the nurse administer?

    1. 0.8 ml

    2. 0.5 ml

    3. 0.6 ml

    4. 0.9 ml

16. Heparin 30,000 units in 1000 ml of normal saline is to be administered IV over 24 hours via microdrip. The nurse should administer how many units of heparin per hour?

    1. 635

    2. 1000

    3. 1250

    4. 125

Answer: 1

Rationale: What volume will the nurse administer?

The order is for 2000 units and available is a 2500 units/ml solution.

Set up a ratio:

$$\frac{2500 \text{ units}}{1 \text{ ml}} = \frac{2000 \text{ units}}{x}$$

$$x = \frac{2000}{2500}$$

x = 4/5 or 0.8 ml

The nurse will administer 0.8 ml.

Nursing process: Implementation

Client need: Pharmacological and Parenteral Therapies

Cognitive level: Application

Subject area: Pharmacologic

Answer: 3

Rationale: Determine the units to be administered per hour.

The rate is 30,000 units over 24 hours.

Note: The mention of "microdrip" does not enter into this calculation at all; you only need to convert units per day to units per hour. The microdrip calculation is only a factor when determining the setting for delivery of the order.

The order is for $\dfrac{30,000 \text{ units}}{24 \text{ hours}} = \dfrac{x}{1 \text{ hour}}$.

$$x = \frac{30,000 \text{ units}}{24 \text{ hours}}$$

x = 1249.9 units per hour, or 1250 units per hour

The nurse will administer 1250 units per hour.

Nursing process: Implementation

Client need: Pharmacological and Parenteral Therapies

Cognitive level: Application

Subject area: Pharmacologic

17. Infuse 2000 ml of lactated Ringer's over 12 hours. The drop factor is 15 gtt/ml. The nurse will regulate the IV to how many gtt per minute?

1. 28

2. 42

3. 56

4. 14

18. Use an electronic regulator to administer 1500 ml of D_5W in 6 hours. The nurse will set the machine for

1. 150 ml/hour.

2. 200 ml/hour.

3. 250 ml/hour.

4. 275 ml/hour.

19. The physician has ordered morphine sulfate (Duramorph) 10 mg s.q. every 4 hours p.r.n. The child weighs 80 Kg. The recommended maximum dose of morphine sulfate (Duramorph) is 0.1 mg to 0.2 mg/kg/dose. The nurse is determining the safety of this dose, what is the safe dose range for this child?

1. 3.6 mg to 7.3 mg/dose

2. 5 mg to 10 mg/dose

3. 36 mg to 73 mg/dose

4. 2.8 mg to 6 mg/dose

Answer: 2

Rationale: Determine the drip rate in gtt/minute.

The order is for 2000 ml/12 hours; the drop factor is 15 gtt/minute.

Convert the prescription to a rate per minute:

$$\frac{2000 \text{ ml}}{12 \text{ hours}} = 167 \text{ ml/hours}$$

$$\frac{167 \text{ ml}}{60 \text{ minutes}} = 2.78 \text{ ml/minute}$$

Now calculate the drip rate:

2.78 ml/minute $\times$ 15 gtt/ml = 41.7 gtt/minute or 42 gtt/minute

The nurse will administer 42 gtt/minute.

Nursing process: Implementation

Client need: Pharmacological and Parenteral Therapies

Cognitive level: Application

Subject area: Pharmacologic

Answer: 3

Rationale: Determine the setting in ml/hour for an electronic regulator.

The order is for 1500 ml/6 hours.

$$x = \frac{1500 \text{ ml}}{6 \text{ hours}} = 250 \text{ ml/hour}$$

The nurse will set the machine to administer 250 ml/hour.

Nursing process: Implementation

Client need: Pharmacological and Parenteral Therapies

Cognitive level: Application

Subject area: Pharmacologic

Answer: 1

Rationale: Determine the safety of this order.

The recommended dose is from 0.1 mg/kg to 0.2 mg/kg; the child's weight is 80 pounds.

Convert the child's weight to kilograms:

1 pound $= \dfrac{1}{2.2}$ kilograms, 80 lb $= \dfrac{80}{2.2}$ kg $= 36.4$ kg

Calculate the recommended upper and lower thresholds for this child.

Lower threshold: 0.1 mg/kg $\times$ 36.4 kg = 3.6 mg

Upper threshold: 0.2 mg/kg $\times$ 36.4 kg = 7.3 mg

10 mg per dose is not within the safe dose range for this child.

Nursing process: Implementation

Client need: Pharmacological and Parenteral Therapies

Cognitive level: Application

Subject area: Pharmacologic

20. The dose ordered by a physician for a child is outside the safe range published by the manufacturer. What should the nurse do? _____

21. The recommended dosage for cefaclor (Ceclor) suspension is 20 to 40 mg/kg/day divided into two or three doses. The child receiving the cefaclor (Ceclor) weighs 22 kg. What is the recommended range for the individual dose ordered as twice daily for this child?

1. 330 to 660 mg

2. 440 to 880 mg

3. 220 to 440 mg

4. 200 to 400 mg

22. The recommended dosage for furosemide (Lasix) oral solution is a single dose of 2 mg/kg, and subsequent doses of 1 to 2 mg/kg every 6 hours until suitable response, up to a maximum of 6 mg/kg/day. What is the minimum to maximum 24-hour dose range for a child weighing 26 kg?

1. 52 mg to 156 mg/24 hours

2. 52 mg to 104 mg/24 hours

3. 26 mg to 52 mg/24 hours

4. 46 mg to 100 mg/24 hours

Answer: Call the physician to question the order

Rationale: If there is reason to believe that the ordered dose is not safe for a client, it should not be administered. The dosage range given by the manufacturer already takes into account height and weight variations in children. The nurse needs to clarify the order with the physician.

Nursing process: Implementation

Client need: Pharmacological and Parenteral Therapies

Cognitive level: Application

Subject area: Pharmacologic

Answer: 3

Rationale: Determine the recommended safety range of this drug.

The recommended dosage is from 20 mg/kg/day to 40 mg/kg/day.

The child's weight is 22 kg; the drug will be administered two times per day.

Calculate the recommended upper and lower thresholds for this child.

Lower threshold: 20 mg/kg/day $\times$ 22 kg = 440 mg/day

2 doses per day, lower threshold per dose = 1/2 $\times$ 440 mg = 220 mg

Upper threshold: 40 mg/kg/day $\times$ 22 kg = 880 mg/day

2 doses per day, upper threshold per dose = 1/2 $\times$ 880 mg = 440 mg

The range for this child is 220 mg to 440 mg.

Nursing process: Implementation

Client need: Pharmacological and Parenteral Therapies

Cognitive level: Application

Subject area: Pharmacologic

Answer: 1

Rationale: Determine the range of daily safe dosages for a 26-kg child.

The safe dosage range has a minimum of 2 mg/kg as a single application, and a maximum of 6 mg/kg/day.

Determine the lower threshold for this child:

If the first 2 mg/kg shows results, there would be no further application.

For a child of 26 kg, the lower threshold is 26 kg $\times$ 2 mg/kg = 52 mg.

Determine the upper threshold:

The daily upper limit is given as 6 mg/kg/day.

For a child of 26 kg, the upper threshold is 26 kg $\times$ 6 mg/kg = 156 mg.

The range for this child is 52 mg to 156 mg.

Nursing process: Implementation

Client need: Pharmacological and Parenteral Therapies

Cognitive level: Application

Subject area: Gerontologic

23. Using the child's weight, determine what the pediatric dose for digoxin (Lanoxin) would be if the usual adult dose is 0.15 mg p.o. every day. The child weighs 13 kg. The nurse will administer

    1. 0.15 mg.

    2. 0.05 mg.

    3. 0.1 mg.

    4. 0.07 mg.

24. An adult dose of doxycycline (Vibramycin) is 100 mg b.i.d. The child who is to take doxycycline (Vibramycin) is 32 inches tall and weighs 48 pounds. Determine the child's dose based on BSA.

    1. 30 mg/dose

    2. 25 mg/dose

    3. 50 mg/dose

    4. 41 mg/dose

Answer: 2

Rationale: Find the amount of digoxin the nurse should administer based on BSA.

The usual adult dose is for 0.15 mg, and the child weighs 13 kg.

$S = \log W \times 0.425 + \log H \times 0.725 + 1.8564$, where

S is in cm^2; W is in kg; and H is in cm

Determine the child's BSA using weight:

$$\frac{(4 \times 13) + 7}{13 + 90} = \frac{52 + 7}{103} = \frac{59}{103} = 0.57 \, m^2 \, BSA$$

Determine the child's dose based on BSA:

$$\frac{0.57 \, m^2}{1.7} \times 0.15 \, mg = 0.34 \times 0.15 = 0.05 \, mg$$

The nurse will administer a 0.05 mg dose.

Nursing process: Implementation

Client need: Pharmacological and Parenteral Therapies

Cognitive level: Application

Subject area: Pharmacologic

Answer: 4

Rationale: Determine a child's dose of Vibramycin using BSA.

An adult dose is 100 mg; the child is 32 inches tall, and weighs 48 pounds.

$S = \log W \times 0.425 + \log H \times 0.725 + 1.8564$,

S is in cm^2; W is in kg; and H is in cm

Determine the child's BSA:

$$\sqrt{\frac{48 \times 32}{3131}} = \sqrt{\frac{1536}{3131}} = \sqrt{0.49} = 0.70 \, m^2$$

Determine the child's dose based on the BSA:

$$\frac{0.70 \, m^2}{1.7} \times 100 \, mg = 41 \, mg/dose$$

The nurse will administer 41 mg per dose.

Nursing process: Implementation

Client need: Pharmacological and Parenteral Therapies

Cognitive level: Application

Subject area: Pharmacologic

25. The recommended adult dose of acyclovir is 200 mg every 4 hours. The nurse should administer what dose for a child weighing 8 kg and standing 57 cm tall?

1. 42 mg

2. 60 mg

3. 30 mg

4. 50 mg

Answer: 1

Rationale: Determine a child's dose of acyclovir using BSA.

The adult dose is 200 mg; the child is 57 cm tall and weighs 8 kg.

Determine the child's BSA:

$$\sqrt{\frac{8 \text{ kg} \times 57 \text{ cm}}{3600}} = \sqrt{\frac{456}{3600}} = \sqrt{0.12} = 0.35 \text{ m}^2$$

Determine the child's dose:

$$\frac{0.35 \text{ m}^2}{1.7} \times 200 \text{ mg} = \text{child's dose}$$

$0.21 \times 200 = 42$ mg

The nurse will administer 42 mg every 4 hours.

Nursing process: Implementation

Client need: Pharmacological and Parenteral Therapies

Cognitive level: Application

Subject area: Pharmacologic

Drugs for Eye, Ear, Nose, and Throat Disorders

16

1. The nurse should question which of the following drugs is for use in a client who has glaucoma.
   1. Acetazolamide (Diamox)
   2. Pilocarpine
   3. Atropine sulfate
   4. Mannitol

2. The nurse is administering an adrenergic blocking agent, such as a beta blocker, to a client with glaucoma. Which of the following would the nurse interpret as indicative of a serious adverse reaction?
   1. Photophobia
   2. Blurred vision
   3. Drop in blood pressure
   4. Exacerbation of asthma

3. The nurse administers which of the following drugs to a client who has keratitis?
   1. Acyclovir (Zovirax)
   2. Acetazolamide (Diamox)
   3. Scopolamine (Isopto Hyoscine)
   4. Idoxuridine (Stoxil)

Answer: 3

Rationale: Atropine sulfate is an anticholinergic drug that is used as a mydriatic to dilate the pupil. This blocks the drainage of aqueous humor. If used by a client who has glaucoma, it could cause an acute attack by increasing the intraocular pressure. Glaucoma is treated by drugs that constrict the pupil to allow for the escape of aqueous humor and that reduce intraocular pressure. Acetazolamide (Diamox) is a carbonic anhydrase inhibitor that decreases the aqueous fluid. Pilocarpine is a cholinergic agonist used in the treatment of glaucoma. Mannitol is an osmotic diuretic that draws the aqueous fluid from the eye by osmosis.

Nursing process: Analysis

Client need: Pharmacological and Parenteral Therapies

Cognitive level: Analysis

Subject area: Pharmacologic

Answer: 4

Rationale: Adrenergic blocking agents (beta blockers) are miotics used in the treatment of glaucoma. They decrease the aqueous production and intraocular pressure. Adverse reactions include stinging, photophobia, burning, tearing, and blurred vision. Although a decrease in blood pressure may occur, the most serious adverse reaction is an exacerbation in a client's asthma.

Nursing process: Analysis

Client need: Pharmacological and Parenteral Therapies

Cognitive level: Analysis

Subject area: Pharmacologic

Answer: 4

Rationale: Keratitis is inflammation of the cornea that is treated with topical idoxuridine (Stoxil), which is an anti-infective. Acyclovir (Zovirax) is an antiviral used in the treatment of herpes zoster ophthalmicus. Acetazolamide (Diamox) is a carbonic anhydrase inhibitor used for a client who has glaucoma to decrease the aqueous fluid. Scopolamine (Isopto Hyoscine) is a mydriatic that is used for cycloplegic refractions and uveitis.

Nursing process: Implementation

Client need: Pharmacological and Parenteral Therapies

Cognitive level: Application

Subject area: Pharmacologic

4. The nurse is to administer timolol (Timoptic) 1 drop in each eye. Which of the following comments by the client indicates the need for further teaching?

1. "I must wash my hand before putting in my drops."

2. "This drug will decrease the fluid in my eye."

3. "I'll need to take this until my eye pressure is normal."

4. "Adverse reactions include dizziness and double vision."

5. The nurse instructs the client that the best position for instilling nose spray is to

1. bend the head forward.

2. push one nare to the side.

3. tilt the head backward.

4. open the mouth to facilitate breathing.

6. The nurse is assigned to administer eyedrops to a client being prepared for cataract surgery. Which of the following type of eyedrop does the nurse expect to administer?

1. An osmotic diuretic

2. A miotic agent

3. A mydriatic agent

4. A thiazide diuretic

7. A child requires administration of eardrops for swimmer's ear. The nurse evaluates another nurse correctly administering the drops when the ear canal is straightened by _____.

Answer: 3
Rationale: Timolol (Timoptic) is an antiglaucoma agent. This is required daily for the rest of the client's life unless surgical intervention is performed. It will decrease the aqueous fluid and decrease the intraocular pressure. Hand washing is an aseptic measure to prevent microorganism transfer. Adverse reactions include dizziness, double vision, and other visual changes.
Nursing process: Evaluation
Client need: Pharmacological and Parenteral Therapies
Cognitive level: Analysis
Subject area: Pharmacologic

Answer: 3
Rationale: Tilting the head backward can facilitate movement of the drug into the nasal passages.
Nursing process: Implementation
Client need: Health Promotion and Maintenance
Cognitive level: Application
Subject area: Pharmacologic

Answer: 3
Rationale: A mydriatic agent produces dilation of the pupil. Mydriatic eyedrops are used preoperatively for cataract surgery. They not only dilate the pupil, but also constrict blood vessels. A miotic agent constricts the pupil. An osmotic diuretic will decrease intraocular pressure. A thiazide diuretic promotes the excretion of body fluid and is not prescribed for cataract surgery.
Nursing process: Planning
Client need: Pharmacological and Parenteral Therapies
Cognitive level: Analysis
Subject area: Pharmacologic

Answer: pulling the earlobe down and back
Rationale: The correct procedure for administering eardrops to a child includes pulling the earlobe down and back. The correct procedure for administering eardrops to an adult is to pull the earlobe up and back.
Nursing process: Evaluation
Client need: Pharmacological and Parenteral Therapies
Cognitive level: Application
Subject area: Pharmacologic

8. A client with Ménière's disease asks the nurse why meclizine hydrochloride (Antivert) is being administered. The most appropriate response by the nurse is

   1. "It will control the vertigo."

   2. "It will help you sleep."

   3. "It will decrease your pain."

   4. "It will alleviate your nausea."

9. When providing care to a client who is receiving phenylephrine HCl (Neo-Synephrine) the nurse should monitor the client for which of the following adverse reactions?
   Select all that apply:

   [   ] **1.** Urinary retention

   [   ] **2.** Dry skin

   [   ] **3.** Hypertension

   [   ] **4.** Tachycardia

   [   ] **5.** Headache

   [   ] **6.** Decreased sensitivity to light

10. The nurse is caring for a client receiving a miotic topical drug for glaucoma. Three adverse reactions that the nurse would evaluate and report that systemic absorption has taken place are _____.

11. The nurse is collecting a medication history from a client with herpes simplex 1 of the eye. The nurse should ask the client if which of the following drugs are taken?

    1. Trifluridine (Viroptic)

    2. Cromolyn (Cromlom)

    3. Idoxuridine (Stoxil)

    4. Acetazolamide (Diamox)

Answer: 4

Rationale: Meclizine hydrochloride (Antivert) is an antiemetic used to alleviate the nausea that occurs in Ménière's disease from the violent vertigo. It does not directly stop the vertigo.

Nursing process: Analysis

Client need: Pharmacological and Parenteral Therapies

Cognitive level: Analysis

Subject area: Pharmacologic

Answer: 3, 4, 5

Rationale: Phenylephrine HCI (Neo-Synephrine) is an adrenergic drug used for a variety of purposes, such as a topical ocular vasoconstrictor in uveitis, open-angle glaucoma, refraction without cycloplegia, and nasal congestion. Adverse reactions include hypertension, tachycardia, and headache.

Nursing process: Assessment

Client need: Pharmacological and Parenteral Therapies

Cognitive level: Application

Subject area: Pharmacologic

Answer: abdominal cramps, diarrhea, and increased salivation

Rationale: Miotic drugs are used in the treatment for glaucoma to constrict the pupil. Topical adverse reactions include blurred vision and eye and brow ache. Systemic adverse reactions include abdominal cramps, diarrhea, and increased salivation.

Nursing process: Analysis

Client need: Pharmacological and Parenteral Therapies

Cognitive level: Analysis

Subject area: Pharmacologic

Answer: 1

Rationale: Trifluridine (Viroptic) is an antiviral drug used to treat herpes simplex 1. Cromolyn (Cromlom) is an antiallergic drug used to treat conjunctivitis by reducing the itching and redness. Idoxuridine (Stoxil) is an anti-infective used topically to treat keratitis. Acetazolamide (Diamox) is a carbonic anhydrase inhibitor used in the treatment of glaucoma, to decrease aqueous fluid.

Nursing process: Assessment

Client need: Pharmacological and Parenteral Therapies

Cognitive level: Application

Subject area: Pharmacologic

12. The nurse should understand that a client is to receive which of the following drugs to paralyze the ciliary body muscles?

   1. Phenylephrine HCl (Neo-Synephrine)

   2. Homatropine

   3. Hydroxyamphetamine-hydrobromide (Paredrine)

   4. Cromolyn (Cromlom)

13. Which of the following discharge instructions should the nurse include on diazepam (Valium) for a client going home after an acute exacerbation of Ménière's disease?
   Select all that apply:

   [   ] **1.** Take on an empty stomach

   [   ] **2.** Use alcohol sparingly

   [   ] **3.** Avoid driving

   [   ] **4.** Report any urinary incontinence

   [   ] **5.** Drowsiness may occur at the beginning of treatment

   [   ] **6.** Get up slowly after lying down

14. The nurse should question which of the following drugs that is ordered to be given prior to an eye refraction?

   1. Scopolamine

   2. Pilocarpine (Pilocar)

   3. Phenylephrine HCl (Neo-Synephrine)

   4. Hydroxyamphetamine (Paredrine)

15. The nurse understands that a client is to receive prednisolone (Pred Forte) for which of the following purposes?

   1. Acts as an antiviral

   2. Decreases aqueous fluid

   3. Decreases intraocular pressure

   4. Is an anti-inflammatory

Answer: 2

Rationale: Homatropine is a cycloplegic mydriatic administered for ciliary muscle paralysis. Phenylephrine HCl (Neo-Synephrine) and hydroxyamphetamine-hydrobromide (Paredrine) are mydriatics used to dilate the pupil. Cromolyn (Cromlom) is used to treat conjunctivitis by reducing itching and redness.

Nursing process: Analysis

Client need: Pharmacological and Parenteral Therapies

Cognitive level: Analysis

Subject area: Pharmacologic

Answer: 3, 5, 6

Rationale: Diazepam (Valium) is an antianxiety, anticonvulsant, and a skeletal muscle relaxant that has been proven to be helpful in the treatment of Ménière's disease. Interventions that should be in the plan of care for a client taking diazepam (Valium) include taking the drug with food to alleviate gastrointestinal upset, being aware that drowsiness may occur at the beginning of treatment, getting up slowly after lying down, and avoiding alcohol and driving.

Nursing process: Planning

Client need: Health Promotion and Maintenance

Cognitive level: Application

Subject area: Pharmacologic

Answer: 2

Rationale: Pilocarpine (Pilocar) is a cholinergic used in the treatment of glaucoma. It should be questioned because it stimulates the iris to contract. Scopolamine is a cycloplegic and phenylephrine HCl (Neo-Synephrine) is a mydriatic used for eye refraction. Hydroxyamphetamine (Paredrine) is a mydriatic used diagnostically to differentiate among postganglionic, central, or preganglionic Horner's syndrome.

Nursing process: Analysis

Client need: Pharmacological and Parenteral Therapies

Cognitive level: Analysis

Subject area: Pharmacologic

Answer: 4

Rationale: Prednisolone (Pred Forte) is a topical corticosteroid used to treat postoperative eye inflammation.

Nursing process: Analysis

Client need: Pharmacological and Parenteral Therapies

Cognitive level: Application

Subject area: Pharmacologic

16. Which of the following interventions is a priority for the nurse to implement when a client with glaucoma receiving betaxolol (Betoptic) experiences bradycardia, headache, and depression?

    1. Report these adverse reactions as systemic

    2. Decrease the dose

    3. Take the vital signs prior to administering

    4. Refer the client for treatment of the depression

17. The nurse assesses a client receiving brinzolamide (Azopt) for which of the following adverse reactions? Select all that apply:

    [ ] **1.** Urinary retention

    [ ] **2.** Constipation

    [ ] **3.** Blurred vision

    [ ] **4.** Loss of appetite

    [ ] **5.** Transient stinging

    [ ] **6.** Redness

18. The nurse is caring for a client with allergic rhinitis and evaluates which of the following drugs to act as a mast cell stabilizer?

    1. Diphenhydramine (Benadryl)

    2. Brompheniramine (Dimetane)

    3. Loratidine (Claritin)

    4. Cromolyn (Nasalcrom)

19. Which of the following drugs should the nurse question in a client with cardiovascular disease and hypertension?

    1. Pseudoephedrine (Sudafed)

    2. Diphenhydramine (Benadryl)

    3. Loratidine (Claritin)

    4. Cetirizine (Zyrtec)

Answer: 1

Rationale: Betaxolol (Betoptic) is a beta-adrenergic blocker given for glaucoma. The adverse reactions are generally considered as being transient discomfort. Adverse reactions, although rare, may include bradycardia, pulmonary distress, headache, depression, and heart block. These indicate a systemic reaction and must be reported.

Nursing process: Implementation

Client need: Pharmacological and Parenteral Therapies

Cognitive level: Analysis

Subject area: Pharmacologic

Answer: 3, 5, 6

Rationale: Brinzolamide (Azopt) is a topical carbonic anhydrase inhibitor that decreases the aqueous humor production. Adverse reactions include blurred vision, transient stinging, redness, and diarrhea.

Nursing process: Assessment

Client need: Pharmacological and Parenteral Therapies

Cognitive level: Application

Subject area: Pharmacologic

Answer: 4

Rationale: Cromolyn (Nasalcrom) is the only mast cell stabilizer. Diphenhydramine (Benadryl), brompheniramine (Dimetane), and loratidine (Claritin) are all antihistamines.

Nursing process: Evaluation

Client need: Pharmacological and Parenteral Therapies

Cognitive level: Comprehension

Subject area: Pharmacologic

Answer: 1

Rationale: Pseudoephedrine (Sudafed) is a nasal decongestant used for temporary relief of nasal congestion from the common cold, hay fever, or other respiratory allergies. Decongestants such as pseudoephedrine (Sudafed) are contraindicated in clients with cardiovascular disease and hypertension. Diphenhydramine (Benadryl), loratidine (Claritin), and cetirizine (Zyrtec) are all antihistamines and are not contraindicated.

Nursing process: Analysis

Client need: Pharmacological and Parenteral Therapies

Cognitive level: Analysis

Subject area: Pharmacologic

20. A client on diazepam (Valium) asks the nurse why the physician said to avoid drinking alcohol while taking this medication. Which of the following responses by the nurse appropriately explains what alcohol will do?

  1. Cause a decrease in vasoconstriction

  2. Increase the sedative effect

  3. Interfere with the absorption of Valium

  4. Promote a decreased sensitivity to Valium

21. When admitting a new client with glaucoma, the nurse notes an order for atropine. The nurse should question this order because atropine

  1. causes a moistening effect.

  2. is likely to cause respiratory depression.

  3. causes an increase in intraocular pressure.

  4. may cause diuresis.

22. Prior to discharge, the nurse instructs the client who is receiving dipivefrin (Propine) to notify the physician if which of the following occurs?

  1. Fatigue

  2. Increase in urinary frequency

  3. Weight gain of five pounds in two weeks

  4. Tachycardia

23. The nurse should administer dipivefrin (Propine) at which of the following times?

  1. Every 12 hours

  2. Daily

  3. One hour after a meal

  4. With food three times a day

Answer: 2

Rationale: Alcohol is a central nervous system depressant and, when taken with Valium, will give an additive effect and increase the sedative value of the Valium. Alcohol causes vasoconstriction, not vasodilation. Alcohol will serve as an additive effect when taken with Valium, yielding an increased sensitivity to the Valium.

Nursing process: Analysis

Client need: Pharmacological and Parenteral Therapies

Cognitive level: Analysis

Subject area: Pharmacologic

Answer: 3

Rationale: Atropine is a cycloplegic mydriatic. It blocks the effects of acetylcholine on the sphincter muscle of the iris and the accommodative muscle of the ciliary body. Atropine causes an increase in intraocular pressure. In the treatment of glaucoma, the goal is to decrease intraocular pressure in order to avoid damage to the optic nerve. Adverse reactions of atropine include a decrease in secretions, urinary hesitancy or retention, but not diuresis.

Nursing process: Analysis

Client need: Pharmacological and Parenteral Therapies

Cognitive level: Analysis

Subject area: Pharmacologic

Answer: 4

Rationale: Dipivefrin (Propine) is a sympathomimetic that can cause tachycardia. An increase in urinary frequency, fatigue, and weight gain are not adverse reactions.

Nursing process: Implementation

Client need: Pharmacological and Parenteral Therapies

Cognitive level: Analysis

Subject area: Pharmacologic

Answer: 1

Rationale: Dipivefrin (Propine) is a sympathomimetic drug used in the treatment of glaucoma. Treatment includes regular administration of the eyedrops every 12 hours. The objective of the treatment is to reduce the intraocular pressure.

Nursing process: Implementation

Client need: Pharmacological and Parenteral Therapies

Cognitive level: Application

Subject area: Pharmacologic

24. Which of the following is essential that the nurse include in the assessment of a client who works evenings and takes pilocarpine (Pilocar)?
    1. Hypotension
    2. Urinary retention
    3. Constipation
    4. Decreased dark adaptation

25. The nurse is collecting a health history from a client who is to begin taking acetazolamide (Diamox). Which of the following questions should the nurse ask to determine the safety of this drug?
    1. "Do you operate dangerous equipment?"
    2. "Have you ever had an allergy to sulfa?"
    3. "Have you had any chest pains or a heart attack?"
    4. "Have you had any frequent diarrhea?"

26. The nurse instructs a client who is prescribed a topical ear medication to
    1. use with earplugs to retain the drops.
    2. avoid using daily.
    3. report a sedative effect.
    4. administer at room temperature.

27. The registered nurse is planning to delegate nursing tasks for the day. Which of the following tasks may be delegated to a licensed practical nurse?
    1. Instruct a client taking antihistamines on the adverse reactions
    2. Assess a client for cardiovascular disease before administering a nasal decongestant
    3. Review an electrolyte panel of a client taking a diuretic ear medication
    4. Cleanse a client's eyelid with plain water to soften and remove crusting

Answer: 4

Rationale: Pilocarpine (Pilocar) is a cholinergic agonist used in the treatment of glaucoma. Due to the contraction of the iris, it causes a decreased adaptation to dark. Other adverse reactions include hypertension, urinary frequency, and diarrhea.

Nursing process: Assessment

Client need: Pharmacological and Parenteral Therapies

Cognitive level: Application

Subject area: Pharmacologic

Answer: 2

Rationale: Acetazolamide (Diamox) is a carbonic anhydrase inhibitor used in the treatment of glaucoma. It should not be used if a prior history to a sulfa allergy is known. It inhibits carbonic anhydrase in the kidney, which decreases the formation of bicarbonate and hydrogen ions from carbon dioxide, thus decreasing the availability of the ions for transport.

Nursing process: Analysis

Client need: Pharmacological and Parenteral Therapies

Cognitive level: Analysis

Subject area: Pharmacologic

Answer: 4

Rationale: Topical ear medications should be administered at room temperature because the cold can cause dizziness. Earplugs are not used to retain drops. Treatment of a fungal infection requires application once or twice daily. Topical ear medication has no sedative effect.

Nursing process: Implementation

Client need: Pharmacological and Parenteral Therapies

Cognitive level: Application

Subject area: Pharmacologic

Answer: 4

Rationale: A registered nurse may delegate cleansing a client's eyelid with plain water to soften and remove crusting to a licensed practical nurse. A licensed practical nurse may not instruct a client taking antihistamines on the adverse reactions, assess a client for cardiovascular disease before administering a nasal decongestant, or review the electrolyte panel of a client taking a diuretic ear medication. These nursing tasks require the knowledge level of a registered nurse.

Nursing process: Planning

Client need: Management of Care

Cognitive level: Analysis

Subject area: Legal and Ethical Issues

Drugs for the Respiratory System

17

1. A client has been receiving intravenous theophylline and the physician writes new orders to discontinue the IV medication and begin an immediate-release oral form of the medication. When should the nurse schedule the first dose of the oral medication to be administered?

   1. Immediately after stopping the intravenous infusion of theophylline
   2. Four to six hours after stopping the intravenous infusion of theophylline
   3. Begin the initial dose at bedtime
   4. Start the oral dose with the morning medications and breakfast

2. A client with acute asthma is treated for inspiratory and expiratory wheezes and a decreased forced expiratory volume. Which class of prescribed drugs should the nurse administer first to this client?

   1. Oral steroids
   2. Bronchodilators
   3. Inhaled steroids
   4. Mucolytics

3. The nurse is admitting a client with asthma who is to be started on theophylline. Which of the following questions would be appropriate to ask this client?

   1. "Are you a diabetic and taking insulin?"
   2. "Do you take cimetidine (Tagamet)?"
   3. "Do you use aspirin on a daily basis?"
   4. "Do you exercise routinely?"

Answer: 2

Rationale: After stopping IV therapy, a period of 4 to 6 hours should elapse before initiating oral therapy. The half-life of the drug is 3 to 15 hours in nonsmoking adults, and 4 to 5 hours in adult heavy smokers. If the oral dose is initiated too soon it could lead to adverse reactions, such as nausea, vomiting, diarrhea, irritability, insomnia, or headache. More serious theophylline toxicity is manifested by cardiac arrhythmias, hypotension and peripheral vascular collapse, tachycardia, hyperglycemia, or seizures. The therapeutic serum level for theophylline is 10 to 20 mcg/ml.

Nursing process: Planning

Client need: Pharmacological and Parenteral Therapies

Cognitive level: Application

Subject area: Pharmacologic

Answer: 2

Rationale: The most immediate need of a client with inspiratory and expiratory wheezes and a decreased forced expiratory volume is to dilate the bronchioles and improve air exchange. Steroids (inhaled or oral) may follow the emergent treatment to reduce the inflammation, but would not be first-line drugs. Mucolytics are not appropriate for the client with asthma, as there is little mucus production associated with asthma.

Nursing process: Planning

Client need: Pharmacological and Parenteral Therapies

Cognitive level: Application

Subject area: Pharmacologic

Answer: 2

Rationale: Cimetidine (Tagamet) will decrease theophylline clearance and may increase serum drug levels. The dose may have to be reduced for this client. Insulin and aspirin do not affect drug clearance.

Nursing process: Assessment

Client need: Pharmacological and Parenteral Therapies

Cognitive level: Application

Subject area: Pharmacologic

4. After instructing a client to use a beclomethasone (Vanceril) inhaler, which of the following statements by the client indicates to the nurse that the teaching has been successful?

    1. "I will limit myself to two cups of coffee per day."

    2. "I will take it before bed each night."

    3. "I will take it with meals to mask the taste."

    4. "I will rinse my mouth after each use."

5. Which of the following statements made by the client indicates to the nurse that the client does not understand how to use cromolyn sodium (Intal) and is in need of further instructions?

    1. "If I don't feel better in two to three weeks, I should stop taking the medication."

    2. "I will call my doctor if this medication causes severe coughing."

    3. "I have to take this medication routinely, even when I feel good."

    4. "I do not stop my other medications just because I'm taking this one."

6. When instructing a client to use a metered dose inhaler, it would be essential for the nurse to include which of the following aspects? Instruct the client to

    1. hold the breath for three seconds after using the inhaler.

    2. take a quick deep breath after activating the canister.

    3. activate the canister at the beginning of a slow deep breath.

    4. place the canister six inches in front of an open mouth.

Answer: 4

Rationale: Inhaled steroids increase the risk of oral candidiasis and irritation. Clients should rinse their mouth out with water or mouthwash after each dose. If other drugs are taken by inhaler at the same time, the steroid should be the last drug given. Many may cause nausea, so they should not be taken around mealtime. The client should be instructed to follow the schedule of dosing intervals. It is not a one time per day drug. Caffeine is not limited and, in fact, has some bronchodilating effect. Inhaled steroids are used for maintenance and prophylactic treatment of asthma.

Nursing process: Evaluation

Client need: Health Promotion and Maintenance

Cognitive level: Application

Subject area: Pharmacologic

Answer: 1

Rationale: Cromolyn sodium (Intal) is a drug used prophylactically for asthma to inhibit the degranulation of sensitized mast cells that occur after exposure to certain antigens and to prevent histamine release. This drug may take four to eight weeks for optimal effect. It may cause bronchospasm in some individuals. Steroids and other drugs are continued along with the cromolyn. If cromolyn is effective, steroids can often be tapered down. Do not stop inhalation or nasal medication abruptly. Rapid withdrawal of the drug may precipitate an asthmatic attack.

Nursing process: Evaluation

Client need: Pharmacological and Parenteral Therapies

Cognitive level: Analysis

Subject area: Pharmacologic

Answer: 3

Rationale: Proper technique for using a metered dose inhaler is to have the client place the canister either in the mouth or two inches in front of an open mouth. The canister must be activated at the beginning of a slow deep inspiratory effort. The inhalation is followed by 5 to 10 seconds of breath holding. Sequence is then repeated if a second puff is ordered.

Nursing process: Implementation

Client need: Health Promotion and Maintenance

Cognitive level: Application

Subject area: Pharmacologic

7. What is the category of drugs and the route of administration for the nurse to administer as a priority to a client to promote the most effective treatment for acute bronchospasm and to prevent exercise-induced bronchospasm? _____

8. A client who has asthma asks the nurse why the preferred route of administration for corticosteroids is inhalation. The appropriate response by the nurse is

   1. "inhaled medications are easier to take."

   2. "the systemic adverse reactions are reduced."

   3. "no weaning is required when stopping the drug."

   4. "oral care is not required."

9. A client with asthma awakens in the middle of the night with an asthma attack. Which of the following inhaler medications should the nurse administer first?

   1. Albuterol (Proventil)

   2. Triamcinolone acetonide (Azmacort)

   3. Fluticasone propionate (Flovent)

   4. Cromolyn (Intal)

10. After a client diagnosed with pneumonia has an episode of respiratory distress, the client is intubated and placed on a ventilator. The breath sounds are diminished and the chest x-ray shows left lower lobe consolidation. The physician orders respiratory treatments with acetylcysteine (Mucomyst). The nurse should monitor the client for which of the following results from this treatment?

   1. Bronchodilation

   2. Increased sputum, removed with suctioning

   3. Decreased level of consciousness

   4. Hypotension

Answer: Inhaled bronchodilators

Rationale: Inhaled bronchodilators are the primary drugs used both to treat acute bronchospasm and to prevent exercise-induced bronchospasm. The most effective route of administration of beta-adrenergic agents is by inhalation.

Nursing process: Implementation

Client need: Pharmacological and Parenteral Therapies

Cognitive level: Application

Subject area: Pharmacologic

Answer: 2

Rationale: The inhaled glucocorticoids are effective on topical administration, and systemic adverse reactions can be reduced when delivered by this route. Instruction is necessary for the client to properly learn the technique of using inhalers. Inhaled steroids should not be stopped suddenly and oral care is necessary after every treatment to reduce oral candidiasis.

Nursing process: Analysis

Client need: Pharmacological and Parenteral Therapies

Cognitive level: Application

Subject area: Pharmacologic

Answer: 1

Rationale: The initial treatment for acute asthma is a bronchodilator. Steroids such as triamcinolone acetonide (Azmacort) and fluticasone propionate (Flovent) may be given after initial bronchospasm is relieved. Cromolyn (Intal) has no immediate effect and is a prophylactic mast cell inhibitor.

Nursing process: Implementation

Client need: Management of Care

Cognitive level: Analysis

Subject area: Pharmacologic

Answer: 2

Rationale: Acetylcysteine (Mucomyst) is a mucolytic agent that breaks down thick secretions and facilitates sputum expectoration. Adverse reactions include nausea and bronchospasm. There is no effect on level of consciousness or vital signs.

Nursing process: Assessment

Client need: Pharmacological and Parenteral Therapies

Cognitive level: Application

Subject area: Pharmacologic

11. The nurse is caring for a client with lung cancer who has an intractable cough and is exhausted from the effort of coughing. Which of the following drugs should the nurse administer to this client?

    1. Rifampin (Rifadin)

    2. Acetylcysteine (Mucomyst)

    3. Fluticasone (Flovent)

    4. Codeine

12. Which of the following treatments is the priority for the nurse to administer to a client who has a positive tuberculosis (TB) skin test but has no other evidence of active disease?

    1. No treatment and repeat skin test in 6 months

    2. Isoniazid (INH) for 12 months

    3. Multidrug therapy for at least 12 months

    4. Streptomycin for 12 months

13. The nurse is developing a medication schedule for a client who is receiving isoniazid (INH). To promote the best absorption, this medication would be administered

    1. on an empty stomach.

    2. with antacids to relieve stomach upset.

    3. with food.

    4. 30 minutes after meals.

14. Which of the following is the priority for the nurse to monitor in a client who has been on a ventilator and on 70% FIO_2 for the past 72 hours?

    1. Atelectasis

    2. Pulmonary fibrosis

    3. Expense to client

    4. Oxygen dependence

Answer: 4

Rationale: Codeine is a narcotic drug that selectively depresses the cough center in the medulla and inhibits coughing. It is typically used in a dry, nonproductive, intractable cough. It is used with caution in combination with other central nervous system depressants. Rifampin (Rifadin) is a drug used to treat tuberculosis. Acetylcysteine (Mucomyst) is a mucolytic that decreases the viscosity of purulent and nonpurulent secretions and facilitates their removal. Fluticasone (Flovent) is an inhaled corticosteroid used in the treatment of asthma.

Nursing process: Implementation

Client need: Pharmacological and Parenteral Therapies

Cognitive level: Application

Subject area: Pharmacologic

Answer: 2

Rationale: A positive skin test with no other evidence of disease indicates exposure to the disease. Isoniazid (INH) therapy for 12 months is the usual protocol. Once a client has a positive skin test, it will always be positive and there is no value in repeating a test. Multidrug therapy is used to treat active disease and streptomycin or Amikacin is often added in the induction phase of treatment.

Nursing process: Implementation

Client need: Pharmacological and Parenteral Therapies

Cognitive level: Application

Subject area: Pharmacologic

Answer: 1

Rationale: Isoniazid (INH) should be taken on an empty stomach, either one hour before or two hours after meals. Avoid antacids with the medication.

Nursing process: Planning

Client need: Pharmacological and Parenteral Therapies

Cognitive level: Application

Subject area: Pharmacologic

Answer: 2

Rationale: Clients on an FIO_2 of 50% or greater for 24 to 48 hours have a higher incidence of pulmonary fibrosis and oxygen toxicity. Atelectasis can occur but is generally reversible and therefore not the greatest concern. Expense is considered, but treatment requirements for the client take priority. Oxygen dependence is related to pulmonary disease.

Nursing process: Assessment

Client need: Management of Care

Cognitive level: Analysis

Subject area: Pharmacologic

15. The nurse is caring for a client who has chronic obstructive lung disease (COPD) and pneumonia. After being extubated, which of the following orders should the nurse question?
    1. Continuation of the current antibiotics
    2. O_2 per nasal cannula at 6 L/min
    3. Out of bed with assistance
    4. Continuation of current nebulizer treatments

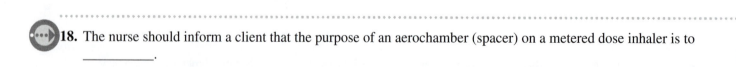

16. It is essential that the nurse provide a client receiving high-dose oxygen therapy and ventilator support through a tracheostomy tube _____.

17. The nurse is preparing to teach a class on the appropriate use of nebulizers and metered dose inhalers. Which of the following should the nurse include in the class?
    1. Metered dose inhalers require a gas flow rate of 6 to 10 L/min
    2. Nebulizers deliver medication through a face mask or mouthpiece
    3. Nebulizers deliver doses in puffs
    4. Metered dose inhalers require refrigeration

18. The nurse should inform a client that the purpose of an aerochamber (spacer) on a metered dose inhaler is to _____.

Answer: 2

Rationale: For a client with chronic obstructive lung disease (COPD), there is an insensitivity to high levels of carbon dioxide and therefore an inspiratory drive that is now triggered by low oxygen levels. Giving higher concentrations of oxygen (greater than 2 to 3 L/min) can decrease the respiratory rate and depth, leading to oxygen-induced hypoventilation, apnea, and respiratory arrest.

Nursing process: Analysis

Client need: Pharmacological and Parenteral Therapies

Cognitive level: Analysis

Subject area: Pharmacologic

Answer: heated and humidified circuit

Rationale: Clients who receive oxygen support via ventilator should have humidification. In addition, if the upper airways are bypassed (endotracheal tube or tracheostomy), a heated circuit is also necessary.

Nursing process: Implementation

Client need: Pharmacological and Parenteral Therapies

Cognitive level: Application

Subject area: Pharmacologic

Answer: 2

Rationale: Nebulizers deliver medication through a face mask or mouthpiece, using compressed air or oxygen with a gas flow of 6 to 10 L/min. Metered dose inhalers deliver medication via puffs. Generally, the standard is 2 puffs per administration, a wait of 2 to 5 minutes between puffs, and no more than 12 puffs in 24 hours for most medications. Metered dose inhalers do not require refrigeration.

Nursing process: Planning

Client need: Pharmacological and Parenteral Therapies

Cognitive level: Analysis

Subject area: Pharmacologic

Answer: improve delivery of the medication to the lungs

Rationale: Spacers can significantly improve the delivery of medication to the lungs and should be used whenever possible. They are particularly helpful for small children who have difficulty synchronizing the breath and the activation of the inhaler canister.

Nursing process: Implementation

Client need: Pharmacological and Parenteral Therapies

Cognitive level: Application

Subject area: Pharmacologic

19. The nurse is instructing a client on the proper use of the pump for nasal spray administration. Which of the following statements by the client indicates a need for further instruction?

    1. "I should clear my nasal passages gently before using the pump."
    2. "I should inhale deeply during administration of the medication."
    3. "I should prime the pump if it hasn't been used for more than 24 hours."
    4. "I should not inhale during administration of the medication."

20. The nurse is admitting a client who was recently diagnosed with asthma and has been taking a long-acting theophylline (Theo-Dur). After reviewing the client's history, the nurse discovered that the client has a manic disorder controlled by lithium (Eskalith). Which of the following is a priority for the nurse to include in this client's treatment plan?

    1. Increase the dose of lithium
    2. Obtain a serum lithium level
    3. Increase the dose of theophylline
    4. Obtain a consult for a psychiatric consultation

21. A client questions a prescription for pyridoxine (B_6) after being started on the triple drug therapy for tuberculosis (ethambutol, rifampin, and isoniazid). The nurse explains that pyridoxine will

    1. prevent skin rash from the ethambutol.
    2. reduce the time the other drugs must be taken.
    3. counter the peripheral neuritis of the isoniazid.
    4. prevent damage to the eighth cranial nerve from the streptomycin.

22. The nurse is collecting a medication history on a client admitted with asthma who has been taking theophylline. Which of the following drugs is a priority for the nurse to notify the physician that the client has also been taking for a urinary tract infection?

    1. Cephradine (Velosef)
    2. Cephapirin sodium (Cefadyl)
    3. Trimethoprim and sulfamethoxazole (Bactrim)
    4. Ciprofloxacin (Cipro)

Answer: 2

Rationale: The client should not inhale during administration, so that the medication can remain in the nasal passages for best absorption. Initially, and if not used for more than seven days, the pump needs to be primed with seven actuations; if not used within 24 hours, prime with two actuations.

Nursing process: Evaluation

Client need: Health Promotion and Maintenance

Cognitive level: Application

Subject area: Pharmacologic

Answer: 2

Rationale: Theophylline may reduce the effects of lithium by increasing its rate of excretion. The client may need to have the dose of lithium increased, but not before the client's current serum lithium level is known. There is no indication to increase the theophylline dose. Obtaining a serum theophylline level would also be appropriate.

Nursing process: Analysis

Client need: Management of Care

Cognitive level: Analysis

Subject area: Pharmacologic

Answer: 3

Rationale: Pyridoxine (B_6) helps counter the peripheral neuritis associated with isoniazid therapy. Skin rash is a possible adverse reaction of ethambutol and clients on streptomycin should be monitored for hearing loss, particularly those with renal insufficiency. The duration of therapy is not shortened by pyridoxine.

Nursing process: Implementation

Client need: Pharmacological and Parenteral Therapies

Cognitive level: Application

Subject area: Pharmacologic

Answer: 4

Rationale: Ciprofloxacin (Cipro) causes a decrease in theophylline clearance and can elevate serum drug levels, causing theophylline toxicity.

Nursing process: Analysis

Client need: Management of Care

Cognitive level: Analysis

Subject area: Pharmacologic

23. A client arrives at the emergency room in status asthmaticus. Which of the following is the priority nursing action?

  1. Administer aminophylline intravenously as ordered

  2. Monitor the respiratory status and for signs of hypoxia

  3. Administer inhaled bronchodilator therapy as ordered

  4. Provide emotional support

24. The nurse evaluates which of the following as the appropriate method of improving oxygenation in a client with chronic airway limitation (CAL) who is lethargic, sleeps with the mouth open, is receiving 2 L/minute of oxygen per nasal cannula, and has a pulse oximetry check of 88%?

  1. Keep the client awake more so deeper breaths can be taken

  2. Turn the oxygen up to 4 L/minute

  3. Obtain an order for a face mask and use nasal cannula during meals

  4. Intubate the client and place the client on a ventilator

25. The nurse reviewing oxygen delivery modes selects which low-flow delivery mode to deliver the highest fraction of inspired oxygen (FIO_2)? _____

26. The nurse is preparing to delegate the nursing tasks for the day. Which of the following tasks should the nurse delegate to a licensed practical nurse?

  1. Monitor a client using a decongestant for the effectiveness of the drug

  2. Develop a teaching plan for effective coughing techniques for a client taking an expectorant

  3. Increase the oxygen flow rate to a client receiving oxygen by a simple face mask

  4. Administer a nasal spray to a client with rhinitis

Answer: 3

Rationale: To administer aminophylline intravenously, monitor the respiratory status and for signs of hypoxia, and provide emotional support are all appropriate interventions, but the initial action should be focused on improving oxygenation (airway, breathing, circulation). An inhalation bronchodilator will act quickly and should be followed by intravenous medications.

Nursing process: Implementation

Client need: Management of Care

Cognitive level: Analysis

Subject area: Pharmacologic

Answer: 3

Rationale: Clients who are mouth breathers may not get the full benefit from nasal cannula administration of oxygen. A face mask may be more effective. Face masks are removed for meals and a nasal cannula would be appropriate at that time. The client's oxygenation may improve when awake, but one cannot be kept awake all the time. Clients with chronic airway limitation (CAL) should not receive oxygen greater than 2 to 3 L/minute because greater oxygen administration may suppress the respiratory drive.

Nursing process: Evaluation

Client need: Pharmacological and Parenteral Therapies

Cognitive level: Analysis

Subject area: Pharmacologic

Answer: Nonrebreather mask

Rationale: A nasal cannula delivers up to 40% FIO_2. A simple face mask delivers up to 60% FIO_2. A partial rebreather mask delivers up to 75% FIO_2 and nonrebreather mask delivers up to 95% FIO_2.

Nursing process: Implementation

Client need: Pharmacological and Parenteral Therapies

Cognitive level: Application

Subject area: Pharmacologic

Answer: 4

Rationale: A licensed practical nurse cannot monitor a drug for its effectiveness or develop a teaching plan. These are job functions reserved for a registered nurse. Neither a registered nurse nor a licensed practical nurse can increase the oxygen flow rate to a client without a physician's order. Once a physician's order is obtained, a registered nurse should increase the flow rate.

Nursing process: Planning

Client need: Management of Care

Cognitive level: Analysis

Subject area: Pharmacologic

Drugs for the Cardiovascular System

18

1. Which of the following is the priority for the nurse to assess before administering digoxin (Lanoxin)?
   1. Auscultate the apical pulse for one full minute
   2. Palpate the radial pulse for 60 seconds
   3. Monitor the renal function tests
   4. Assess the serum potassium

2. Upon finding a client in cardiac arrest, the nurse should administer which of the following drugs first?
   1. Atropine
   2. Epinephrine
   3. Lidocaine
   4. Atenolol (Tenormin)

3. After medication teaching on atenolol (Tenormin), which of the following statements by a client with diabetes mellitus demonstrates an understanding of the atenolol? "It may
   1. cause hyperglycemia."
   2. mask an early indication of hypoglycemia."
   3. increase the action of insulin."
   4. diminish the action of insulin."

4. The nurse is caring for a client with hypertension. Which of the following drugs should the nurse administer?
   1. Mexiletine (Mexitil)
   2. Triamterene and hydrochlorothiazide (Dyazide)
   3. Digoxin (Lanoxin)
   4. Warfarin

Answer: 1

Rationale: A long-standing hallmark in the nursing interventions of the plan of care for a client taking digoxin (Lanoxin) is to take the apical pulse for a full minute. This is the priority nursing action. Bradycardia, in which the pulse is less than 60 beats per minute for one full minute, is one potential sign of digoxin toxicity. Although monitoring the renal function tests and serum potassium are appropriate interventions in the plan of care for a client taking Lanoxin, they are not the priority.

Nursing process: Assessment

Client need: Management of Care

Cognitive level: Application

Subject area: Pharmacologic

Answer: 2

Rationale: Epinephrine is the initial drug administered for cardiac arrest using the advanced cardiac life support (ACLS) algorithm. Atropine is used to restore cardiac rate in a client experiencing symptomatic sinus bradycardia. Lidocaine is used in the treatment of arrhythmias. Atenolol (Tenormin) is a beta-adrenergic blocking drug used for hypertension.

Nursing process: Implementation

Client need: Management of Care

Cognitive level: Analysis

Subject area: Pharmacologic

Answer: 2

Rationale: Beta blockers, such as atenolol (Tenormin), depress the heart rate and prevent tachycardia, one of the early indications of hypoglycemia.

Nursing process: Evaluation

Client need: Health Promotion and Maintenance

Cognitive level: Application

Subject area: Pharmacologic

Answer: 2

Rationale: Dyazide contains a combination of potassium-sparing diuretic and thiazide diuretic, triamterene and hydrochlorothiazide, to induce antihypertension by diminishing blood volume. Mexiletine (Mexitil) is an antiarrhythmic used in the treatment of ventricular arrhythmias. Digoxin (Lanoxin) is a cardiac glycoside used in the treatment of congestive heart failure and to slow the heart rate in a client with sinus tachycardia. Warfarin (Coumadin) is an anticoagulant.

Nursing process: Planning

Client need: Pharmacological and Parenteral Therapies

Cognitive level: Analysis

Subject area: Pharmacologic

5. Based on an understanding of nitroglycerin, the nurse administers it for which of the following reasons to a client with angina?

   1. Increase afterload

   2. Increase preload

   3. Constrict the arteries

   4. Dilate the veins

6. The nurse is caring for a client with atrial fibrillation who is being treated with a variety of drugs. The nurse administers which of the following drugs in combination with quinidine that may result in an increased level of the drug?

   1. Furosemide (Lasix)

   2. Digoxin (Lanoxin)

   3. Propranolol (Inderal)

   4. Triamterene and hydrochlorothiazide (Dyazide)

7. The nurse should administer amiodarone (Cordarone) to treat which of the following arrhythmias?

   1. Sinus bradycardia

   2. Bundle branch block

   3. Ventricular tachycardia

   4. Junctional rhythm

Answer: 4

Rationale: Nitroglycerin is a coronary vasodilator used in the treatment of angina. The venodilation decreases preload by decreasing blood return to the heart. Decreased preload diminishes the work of the heart, which reduces the oxygen needs and diminishes the anginal pain.

Nursing process: Analysis

Client need: Pharmacological and Parenteral Therapies

Cognitive level: Analysis

Subject area: Pharmacologic

Answer: 2

Rationale: Quinidine is an antiarrhythmic used in combination with digoxin and may potentially double digoxin levels. Furosemide (Lasix) is a loop diuretic. Digoxin (Lanoxin) is a cardiac glycoside used to control the rapid ventricular contraction rate in atrial fibrillation or atrial flutter, slow the heart rate in sinus tachycardia, and in the treatment of recurrent paroxysmal atrial tachycardia with paroxysmal A-V junctional rhythm. Propranolol (Inderal) is a beta-adrenergic blocking drug used in the treatment of hypertension. Triamterene and hydrochlorothiazide (Dyazide) is a combination antihypertensive drug.

Nursing process: Analysis

Client need: Pharmacological and Parenteral Therapies

Cognitive level: Analysis

Subject area: Pharmacologic

Answer: 3

Rationale: Amiodarone (Cordarone) is an antiarrhythmic that prolongs the duration of the action potential and refractory period, thus preventing life-threatening ventricular arrhythmias such as ventricular tachycardia by decreasing the sinus rate. Sinus bradycardia, bundle branch block, and junctional rhythm are all arrhythmias in which there is a slow heart rate.

Nursing process: Implementation

Client need: Pharmacological and Parenteral Therapies

Cognitive level: Analysis

Subject area: Pharmacologic

8. Which of the following is the priority nursing intervention for a client who is receiving adenosine (Adenocard) for supraventricular tachycardia (SVT)?

   1. Document the presence of peripheral pulses
   2. Monitor the pulse oximetry
   3. Assure a patent IV in the antecubital vein
   4. Prepare for emergency defibrillation

9. A client has been taking Viagra and is now experiencing angina. The physician has prescribed nitroglycerin p.r.n. for the angina. Which of the following should the nurse include in the discharge instructions?

   1. Viagra should not be used within 24 hours of taking nitroglycerin
   2. Nitroglycerin and Viagra should be taken at the same time
   3. Viagra is not effective when used in combination with nitroglycerin
   4. The effect of nitroglycerin is impaired by concurrent use with Viagra

10. Which of the following adverse reactions should the nurse assess in a 70-year-old adult who is receiving a continuous infusion of lidocaine?

   1. Hypertension
   2. Osteoarthritis
   3. Confusion
   4. Decreased visual acuity

11. Based on an understanding of beta blockers used for unstable angina, the nurse administers a beta blocker because of which of the following actions?

   1. To increase myocardial contractility
   2. To decrease heart rate
   3. To promote cardiovascular fluid shift
   4. Coronary artery vasodilation

Answer: 3

Rationale: Adenosine (Adenocard) is an antiarrhythmic that must be given in a large vessel, closest to the heart, due to its extremely short half-life. Documenting the presence of peripheral pulses, monitoring the pulse oximetry, and preparing for emergency defibrillation are all appropriate interventions, but the drug cannot be administered without IV access so this is the priority.

Nursing process: Analysis

Client need: Management of Care

Cognitive level: Analysis

Subject area: Pharmacologic

Answer: 1

Rationale: When used in combination, Viagra and nitroglycerin may cause life-threatening hypotension. Manufacturer's recommendations state that Viagra should not be used within 24 hours of taking nitroglycerin.

Nursing process: Planning

Client need: Health Promotion and Maintenance

Cognitive level: Application

Subject area: Pharmacologic

Answer: 3

Rationale: Lidocaine is an antiarrhythmic used in the treatment of ventricular arrhythmias. Confusion is a potential adverse reaction of a lidocaine infusion and is more common in the older adult.

Nursing process: Assessment

Client need: Pharmacological and Parenteral Therapies

Cognitive level: Analysis

Subject area: Pharmacologic

Answer: 2

Rationale: Beta blockers decrease the heart rate, diminishing the work of the heart and the oxygen needs, which results in a decrease in the anginal pain.

Nursing process: Implementation

Client need: Pharmacological and Parenteral Therapies

Cognitive level: Analysis

Subject area: Pharmacologic

12. Which of the following interventions should the nurse include in the plan of care for a client taking an ACE inhibitor?

    1. Monitor the blood pressure closely for two hours after the first dose

    2. Begin with a high dose and gradually decrease the dose

    3. Administer potassium supplements to the client

    4. Begin with daily dosing followed by dosing every other day

13. The nurse administers what drug to a client who is experiencing symptomatic sinus bradycardia?
    _____

14. A client's family member asks the nurse how to know if the client is improving while receiving furosemide (Lasix) for congestive heart failure. The nurse's response should be based on the understanding that improvement in the client's condition is characterized by

    1. diminishing oxygen needs.

    2. increased thirst.

    3. weight gain.

    4. intake greater than output.

15. A client with congestive heart disease returns to the clinic with muscle aching. The physician orders a potassium level, which shows hypokalemia. The drug regimen includes furosemide (Lasix) 80 mg b.i.d. In addition to treatment with a potassium supplement, the nurse administers which of the following prescribed drugs?

    1. Bumetanide (Bumex)

    2. Torsemide (Demadex)

    3. Spironolactone (Aldactone)

    4. Clonidine (Catapres)

Answer: 1

Rationale: ACE inhibitors used in the treatment of hypertension have a high potential for "first dose" hypotension, necessitating precautionary blood pressure monitoring.

Nursing process: Planning

Client need: Pharmacological and Parenteral Therapies

Cognitive level: Application

Subject area: Pharmacologic

Answer: Atropine

Rationale: Atropine is a cholinergic blocking drug that blocks vagal impulses to the heart, resulting in an increased heart rate and cardiac output. This increases blood pressure and heart rate.

Nursing process: Implementation

Client need: Pharmacological and Parenteral Therapies

Cognitive level: Analysis

Subject area: Pharmacologic

Answer: 1

Rationale: With congestive heart failure (CHF), fluid accumulates in the lung tissue due to ineffective pump action by the heart. As a diuretic, furosemide (Lasix) works to remove excess bodily fluids via the kidneys. The fluid shifts out of the lung tissue and therefore diminishes oxygen needs.

Nursing process: Analysis

Client need: Pharmacological and Parenteral Therapies

Cognitive level: Analysis

Subject area: Pharmacologic

Answer: 3

Rationale: Spironolactone (Aldactone) is a potassium-sparing diuretic. Its diuretic action is scant and it works to retain potassium. It is very often used in combination with the more powerful loop diuretics, like furosemide (Lasix), to counteract their potassium-wasting effects. Bumetanide (Bumex) and torsemide (Demadex) are loop diuretics, which deplete the body of potassium. Clonidine (Catapres) is an antihypertensive.

Nursing process: Implementation

Client need: Pharmacological and Parenteral Therapies

Cognitive level: Analysis

Subject area: Pharmacologic

16. While providing care to a client on cholestyramine (Questran), the nurse should monitor the client for which of the following?

Select all that apply:

[   ] **1.** Urinary retention

[   ] **2.** Abdominal pain

[   ] **3.** Bradycardia

[   ] **4.** Flatulence

[   ] **5.** Constipation

[   ] **6.** Confusion

17. The nurse is caring for a client on a heparin infusion when the client expresses concern over a progressively painful headache. Which of the following is the priority nursing action?

1. Stop the heparin infusion

2. Administer protamine

3. Notify the physician

4. Administer morphine

18. A client has been taking warfarin sodium (Coumadin) for the prevention of deep vein thrombosis. When the home care nurse arrives for a weekly visit, the client reports having been using aspirin (acetylsalicylic acid) daily for arthritic pain since hearing a commercial on television bolstering its benefits. Which of the following is the most appropriate response by the nurse, based on an understanding of the effect of combining Coumadin with aspirin?

1. "As long as you use aspirin only once a day, there will be no problems."

2. "Coumadin and aspirin used in combination increase the potential for bleeding."

3. "Aspirin and Coumadin may be used safely together."

4. "Coumadin may be used with aspirin without problem if vitamin K is taken with each dose."

19. The nurse is instructing a client on clopidogrel bisulfate (Plavix). Which of the following statements by the client indicates an understanding of the effect of this drug?

1. "I should ambulate slowly."

2. "I may experience hypotension."

3. "I should use caution taking other drugs that cause bleeding."

4. "I should take a stool softener while on this drug."

Answer: 2, 4, 5

Rationale: Cholestyramine (Questran) is an antihyperlipidemic. It absorbs and combines with intestinal bile acids, forming an insoluble, nonabsorbable complex that is excreted in the feces. Adverse reactions include abdominal pain, flatulence, and constipation.

Nursing process: Assessment

Client need: Pharmacological and Parenteral Therapies

Cognitive level: Application

Subject area: Pharmacologic

Answer: 3

Rationale: The priority nursing action is to notify the physician. Headache, although rare, is an adverse reaction to a heparin hypersensitivity. The nurse may anticipate stopping the heparin infusion or administering protamine sulfate, a heparin antagonist, but the priority intervention is to notify the physician of a potential hypersensitivity.

Nursing process: Planning

Client need: Management of Care

Cognitive level: Analysis

Subject area: Pharmacologic

Answer: 2

Rationale: Aspirin inhibits platelet aggregation, diminishing the potential for clot formation. Warfarin (Coumadin) is an anticoagulant that interferes with blood clot formation by interfering with the synthesis of vitamin K clotting factors, resulting in depletion of the clotting factors. The combination of Coumadin and aspirin increases the potential for bleeding.

Nursing process: Analysis

Client need: Pharmacological and Parenteral Therapies

Cognitive level: Analysis

Subject area: Pharmacologic

Answer: 3

Rationale: Clopidogrel bisulfate (Plavix) is an antiplatelet drug that inhibits platelet aggregation, diminishing the potential for clot formation. Caution should be used when taking other drugs that may increase bleeding. Plavix may cause the adverse reactions of hypertension and diarrhea.

Nursing process: Evaluation

Client need: Health Promotion and Maintenance

Cognitive level: Analysis

Subject area: Pharmacologic

20. The nurse should monitor a client with an acute myocardial infarction who is receiving intravenous streptokinase (Streptase) for which of the following serious adverse reactions?

    1. Intracranial hemorrhage

    2. Intractable nausea

    3. Extension of myocardial damage

    4. Pulmonary embolus

21. The nurse is caring for a client taking atorvastatin [Lipitor]. The client admits to consuming 6 to 12 beers daily. The nurse should monitor the client for what potentially serious adverse reaction to Lipitor?

    1. Nephrotoxicity

    2. Hypertension

    3. Hepatotoxicity

    4. Dyspepsia

22. The nurse is developing a medication schedule for a client receiving simvastatin (Zocor). To promote maximal effectiveness, the nurse should administer the drug

    1. 30 minutes before a meal.

    2. with meals.

    3. at bedtime.

    4. early in the morning.

23. The nurse is caring for a client receiving gemfibrozil (Lopid). The nurse understands that this medication is given for what purpose? _____

Answer: 1

Rationale: Streptokinase (Streptase) is a thrombolytic enzyme used in the treatment of deep vein thrombosis, arterial thrombosis, acute evolving myocardial infarction, pulmonary embolism, and to clear an occluded arteriovenous and IV cannula. It is a priority that the client is monitored for an intracranial hemorrhage that could potentially lead to coma and death.

Nursing process: Assessment

Client need: Pharmacological and Parenteral Therapies

Cognitive level: Analysis

Subject area: Pharmacologic

Answer: 3

Rationale: Atorvastatin (Lipitor) is an antihyperlipidemic and HMG-CoA reduction inhibitor. The risk for hepatotoxicity while using Lipitor is increased by excessive alcohol ingestion.

Nursing process: Assessment

Client need: Pharmacological and Parenteral Therapies

Cognitive level: Analysis

Subject area: Pharmacologic

Answer: 3

Rationale: Simvastatin (Zocor) is an antihyperlipidemic. Because cholesterol synthesis normally increases during the night, statins, like Zocor, are most effective when given in the evening.

Nursing process: Implementation

Client need: Pharmacological and Parenteral Therapies

Cognitive level: Analysis

Subject area: Pharmacologic

Answer: To lower levels of plasma triglycerides

Rationale: Gemfibrozil (Lopid) is an antihyperlipidemic that decreases VLDL (triglyceride) synthesis and secretion, resulting in lowering levels of plasma triglycerides.

Nursing process: Analysis

Client need: Pharmacological and Parenteral Therapies

Cognitive level: Comprehension

Subject area: Pharmacologic

24. The nurse is caring for a client admitted with severe rectal bleeding who is receiving warfarin (Coumadin) therapy. Which of the following interventions should have priority in the plan of care?

1. Accurate intake and output

2. Discontinue the warfarin

3. Assure a patent 18-gauge IV

4. Administer vitamin K

25. The registered nurse is preparing to delegate assignments for the day. Which of the following assignments would be appropriate to delegate to a licensed practical nurse?

1. Contact a client's physician when the blood pressure is lower than 100 mm Hg before administering a beta$_2$-adrenergic blocker

2. Monitor the heparin level daily before administering heparin

3. Question administration of streptokinase (Streptase) to a client admitted and suspected of an intracranial hemorrhage

4. Take the blood pressure before administering a dose of verapamil (Calan)

Answer: 3

Rationale: Although maintaining an accurate intake and output, discontinuing the Coumadin, and administering vitamin K may be anticipated, the priority intervention is to assure an 18-gauge IV needed for potential transfusion of blood, if bleeding causes hypovolemia and low hemoglobin.

Nursing process: Planning

Client need: Management of Care

Cognitive level: Analysis

Subject area: Pharmacologic

Answer: 4

Rationale: Contacting a client's physician, monitoring the heparin level, and questioning the administration of a drug are all nursing tasks that should be performed by a registered nurse. A licensed practical nurse (LPN) may take a blood pressure before administering a drug. LPNs are trained to take the blood pressure; if the blood pressure is too low or too high, it becomes the responsibility of the registered nurse to notify the physician.

Nursing process: Planning

Client need: Management of Care

Cognitive level: Analysis

Subject area: Legal and Ethical Issues

Drugs for the Gastrointestinal System

19

1. The nurse evaluates that medication teaching has been effective when the client states that ranitidine (Zantac)
   1. decreases gastric acid levels.
   2. changes hormonal levels.
   3. increases pepsin levels.
   4. decreases pH levels.

2. Which of the following should the nurse include in the teaching plan the nurse is preparing for a client taking sucralfate (Carafate)?
   1. Sucralfate reduces gastric acid production
   2. Administer sucralfate with breakfast
   3. Separate administration of sucralfate with other drugs by two hours
   4. Sucralfate works against *H. pylori*

3. Which of the following is a priority for the nurse to administer to a client with gastroesophageal reflux disease (GERD)?
   1. Cytoprotectors
   2. Antibiotics
   3. Proton pump inhibitors
   4. Anticholinergics

4. The nurse should assess which of the following body systems while administering intravenous cimetidine (Tagamet) to a client?
   1. Urinary
   2. Immune
   3. Respiratory
   4. Cardiovascular

Answer: 1

Rationale: Ranitidine (Zantac) is a histamine 2-receptor antagonist, which suppresses gastric acid secretion. Changing hormonal levels is not a primary action of ranitidine. Cimetidine (Tagamet) suppresses pepsin production. Zantac also reduces hydrogen ion concentration, which will increase pH levels.

Nursing process: Evaluation

Client need: Health Promotion and Maintenance

Cognitive level: Application

Subject area: Pharmacologic

Answer: 3

Rationale: The administration of sucralfate (Carafate) should be separated from other drug administration by two hours to protect those drugs from binding to the protective adhesive that forms. Sucralfate is an antipeptic/cytoprotective gastrointestinal drug used to protect eroded ulcer sites from further acidic damage. Sucralfate should be administered one hour before meals. Antibiotics are used in peptic ulcer disease to fight against *H. pylori*.

Nursing process: Planning

Client need: Health Promotion and Maintenance

Cognitive level: Application

Subject area: Pharmacologic

Answer: 3

Rationale: Drugs used to promote healing the tissues damaged by acid reflux include antacids and antisecretory drugs, such as proton pump inhibitors and histamine 2-receptor antagonists. Cytoprotective/antipeptics and antibiotics (and anticholinergics) are primarily used for peptic ulcer disease. Cholinergics are used on rare occasions for gastroesophageal reflux to increase the rate of gastric emptying.

Nursing process: Planning

Client need: Management of Care

Cognitive level: Application

Subject area: Pharmacologic

Answer: 4

Rationale: Cimetidine (Tagamet) is a histamine 2-receptor blocking drug used in the treatment of ulcers and gastroesophageal reflux disease. The cardiovascular system needs to be assessed. Intravenous cimetidine (Tagamet) can cause dysrhythmias and hypotension. Other body systems that need to be assessed include the gastrointestinal, hematologic, metabolic, central nervous system, and genital systems. Tagamet does not affect the urinary, immune, or respiratory system.

Nursing process: Assessment

Client need: Pharmacological and Parenteral Therapies

Cognitive level: Application

Subject area: Pharmacologic

5. The nurse should monitor a client taking lansoprazole (Prevacid) for which of the following adverse reactions?

Select all that apply:

[ ] 1. Headache

[ ] 2. Oliguria

[ ] 3. Anxiety

[ ] 4. Dry mouth

[ ] 5. Diarrhea

[ ] 6. Decreased appetite

6. A client is experiencing peptic ulcer disease caused by *Helicobacter pylori.* The nurse should plan to administer which of the following oral drug combinations? Clarithromycin (Biaxin) with

1. tetracycline (Achromycin) with sodium bicarbonate (baking soda).

2. metronidazole (Flagyl) and aluminum hydroxide (Amphogel).

3. amoxicillin (Amoxil) and omeprazole (Prilosec).

4. penicillin (Pen-G) and nizatidine (Axid).

7. The nurse should instruct a client that taking which antacid may result in constipation? A client taking

1. magaldrate (Riopan).

2. magnesium and aluminum (Maalox).

3. aluminum carbonate (Basaljel).

4. magnesium hydroxide (milk of magnesia).

8. The nurse is caring for a client who admits to a 15-year history of gastric ulcers. The nurse instructs this client to take which of the following drugs for minor aches and pains?

1. Acetaminophen (Tylenol)

2. Buffered aspirin

3. Plain aspirin

4. Ibuprofen (Motrin)

Answer: 1, 3, 4, 5

Rationale: Lansoprazole (Prevacid) is a proton pump inhibitor used in the treatment of ulcers and gastroesophageal reflux disease. Adverse reactions associated with Prevacid include headache, anxiety, dry mouth, and diarrhea.

Nursing process: Assessment

Client need: Pharmacological and Parenteral Therapies

Cognitive level: Application

Subject area: Pharmacologic

Answer: 3

Rationale: Clarithromycin (Biaxin) is used in combination with amoxicillin (Amoxil) and omeprazole (Prilosec) as an effective combination to combat *H. pylori.*

Nursing process: Planning

Client need: Pharmacological and Parenteral Therapies

Cognitive level: Analysis

Subject area: Pharmacologic

Answer: 3

Rationale: Most antacids affect the bowel. Some promote constipation, such as aluminum carbonate (Basaljel), and others promote diarrhea, such as magnesium. Effects can be minimized by combining aluminum and magnesium.

Nursing process: Planning

Client need: Health Promotion and Maintenance

Cognitive level: Application

Subject area: Pharmacologic

Answer: 1

Rationale: Acetaminophen (Tylenol) has no adverse effect on the gastric mucosa and produces no ulcerative effects when administered for pain. Buffered aspirin does not reduce the incidence of gastric ulcers, although enteric-coated aspirin dissolves in the intestine rather than the stomach. Plain aspirin is associated with development of gastric ulcers. Nonsteroidal anti-inflammatory drugs, such as ibuprofen (Motrin), may cause gastric ulceration.

Nursing process: Implementation

Client need: Pharmacological and Parenteral Therapies

Cognitive level: Application

Subject area: Pharmacologic

9. Which of the following antacids should the nurse question administering to the client with a gastric ulcer and congestive heart failure?

1. Magaldrate (Riopan)

2. Calcium carbonate (Tums)

3. Magnesium hydroxide (milk of magnesia)

4. Sodium bicarbonate (baking soda)

10. The nurse is developing a medication schedule for a client who is receiving magnesium and aluminum (Mylanta) for gastritis. To promote the best absorption, when should this drug be administered?

Select all that apply:

[   ] 1. At bedtime

[   ] 2. One hour before meals

[   ] 3. Immediately after meals

[   ] 4. Upon arising in the morning

[   ] 5. One hour after meals

[   ] 6. 30 minutes after meals

11. After obtaining a medication history from a client who informs the nurse of her early pregnancy, which of the following drugs is a priority for the nurse to obtain an order to discontinue?

1. Misoprostol (Cytotec)

2. Docusate (Surfak)

3. Magnesium hydroxide (milk of magnesia)

4. Bismuth subsalicylate (Pepto-Bismol)

12. When administering cimetidine (Tagamet), the nurse assesses the client for which of the following adverse reactions?

Select all that apply:

[   ] 1. Tinnitus

[   ] 2. Alopecia

[   ] 3. Diarrhea

[   ] 4. Mental confusion

[   ] 5. Dizziness

[   ] 6. Dyspepsia

Answer: 4

Rationale: Sodium bicarbonate has higher sodium levels than other antacids and is contraindicated for clients with ulcerative disease and heart failure. Magnesium-based and calcium-based antacids, such as magaldrate (Riopan), calcium carbonate (Tums), and magnesium hydroxide (milk of magnesia), are often chosen for clients with heart failure because of their low sodium content.

Nursing process: Analysis

Client need: Pharmacological and Parenteral Therapies

Cognitive level: Analysis

Subject area: Pharmacologic

Answer: 1, 2, 5

Rationale: Ideally antacids should be administered one hour before meals, one hour after meals, and at bedtime to reduce gastric acid secretion and promote ulcer healing. Administering an antacid first thing in the morning is not appropriate because the neutralizing action lasts only approximately 30 minutes and there is nothing in the stomach to slow its emptying.

Nursing process: Planning

Client need: Pharmacological and Parenteral Therapies

Cognitive level: Application

Subject area: Pharmacologic

Answer: 1

Rationale: Although all drug use needs to be questioned in the first trimester of pregnancy, misoprostol (Cytotec), which may be used in peptic ulcer prevention as a prostaglandin and cytoprotective agent, is known to cause miscarriages. Docusate (Surfak) is a mild surfactant laxative, which has no adverse effects. Magnesium hydroxide (milk of magnesia) and bismuth subsalicylate are mild antacids with no teratogenic effects.

Nursing process: Analysis

Client need: Management of Care

Cognitive level: Analysis

Subject area: Pharmacologic

Answer: 3, 4, 5

Rationale: Cimetidine (Tagamet) is a histamine 2-receptor blocking drug used in the treatment of ulcers and gastroesophageal reflux disease. Adverse reactions include diarrhea, mental confusion (especially in the older adult), and dizziness.

Nursing process: Assessment

Client need: Pharmacological and Parenteral Therapies

Cognitive level: Application

Subject area: Pharmacologic

13. The client is to begin taking methylcellulose (Citrucel) daily. The nurse will include which of the following instructions in the teaching plan?

   1. Administer with at least 8 ounces of liquid

   2. Administer at hour of sleep

   3. Discontinue if no bowel movement in five days

   4. Discontinue if taking docusate (Colace)

14. The nurse should include which of the following in the medication instructions given to a client who is being started on antiemetics?

   1. Take the antiemetic within one hour after activity that promotes nausea

   2. Stop taking the antiemetic when the activity that induces the nausea ceases

   3. The urine may turn an orangish color

   4. Avoid activities that require mental alertness

15. The nurse informs a student nurse that the loperamide (Imodium) prescribed for a client who is experiencing diarrhea has which of the following actions?

   1. Inhibits the peristaltic activity of intestinal muscles

   2. Consolidates the stool in the intestine

   3. Lowers the surface tension, allowing more water into stool

   4. Distends the intestine by osmotic retention of fluid

Answer: 1

Rationale: Methylcellulose is a bulk laxative. Bulk laxatives must be given with at least 8 ounces of liquid to provide enough water to increase the size of the stool mass and stretch the intestinal wall promoting peristalsis. Bulk laxatives should be taken when the client is most active. The therapeutic effect occurs within two to three days. Stool softeners are not contraindicated with bulk laxative use.

Nursing process: Planning

Client need: Health Promotion and Maintenance

Cognitive level: Application

Subject area: Pharmacologic

Answer: 4

Rationale: A client taking an antiemetic should be instructed to avoid activities that require mental alertness because all antiemetics cause varying degrees of drowsiness that will affect the ability to perform a task.

Nursing process: Planning

Client need: Health Promotion and Maintenance

Cognitive level: Application

Subject area: Pharmacologic

Answer: 1

Rationale: Loperamide (Imodium) directly inhibits peristaltic activity of the intestinal muscle, which results in decreased gastrointestinal motility. Consolidating stool in the intestine describes pectin, which is a component of the antidiarrheal Kaopectate. Lowering the surface tension allows more water into the stool, which describes surfactant laxatives or stool softeners. Distending the intestine by osmotic retention of fluid describes the action of saline or osmotic laxatives.

Nursing process: Implementation

Client need: Pharmacological and Parenteral Therapies

Cognitive level: Comprehension

Subject area: Pharmacologic

16. Which of the following is a priority for the nurse to include in the plan of care for a client taking ondansetron (Zofran) for chemotherapy?

    1. Monitor the client for fluid and electrolyte imbalance

    2. Instruct the client to take the Zofran 30 minutes before the chemotherapy

    3. Instruct the client to take an analgesic for the adverse reaction to a headache

    4. Encourage the client to avoid activities that may cause drowsiness

17. Which of the following is the priority for the nurse to include in the plan of care for a client receiving metoclopramide (Reglan) with chemotherapy in a clinic?

    1. Instruct the client to avoid driving home

    2. Offer gum or hard candy for dry mouth

    3. Administer 1/2 to 1 hour before the chemotherapy treatment

    4. Assess the client for extrapyramidal clinical manifestations

18. The nurse should question which of the following medication administration orders?

    1. Cimetidine (Tagamet) 300 mg orally four times a day to an 86-year-old client with gastroesophageal reflux disease

    2. Famotidine (Pepcid) 20 mg and Maalox 30 ml orally at bedtime to a 23-year-old client with a peptic ulcer

    3. Lansoprazole (Prevacid) 15 mg orally daily to a 51-year-old client with a duodenal ulcer

    4. Omeprazole (Prilosec) 20 mg orally three times a day to a 40-year-old client with a pathological hypersecretion condition

Answer: 1

Rationale: Ondansetron (Zofran) is a serotonin receptor antagonist, which suppresses the vomiting reflex and chemotherapy-induced emesis. Because diarrhea is the most common adverse reaction of Zofran and the client may be experiencing vomiting from the chemotherapy, the client may become dehydrated. The client should be monitored for fluid and electrolyte imbalances. Although it is appropriate to tell the client to take the Zofran 30 minutes before the chemotherapy, to avoid activities that may cause drowsiness, and to take an analgesic if a headache occurs, they are not the priority interventions.

Nursing process: Planning

Client need: Management of Care

Cognitive level: Analysis

Subject area: Pharmacologic

Answer: 1

Rationale: Although it is appropriate to offer a client receiving metoclopramide (Reglan) gum or hard candy, administer the Reglan 1/2 to 1 hour before the chemotherapy, and assess the client for extrapyramidal clinical manifestations, the priority nursing intervention is to instruct the client to avoid driving home.

Nursing process: Planning

Client need: Management of Care

Cognitive level: Analysis

Subject area: Pharmacologic

Answer: 1

Rationale: Cimetidine (Tagamet), a histamine 2-receptor blocking agent, should be avoided in the older adult because it causes confusion.

Nursing process: Analysis

Client need: Pharmacological and Parenteral Therapies

Cognitive level: Analysis

Subject area: Pharmacologic

19. The nurse selects the ideal antacid for a client because of which of the following characteristics?

    1. Sweet to taste, cathartic in nature, and effective for a prolonged period of time

    2. Short acting and readily absorbed

    3. Not absorbed by the body and acts as a laxative

    4. Decreases acidity without constipating or cathartic properties

20. After administering ursodiol (Actigall) to the client with gallbladder disease, the nurse evaluates the priority outcome to be

    1. decreased vomiting.

    2. increased comfort.

    3. reduced stone formation.

    4. decreased bile production.

21. The nurse has administered prochlorperazine (Compazine) on several occasions over the past week to the client experiencing severe vomiting. The nurse should assess this client for which of the following adverse reactions?

    Select all that apply:

    [ ] **1.** Bradycardia

    [ ] **2.** Weight loss

    [ ] **3.** Akathisia

    [ ] **4.** Orthostatic hypotension

    [ ] **5.** Acute dystonia

    [ ] **6.** Oliguria

22. The nurse is collecting a nursing history from a client admitted on pancreatin. Which of the following diseases should the nurse question in the client's medical history?

    1. Hepatitis

    2. Cirrhosis

    3. Gallbladder cancer

    4. Cystic fibrosis

Answer: 4

Rationale: The ideal antacid would decrease the acidity of the gastric secretions without either constipating or cathartic effects.

Nursing process: Implementation

Client need: Pharmacological and Parenteral Therapies

Cognitive level: Analysis

Subject area: Pharmacologic

Answer: 3

Rationale: Gallstone dissolvers, such as ursodiol, are bile acids that reduce the cholesterol content in bile and allow for the dissolution of cholesterol-type gallstones. Decreased vomiting may result from a decrease in pain, which more likely will occur with analgesic use. Increased comfort will primarily occur with analgesic use and may be a secondary effect of stone dissolution. Ursodiol reduces the cholesterol content of bile, but hepatic production of bile is not affected.

Nursing process: Evaluation

Client need: Management of Care

Cognitive level: Analysis

Subject area: Pharmacologic

Answer: 3, 4, 5

Rationale: Prochlorperazine (Compazine) is a phenothiazine-type antiemetic that results in extrapyramidal effects, such as akathisia and acute dystonia. Other adverse reactions include tachycardia, weight gain, orthostatic hypotension, and urinary difficulties such as loss of bladder control.

Nursing process: Assessment

Client need: Pharmacological and Parenteral Therapies

Cognitive level: Application

Subject area: Pharmacologic

Answer: 4

Rationale: Pancreatin is a pancreatic enzyme used to replace enzyme deficiencies caused by disorders such as cystic fibrosis. Hepatitis and cirrhosis may cause vitamin and other hepatic deficiencies, but not pancreatic enzyme deficiencies. Enzyme replacement is generally not indicated for gallbladder cancer.

Nursing process: Analysis

Client need: Pharmacological and Parenteral Therapies

Cognitive level: Analysis

Subject area: Pharmacologic

23. When providing care to a client who is on propantheline (Pro-Banthine), the nurse should assess the client for which of the following?

    Select all that apply:

    [   ] 1. Dry mouth

    [   ] 2. Diarrhea

    [   ] 3. Blurred vision

    [   ] 4. Hypertension

    [   ] 5. Urinary frequency

    [   ] 6. Tachycardia

24. The nurse has instructed the client about sulfasalazine (Azulfidine), which was prescribed for her ulcerative colitis. The nurse evaluates which of the following statements by the client to indicate that the client understood the instructions?

    1. "Nausea, vomiting, and abdominal pain are adverse reactions of Azulfidine."

    2. "I should chew the tablets thoroughly and follow with a sip of water."

    3. "I may notice my urine turns blue."

    4. "Azulfidine will decrease intestinal gas production."

25. The client was recently diagnosed with chronic hepatitis C. The nurse plans to instruct the client about which of the following drugs that is used in combination with oral ribavirin?

    1. Lamivudine (Epivir HBV)

    2. Interferon alfa

    3. Interferon gamma

    4. Ganciclovir (Cytovene)

26. The nurse is preparing to delegate which of the following nursing tasks to a licensed practical nurse?

    1. Administer IV ondansetron (Zofran) to a client experiencing nausea from chemotherapy

    2. Instruct a client on the adverse reactions of propantheline (Pro-Banthine)

    3. Administer trimethobenzamide (Tigan) Z-track to a client prior to chemotherapy

    4. Develop a medication schedule for a client taking an antacid and several other drugs

Answer: 1, 3, 6

Rationale: Anticholinergic agents, such as propantheline (Pro-Banthine), cause dry mouth, constipation, urinary retention, blurred vision, tachycardia, and orthostatic hypotension.

Nursing process: Assessment

Client need: Pharmacological and Parenteral Therapies

Cognitive level: Application

Subject area: Pharmacologic

Answer: 1

Rationale: Sulfasalazine (Azulfidine) is an anti-inflammatory agent and sulfonamide, which reduces gastrointestinal motility, inflammation, and microbial flora such as *E. coli.* Nausea, vomiting, and abdominal pain are adverse reactions. Decreasing gas formation is the action of simethicone. The tablets are not chewed and Azulfidine should be administered with a full glass of water. The skin and urine may turn yellow-orange.

Nursing process: Evaluation

Client need: Pharmacological and Parenteral Therapies

Cognitive level: Analysis

Subject area: Pharmacologic

Answer: 2

Rationale: In clients with chronic hepatitis C, modest responses have occurred with combining ribavirin with interferon alfa. All interferons of the alfa class are used to treat hepatitis. Lamivudine is used only in the treatment of hepatitis B virus. Interferons of the gamma class are not utilized for hepatitis. Ganciclovir is utilized to treat herpes viruses.

Nursing process: Planning

Client need: Pharmacological and Parenteral Therapies

Cognitive level: Application

Subject area: Pharmacologic

Answer: 3

Rationale: A licensed practical nurse may administer a drug by Z-track. Administering a drug IV, instructing a client on the adverse reactions of a drug, and developing a medication schedule for a client taking an antacid and several other drugs are nursing tasks reserved for a registered nurse.

Nursing process: Planning

Client need: Management of Care

Cognitive level: Analysis

Subject area: Legal and Ethical Issues

Drugs for the Endocrine System

20

1. Which of the following should the nurse include in the instructions given to a client receiving somatropin (Humatrope)?

    1. Get an annual bone age assessment

    2. Schedule a fasting blood sugar once a year if there is a family history of diabetes mellitus

    3. Record height weekly and report linear growth of 7 to 15 cm in the first year

    4. Notify the physician if urine output increases

2. Which of the following assessment data is an anticipated outcome for a client with diabetes insipidus who is receiving vasopressin (Pitressin) injections?

    1. Urine output of 2500 ml/day

    2. Weight loss of 4 pounds in one week

    3. Urine specific gravity of 1.005

    4. Oral intake of 4500 ml/day

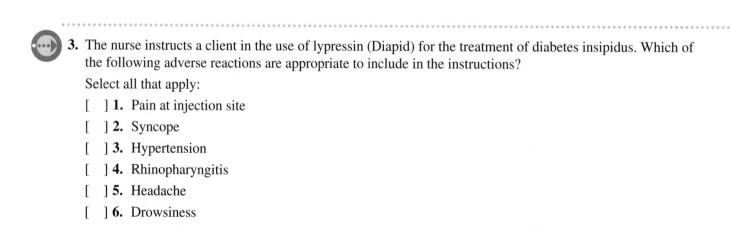

3. The nurse instructs a client in the use of lypressin (Diapid) for the treatment of diabetes insipidus. Which of the following adverse reactions are appropriate to include in the instructions?

    Select all that apply:

    [   ] **1.** Pain at injection site

    [   ] **2.** Syncope

    [   ] **3.** Hypertension

    [   ] **4.** Rhinopharyngitis

    [   ] **5.** Headache

    [   ] **6.** Drowsiness

Answer: 1

Rationale: Somatropin (growth hormone) is given when there is growth failure prior to epiphyseal closure. Annual bone assessment is necessary to make certain that epiphyseal closure has not occurred. Growth hormone increases the glucose level in the blood, so that those with a family history of diabetes are likely to develop diabetes mellitus. Fasting blood sugars should be done more frequently than once a year to detect development of diabetes mellitus. Linear growth of 7 to 20 cm in the first year is normal and not necessary to report. Growth hormone does not affect urinary output.

Nursing process: Planning

Client need: Health Promotion and Maintenance

Cognitive level: Application

Subject area: Pharmacologic

Answer: 1

Rationale: The client with diabetes insipidus who is receiving vasopressin injections should have an improvement in the clinical manifestations of diabetes insipidus (polyuria and polydipsia). The client should notice an increase in weight and a decrease in urine output. The urine output of 2500 ml is in the normal range. Urine specific gravity of 1.005 and an oral intake of 4500 ml/day are characteristic of untreated diabetes insipidus.

Nursing process: Evaluation

Client need: Pharmacological and Parenteral Therapies

Cognitive level: Analysis

Subject area: Pharmacologic

Answer: 3, 4, 5, 6

Rationale: Lypressin (Diapid) is an antidiuretic hormone used to treat diabetes insipidus. It is only administered intranasally, not by injection. Adverse reactions include intranasal congestion, rhinorrhea, irritation, hypertension, headache, and drowsiness.

Nursing process: Planning

Client need: Health Promotion and Maintenance

Cognitive level: Application

Subject area: Pharmacologic

4. The client starting on vasopressin asks the nurse, "Why did the physician say to avoid drinking alcohol while taking this medication?" Which of the following responses by the nurse is appropriate? "Alcohol will

   1. cause an increase in vasoconstriction."
   2. decrease the antidiuretic effect."
   3. interfere with the absorption of vasopressin in the stomach."
   4. promote a hypersensitivity to vasopressin."

5. When admitting a new client with hypothyroidism (myxedema), the nurse notices an order for a sedative at bedtime. The nurse should question this order because sedatives _____.

6. Prior to discharge, the nurse instructs a client who is receiving liothyronine (Cytomel) to notify the physician if which of the following occurs?

   1. A pulse rate of more than 100 beats per minute
   2. A weight loss of five pounds in two weeks
   3. More frequent urination
   4. Excessive sleepiness

7. The nurse instructs a client who is started on levothyroxine sodium (Synthroid) that the best time to take the medication is

   1. one hour after a meal.
   2. with a bedtime snack.
   3. 30 minutes before breakfast.
   4. once a day with any meal.

Answer: 2

Rationale: Alcohol causes vasodilatation, not vasoconstriction, in a client taking vasopressin. Alcohol does decrease the antidiuretic effect of vasopressin from its action on the kidneys. Vasopressin is injected and absorbed intramuscularly. Hypersensitivity reactions occur with vasopressin, but are not related to the ingestion of alcohol.

Nursing process: Analysis

Client need: Pharmacological and Parenteral Therapies

Cognitive level: Analysis

Subject area: Pharmacologic

Answer: cause respiratory depression

Rationale: Clients with hypothyroidism have depressed respirations and are very susceptible to respiratory depression when given hypnotic and sedative agents. These drugs decrease the rate and depth of respirations. These clients are prescribed thyroid drugs.

Nursing process: Analysis

Client need: Pharmacological and Parenteral Therapies

Cognitive level: Analysis

Subject area: Pharmacologic

Answer: 1

Rationale: Liothyronine (Cytomel) is a thyroid drug used in the treatment of hypothyroidism. It increases the metabolic rate, but a rate of more than 100 beats per minute is an indication that the dosage needs to be decreased. A weight loss and diuresis would be expected therapy outcomes. A client with hypothyroidism would be very lethargic and sleep most of the day. The activity level should increase as a response to the drug, and a nap during the day would improve the condition.

Nursing process: Implementation

Client need: Health Promotion and Maintenance

Cognitive level: Analysis

Subject area: Pharmacologic

Answer: 3

Rationale: Food interferes with the absorption of levothyroxine (Synthroid). The client should take the drug at the same time of day, preferably before breakfast.

Nursing process: Implementation

Client need: Pharmacological and Parenteral Therapies

Cognitive level: Application

Subject area: Pharmacologic

8. Which of the following is essential that the nurse include in the assessment of a client receiving methimazole (Tapazole)?

   1. Serum sodium levels

   2. White blood cell count and differential

   3. Platelet count

   4. Serum lipid levels

9. The nurse instructs a client who has been prescribed Lugol's solution to notify the physician if which of the following occurs?

   1. Blurred vision

   2. Weight gain

   3. Increased urinary output

   4. Brassy taste in mouth

10. When a client experiencing thyrotoxicosis arrives at the emergency room, the nurse should administer which of the following drugs intravenously?

    1. 50% dextrose

    2. Saturated solution of potassium iodide

    3. Calcium gluconate

    4. Theophylline

Answer: 2

Rationale: A serious adverse reaction to antithyroid drugs is agranulocytosis, a severe reduction in the number of granulocytes (basophils, eosinophils, and neutrophils). Antithyroid drugs do not affect serum sodium and lipid levels or platelet count.

Nursing process: Assessment

Client need: Pharmacological and Parenteral Therapies

Cognitive level: Application

Subject area: Pharmacologic

Answer: 4

Rationale: Clients receiving iodine preparations, such as Lugol's solution, are advised to notify the physician if they experience a brassy taste in the mouth, which may be significant for iodism (excessive amounts of iodine in the body). Blurred vision, weight gain, and increased urinary output are clinical manifestations of endocrine disorders, but are not attributed to iodine preparations.

Nursing process: Implementation

Client need: Health Promotion and Maintenance

Cognitive level: Analysis

Subject area: Pharmacologic

Answer: 2

Rationale: The client with thyrotoxicosis (thyroid storm) is experiencing severe hyperthyroidism. Saturated solution of potassium iodide is given IV, because it acts quickly to reduce the metabolic rate. Dextrose 50% is an emergency drug for the treatment of hypoglycemia. Calcium gluconate is used for hypoparathyroidism in clients who are experiencing tetany. Theophylline is an emergency drug for clients experiencing breathing difficulties.

Nursing process: Implementation

Client need: Pharmacological and Parenteral Therapies

Cognitive level: Application

Subject area: Pharmacologic

11. The nurse is caring for a client who developed tetany postoperatively. The client is to receive aluminum hydroxide gel (Gelusil) and calcium gluconate (Kalcinate). The nurse should understand that the client is to receive aluminum hydroxide gel (Gelusil) for which of the following purposes?

    1. To neutralize the hydrochloric acid in the stomach so that the calcium can be absorbed

    2. To coat the esophagus and stomach linings from the irritation of the calcium salts

    3. To bind dietary phosphorus and promote the elimination of insoluble aluminum phosphate by the GI tract

    4. To increase the rate of gastric emptying to enhance absorption of calcium in the small intestine

12. The nurse is collecting a health history from a client who is to begin taking calcium lactate. Which of the following questions should the nurse ask to determine the safety of taking calcium supplements?

    1. "Have you had any kidney stones within the past year?"

    2. "Have you ever been told that you have high blood pressure?"

    3. "Have you had any chest pains or a heart attack?"

    4. "Have you had any problems with frequent diarrhea?"

13. A client with Addison's disease is scheduled for hernia surgery in the morning. Which of the following drugs should the nurse expect to give with a sip of water the morning of surgery?

    1. Micronase

    2. Prednisone

    3. Synthroid

    4. Furosemide (Lasix)

Answer: 3

Rationale: Aluminum hydroxide gel (Gelusil) is given in conjunction with calcium gluconate to bind dietary phosphorus and promote the elimination of insoluble aluminum phosphate in the feces in a client who is experiencing tetany. The client with tetany has decreased serum calcium and an increase in serum phosphate levels. The neutralization of hydrochloric acid in the stomach does not affect the absorption of calcium. Calcium gluconate is not irritating to the mucosa of the esophagus and stomach. Aluminum hydroxide gel decreases, rather than increases, the rate of gastric emptying.

Nursing process: Implementation

Client need: Pharmacological and Parenteral Therapies

Cognitive level: Application

Subject area: Pharmacologic

Answer: 1

Rationale: Calcium salts cause an increase in serum calcium, which can lead to calcium deposits in the kidneys; therefore, calcium salts are contraindicated for the client with a history of renal calculi. A history of hypertension and myocardial infarction are not cardiovascular changes that would be contraindications. Calcium salts may cause constipation.

Nursing process: Assessment

Client need: Pharmacological and Parenteral Therapies

Cognitive level: Analysis

Subject area: Pharmacologic

Answer: 2

Rationale: The client with Addison's disease has a deficiency in glucocorticoids and mineralocorticoids. The treatment is life-long replacement therapy with prednisone. Glucocorticoids must never be withdrawn abruptly and are therefore given the morning of surgery. A client receiving Micronase would have type 2 diabetes mellitus and the drug could be administered later in the day. A client receiving Synthroid for the treatment of hypothyroidism could also miss the morning dose without consequence. Furosemide (Lasix), a loop diuretic, would not be given to a client with Addison's disease because clients with Addison's disease have low sodium levels.

Nursing process: Planning

Client need: Pharmacological and Parenteral Therapies

Cognitive level: Analysis

Subject area: Pharmacologic

14. The nurse is caring for a client taking prednisone. The nurse instructs the client that the best time to take the drug to promote absorption is
    1. at bedtime with a full glass of water.
    2. on an empty stomach.
    3. in the morning with breakfast.
    4. two hours after a meal.

15. The nurse should monitor which of the following laboratory reports for a client receiving long-term corticosteroid therapy?
    1. Magnesium and calcium
    2. Cholesterol and sodium
    3. Hemoglobin and hematocrit
    4. Glucose and potassium

16. The nurse should monitor a client who has been taking fludrocortisone acetate for several months for which of the following adverse reactions of this drug?
    1. Pedal edema
    2. Hyperkalemia
    3. Episodes of hypoglycemia
    4. Weight loss

17. The nurse instructs a female client who has been prescribed testosterone to notify the physician if which of the following is experienced?
    1. Irregular menses
    2. Decreased libido
    3. Engorged breasts
    4. Low-pitched voice

Answer: 3

Rationale: Prednisone is irritating to the gastric mucosa and should be given with food or fluid in the morning with breakfast. The client needs the higher cortisol levels in the daytime, when one is more active. It should not be given on an empty stomach or two hours after a meal.

Nursing process: Implementation

Client need: Pharmacological and Parenteral Therapies

Cognitive level: Application

Subject area: Pharmacologic

Answer: 4

Rationale: Corticosteroids increase glucose metabolism (effect of glucocorticoids) and the absorption of sodium and elimination of potassium (effect of mineralocorticoids). Thus, clients receiving long-term corticosteroid therapy need to be monitored for increased blood glucose levels and low serum potassium. Corticosteroids do not affect calcium, magnesium, cholesterol levels, or hemoglobin and hematocrit levels.

Nursing process: Assessment

Client need: Reduction of Risk Potential

Cognitive level: Analysis

Subject area: Pharmacologic

Answer: 1

Rationale: Fludrocortisone acetate, a mineralocorticoid, promotes sodium ion absorption and potassium ion excretion by the kidneys. A major side effect of the drug is sodium retention, which would contribute to the development of pedal edema. Other adverse reactions are hypokalemia, hyperglycemia, and weight gain.

Nursing process: Assessment

Client need: Pharmacological and Parenteral Therapies

Cognitive level: Application

Subject area: Pharmacologic

Answer: 4

Rationale: Females receiving testosterone should notify the physician if any signs of virilism appear. Testosterone antagonizes the effects of estrogen on the endometrium, so that it is expected that menstruation will become irregular. It is also expected that libido will decrease. Testosterone is given to treat engorged breasts.

Nursing process: Implementation

Client need: Pharmacological and Parenteral Therapies

Cognitive level: Analysis

Subject area: Pharmacologic

18. The nurse should assess a client who received Humulin N insulin at 0730 for hypoglycemia at

    1. 2000 hours.

    2. 1600 hours.

    3. 2400 hours.

    4. 1000 hours.

19. Which of the following should the nurse include in the medication instructions for a client taking chlorpropamide (Diabinese)?

    1. Avoid drinking alcohol

    2. Take on an empty stomach each morning

    3. Take once a day at bedtime with milk or juice

    4. Avoid food products that contain aspartame (NutraSweet)

20. Which of the following should the nurse include in the insulin administration instructions for a client being discharged on insulin?

    1. Inject into the extremity to be exercised to enhance absorption

    2. The muscles in the abdomen and thigh are the easiest to use for self-administration

    3. Insert the needle and then aspirate prior to injecting

    4. Sites should be rotated systematically and not used again for two to three weeks

21. After administering five units of regular insulin per minute to a client in diabetic ketoacidosis, the nurse should add dextrose to the intravenous fluids when the blood glucose reaches which of the following levels?

    1. 350 mg/dl

    2. 300 mg/dl

    3. 400 mg/dl

    4. 450 mg/dl

Answer: 2

Rationale: Hypoglycemia occurs during the peak action time of specific insulin. Humulin N insulin peaks in 4 to 12 hours after administration. The peak time is too early at 1000 hours and too late at 2000 hours and 2400 hours.

Nursing process: Assessment

Client need: Pharmacological and Parenteral Therapies

Cognitive level: Application

Subject area: Pharmacologic

Answer: 1

Rationale: When clients take chlorpropamide (Diabinese), an antidiabetic agent, there is an additional adverse reaction, which is an antabuse type reaction, when alcohol is ingested. To prevent gastrointestinal adverse reactions, the drug should be taken with breakfast. Antidiabetic agents are given daily each morning and aspartame is not contraindicated for this category of antidiabetic drugs.

Nursing process: Planning

Client need: Health Promotion and Maintenance

Cognitive level: Application

Subject area: Pharmacologic

Answer: 4

Rationale: The client needs to develop a systematic plan for rotating injection sites. Once a site is injected, it should not be used again for two to three weeks. If an injection were to be given into an extremity to be exercised, it would cause rapid absorption of the insulin and cause hypoglycemia. Insulin injections are given into subcutaneous tissue, not into muscles. It is not recommended that clients aspirate prior to injecting insulin.

Nursing process: Planning

Client need: Health Promotion and Maintenance

Cognitive level: Application

Subject area: Pharmacologic

Answer: 2

Rationale: Dextrose is added to the intravenous fluids when the blood glucose level reaches 250 to 300 mg/dl, so that the blood sugar doesn't drop too rapidly and put the client at risk for hypoglycemia. The values of 350 mg/dl, 400 mg/dl, and 450 mg/dl are not low enough to add dextrose.

Nursing process: Implementation

Client need: Pharmacological and Parenteral Therapies

Cognitive level: Analysis

Subject area: Pharmacologic

22. After receiving blood glucose monitoring instructions from the nurse, which of the following client statements indicates an understanding of when more frequent monitoring is necessary?
    1. "I should check my glucose level after each additional period of exercise."
    2. "I will need to take more insulin and monitor my glucose more when I go to the dentist."
    3. "I should monitor my glucose more when I am under stress."
    4. "I will need to check my glucose level more frequently when I go on vacation."

23. The nurse instructs a type 1 diabetic client to avoid which of the following while taking insulin?
    1. Furosemide (Lasix)
    2. Dicumarol (Bishydroxycoumarin)
    3. Reserpine (Serpasil)
    4. Cimetidine (Tagamet)

24. The nurse instructs the family of a diabetic client to administer glucagon by which of the following routes?
    1. Sublingually
    2. Rectally
    3. Intravenously
    4. Subcutaneously

Answer: 3

Rationale: Stressful situations, whether they be physiological or emotional, precipitate the release of hormones, which elevate the blood sugar levels and alter the body's need for insulin. Exercising should be part of the daily routine and would not be an indication for more frequent blood glucose monitoring. A dental examination would not normally cause a significant rise in blood glucose level. Vacationing should not impact the blood sugar level, unless the daily routines of insulin injections or oral antidiabetic agents, nutrition, and exercise were changed substantially.

Nursing process: Evaluation

Client need: Pharmacological and Parenteral Therapies

Cognitive level: Analysis

Subject area: Pharmacologic

Answer: 1

Rationale: Furosemide (Lasix), a loop diuretic, is one of several drugs that increases serum glucose levels and is therefore contraindicated if one is taking insulin. Dicumarol, an anticoagulant, reserpine, an antihypertensive agent, and cimetidine, an H_2-receptor antagonist, do not affect blood sugar levels.

Nursing process: Implementation

Client need: Pharmacological and Parenteral Therapies

Cognitive level: Analysis

Subject area: Pharmacologic

Answer: 4

Rationale: Family members are taught to give glucagon either subcutaneously or intramuscularly to clients in hypoglycemia who are unresponsive. It is only available in injectable form, so it cannot be given sublingually or rectally. Family members would not routinely be taught to administer a drug intravenously.

Nursing process: Implementation

Client need: Pharmacological and Parenteral Therapies

Cognitive level: Application

Subject area: Pharmacologic

25. The nurse instructs the family that after the administration of the drug glucagon, the client's blood sugar should begin to rise and the client should regain consciousness. The nurse should tell the family members to wait for how long for the client to respond before summoning emergency assistance?

 1. 4 minutes

 2. 20 minutes

 3. 30 minutes

 4. 40 minutes

26. The registered nurse is preparing to delegate the nursing tasks for the day. Which of the following nursing tasks should the nurse delegate to a licensed practical nurse?

 1. Administer intravenous insulin to a client in diabetic ketoacidosis

 2. Administer an oral calcium supplement one hour after meals

 3. Develop a medication schedule for a client with diabetes mellitus and congestive heart failure

 4. Assess a client taking iodine for signs of iodine poisoning

Answer: 2

Rationale: The blood glucose level should begin to rise in approximately 5 to 20 minutes after an injection of glucagon. It would take more than 4 minutes for the client to respond. If the client doesn't respond in 20 to 30 minutes, emergency personnel need to be summoned to administer dextrose intravenously.

Nursing process: Implementation

Client need: Pharmacological and Parenteral Therapies

Cognitive level: Application

Subject area: Pharmacologic

Answer: 2

Rationale: A licensed practical nurse may administer a calcium supplement one hour after meals. Developing a medication schedule, administering intravenous insulin, and assessing a client taking iodine for signs of iodine poisoning are tasks that should be performed by a registered nurse.

Nursing process: Planning

Client need: Management of Care

Cognitive level: Analysis

Subject area: Legal and Ethical Issues

Drugs for the Neurological System

21

1. The nurse should monitor a client receiving pyridostigmine (Mestinon) for which of the following adverse reactions?

   1. Constipation

   2. Decreased heart rate

   3. Hypertension

   4. Increased intraocular pressure

2. The nurse should assess for which of the following after slowly administering lorazepam (Ativan) intravenously to a client who has been experiencing seizures in rapid succession?

   1. Tachycardia

   2. Hypertension

   3. Tissue hypoxia

   4. Respiratory depression

3. A client is taking phenytoin (Dilantin) 200 mg daily. The nurse monitors the client for which of the following adverse reactions?

   1. Diarrhea

   2. Pruritis

   3. Sedation

   4. Hypertension

4. The nurse infuses phenytoin (Dilantin) with which of the following solutions to control seizures?

   1. Normal saline

   2. D$_5$W

   3. Lactated Ringer's

   4. D$_5$W 0.5 normal saline

Answer: 2

Rationale: Pyridostigmine (Mestinon) is a cholinergic drug in the treatment of myasthenia gravis. Adverse reactions include bradycardia, diarrhea, and hypotension.

Nursing process: Assessment

Client need: Pharmacological and Parenteral Therapies

Cognitive level: Application

Subject area: Pharmacologic

Answer: 4

Rationale: Lorazepam (Ativan) is given intravenously in the treatment of status epilepticus. A client receiving Ativan for status epilepticus must be closely monitored for respiratory depression.

Nursing process: Assessment

Client need: Pharmacological and Parenteral Therapies

Cognitive level: Application

Subject area: Pharmacologic

Answer: 3

Rationale: Phenytoin (Dilantin) is an anticonvulsant used in the treatment of seizures. Adverse reactions include sedation, hypotension, and constipation.

Nursing process: Assessment

Client need: Pharmacological and Parenteral Therapies

Cognitive level: Application

Subject area: Pharmacologic

Answer: 1

Rationale: Phenytoin (Dilantin) should not be used intravenously with dextrose because it forms a precipitate. Dilantin should only be infused intravenously with normal saline.

Nursing process: Implementation

Client need: Pharmacological and Parenteral Therapies

Cognitive level: Analysis

Subject area: Pharmacologic

5. Phenytoin (Dilantin) has been prescribed for a client. Based on an understanding of medication, the nurse caring for the client should

   1. maintain a Dilantin level of 30 to 50 µg/ml.

   2. dilute IV Dilantin with 5% dextrose.

   3. administer good oral hygiene.

   4. give intramuscularly.

6. The nurse is caring for a client who is receiving phenobarbital for epilepsy. The nurse identifies the nursing diagnosis "High risk for injury related to unpredictable intermittent neurological dysfunction." Which of the following is a priority to include in this client's plan of care?

   1. Consume alcohol in moderation

   2. Drive a car only during the day

   3. Lie down at the first sign of an aura

   4. Increase fiber in the diet and fluids

7. The nurse obtains a subtherapeutic serum level for a client who is receiving phenytoin (Dilantin) with seizure activity under control. Based on the results of the Dilantin level, the appropriate nursing action is to

   1. change the medication to carbamazepine (Tegretol).

   2. increase the dose of the phenytoin (Dilantin).

   3. add phenobarbital to the drug regimen.

   4. continue the phenytoin (Dilantin) as ordered.

8. The nurse is caring for a client who has cerebral edema following a cerebrovascular accident. The nurse should understand that the client is to receive mannitol IV for which of the following purposes?

   1. Inhibit prothrombin formation

   2. Prevent platelet aggregation

   3. Decrease intracranial pressure

   4. Perfusion of occluded intracranial arteries

Answer: 3

Rationale: Gingival hyperplasia is an adverse reaction to phenytoin (Dilantin). Administering good oral hygiene is the appropriate intervention. The normal therapeutic Dilantin level is 7.5 to 20 µg/ml. Dilantin should not be administered with dextrose because it forms precipitates. It should only be infused with normal saline. Dilantin is not administered intramuscularly.

Nursing process: Analysis

Client need: Pharmacological and Parenteral Therapies

Cognitive level: Analysis

Subject area: Pharmacologic

Answer: 3

Rationale: The priority nursing intervention for a client with epilepsy and a nursing diagnosis of "High risk for injury related to unpredictable intermittent neurological dysfunction" is to lie down at the first sign of an aura. Safety is always the priority. The client should be advised to avoid alcohol with phenobarbital because of the combined sedative effect. Because of this client's neurological nursing diagnosis, the client should not be driving at a time of unpredictability. Increasing fiber and fluids in the diet have no impact on safety.

Nursing process: Planning

Client need: Management of Care

Cognitive level: Analysis

Subject area: Pharmacologic

Answer: 4

Rationale: Therapeutic ranges for drugs serve only as a guide. The therapeutic drug range excludes a serum level lower than where the client continues to have seizures and higher than where the client experiences toxic effects. If a client's seizures are well controlled at a subtherapeutic level, the dose does not need to be increased because it appears to be stabilizing the client's seizures, which is the goal of therapy.

Nursing process: Planning

Client need: Pharmacological and Parenteral Therapies

Cognitive level: Analysis

Subject area: Pharmacologic

Answer: 3

Rationale: Mannitol is an osmotic diuretic used to promote systemic diuresis in cerebral edema and to decrease intracranial pressure.

Nursing process: Analysis

Client need: Pharmacological and Parenteral Therapies

Cognitive level: Application

Subject area: Pharmacologic

9. Which of the following would the nurse recognize as the appropriate rationale for the administration of the drug levodopa (L-dopa) to a client with Parkinson's disease? The drug
   1. activates enzymes to degrade dopamine
   2. blocks the release of dopamine
   3. provides the precursor of dopamine
   4. inhibits the synthesis of dopamine

10. The nurse is caring for a client who has tetanus and is experiencing seizures unrelieved by sedation. Which of the following drugs should the nurse administer?
    1. Diazepam (Valium)
    2. D-tubocurarine (Curate)
    3. Chlorpromazine (Thorazine)
    4. Phenytoin (Dilantin)

11. The nurse is caring for a client who is receiving dexamethasone (Decadron) for a spinal cord tumor. The nurse should assess for which of the following adverse reactions?
    1. Hypoglycemia
    2. Nausea
    3. Constipation
    4. Hypotension

12. The nurse is caring for a client who is experiencing an overdose of atropine. The nurse should prepare to administer which of the following drugs?
    1. Diazepam (Valium)
    2. Dexamethasone (Decadron)
    3. Physostigmine salicylate (Antilirium)
    4. Epinephrine

Answer: 3
Rationale: Levodopa (L-dopa) is an antiparkinsonian drug. When L-dopa enters the bloodstream, it is converted to dopamine by the enzyme dopadecarboxylase and increases the dopamine available to the brain.
Nursing process: Analysis
Client need: Pharmacological and Parenteral Therapies
Cognitive level: Analysis
Subject area: Pharmacologic

Answer: 2
Rationale: When seizures are not controlled by sedation, d-tubocurarine (Curate) is a skeletal muscle–paralyzing drug that is used.
Nursing process: Implementation
Client need: Pharmacological and Parenteral Therapies
Cognitive level: Analysis
Subject area: Pharmacologic

Answer: 2
Rationale: Adverse reactions to dexamethasone (Decadron) include hypertension, hyperglycemia, nausea, and diarrhea.
Nursing process: Assessment
Client need: Pharmacological and Parenteral Therapies
Cognitive level: Application
Subject area: Pharmacologic

Answer: 3
Rationale: Physostigmine salicylate (Antilirium) is a specific antidote for atropine overdose. A client exhibiting an atropine overdose would present with flushing, warm, dry skin, decreased salivation, tachycardia, and urinary retention.
Nursing process: Planning
Client need: Pharmacological and Parenteral Therapies
Cognitive level: Analysis
Subject area: Pharmacologic

13. Benztropine (Cogentin) has been prescribed for a client. Based on an understanding of the adverse reactions, the nurse caring for the client should
    1. inform the client that diarrhea is a common adverse reaction.
    2. instruct the client to drink alcohol in moderation.
    3. turn and position the client frequently.
    4. monitor the client for urinary retention.

14. The nurse is caring for a client with myasthenia gravis who has become progressively weaker. Edrophonium (Tensilon) has been prescribed for which of the following purposes?
    1. Treat the client's muscle weakness
    2. Differentiate between a cholinergic crisis and myasthenic crisis
    3. Increase skeletal muscle relaxation
    4. Decrease difficulty breathing

15. When providing care for a client who is receiving methylphenidate (Ritalin), the nurse should monitor the client for which of the following?

    Select all that apply:
    [   ] 1. Constipation
    [   ] 2. Weight gain
    [   ] 3. Tachycardia
    [   ] 4. Nervousness
    [   ] 5. Gingival hyperplasia
    [   ] 6. Palpitation

16. The nurse should evaluate a client's muscle strength following the administration of what drug that is used to diagnose myasthenia gravis? _____

Answer: 4

Rationale: Urinary retention is a common adverse reaction to benztropine (Cogentin), which is an anticholinergic drug used in the treatment of Parkinson's disease. Other common adverse reactions include constipation, dry mouth, blurry vision, and tachycardia. The client should be instructed to avoid driving or operating heavy machinery.

Nursing process: Planning

Client need: Pharmacological and Parenteral Therapies

Cognitive level: Application

Subject area: Pharmacologic

Answer: 2

Rationale: Edrophonium (Tensilon) is used to differentiate between a cholinergic crisis and a myasthenic crisis. If a client is experiencing a cholinergic crisis, edrophonium (Tensilon) will result in an increase in the muscle weakness. If a client is experiencing a myasthenic crisis, edrophonium (Tensilon) will result in an improvement of the client's clinical manifestations.

Nursing process: Analysis

Client need: Pharmacological and Parenteral Therapies

Cognitive level: Analysis

Subject area: Pharmacologic

Answer: 3, 4, 6

Rationale: Methylphenidate hydrochloride (Ritalin) is a central nervous system stimulant used in the treatment of an attention deficit disorder. Adverse reactions to Ritalin include tachycardia, palpitations, nervousness, agitation, hyperexcitability, insomnia, dizziness, and weight loss.

Nursing process: Assessment

Client need: Pharmacological and Parenteral Therapies

Cognitive level: Application

Subject area: Pharmacologic

Answer: Edrophonium (Tensilon)

Rationale: Edrophonium (Tensilon) is a short-acting cholinergic drug used to establish a differential diagnosis of myasthenia gravis. After the administration of Tensilon, the client's muscle contractility is significantly improved.

Nursing process: Evaluation

Client need: Pharmacological and Parenteral Therapies

Cognitive level: Application

Subject area: Pharmacologic

17. The nurse should monitor which of the following laboratory tests in a client receiving ethosuximide (Zarontin)?

1. Thyroid profile and follicle stimulating hormone

2. Calcium and magnesium

3. Potassium and sodium

4. Complete blood count and liver function studies

18. The nurse is teaching a class on drugs used in the treatment of neurological disorders. Which of the following should the nurse include in the class?

1. Allergic reactions, hepatitis, and bone marrow depression are common adverse reactions to anticonvulsants

2. Antihistamines and antipsychotic drugs decrease the effect of anticholinergic drugs

3. Narrow-angle glaucoma is a contraindication in the use of anti-Parkinson drugs

4. Cushing's syndrome occurs with short-term corticosteroid use

19. The nurse should assess a client receiving ergotamine tartrate (Ergomar) for which of the following adverse reactions?

Select all that apply:

[   ] **1.** Nausea

[   ] **2.** Urinary retention

[   ] **3.** Hypertension

[   ] **4.** Constipation

[   ] **5.** Dry mouth

[   ] **6.** Tachycardia

Answer: 4

Rationale: Ethosuximide (Zarontin) is an anticonvulsant drug used to treat absence seizures. Complete blood count and liver function studies should be monitored. Anticonvulsants are contraindicated in hepatic dysfunction and bleeding disorders.

Nursing process: Assessment

Client need: Pharmacological and Parenteral Therapies

Cognitive level: Analysis

Subject area: Pharmacologic

Answer: 3

Rationale: Narrow-angle glaucoma is a contraindication in the use of anti-Parkinson drugs. Allergic reactions, hepatitis, and bone marrow depression are uncommon adverse reactions to anticonvulsants. Common adverse reactions include central nervous system effects such as drowsiness, nervousness, ataxia, and dizziness. Common gastrointestinal adverse reactions include gingival hyperplasia, nausea, vomiting, and epigastric discomfort. Antihistamines and antipsychotic drugs increase the effects of anti-Parkinson drugs. Clinical manifestations of Cushing's syndrome include buffalo hump, moon face, abdominal distention, ecchymosis, hypertension, weakness, osteoporosis, amenorrhea, and impotence, and are the result of long-term corticosteroid use.

Nursing process: Planning

Client need: Pharmacological and Parenteral Therapies

Cognitive level: Application

Subject area: Pharmacologic

Answer: 1, 3, 6

Rationale: Ergotamine tartrate (Ergomar) is an alpha-adrenergic blocking agent used in the treatment of migraine, cluster, and other vascular headaches. Adverse reactions include nausea, vomiting, diarrhea, abdominal pain, tachycardia, hypertension or hypotension, paresthesia, weakness, and itching.

Nursing process: Assessment

Client need: Pharmacological and Parenteral Therapies

Cognitive level: Application

Subject area: Pharmacologic

20. Methysergide maleate (Sansert) has been prescribed for a client experiencing cluster headaches. Which of the following should the nurse include in the medication instructions?

    1. Sansert may be safely used in the management of acute migraine attacks
    2. Administer the medication sublingually
    3. Discontinue the medication for one month after every four months
    4. One additional tablet may be taken after 30 minutes if the headache has not subsided

21. The nurse questions an order to administer rizatriptan (Maxalt) to which of the following clients? A client with

    1. gastroesophageal reflux disease.
    2. Parkinson's disease.
    3. hypertension.
    4. osteoarthritis.

22. The registered nurse is preparing to delegate nursing tasks for the day. Which of the following tasks should the nurse delegate to a licensed practical nurse?

    1. Administration of intravenous phenytoin (Dilantin) to a client with partial seizures
    2. Develop a nutritional plan for a client experiencing migraine headaches
    3. Monitor a client taking carbidopa (Lodosyn) for adverse reactions
    4. Offer a client taking trihexyphenidyl (Artane) increased fluids

Answer: 3

Rationale: Methysergide maleate (Sansert) is a synthetic ergot derivative used to prevent but not manage acute migraine attacks because of the serious adverse reactions. It is recommended to discontinue Sansert for one month after every four to six months. This too is part of the prescription protocol to prevent serious adverse reactions. The client should never take an additional tablet if the first does not provide relief. This is likely an indication that the drug is not effective for this client. Sansert is taken orally, not sublingually. Ergotamine tartrate (Ergomar) is administered sublingually in the treatment of vascular headaches.

Nursing process: Planning

Client need: Health Promotion and Maintenance

Cognitive level: Analysis

Subject area: Pharmacologic

Answer: 3

Rationale: Rizatriptan (Maxalt) is used in the treatment of migraine headaches. It is contraindicated for a client with hypertension because hypertension is also an adverse reaction to the drug.

Nursing process: Implementation

Client need: Pharmacological and Parenteral Therapies

Cognitive level: Analysis

Subject area: Pharmacologic

Answer: 4

Rationale: It would be appropriate to delegate increasing fluids to a client taking trihexyphenidyl (Artane) to a licensed practical nurse. Artane is an anticholinergic drug that causes constipation. A licensed practical nurse may not administer intravenous drugs, develop a nutritional plan, or monitor a client for adverse reactions.

Nursing process: Planning

Client need: Management of Care

Cognitive level: Analysis

Subject area: Legal and Ethical Issues

23. The nurse is caring for a client admitted to the emergency room who is experiencing status epilepticus. What is the drug of choice for the nurse to administer to this client? _____

24. The nurse is caring for a client taking felbamate (Felbatol) for partial seizures. Which of the following actions should the nurse include in the plan of care for this client?

1. Monitor the client for an increased appetite and weight gain

2. Instruct the client that hyperkalemia and hypernatremia are adverse reactions

3. Have the client sign a consent form acknowledging the increased risk of aplastic anemia and liver failure

4. Monitor the serum sodium level

25. The nurse should monitor a client carefully and use extreme caution when administering phenobarbital with what additional drug?

1. Valproic acid (Depakene)

2. Phenytoin (Dilantin)

3. Carbamazepine (Tegretol)

4. Ethosuximide (Zarontin)

Answer: Lorazepam (Ativan)

Rationale: Lorazepam (Ativan) is the drug of choice to terminate tonic-clonic seizures. Lorazepam is chosen over diazepam (Valium) because of the longer duration of its effect.

Nursing process: Implementation

Client need: Pharmacological and Parenteral Therapies

Cognitive level: Analysis

Subject area: Pharmacologic

Answer: 3

Rationale: Felbamate (Felbatol) is a second-line drug used for intractable atonic or partial seizures. It may be appropriate to have a client sign a consent form acknowledging the increased risk of aplastic anemia and liver failure. Weight loss, decreased appetite, hypokalemia, and hyponatremia are adverse reactions. Complete blood count and liver function studies should be monitored. The serum sodium level would be monitored with carbamazepine (Tegretol).

Nursing process: Planning

Client need: Pharmacological and Parenteral Therapies

Cognitive level: Application

Subject area: Pharmacologic

Answer: 1

Rationale: The combination of phenobarbital and valproic acid (Depakene) may increase the risk of phenobarbital toxicity.

Nursing process: Assessment

Client need: Reduction of Risk Potential

Cognitive level: Analysis

Subject area: Pharmacologic

Drugs for the Integumentary System

22

1. How should the nurse prepare the skin for application of a topical drug? _____

2. The nurse instructs a client taking an oral retinoid to avoid which of the following?
 1. Dairy products
 2. Carbonated drinks
 3. Extremely cold air
 4. Vitamin A supplements

3. The nurse is caring for a client who has been taking isotretinoin (Accutane) for the past two months. Which of the following is a priority for the nurse to report?
 1. Pruritus
 2. Depression
 3. Dry skin
 4. Headache

4. The nurse instructs a client with pruritis to take an oral antihistamine to relieve the itching. Which of the following should be included in this instruction?
 1. "The effects will be best if you take the medication around the clock."
 2. "Take the medication only when the itching is at its worst."
 3. "Use the oral medication in combination with a topical antihistamine."
 4. "Increase the dosage of the oral medication as needed if the itching is severe."

Answer: Wash the skin and pat dry

Rationale: Any skin surfaces that are to receive topical medications should be clean and dry to allow for best absorption of the medication. The appropriate method to prepare the skin is to wash the skin and pat dry. Simply rinsing will not remove oil or dirt from the skin. Cold water causes local vasoconstriction, which impedes the absorption of topical medication. Scrubbing the skin can cause irritation, as can rubbing it dry.

Nursing process: Implementation

Client need: Pharmacological and Parenteral Therapies

Cognitive level: Application

Subject area: Pharmacologic

Answer: 4

Rationale: Oral retinoids are derived from vitamin A; hence, taking supplemental vitamin A could cause an overdose of this fat-soluble vitamin.

Nursing process: Implementation

Client need: Health Promotion and Maintenance

Cognitive level: Application

Subject area: Pharmacologic

Answer: 2

Rationale: Isotretinoin (Accutane) is a retinoid used in the treatment of acne. Adverse reactions include pruritus, dry skin, and headache and should be reported, but the priority adverse reaction to report is depression. There have been reports of depression and possibly suicidal ideation associated with the use of isotretinoin.

Nursing process: Analysis

Client need: Management of Care

Cognitive level: Analysis

Subject area: Pharmacologic

Answer: 1

Rationale: Oral antihistamines have their maximal effect when taken regularly around the clock. Drowsiness is an adverse reaction that is also minimized by this dosing.

Nursing process: Implementation

Client need: Health Promotion and Maintenance

Cognitive level: Application

Subject area: Pharmacologic

5. The nurse is discharging a client who has second-degree burns on the hands and arms. Treatment includes application of silver sulfadiazine (Silvadene) to the burn area twice a day. Which of the following must be included in wound care instructions for this client?

    1. "Wash the area with warm water before the application of Silvadene."

    2. "Apply salve after the Silvadene to seal the medication into the burned area."

    3. "Apply the Silvadene using sterile technique."

    4. "Apply the medication only at bedtime."

6. A 22-year-old has been diagnosed with acne vulgaris and is to start on tetracycline. Which of the following is a priority question to ask this client before therapy is started?

    1. "How long have you had the cystlike nodules on your face?"

    2. "When was your last menstrual period?"

    3. "How many times a day do you scrub your face?"

    4. "Have you been taking any oral medication for acne?"

7. The nurse is instructing a client about use of benzoyl peroxide to treat acne. Which of the following should be included?

    1. Overuse can cause extreme dryness of the skin

    2. Use caution when driving or operating heavy machinery

    3. Nausea and vomiting may occur

    4. A decrease in appetite may occur

8. The nurse is providing instruction to a client about use of lindane (Kwell) shampoo for treatment of *Pediculus humanus capitis* (head lice). Which of the following should be included in the teaching?

    1. Apply the shampoo to dry hair and leave on for 4 to 5 minutes

    2. Wet the hair first and massage the shampoo in for one minute

    3. Use the shampoo on dry hair, rinse and shampoo with regular shampoo

    4. Apply the shampoo to wet hair and rinse thoroughly

Answer: 1

Rationale: Burn wounds should be cleansed prior to application of Silvadene cream. This helps remove dead tissue and old cream. There is no need to apply salve over the Silvadene. Silvadene provides a protective cover by itself. The client should use a clean technique at home rather than a sterile technique. The treatment must be twice a day, generally in the morning and evening.

Nursing process: Planning

Client need: Health Promotion and Maintenance

Cognitive level: Application

Subject area: Pharmacologic

Answer: 2

Rationale: Because tetracycline is teratogenic, it is a priority to establish that the client is not pregnant before starting the drug. Tetracycline is not the drug of choice for a cystlike type of acne. Scrubbing of the face has no impact on the use of tetracycline systemically. Although asking a client if an oral medication for acne has been taken is appropriate, it is not the priority because of the teratogenic effects of the tetracycline.

Nursing process: Assessment

Client need: Management of Care

Cognitive level: Analysis

Subject area: Pharmacologic

Answer: 1

Rationale: Benzoyl is an effective drying agent that can cause too much drying if overused. Benzoyl peroxide is topical and does not have systemic adverse reactions. Benzoyl peroxide is not associated with the adverse reactions of nausea, vomiting, or a decrease in appetite.

Nursing process: Implementation

Client need: Health Promotion and Maintenance

Cognitive level: Application

Subject area: Pharmacologic

Answer: 1

Rationale: The Kwell shampoo should be applied to dry hair and left on the scalp for 4 to 5 minutes to allow for maximal effect. Treatment should be repeated in a week.

Nursing process: Implementation

Client need: Pharmacological and Parenteral Therapies

Cognitive level: Application

Subject area: Pharmacologic

9. The nurse is instructing the mother of four children on how to treat all of the children for *Pediculus humanus capitis* (head lice) with Kwell shampoo. The ages of the children are 8 years, 5 years, 2 years, and a premature infant who now weighs six pounds. Which one of the following is the priority to include in the instructions given to this mother?

   1. The cost associated with purchasing shampoo for four children may lead to undertreatment

   2. Lindane (Kwell) may cause seizures in premature babies

   3. There is an increased incidence of reinfection from one child to another

   4. Help should be sought to help apply the shampoo

10. The physician prescribes ketoconazole (Nizoral) to treat a systemic candidiasis. The client asks, "What are the main advantages of this drug?" The nurse's best response is

    1. "It can be given orally and is safer than amphotericin B."

    2. "It is less expensive than other medications."

    3. "It is the physician's choice."

    4. "It can be used once a week instead of daily."

11. The nurse identifies what as the goal of therapy for a client who is to receive topical corticosteroids for a skin condition? _____

12. When teaching a client about using salicylic acid as a drug to promote shedding of the horny layer of skin, the nurse should explain which of the following about salicylic acid?

    1. It is not absorbed through the skin

    2. It may burn the skin

    3. It is not advised for dandruff

    4. It may cause acne

Answer: 2

Rationale: It is a priority to inform the parent that applying Kwell shampoo to premature infants may cause seizures. Purchasing Kwell shampoo for three children may be costly, but it is essential to prevent the spread of *Pediculus humanus capitis* (head lice). Although an increased incidence of reinfection of the children from one child to another is a minor concern, it is not the priority. Securing help to apply the shampoo may be beneficial, but it is not the priority.

Nursing process: Planning

Client need: Health Promotion and Maintenance

Cognitive level: Analysis

Subject area: Pharmacologic

Answer: 1

Rationale: Ketoconazole (Nizoral) is just as effective to treat systemic candidiasis and not as dangerous as amphotericin B. Amphotericin B is highly toxic and used for progressive and potentially fatal infections. Although expense is a consideration, safety is the most important factor.

Nursing process: Analysis

Client need: Pharmacological and Parenteral Therapies

Cognitive level: Analysis

Subject area: Pharmacologic

Answer: Relief of inflammation and itching

Rationale: Corticosteroids reduce inflammation and reduce the histamine response that causes itching.

Nursing process: Implementation

Client need: Pharmacological and Parenteral Therapies

Cognitive level: Application

Subject area: Pharmacologic

Answer: 1

Rationale: Salicylic acid has its effect on the keratin layer of the skin. The acid is too mild to burn the skin. It can be used for dandruff. It may also be used to treat acne, since it causes drying and sloughing.

Nursing process: Planning

Client need: Health Promotion and Maintenance

Cognitive level: Application

Subject area: Pharmacologic

13. The nurse is caring for a pressure ulcer using a topical debriding agent. Another nurse asks the nurse the type of drug typically used for this purpose. Which of the following is the best response?

   1. An enzyme ointment

   2. A corticosteroid cream

   3. An antipsoriatic lotion

   4. A topical antihistamine

14. The nurse should monitor a client taking betamethasone for which of the following adverse reactions? Select all that apply:

   [　] **1.** Weight loss

   [　] **2.** Decreased appetite

   [　] **3.** Hypotension

   [　] **4.** Muscle wasting

   [　] **5.** Edema

   [　] **6.** Skin thinning

15. The registered nurse is preparing to make out the clinical assignments for the day. Which of the following nursing tasks may the nurse delegate to a licensed practical nurse?

   1. Inform a client taking etretinate (Tegison) to use birth control when taking the drug

   2. Instruct client on how to use isotretinoin (Accutane)

   3. Administer acyclovir (Zovirax) intravenously to a client

   4. Ask the client if stinging occurs when applying topical acyclovir (Zovirax)

Answer: 1

Rationale: An enzyme ointment best describes the classification of agents used for debriding pressure ulcers. Corticosteroids do not have debridement properties. Drugs used for psoriasis do not debride. Topical antihistamines are used for itching and inflammation rather than debridement.

Nursing process: Analysis

Client need: Pharmacological and Parenteral Therapies

Cognitive level: Application

Subject area: Pharmacologic

Answer: 4, 5, 6

Rationale: Betamethasone (Diprolene) is a superhigh-potency corticosteroid that causes weight gain, increased appetite, hypertension, muscle wasting, edema, and skin thinning.

Nursing process: Assessment

Client need: Pharmacological and Parenteral Therapies

Cognitive level: Application

Subject area: Pharmacologic

Answer: 4

Rationale: A licensed practical nurse may ask a client if stinging occurs when a topical drug is applied. Informing or instructing a client about certain effects of a drug are nursing tasks that should be performed by a registered nurse. Administering a drug intravenously is also a task that belongs to a registered nurse.

Nursing process: Planning

Client need: Management of Care

Cognitive level: Analysis

Subject area: Legal and Ethical Issues

16. The nurse is teaching the client about using tretinoin (Retin-A) for treatment of acne vulgaris. Which of the following indicates that the teaching has been successful? The client

   1. avoids washing the skin with drying soap

   2. limits exposure to sunlight

   3. reduces the intake of caffeine-containing foods

   4. stops using the medication if a stinging feeling occurs

17. The nurse should inform a client taking fluconazole (Diflucan) to be aware of which of the following adverse reactions?

   Select all that apply:

   [　] **1.** Tremors

   [　] **2.** Headache

   [　] **3.** Constipation

   [　] **4.** Skin rash

   [　] **5.** Pruritus

   [　] **6.** Abdominal pain

18. After instructing a client on the application of anthralin, the client states, "I want to apply the medication to the nonaffected areas to prevent other lesions from developing." Which of the following responses by the nurse is most appropriate?

   1. "The medication can cause chemical burns, so it should be used on the psoriatic lesions only."

   2. "Anthralin is very expensive, so limit its use to the psoriatic lesions."

   3. "As long as you leave it on for a maximum of two hours, it should be all right."

   4. "Because anthralin promotes fluid and electrolyte loss, you should limit the areas that are treated."

Answer: 2

Rationale: Tretinoin (Retin-A) is a retinoid that causes sensitivity to sunlight and susceptibility to sunburn, so limiting exposure and using sunscreen of at least 15 SPF are advised. The use of a drying soap assists the client in treating the acne. Although the use of caffeine has no relationship to the medication itself, some clients find that certain foods aggravate their acne and are advised to avoid them or reduce the amount consumed. A stinging sensation is normal for clients with sensitive skin. Avoiding abrasive soaps and keratolytic agents, like benzoyl peroxide and salicylic acid, can reduce this sensation.

Nursing process: Evaluation

Client need: Pharmacological and Parenteral Therapies

Cognitive level: Application

Subject area: Pharmacologic

Answer: 2, 4, 6

Rationale: Fluconazole (Diflucan) is an antifungal used in the treatment of candidiasis. Adverse reactions include diarrhea, headache, skin rash, and abdominal pain.

Nursing process: Implementation

Client need: Pharmacological and Parenteral Therapies

Cognitive level: Application

Subject area: Pharmacologic

Answer: 1

Rationale: Anthralin may be used in the treatment of psoriasis. It inhibits the DNA synthesis to suppress the overgrowth of epidermal cells. It is a strong irritant and should be applied only to affected skin. It may be very irritating to unaffected skin. It also stains clothing, skin, and hair.

Nursing process: Analysis

Client need: Pharmacological and Parenteral Therapies

Cognitive level: Analysis

Subject area: Pharmacologic

19. The client is being treated with haloprogin (Halotex) for tinea pedis (athlete's feet). Which of the following statements by the client indicates the client understands the teaching about the medication?

   1. "I will apply the ointment daily for six weeks."
   2. "I will use the powder three times a day."
   3. "I will soak my feet in cold water before each application."
   4. "I will apply the medication morning and evening for two to four weeks."

20. The client with a rash in the axilla is prescribed amcinonide (Cyclocort) topical. For which of the following adverse reactions should the nurse monitor the client?

   1. Gastrointestinal manifestations
   2. Cracking and splitting of the skin
   3. Thinning of the skin
   4. Loss of pigmentation

21. A female client with herpes genitalis is receiving education about the medication regimen. Which of the following would be most appropriate to include in the teaching?

   1. Use one applicator of terconazole intravaginally at bedtime for seven days
   2. Use topical acyclovir every four hours five times a day for 10 days
   3. Use sulconazole nitrate twice a day and massage in
   4. Use one applicator of tioconazole intravaginally at bedtime for seven days

22. During the early emergent phase of a burn injury, clients are at risk for infection. Which of the following prescribed drugs would the nurse anticipate to administer to prevent infection?

   1. Mafenide acetate (Sulfamylon)
   2. Lindane (Kwell)
   3. Acitretin (Soriatane)
   4. Azelaic acid (Azelex)

Answer: 4

Rationale: Haloprogin (Halotex) is an antifungal. Treatment for tinea pedis (athlete's foot) requires twice a day application of Halotex. Soaking the feet in cold water will not improve absorption of the medication.

Nursing process: Evaluation

Client need: Health Promotion and Maintenance

Cognitive level: Application

Subject area: Pharmacologic

Answer: 3

Rationale: Amcinonide (Cyclocort) is a topical steroid. Regular use of topical steroids is associated with the adverse effect of thinning of the skin and appearance of "stretch marks."

Nursing process: Assessment

Client need: Pharmacological and Parenteral Therapies

Cognitive level: Application

Subject area: Pharmacologic

Answer: 2

Rationale: Acyclovir (Zovirax) is an antiviral used in the treatment of genital herpes. It is used every four hours five times a day for 10 days. Terconazole, sulconazole nitrate, and tioconazole are all antifungal drugs.

Nursing process: Planning

Client need: Health Promotion and Maintenance

Cognitive level: Analysis

Subject area: Pharmacologic

Answer: 1

Rationale: Sulfamylon is a topical anti-infective that is used to prevent infections in burn wounds. Lindane (Kwell) is used to treat pediculosis. Acitretin (Soriatane) is a retinoid used in the treatment of psoriasis. Azelaic acid (Azelex) is used in the treatment of acne.

Nursing process: Analysis

Client need: Pharmacological and Parenteral Therapies

Cognitive level: Application

Subject area: Pharmacologic

23. The nurse should monitor a client receiving mafenide acetate (Sulfamylon) for which of the following adverse reactions?

Select all that apply:

[   ] **1.** Petechiae

[   ] **2.** Constipation

[   ] **3.** Pain

[   ] **4.** Acidosis

[   ] **5.** Rash

[   ] **6.** Erythema

24. A client with sebhorrheic dermatitis of the face is being treated with topical ketoconazole (Nizoral). Which of the following behaviors by the client indicate that teaching has been effective?

1. Application of a thick layer of cream, washing the area once a week

2. Removal of any dry scales prior to application of the cream to aid absorption

3. Applying an emollient before applying the ketoconazole

4. Applying moisturizing cream sparingly after applying the ketoconazole

Answer: 3, 4, 5, 6

Rationale: Mafenide acetate (Sulfamylon) is a sulfonamide used in the treatment of burns. The topical application is painful and may result in acidosis. Rash and erythema are other adverse reactions.

Nursing process: Assessment

Client need: Pharmacological and Parenteral Therapies

Cognitive level: Application

Subject area: Pharmacologic

Answer: 2

Rationale: Topical ketoconazole (Nizoral) is best absorbed through skin that is free of scales. Gentle washing with soap and water to remove scales will aid in absorption of the topical antifungal. A thin layer that is rubbed in will be more effectively absorbed. The old cream and dead skin must be removed daily. Application of an emollient prior to application of the antifungal will reduce absorption of the antifungal. Moisturizing creams are of no value in treating the fungal infection that caused the dermatitis to begin with.

Nursing process: Evaluation

Client need: Health Promotion and Maintenance

Cognitive level: Analysis

Subject area: Pharmacologic

Drugs for the Musculoskeletal System

23

1. The nurse explains to the client that the following drug is the drug of choice in Raynaud's phenomenon.
   1. Nonsteroidal anti-inflammatories
   2. Corticosteroids
   3. Aspirin
   4. Calcium channel blockers

2. Allopurinol (Zyloprim) and colchicine have been prescribed for a client with gout and diabetes mellitus. Which of the following instructions should be given to this client?
   1. Blood glucose tests may not be valid
   2. Urine sugar tests may not be valid
   3. Protein restrictions can cause diabetic ketoacidosis
   4. Protein cannot be restricted so increased dosing of allopurinol may be required

3. The nurse should administer which of the following prescribed drugs to a client with rheumatoid arthritis who has severe joint involvement and a positive rheumatoid factor?
   1. Methotrexate
   2. Naproxen (Naprosyn)
   3. Acetylsalicylic acid (aspirin)
   4. Hydroxychloroquine sulfate (Plaquenil)

4. Which of the following should the nurse consider before administering an opioid analgesic to a child?
   1. The child's age, weight, height, and respiratory status
   2. Children are less susceptible to adverse reactions
   3. Addiction is increased in children
   4. Sedation is increased in children

Answer: 4
Rationale: The drugs of choice to treat Raynaud's phenomenon are calcium channel blockers, such as diltiazem (Cardizem) and nifedipine (Procardia). They are particularly useful in treating acute episodes, but are also used in chronic episodes. They relieve vasospastic attacks by relaxing the smooth muscles of the arterioles.
Nursing process: Implementation
Client need: Pharmacological and Parenteral Therapies
Cognitive level: Application
Subject area: Pharmacologic

Answer: 2
Rationale: Urine sugar tests may indicate false positives when taking gout medications. Blood glucose testing is still accurate. Protein restrictions do not cause diabetic ketoacidosis and protein is not restricted for diabetic clients.
Nursing process: Planning
Client need: Health Promotion and Maintenance
Cognitive level: Application
Subject area: Pharmacologic

Answer: 1
Rationale: Because of the serious adverse reactions, such as hepatotoxicity and bone marrow depression, methotrexate is reserved for severe rheumatoid arthritis with severe systemic involvement and a positive rheumatoid factor. Laboratory monitoring must be obtained periodically throughout treatment. Methotrexate acts by facilitating a rapid anti-inflammatory response within days to weeks.
Nursing process: Implementation
Client need: Pharmacological and Parenteral Therapies
Cognitive level: Application
Subject area: Pharmacologic

Answer: 1
Rationale: Age, weight, height, and respiratory status must be considered before administering an opioid analgesic to children. There is no evidence to support that addiction or sedation are increased risks in children.
Nursing process: Analysis
Client need: Pharmacological and Parenteral Therapies
Cognitive level: Application
Subject area: Pharmacologic

5. The nurse instructs a client who has salsalate (Disalcid) prescribed for a sprained ankle. Which of the following statements by the client indicates the client understood the instructions?

   1. "It may cause me to have a headache and I should report this to my physician."

   2. "It can be purchased at the drug store without a prescription, because there are few adverse reactions."

   3. "There are some adverse reactions associated with Disalcid, but none that I need to report to the doctor."

   4. "If I get dizzy after taking Disalcid, I should lie down and let the drug wear off before I resume my activities."

6. The nurse is collecting a medication history for a client who has meloxicam (Mobic) prescribed. Which of the following drugs that the client is taking should the nurse question?

   1. Atorvastatin calcium (Lipitor)

   2. Alendronate sodium (Fosamax)

   3. Omeprazole (Prilosec)

   4. Diclofenac potassium (Cataflam)

7. A client who has osteoarthritis and is taking acetaminophen (Tylenol) orally and capsaicin cream topically to the knees develops a rash. Based on an understanding of the action of the drugs, which of the following is most likely the cause of the rash?

   1. The rash is an allergic reaction to acetaminophen (Tylenol) but not to the capsaicin

   2. The rash is an allergic reaction to capsaicin but not to the acetaminophen (Tylenol)

   3. A rash is not an adverse reaction to either the acetaminophen (Tylenol) or the capsaicin

   4. A rash is an adverse reaction to both the acetaminophen (Tylenol) and capsaicin

8. The nurse is admitting a client with fibromyalgia and a fractured hip who is taking sertraline (Zoloft) and diazepam (Valium). The physician orders morphine 10 mg IV push for the acute pain. Which of the following adverse reactions is a priority for the nurse to consider before administering the morphine?

   1. Sedation

   2. Gastrointestinal upset

   3. Constipation

   4. Dizziness

Answer: 1

Rationale: Salsalate (Disalcid) is a nonacetylated salicylate prescription drug. All adverse reactions should be reported to the physician. If the client becomes dizzy, lying down is appropriate, but the physician should be notified before resuming normal activities.

Nursing process: Evaluation

Client need: Pharmacological and Parenteral Therapies

Cognitive level: Analysis

Subject area: Pharmacologic

Answer: 4

Rationale: Diclofenac potassium (Cataflam) is a nonsteroidal anti-inflammatory. Because the client is already taking meloxicam (Mobic), taking two anti-inflammatories at the same time is contraindicated. Taking two anti-inflammatory drugs increases the incidence of adverse reactions. Atorvastatin calcium (Lipitor) is an antihyperlipidemic. Alendronate sodium (Fosamax) is a bone growth regulator used in the treatment of osteoporosis. Omeprazole (Prilosec) is a proton pump inhibitor used in the treatment of ulcers and gastroesophageal reflux disease.

Nursing process: Analysis

Client need: Pharmacological and Parenteral Therapies

Cognitive level: Analysis

Subject area: Pharmacologic

Answer: 4

Rationale: Both acetaminophen (Tylenol) and capsaicin may cause a rash.

Nursing process: Analysis

Client need: Pharmacological and Parenteral Therapies

Cognitive level: Analysis

Subject area: Pharmacologic

Answer: 1

Rationale: Sedation is an adverse reaction to sertraline (Zoloft), diazepam (Valium), and morphine.

Nursing process: Analysis

Client need: Management of Care

Cognitive level: Analysis

Subject area: Pharmacologic

9. The nurse is caring for a client who is receiving salicylate (Disalcid) to manage arthritis pain. Which statement would indicate the client has a good understanding of this drug?

   1. "I should take this drug on an empty stomach and not eat for 30 minutes."

   2. "To work well on my pain, I should make sure to take all the doses every day."

   3. "I only need to take this drug when I am in pain."

   4. "I can take this drug and Naprosyn together to help my pain."

10. Which of the following adverse reactions of infliximab (Remicade) should the nurse include in the medication instructions given to a client?

    Select all that apply:

    [ ] **1.** Hypertension

    [ ] **2.** Headache

    [ ] **3.** Urinary retention

    [ ] **4.** Fever

    [ ] **5.** Rash

    [ ] **6.** Hearing loss

11. When the first class of drugs prescribed for rheumatoid arthritis fails, the nurse anticipates which category of drugs will be prescribed?

    1. Nonsteroidal anti-inflammatory

    2. Disease-modifying antirheumatic

    3. Salicylates

    4. Biologic response modulators

12. Which of the following would be the best indicators to the nurse that a client receiving Naprosyn for rheumatoid arthritis is experiencing adverse reactions from this drug?

    Select all that apply:

    [ ] **1.** Tinnitus

    [ ] **2.** Blurred vision

    [ ] **3.** Confusion

    [ ] **4.** Headache

    [ ] **5.** Vasoconstriction

    [ ] **6.** Hypokalemia

Answer: 2

Rationale: Salicylate (Disalcid) should be taken with food and on a regular schedule. Disalcid should not be taken with an anti-inflammatory drug such as Naprosyn.

Nursing process: Evaluation

Client need: Pharmacological and Parenteral Therapies

Cognitive level: Analysis

Subject area: Pharmacologic

Answer: 2, 4, 5

Rationale: Infliximab (Remicade) may be used with methotrexate for inhibition of the progression of the structural damage in clients with rheumatoid arthritis who have been unsuccessfully treated with methotrexate alone. Adverse reactions include fever, fatigue, headache, dizziness, depression, rash, and urticaria.

Nursing process: Planning

Client need: Pharmacological and Parenteral Therapies

Cognitive level: Application

Subject area: Pharmacologic

Answer: 4

Rationale: Disease-modifying antirheumatic drugs (DMARDs) are the first drugs used to try to reduce joint clinical manifestations in rheumatoid arthritis. Biologic response modulators have a 66% success rate after failure with DMARDs.

Nursing process: Analysis

Client need: Pharmacological and Parenteral Therapies

Cognitive level: Analysis

Subject area: Pharmacologic

Answer: 1, 2, 3, 4

Rationale: Naprosyn is a nonsteroidal anti-inflammatory drug used in the treatment of musculoskeletal and soft tissue inflammatory disorders, such as rheumatoid arthritis. Adverse reactions include headache, dizziness, blurred vision, confusion, tinnitus, and gastrointestinal upset. Naprosyn results in vasodilation and hyperkalemia.

Nursing process: Evaluation

Client need: Pharmacological and Parenteral Therapies

Cognitive level: Application

Subject area: Pharmacologic

13. A client who had an osteoarthritic knee replacement has been receiving ibuprofen (Motrin) and experiencing excellent pain relief with this drug. Recently the client has been experiencing amblyopia, heartburn, nausea, and diarrhea. Which of the following would be the best nursing action for the nurse to include in this client's plan of care?

   1. Administer the Motrin with milk

   2. Give the Motrin two hours before meals

   3. Administer the Motrin with prescribed misoprostol (Cytotec)

   4. Give the Motrin with aspirin two hours after meals

14. A client with rheumatoid arthritis is being treated with etanercept (Enbrel). Which of the following statements by the nurse indicates the nurse understands the proper handling of this medication?

   1. "I will mix the drug by injecting liquid into the vial of powder, swirl it, and inject the drug into the client's upper arm."

   2. "I will take the prefilled syringe and warm it before injecting it into the client's upper arm."

   3. "I will infuse the drug through a peripheral IV over a period of two hours."

   4. "I will shake the prefilled syringe and inject it into the client's thigh."

15. The nurse is caring for a client with systemic scleroderma. The nurse understands that the client is to receive penicillamine (Cuprimine) for which of the following purposes?

   1. Inhibits the accumulation of collagen

   2. Prevents infection

   3. Causes thinning of the skin

   4. Decreases inflammation

Answer: 3

Rationale: The most appropriate nursing action for a client who verbalizes effective pain relief from a nonsteroidal anti-inflammatory medication such as ibuprofen (Motrin) for osteoarthritis but is now complaining of gastrointestinal upset is to administer misoprostol (Cytotec) in conjunction with the Motrin. Cytotec is frequently given in conjunction with a nonsteroidal anti-inflammatory drug that is causing gastrointestinal upset. Cytotec inhibits gastric acid secretion, has mucosal protective properties, and does not interfere with the efficacy of the Motrin. It is given for the duration that the nonsteroidal anti-inflammatory drug is taken. Amblyopia (blurred vision) has no impact on the gastrointestinal upset. If a client experiences heartburn, nausea, and diarrhea, the NSAID may be administered with food and milk. If no gastrointestinal upset is experienced, the NSAID is given on an empty stomach.

Nursing process: Planning

Client need: Pharmacological and Parenteral Therapies

Cognitive level: Application

Subject area: Pharmacologic

Answer: 1

Rationale: Etanercept (Enbrel) is an immunomodulator used in the treatment of moderate to severe rheumatoid arthritis for clients who have been unsuccessfully treated with one or more antirheumatic drugs. It comes in a vial as a powder. It must be liquefied by adding liquid and swirling to mix. It should not be shaken. It is injected into the upper arm, abdomen, or thigh.

Nursing process: Evaluation

Client need: Pharmacological and Parenteral Therapies

Cognitive level: Application

Subject area: Pharmacologic

Answer: 3

Rationale: Systemic sclerosis or scleroderma is a connective tissue disorder that results in degenerative, fibrotic, and inflammatory changes of the skin, blood vessels, skeletal muscles, and internal organs. Penicillamine (Cuprimine) is an antirheumatic drug that is investigationally used. It acts by thinning the skin.

Nursing process: Analysis

Client need: Pharmacological and Parenteral Therapies

Cognitive level: Application

Subject area: Pharmacologic

16. Which of the following should the nurse consider before administering anakinra (Kineret) to a client with rheumatoid arthritis?

　1. Live vaccines should never be given to this client

　2. Oral doses must be taken with a full glass of water on an empty stomach

　3. Flu vaccines should be given annually to avoid complications from the flu

　4. Biologic response modifiers must be infused in the physician's office

17. The nurse is admitting a client with fibromyalgia who is tearful and states, "I am in so much pain that I can't sleep. I just don't know what can be done for me." Which of the following should the nurse include in the instructions given to this client?

　1. The Food and Drug Administration has approved many drugs for the treatment of fibromyalgia

　2. Anticholinergics have been proven to be beneficial with painful muscles and tissues

　3. Treatment will focus on relieving both pain and sleep disturbances

　4. Medications that are used in the treatment of fibromyalgia do not relieve sleep disturbances

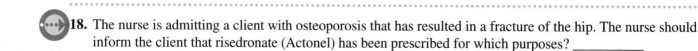

18. The nurse is admitting a client with osteoporosis that has resulted in a fracture of the hip. The nurse should inform the client that risedronate (Actonel) has been prescribed for which purposes? _____

19. The nurse is caring for a client with fibromyalgia who is experiencing pain and insomnia. Which of the following prescribed drugs should the nurse administer to relieve pain and insomnia?

　1. Cyclobenzaprine (Flexeril)

　2. Acetaminophen (Tylenol)

　3. Trazodone (Desyrel)

　4. Clonazepam (Klonopin)

Answer: 1

Rationale: Anakinra (Kineret) is a biologic response modifier that acts by inhibiting cytokines. Administering a live vaccine will manifest the disease process. Flu vaccines should be given each year, but not in the live virus form such as FluMist. Currently, there is no oral dosing of these medications. All biologic response modifiers are expensive, but only infliximab (Remicade) is infused through an IV.

Nursing process: Analysis

Client need: Pharmacological and Parenteral Therapies

Cognitive level: Analysis

Subject area: Pharmacologic

Answer: 3

Rationale: The Food and Drug Administration has approved no drugs specifically for the treatment of fibromyalgia. However, many classes of drugs have proven to be beneficial in relieving pain and sleep disturbances for these clients. Treatment will focus on relieving the pain and facilitating sleep. Anticholinergics are not used to treat clinical manifestations of fibromyalgia.

Nursing process: Planning

Client need: Health Promotion and Maintenance

Cognitive level: Analysis

Subject area: Pharmacologic

Answer: To prevent further bone loss

Rationale: Risedronate (Actonel) is a bisphosphonate that is administered to prevent further bone loss in osteoporosis.

Nursing process: Implementation

Client need: Pharmacological and Parenteral Therapies

Cognitive level: Application

Subject area: Pharmacologic

Answer: 1

Rationale: Cyclobenzaprine (Flexeril) is a skeletal muscle relaxant that is administered to a client with fibromyalgia who is experiencing both pain and insomnia (sleeplessness). Acetaminophen (Tylenol) is a nonopioid analgesic and is administered for pain. Trazodone (Desyrel) is an antidepressant prescribed for depression with or without anxiety. Clonazepam (Klonopin) is a benzodiazepine used in the treatment of depression.

Nursing process: Implementation

Client need: Pharmacological and Parenteral Therapies

Cognitive level: Application

Subject area: Pharmacologic

20. The nurse should include which of the following in the plan of care for a client who has rheumatoid arthritis for which methotrexate (Rheumatrex) has been prescribed?

1. Instruct the client to avoid sunlight
2. Instruct the client to avoid engaging in strenuous exercise
3. Monitor the client for respiratory depression
4. Restrict the client's fluid intake

21. When providing care to a client who is on dexamethasone (Decadron), the nurse should monitor the client for which of the following adverse reactions?

Select all that apply:

[   ] **1.** Hyperglycemia
[   ] **2.** Acne
[   ] **3.** Hypotension
[   ] **4.** Dehydration
[   ] **5.** Menstrual irregularities
[   ] **6.** Depression

22. The nurse should prepare to administer adalimumab (Humira) by which route to a client who has rheumatoid arthritis? _____

Answer: 1

Rationale: Methotrexate (Rheumatrex) is a disease-modifying antirheumatic drug (DMARD). Exposure to sunlight makes the skin more susceptible to adverse reactions of the sun, such as damage to the eye and sunburn, so the client should be advised to avoid sunlight and wear sunscreen and sunglasses. There are no indications that aerobic exercise causes any adverse events to occur with DMARD therapy. Respiratory depression is not an adverse reaction to DMARDs. Fluids should be encouraged to at least 2000 ml daily to ensure adequate hydration and prevent nephrotoxicity.

Nursing process: Planning

Client need: Pharmacological and Parenteral Therapies

Cognitive level: Application

Subject area: Pharmacologic

Answer: 1, 2, 5

Rationale: Adverse reactions to corticosteroids, such as dexamethasone (Decadron), include hyperglycemia, acne, menstrual irregularities, hypertension, edema, and euphoria.

Nursing process: Assessment

Client need: Pharmacological and Parenteral Therapies

Cognitive level: Application

Subject area: Pharmacologic

Answer: Subcutaneously

Rationale: Adalimumab (Humira) is a biologic response modifier (BRM) that blocks the tumor necrosis factor and is useful in the treatment of inflammation and tissue destruction in rheumatoid arthritis. It is administered subcutaneously.

Nursing process: Planning

Client need: Pharmacological and Parenteral Therapies

Cognitive level: Application

Subject area: Pharmacologic

23. The nurse is caring for a client with a history of chronic gout. The nurse should understand that the client is to receive probenecid (Benemid) for which of the following purposes?

    1. Slows uric acid production

    2. Decreases inflammation

    3. Increases uric acid excretion

    4. Reduces pain

24. The nurse is developing a medication schedule for a client who is receiving prednisone. Based on an understanding of this medication, the nurse should administer the medication at what time? _____

25. The nurse is discharging a client with osteoporosis who is to begin on alendronate (Fosamax). Which of the following should the nurse include in the medication instructions?

    1. Take with food or within 30 minutes of eating

    2. Notify the physician if urinary retention develops

    3. Avoid taking within two hours of calcium foods

    4. Avoid driving while taking the medication

26. The nurse is preparing to delegate clinical assignments to a licensed practical nurse. Which of the following assignments may the nurse delegate?

    1. Instruct a client taking an opioid analgesic on the effects of sedation on reactive time

    2. Monitor the white blood count and platelets in a client receiving interleukin-1 anakinra (Kineret)

    3. Evaluate a client with rheumatoid arthritis on compliance with drug therapy

    4. Administer prednisolone (Prelone) with food to a client with rheumatoid arthritis

Answer: 3

Rationale: Probenecid (Benemid) is an antigout drug that acts by inhibiting renal tubular reabsorption of uric acid, promoting uric acid excretion and decreasing serum urate levels. Allopurinol (Zyloprim) slows uric acid production. Colchicine acts by reducing the pain and inflammation.

Nursing process: Analysis

Client need: Pharmacological and Parenteral Therapies

Cognitive level: Comprehension

Subject area: Pharmacologic

Answer: At mealtime

Rationale: Prednisone is a corticosteroid and should be administered at mealtime. Administering the medication with food decreases the incidence of gastrointestinal upset.

Nursing process: Planning

Client need: Pharmacological and Parenteral Therapies

Cognitive level: Analysis

Subject area: Pharmacologic

Answer: 3

Rationale: Alendronate (Fosamax) should not be taken with food or within two hours of calcium-rich foods. It is best if it is taken 30 minutes before food. Urinary retention and sedation are not adverse reactions to Fosamax.

Nursing process: Planning

Client need: Health Promotion and Maintenance

Cognitive level: Application

Subject area: Pharmacologic

Answer: 4

Rationale: It is within the job description of a licensed practical nurse to administer prednisolone (Prelone) with food. Instructing a client taking an opioid analgesic on the effects of sedation, monitoring the white blood count and platelets of a client receiving interleukin-1 anakinra (Kineret), and evaluating compliance with drug therapy are all clinical assignments that require the expertise of a registered nurse.

Nursing process: Planning

Client need: Management of Care

Cognitive level: Analysis

Subject area: Legal and Ethical Issues

Drugs for the Genitourinary System

24

1. When providing care to a client who is on amoxicillin and potassium clavulanate (Augmentin), the nurse should monitor the client for

    1. constipation.

    2. polyuria.

    3. decreased temperature.

    4. increased bleeding.

2. Which of the following should the nurse consider before administering glyburide (Micronase) and chlorthalidone (Hygroton) to a client with diabetes mellitus, hypertension, and edema?

    1. The combination of an oral hypoglycemic agent and a diuretic increases the adverse reactions

    2. A thiazide diuretic decreases the action of glyburide

    3. There is no drug interaction between Hygroton and Micronase

    4. A second-generation oral hypoglycemic agent increases the action of diuretics

3. The nurse is teaching a class on anti-infectives used to treat urinary tract infections. Which of the following should the nurse include in the class?

    1. *E. coli* has developed a resistance to penicillin anti-infectives

    2. Sulfonamides are frequently prescribed for *Pseudomonas* infections

    3. Fluoroquinolones have a limited use in the treatment of urinary tract infections

    4. Cephalosporins are the anti-infective of choice for clients sensitive to penicillin

4. Which of the following should the nurse include in the plan of care for a client with diabetes mellitus and congestive heart failure who is receiving NPH insulin, cefuroxime (Zinacef), and triamterene (Dyrenium)?

    1. Encourage the client to choose foods high in potassium

    2. Monitor the client for clinical manifestations of hypernatremia

    3. Test the client's urine with a Clinistix or Ketodiastix

    4. Notify the physician that the client has a hypersensitivity to quinolones

Answer: 4
Rationale: Amoxicillin and potassium clavulanate (Augmentin) are penicillin anti-infectives. Diarrhea, fever, and increased bleeding time are adverse reactions.
Nursing process: Assessment
Client need: Pharmacological and Parenteral Therapies
Cognitive level: Application
Subject area: Pharmacologic

Answer: 2
Rationale: Glyburide (Micronase) is a sulfonylurea (second-generation) oral hypoglycemic agent. Chlorthalidone (Hygroton) is a thiazide diuretic. The thiazide diuretic decreases the action of the oral hypoglycemic agent and should be administered with caution to a client with diabetes mellitus.
Nursing process: Analysis
Client need: Pharmacological and Parenteral Therapies
Cognitive level: Analysis
Subject area: Pharmacologic

Answer: 1
Rationale: There is an increasing resistance to *E. coli* infections with penicillin anti-infectives. Sulfonamides are effective against aerobic bacteria, except *Pseudomonas*. Fluoroquinolones are effective broad-spectrum antibiotics used in the treatment of urinary tract infections caused by most organisms. Cephalosporins are chemically similar to penicillin and may result in a cross sensitivity in clients with a known allergy to penicillin.
Nursing process: Planning
Client need: Health Promotion and Maintenance
Cognitive level: Application
Subject area: Pharmacologic

Answer: 3
Rationale: It is appropriate to test the urine of a client with diabetes mellitus with a Clinistix or Ketodiastix to avoid a false positive when administering cefuroxime (Zinacef), a cephalosporin. Triamterene is a potassium-sparing diuretic and foods high in potassium do not need to be encouraged. Encouraging foods high in potassium could lead to hyperkalemia. Triamterene results in hyponatremia, not hypernatremia.
Nursing process: Planning
Client need: Pharmacological and Parenteral Therapies
Cognitive level: Application
Subject area: Pharmacologic

5. Phenazopyridine hydrochloride (Pyridium) is prescribed for a client with acute cystitis. Which of the following should the nurse explain to the client?

   1. Dry mouth is a common anticipated adverse reaction

   2. Gastrointestinal adverse reactions are eliminated when taken on an empty stomach

   3. The color of the urine will turn reddish-orange

   4. Exposure to sunlight enhances the effects of the drug

6. Ciprofloxacin (Cipro) has been prescribed for a client with a urinary tract infection who is also receiving theophylline. Based on an understanding of the effects of the two drugs, the nurse should monitor the client for which of the following?

   Select all that apply:

   [　] **1.** Visual disturbances

   [　] **2.** Tachycardia

   [　] **3.** Seizures

   [　] **4.** Oliguria

   [　] **5.** Nausea

   [　] **6.** Flaccid paralysis

7. The nurse evaluates the urine of a client who is taking methenamine mandelate (Mandelamine) to be what color? _____

Answer: 3

Rationale: Phenazopyridine hydrochloride (Pyridium) is a urinary analgesic that exerts a topical analgesic effect on the mucosa lining of the urinary tract. It is normal for the urine to turn reddish-orange. Gastrointestinal adverse reactions are decreased by taking the drug with food.

Nursing process: Analysis

Client need: Pharmacological and Parenteral Therapies

Cognitive level: Application

Subject area: Pharmacologic

Answer: 2, 3, 5

Rationale: Ciprofloxacin (Cipro) and theophylline result in increased plasma theophylline concentrations, prolonged theophylline half-life, and decreased hepatic clearance of the theophylline. The onset of toxicity may be sudden and severe, with arrhythmia and seizures as the first signs. Other indications of toxicity include nausea, vomiting, and irritability. Extreme caution must be used when administering Cipro and theophylline together. The theophylline levels should be closely monitored and the dose adjusted accordingly.

Nursing process: Assessment

Client need: Pharmacological and Parenteral Therapies

Cognitive level: Analysis

Subject area: Pharmacologic

Answer: Blue

Rationale: Methenamine mandelate (Mandelamine) is a urinary anti-infective. It is normal and harmless for the urine to turn blue.

Nursing process: Evaluation

Client need: Pharmacological and Parenteral Therapies

Cognitive level: Application

Subject area: Pharmacologic

8. The nurse is caring for a client who has sustained a traumatic brain injury and is experiencing a neurogenic bladder. The nurse should understand that the client is to receive which of the following drugs in the treatment of neurogenic bladder?

   1. Phenazopyridine HCl (Pyridium)

   2. Nalidixic acid (NegGram)

   3. Methenamine, phenylsalicylate, atropine, and hyoscyamine (Urised)

   4. Probanthine bromide (Pro-Banthine)

9. The nurse is caring for a client with congestive heart failure. The nurse should understand that the client is to receive furosemide (Lasix) for which of the following purposes?

   1. Acts in the renal tubule to decrease the reabsorption of water, sodium, and potassium

   2. Inhibits sodium and chloride reabsorption in the distal tubule while blocking chloride reabsorption in the ascending loop of Henle

   3. Competes with aldosterone in the distal renal tubule, promoting the excretion of water, sodium, chloride, and bicarbonate while sparing potassium

   4. Inhibits the reabsorption of sodium and chloride in the ascending loop of Henle

10. The nurse should montitor a client receiving nalidixic acid (NegGram) for which of the following adverse reactions?

    Select all that apply:

    [   ] **1.** Drowsiness

    [   ] **2.** Sensitivity to light

    [   ] **3.** Headache

    [   ] **4.** Urinary frequency

    [   ] **5.** Bradycardia

    [   ] **6.** Constipation

Answer: 4

Rationale: Probanthine bromide (Pro-Banthine) is an antimuscarinic, also known as an anticholinergic or antispasmodic. It is used to relax the urinary tract smooth muscles by inhibiting acetylcholine in the treatment of bladder spasms or a neurogenic bladder. With a neurogenic bladder, urgency, frequency, incontinence, inability to void, and reflux are common clinical manifestations. Phenazopyridine HCL (Pyridium) is a urinary analgesic used for dysuria. Nalidixic acid (NegGram) and methenamine, phenylsalicylate, atropine, and hyoscyamine (Urised) are urinary anti-infectives used in the treatment of urinary tract infections.

Nursing process: Analysis

Client need: Pharmacological and Parenteral Therapies

Cognitive level: Analysis

Subject area: Pharmacologic

Answer: 4

Rationale: Furosemide (Lasix) is a loop diuretic that inhibits the reabsortion of sodium and chloride in the ascending loop of Henle. A carbonic anhydrase inhibitor acts in the renal tubule to decrease water, sodium, and potassium. A thiazide diuretic inhibits sodium and chloride reabsorption in the distal tubule while blocking chloride reabsorption in the ascending loop of Henle. A potassium-sparing diuretic competes with aldosterone in the distal renal tubule, promoting the excretion of water, sodium, chloride, and bicarbonate while sparing potassium.

Nursing process: Analysis

Client need: Pharmacological and Parenteral Therapies

Cognitive level: Application

Subject area: Pharmacologic

Answer: 1, 2, 3

Rationale: Nalidixic acid (NegGram) is a urinary tract anti-infective with a bactericidal action used in the treatment of urinary tract infections. Adverse reactions include drowsiness, headache, sensitivity to light, and diarrhea.

Nursing process: Assessment

Client need: Pharmacological and Parenteral Therapies

Cognitive level: Application

Subject area: Pharmacologic

11. Tolterodine (Detrol) has been prescribed for an older adult client who has dementia and is experiencing incontinence. The client's medical history reveals congestive heart failure, edema, and hypertension. Which of the following adverse reactions is a priority to report for this client?

    1. Dry mouth

    2. Restlessness

    3. Urinary retention

    4. Nausea

12. The nurse assists a client receiving furosemide (Lasix) to make which of the following dietary selections that are high in potassium?

    Select all that apply:

    [   ] **1.** Raisins

    [   ] **2.** Spinach

    [   ] **3.** White bread

    [   ] **4.** Corn flakes cereal

    [   ] **5.** Salmon

    [   ] **6.** Avocado

13. The nurse is caring for a client who is receiving chlorothiazide (Diuril) who is complaining of forgetfulness, lethargy, weakness, nausea, and vomiting. The nurse assesses the client to have decreased reflexes and polyuria. The nurse should report this as

    1. hypercalcemia.

    2. hypermagnesemia.

    3. hyperkalemia.

    4. hypernatremia.

14. A client with a urinary tract infection has received medication instructions on Levofloxacin (Levaquin). Which of the following statements by the client indicates a need for further instructions?

    1. "I will increase my daily intake of fluids."

    2. "I will take my medication with an antacid to decrease stomach upset."

    3. "I will stay out of the direct sunlight."

    4. "I will ask for assistance walking if I get dizzy."

Answer: 3

Rationale: Although dry mouth, restlessness, urinary retention, and nausea are all adverse reactions to tolterodine (Detrol), urinary retention is the priority to report for a client with congestive heart failure and edema. Urinary retention is a potentially serious adverse reaction for a client already experiencing fluid retention with congestive heart failure.

Nursing process: Analysis

Client need: Pharmacological and Parenteral Therapies

Cognitive level: Analysis

Subject area: Pharmacologic

Answer: 1, 2, 5, 6

Rationale: Furosemide (Lasix) is a potent loop diuretic that often causes a low potassium level. Clients should be instructed to choose foods high in potassium to make appropriate food choices. Raisins, spinach, salmon, and avocado are all foods high in potassium. White bread and corn flakes are low in potassium. Wheat bread and oatmeal, although still low, are better selections.

Nursing process: Implementation

Client need: Basic Care and Comfort

Cognitive level: Application

Subject area: Pharmacologic

Answer: 1

Rationale: Hypercalcemia may be an adverse reaction of a client taking a thiazide diuretic such as chlorothiazide. Normal serum calcium is 9 to 11 mg/dl. Clinical manifestations of hypercalcemia include lethargy, weakness, anorexia, nausea, vomiting, confusion, personality changes, polyuria, dehydration, stupor, and coma.

Nursing process: Analysis

Client need: Pharmacological and Parenteral Therapies

Cognitive level: Application

Subject area: Pharmacologic

Answer: 2

Rationale: Levofloxacin (Levaquin) is a fluoroquinolone. It may or may not be administered with food but should never be administered with an antacid. An antacid decreases the absorption of Levaquin. Fluids should be increased to prevent crystalluria. Direct sunlight should be avoided because of a photosensitivity. Dizziness is an adverse reaction and assistance with ambulation may be required.

Nursing process: Evaluation

Client need: Pharmacological and Parenteral Therapies

Cognitive level: Application

Subject area: Pharmacologic

15. The nurse administers which of the following prescribed diuretics for the purpose of decreasing the adverse effects of hypokalemia and hyperkalemia?

1. Quinethazone (Hydromox)

2. Ethacrynic acid (Edecrin)

3. Triameterene and hydrochlorothiazide (Dyazide)

4. Acetazolamide (Diamox)

16. Which of the following questions is a priority for the nurse to ask a client before administering ceftriaxone (Rocephin)?

1. "Do you have an allergy to penicillin?"

2. "Are you sensitive to the sunlight?"

3. "Do you have a known bleeding disorder?"

4. "Are you prone to gastrointestinal upset?"

17. The nurse is developing a medication schedule for a client who is to receive cefadroxil (Duricef) orally. Based on an understanding of the drug, which of the following administration methods would promote the best absorption?

1. On an empty stomach

2. At bedtime

3. With food

4. Duricef cannot be administered orally

18. Which of the following would be the best indication to the nurse that an antimicrobial given repeatedly in the treatment of chronic urinary tract infections has resulted in a superinfection?

Select all that apply:

[ ] 1. Stomatitis

[ ] 2. Urinary retention

[ ] 3. Loose foul-smelling stools

[ ] 4. Ecchymosis

[ ] 5. Vaginal itching

[ ] 6. Fever

Answer: 3

Rationale: Triameterene and hydrochlorothiazide (Dyazide) is an antihypertensive combination drug used for the purpose of decreasing the effects of both hypokalemia and hyperkalemia. Quinethazone (Hydromox) is a thiazide diuretic, ethacrynic acid (Edecrin) is a loop diuretic, and acetazolamide (Diamox) is a carbonic anhydrase inhibitor. All of these diuretics cause hypokalemia.

Nursing process: Implementation

Client need: Pharmacological and Parenteral Therapies

Cognitive level: Application

Subject area: Pharmacologic

Answer: 1

Rationale: Ceftriaxone (Rocephin) is a cephalosporin that is chemically and pharmacologically related to penicillin. Because of this chemical similarity, there may be a cross-sensitivity in clients with a known allergy to penicillin.

Nursing process: Assessment

Client need: Management of Care

Cognitive level: Application

Subject area: Pharmacologic

Answer: 3

Rationale: Cefadroxil (Duricef) is a cephalosporin given in the treatment of acute urinary tract infections. The usual oral dose is one to two grams twice a day. Oral absorption is increased when taken with food.

Nursing process: Planning

Client need: Pharmacological and Parenteral Therapies

Cognitive level: Application

Subject area: Pharmacologic

Answer: 1, 3, 5, 6

Rationale: A superinfection is the development of a new infection by an organism different from the organism causing the initial infection. The risk of a superinfection may increase with repeated antimicrobial therapy. Indications of a superinfection include a black hairy tongue, glossitis, stomatitis, loose foul-smelling stools, anal itching, vaginal itching, cough, and fever.

Nursing process: Evaluation

Client need: Pharmacological and Parenteral Therapies

Cognitive level: Application

Subject area: Pharmacologic

19. The nurse should monitor a client taking dichlorphenamide (Daranide) for which of the following adverse reactions?

Select all that apply:

[ ] **1.** Tinnitus

[ ] **2.** Hyperglycemia

[ ] **3.** Hypercalcemia

[ ] **4.** Myopia

[ ] **5.** Urinary retention

[ ] **6.** Anxiety

20. Which of the following is a priority to include in the plan of care when starting antimicrobial therapy?

1. Encourage the client to increase fluids

2. Stay with the client for 30 minutes after the initial dose

3. Maintain an accurate intake and output

4. Monitor the client's blood and liver function tests

21. The registered nurse making out clinical assignments for the day may delegate which of the following nursing skills to a licensed practical nurse?

1. Assess a client taking trimethoprim-sulfamethoxazole (Bactrim) for an allergy before initiating therapy

2. Notify the physician that a client taking ciprofloxacin (Cipro) is taking theophylline

3. Assess the BUN and creatinine in a client taking cefadroxil (Duricef)

4. Maintain an accurate intake and output in a client taking spironolactone (Aldactone)

22. The nurse is reviewing the medical history of a client taking dichlorphenamide (Daranide). For which of the following conditions is Daranide contraindicated or to be used with extreme caution?

1. Hyperkalemia

2. Osteoporosis

3. Diabetes mellitus

4. Scleroderma

Answer: 1, 2, 4

Rationale: Dichlorphenamide (Daranide) is a carbonic anhydrase inhibitor that acts in the renal tubule to decrease the reabsorption of water, sodium, and potassium. Adverse reactions include tinnitus, hyperglycemia, hypocalcemia, myopia, polyuria, and drowsiness.

Nursing process: Assessment

Client need: Pharmacological and Parenteral Therapies

Cognitive level: Application

Subject area: Pharmacologic

Answer: 2

Rationale: It is a priority to stay with the client for the first 30 minutes when initiating antimicrobial therapy to monitor the client for a severe reaction, such as anaphylactoid reaction. Encouraging an increased fluid intake, monitoring the liver and blood studies, and maintaining an accurate intake and output are all appropriate interventions, but not the priority.

Nursing process: Planning

Client need: Management of Care

Cognitive level: Application

Subject area: Pharmacologic

Answer: 4

Rationale: Nursing skills that involve assessment, monitoring, or notifying are skills that must be performed by a registered nurse. A licensed practical nurse does have the skill to maintain an accurate intake and output.

Nursing process: Planning

Client need: Management of Care

Cognitive level: Analysis

Subject area: Legal and Ethical Issues

Answer: 1

Rationale: Dichlorphenamide (Daranide) is a potassium-sparing diuretic that is contraindicated or should be used only with extreme caution for a client in renal disease or with an electrolyte imbalance such as hyperkalemia.

Nursing process: Analysis

Client need: Pharmacological and Parenteral Therapies

Cognitive level: Analysis

Subject area: Pharmacologic

23. Based on an understanding of the drug interactions for a client taking a loop diuretic and an aminoglyceride, for which of the following should the nurse monitor the client?

   1. Hypokalemia

   2. Orthostatic hypotension

   3. Ototoxicity

   4. Decreased diuretic effects

24. The nurse should monitor a client taking bumetanide (Bumex) for which of the following adverse reactions? Select all that apply:

   [ ] **1.** Hypertension

   [ ] **2.** Polyuria

   [ ] **3.** Hypokalemia

   [ ] **4.** Weakness

   [ ] **5.** Constipation

   [ ] **6.** Hyponatremia

25. Which of the following nursing actions should the nurse include in the plan of care for a client taking nalidixic acid (NegGram)?

   1. Administer with food

   2. Instruct the client to take with an antacid

   3. Instruct the client to avoid activities that promote fluid loss

   4. Monitor the blood pressure

Answer: 3

Rationale: There is a drug interaction between a loop diuretic and an aminoglyceride that may result in ototoxicity. If a medical necessity to have the client on both, it is essential that the client be monitored for manifestations of ototoxicity. A loop diuretic and corticosteroid interaction may result in hypokalemia. A drug interaction between a loop diuretic and an opiate may result in orthostatic hypotension. A drug interaction between a loop diuretic and a salicylate may decrease the diuretic effects.

Nursing process: Assessment

Client need: Pharmacological and Parenteral Therapies

Cognitive level: Analysis

Subject area: Pharmacologic

Answer: 2, 3, 4, 6

Rationale: Bumetanide (Bumex) is a potent loop diuretic that may result in severe hypokalemia. Other adverse reactions include weakness, orthostatic hypotension, hyponatremia, polyuria, diarrhea, and abdominal cramps.

Nursing process: Assessment

Client need: Pharmacological and Parenteral Therapies

Cognitive level: Application

Subject area: Pharmacologic

Answer: 1

Rationale: Nalidixic acid (NegGram) is a urinary anti-infective with bacteriocidal action used in the treatment of urinary tract infections. It should be administered with food to decrease the gastrointestinal effects. NegGram should not be administered with an antacid. An antacid should be administered two hours before or two hours after an antacid. NegGram has no bearing on fluid loss or blood pressure.

Nursing process: Planning

Client need: Pharmacological and Parenteral Therapies

Cognitive level: Application

Subject area: Pharmacologic

Drugs for the Reproductive System

25

1. Which of the following is a priority for the nurse to include in the instructions for a client starting estrogen hormone replacement therapy for menopause?

    1. Report an increase in weight of three pounds or more to your doctor

    2. Take extra safety precautions to protect yourself from injury and falls

    3. You may have greater frequency and urgency in urination

    4. Remember to do breast self-examination every month

2. After receiving instructions from the nurse regarding the drug alendronate (Fosamax), which of the following statements from a postmenopausal client indicates an understanding of the purpose of the drug?

    1. "This drug should help my mood swings."

    2. "This drug should eliminate my stress incontinence."

    3. "This drug should make my bones stronger."

    4. "This drug should relieve my hot flashes."

 3. The nurse monitors a client receiving hormone replacement therapy for which of the following adverse reactions?

    Select all that apply:

    [ ] **1.** Increase in weight

    [ ] **2.** Menorrhagia

    [ ] **3.** Hypertension

    [ ] **4.** Virilization

    [ ] **5.** Breast tenderness

    [ ] **6.** Decreased libido

4. The nurse instructs the perimenopausal client that it is a priority to stop taking the prescribed estrogen if which of the following occurs?

    1. Spotting between menstrual periods

    2. Painful intercourse

    3. Breast tenderness

    4. Nausea and vomiting

Answer: 4

Rationale: Menopausal women who take estrogen hormone replacement therapy (HRT) are at risk for developing breast cancer; thus, monthly breast self-examinations are very important. It is normal for women who start HRT to gain weight. Menopausal women who do not start HRT will be at risk for osteoporosis and prone to fractures and will have greater frequency and urgency in urination.

Nursing process: Planning

Client need: Management of Care

Cognitive level: Analysis

Subject area: Pharmacologic

Answer: 3

Rationale: Alendronate (Fosamax) is a drug that decreases the rate of bone resorption and is used to prevent or treat osteoporosis in postmenopausal women. Fosamax is not helpful for other clinical manifestations of menopause, which include mood swings, stress incontinence, and hot flashes.

Nursing process: Evaluation

Client need: Pharmacological and Parenteral Therapies

Cognitive level: Analysis

Subject area: Pharmacologic

Answer: 1, 3, 5

Rationale: The adverse reactions of hormone replacement therapy include increase in weight, fluid retention, hypertension, breast tenderness, spotting between periods, and dark skin patches that darken when exposed to sunlight. Women on HRT who do menstruate have normal menstrual cycles without excessive bleeding. Virilization and decreased libido do not normally occur with HRT.

Nursing process: Assessment

Client need: Pharmacological and Parenteral Therapies

Cognitive level: Application

Subject area: Pharmacologic

Answer: 4

Rationale: Hormone replacement therapy should not be taken if one is pregnant; if a woman begins to experience nausea and vomiting, it could indicate morning sickness accompanying a pregnancy. Spotting between menstrual periods and breast tenderness are adverse reactions to HRT. Painful intercourse may be due to vaginal dryness, which commonly occurs in menopause with the absence of estrogen.

Nursing process: Implementation

Client need: Management of Care

Cognitive level: Application

Subject area: Pharmacologic

5. Which of the following should the nurse include in the administration instructions for a client using estrogen vaginal cream?
   1. Insert a tampon afterward to protect your clothing
   2. Remain in bed for 30 minutes after inserting the drug
   3. Apply the drug topically every 10 days throughout the month
   4. Soak the applicator in bleach after each use

6. Based on an understanding of drugs, the nurse plans to instruct a client with amenorrhea to use which of the following drugs?
   1. Danazol (Danocrine)
   2. Progesterone (Progestin)
   3. Estrogen (Premarin)
   4. Naproxen (Naprosyn)

7. Which of the following should the nurse include in the instructions to a client receiving a nonsteroidal anti-inflammatory drug?
   1. Do not take with the drug lithium
   2. Avoid the use of products with caffeine
   3. Notify your physician if you become pregnant
   4. Take on an empty stomach

8. Which of the following allergies should the nurse assess for a client who is taking naproxen (Naprosyn) for the treatment of dysmenorrhea?
   1. Morphine
   2. Penicillin
   3. Aspirin
   4. Tylenol

Answer: 2

Rationale: For proper absorption of the vaginal cream, the client should remain in bed for 30 minutes after insertion. A tampon would absorb the cream and reduce its effectiveness. Application schedules vary, but the cream should be applied at least one to three times per week. The applicator should be cleaned with soap and water after use.

Nursing process: Planning

Client need: Health Promotion and Maintenance

Cognitive level: Application

Subject area: Pharmacologic

Answer: 3

Rationale: Amenorrhea is treated with drugs such as estrogen (Premarin) to stimulate ovulation. Danazol (Danocrine) is used to suppress ovulation. Progesterone (Progestin) causes the uterine lining to shed with menses. Naproxen (Naprosyn) is a nonsteroidal anti-inflammatory drug used in the treatment of dysmenorrhea.

Nursing process: Analysis

Client need: Health Promotion and Maintenance

Cognitive level: Analysis

Subject area: Pharmacologic

Answer: 1

Rationale: Nonsteroidal anti-inflammatory drugs interact with lithium to increase lithium toxicity. Caffeine is not contraindicated with the use of NSAIDs. NSAIDs are not hormones and would not affect pregnancy. NSAIDs should be taken with food or milk to minimize gastric irritation.

Nursing process: Planning

Client need: Health Promotion and Maintenance

Cognitive level: Application

Subject area: Pharmacologic

Answer: 3

Rationale: Naproxen (Naprosyn) and acetylsalicylic acid (aspirin) are both nonsteroidal anti-inflammatory drugs and a hypersensitivity to any NSAID creates a hypersensitivity to all of the others in the group. Allergies to morphine and penicillin would not affect the use of NSAIDs. Tylenol is a nonnarcotic analgesic that does not have the same bleeding tendencies as aspirin and is often used as a substitute for aspirin when aspirin is contraindicated.

Nursing process: Assessment

Client need: Pharmacological and Parenteral Therapies

Cognitive level: Analysis

Subject area: Pharmacologic

9. Which of the following assessment data is expected in a client with premenstrual syndrome (PMS) who is receiving danazol (Danocrine)?

    1. Breast tenderness

    2. Hirsutism

    3. Increased libido

    4. Amenorrhea

10. The nurse instructs a client who is prescribed danazol (Danocrine) for the treatment of premenstrual syndrome (PMS) to take the first dose

    1. two weeks after the next menstrual period.

    2. during the next menstrual period.

    3. the next time thick vaginal mucus is discharged.

    4. a week prior to the beginning of the next menses.

11. The best time to insert (Monistat) a miconazole nitrate vaginal suppository to a client for maximum effectiveness is _____?

12. The nurse instructs the client taking miconazole nitrate (Monistat) to avoid which of the following drugs?

    1. Coumadin

    2. Isoniazid (Nydrazid)

    3. Probenecid (Benemid)

    4. Hydrochlorothiazide (Hydrodiuril)

Answer: 4

Rationale: Danazol (Danocrine) is an ovulatory suppression drug used to create anovulation and amenorrhea in the treatment of premenstrual syndrome (PMS). It does not cause breast tenderness or hirsutism. Danazol is known to decrease libido rather than increase it.

Nursing process: Assessment

Client need: Pharmacological and Parenteral Therapies

Cognitive level: Analysis

Subject area: Pharmacologic

Answer: 2

Rationale: Danazol (Danocrine) is started during the menses to ensure that the client is not pregnant. The client could be pregnant two weeks after her menstrual period and a week prior to the start of the next menses. Thick mucus discharge could indicate that the client has ovulated and possibly conceived.

Nursing process: Implementation

Client need: Health Promotion and Maintenance

Cognitive level: Analysis

Subject area: Pharmacologic

Answer: at bedtime

Rationale: Bedtime is the best time for the insertion of vaginal suppositories, as they are absorbed better when the client remains in the recumbent position for a period of time. Morning insertions do not usually provide sufficient time for complete absorption. Miconazole (Monistat) suppositories are used once a day.

Nursing process: Implementation

Client need: Pharmacological and Parenteral Therapies

Cognitive level: Analysis

Subject area: Pharmacologic

Answer: 2

Rationale: Isoniazid (Nydrazid) is an antitubercular drug that decreases the effectiveness and blood levels of the antifungal drug miconazole nitrate (Monistat). Coumadin, probenecid (Benemid), and hydrochlorothiazide (Hydrodiuril) are not contraindicated when Monistat is prescribed.

Nursing process: Implementation

Client need: Health Promotion and Maintenance

Cognitive level: Analysis

Subject area: Pharmacologic

13. Which of the following should the nurse include in the teaching plan for a client who has a recurrent gonorrheal infection and is treated with ciprofloxacin hydrochloride (Cipro)?

1. The drug should be taken with meals or with a glass of milk

2. Weekly cultures are necessary until two are negative

3. The drug should not be discontinued until all the pills have been taken

4. The drug will be started when the diagnostic culture and sensitivity results are obtained

14. Which of the following should the nurse include in the medication instructions for a client with gonorrhea who is prescribed tetracycline hydrochloride (Achromycin V)?

1. Continue taking birth control pills

2. Take two or three times during the day as prescribed

3. Start the first dose after the results of the culture and sensitivity are determined

4. Use sun protection and cover your body if going outdoors

15. The nurse administers ceftriaxone sodium (Rocephin) to a pregnant client with gonorrhea by what route? _____

Answer: 2

Rationale: The effectiveness of antibiotic therapy in the treatment of recurrent gonorrhea is determined by vaginal cultures done weekly and is considered successful when two cultures are negative. Ciprofloxacin hydrochloride (Cipro) should be taken on an empty stomach, as food affects peak serum levels. Cipro is given as a single dose for the treatment of gonorrhea. When the clinical manifestations are obvious for a diagnosis of a specific infectious disease, the drug is started once the culture has been obtained but before the results are available.

Nursing process: Planning

Client need: Health Promotion and Maintenance

Cognitive level: Application

Subject area: Pharmacologic

Answer: 4

Rationale: A major adverse reaction of most antibiotics including tetracycline hydrochloride (Achromycin V) is photosensitivity; thus, clients should use sun protection and cover their bodies when going outdoors. Clients taking Achromycin V should use a nonhormonal type of contraceptive, as there is decreased effectiveness of hormonal contraceptives and a possibility of breakthrough bleeding. This drug should be taken around the clock to maintain blood levels. The first dose of any antibiotic can be started after the specimen for culture and sensitivity has been obtained but before the results are known.

Nursing process: Planning

Client need: Health Promotion and Maintenance

Cognitive level: Application

Subject area: Pharmacologic

Answer: Intramuscularly

Rationale: Ceftriaxone sodium (Rocephin) is only administered intravenously or intramuscularly. It is not available in transdermal or oral forms. Ceftriaxone sodium must be administered deeply into a large muscle mass such as the gluteal or thigh muscles.

Nursing process: Implementation

Client need: Pharmacological and Parenteral Therapies

Cognitive level: Application

Subject area: Pharmacologic

16. The nurse should notify the physician if which of the following occurs when treating a client receiving antibiotics for gonorrhea?

    1. Perineal lesions fail to clear in two to three days
    2. Sexual intercourse is painful
    3. A black furry growth appears on the tongue
    4. Spotting occurs between periods

17. The nurse is creating a medication schedule for erythromycin prescribed for a client with pelvic inflammatory disease. Which of the following times for administration should the nurse include in the schedule? Administer with

    1. a full glass of water between meals.
    2. fruit juice prior to each meal.
    3. an antacid 30 minutes before each meal.
    4. a glass of milk at each meal.

18. The nurse informs a client with bacterial vaginosis who has been taking metronidazole (Flagyl) that which of the following would indicate an expected response to the drug?

    1. Weight gain
    2. Metallic taste
    3. Reddish-brown urine
    4. Diarrhea

19. The nurse instructs a client who has trichomoniasis to avoid which of the following while taking metronidazole (Flagyl)?

    1. Lithium
    2. Alcohol
    3. Caffeine
    4. Diazepam

Answer: 3

Rationale: A black furry growth that appears on the tongue is an indication of the presence of a superinfection. Herpesvirus type 2 has lesions on the perineal area but gonorrhea does not. Clients with gonorrhea may have painful sexual intercourse and spotting between periods as part of the disease process.

Nursing process: Analysis

Client need: Pharmacological and Parenteral Therapies

Cognitive level: Analysis

Subject area: Pharmacologic

Answer: 1

Rationale: Erythromycin is an antibiotic used in the treatment of pelvic inflammatory disease. It should be taken with a full glass of water one hour before or two hours after a meal. It should not be taken with fruit juices. It is not necessary to take it with an antacid and 30 minutes prior to a meal would interfere with absorption. Erythromycin should be taken on an empty stomach, so milk and meals would both interfere with absorption.

Nursing process: Planning

Client need: Pharmacological and Parenteral Therapies

Cognitive level: Application

Subject area: Pharmacologic

Answer: 3

Rationale: Metronidazole (Flagyl) is an antifungal drug used to treat bacterial vaginosis. It may cause reddish-brown urine, which is of no clinical significance. Weight gain, a metallic taste, and diarrhea are adverse reactions that are not considered to be normal.

Nursing process: Evaluation

Client need: Pharmacological and Parenteral Therapies

Cognitive level: Analysis

Subject area: Pharmacologic

Answer: 2

Rationale: A disulfiram-like reaction may occur when alcohol is ingested while one is taking metronidazole (Flagyl). Lithium, caffeine, and diazepam are not known to be contraindicated with Flagyl.

Nursing process: Implementation

Client need: Health Promotion and Maintenance

Cognitive level: Analysis

Subject area: Pharmacologic

20. Which of the following is correct to include in the procedure for a client with herpesvirus type 2 who is being treated with acyclovir (Zovirax)?

    1. Wash the lesions with bar soap and water and dry well
    2. Apply ointment to the lesions with a nonsterile glove
    3. Apply the medicated patch over a cluster of lesions
    4. Cover the lesions with an occlusive dressing

21. Which of the following laboratory tests would be most important for the nurse to monitor in a client with herpesvirus type 2 who has been taking acyclovir (Zovirax)?

    1. Alkaline phosphatase
    2. White blood cell count
    3. Prothrombin time
    4. Serum creatinine

22. The nurse instructs a client with a history of herpesvirus type 2 to take the prescribed acyclovir (Zovirax)

    1. for up to one year whenever the lesions return.
    2. at the first sign of clinical manifestations returning.
    3. when over-the-counter ointments fail to control itching.
    4. daily for two weeks to prevent reinfection.

23. A client who is prescribed danazol (Danocrine) for endometriosis asks the nurse, "What happens when I stop taking this drug?" The best response of the nurse would be

    1. "You will be cured of your endometriosis."
    2. "You will no longer have dysmenorrhea with your periods."
    3. "You will ovulate and start menstruating in two to three months."
    4. "You will have more regular periods."

Answer: 2

Rationale: Acyclovir (Zovirax) is supplied as an ointment, which is applied topically to the lesions of a client with herpesvirus type 2. A nonsterile glove or finger cot should be used in applying the ointment to prevent cross-contamination. Liquid soap should be used rather than bar soap, as the bar soap would become contaminated for use by others. Acyclovir is not supplied as a transdermal patch and the lesions should be left open to air.

Nursing process: Planning

Client need: Pharmacological and Parenteral Therapies

Cognitive level: Application

Subject area: Pharmacologic

Answer: 4

Rationale: Acyclovir (Zovirax) is an antiviral used in the treatment of herpes. Clients receiving acyclovir (Zovirax) for herpesvirus type 2 need to be assessed frequently to detect changes in renal function, as the drug can be nephrotoxic. Serum creatinine is a good laboratory test to monitor renal function. Zovirax is not known to affect liver function, white cell count, or bleeding and clotting time.

Nursing process: Assessment

Client need: Pharmacological and Parenteral Therapies

Cognitive level: Analysis

Subject area: Pharmacologic

Answer: 2

Rationale: Acyclovir (Zovirax) should be taken as soon as the client notices the clinical manifestations are reappearing. Acyclovir is not recommended to be taken for longer than a six-month period. Over-the-counter ointment and creams should not be used, as they may delay healing and spread infection. Acyclovir should not be taken before clinical manifestations appear and it does not prevent reinfection.

Nursing process: Implementation

Client need: Health Promotion and Maintenance

Cognitive level: Application

Subject area: Pharmacologic

Answer: 3

Rationale: Danazol (Danocrine) is a synthetic androgen that is used to cause atrophy of the endometrium, resulting in amenorrhea. When the drug is stopped, the reactions are reversible and ovulation and menses will return in two to three months. These drugs do not cure endometriosis, but alleviate the clinical manifestations during drug therapy. A client taking this drug may still have some endometrial cells, which are stimulated by estrogen, so the dysmenorrhea may return. Danazol does not affect regularity of menstrual periods.

Nursing process: Analysis

Client need: Pharmacological and Parenteral Therapies

Cognitive level: Analysis

Subject area: Pharmacologic

24. The nurse informs a client taking oral contraceptives for birth control that which of the following is a priority to immediately report?

   1. Spotting between periods

   2. Breast enlargement

   3. Increase in growth of body hair

   4. Calf pain with dorsiflexion of the foot

25. The nurse instructs a client who is prescribed a progestin-only contraceptive for birth control to

   1. take the drug the 5th to 30th day of each monthly menstrual cycle.

   2. use a barrier method of contraception for four months after starting the drug.

   3. wait three months to get pregnant after she stops taking the drug.

   4. stop taking the drug if she experiences a menstrual period.

26. Which of the following nursing tasks may the registered nurse safely delegate to a licensed practical nurse?

   1. Inform a client who is going through menopause on the pros and cons of using hormonal replacement therapy

   2. Advise a client taking estrogen to weigh one to two times per week and report any sudden weight gain or fluid retention in the ankles and feet

   3. Instruct a client on the purpose of ovulation suppression drugs

   4. Question a client taking a nonsteroidal anti-inflammatory drug about the presence of dark tarry stools or a coffee-ground emesis.

Answer: 4

Rationale: Clients taking oral contraceptives are at risk for developing thrombophlebitis as evidenced by calf pain with dorsiflexion of the foot. Spotting between periods, breast enlargement, and an increase in growth of body hair are adverse reactions that occur with the use of oral contraceptives.

Nursing process: Implementation

Client need: Pharmacological and Parenteral Therapies

Cognitive level: Analysis

Subject area: Pharmacologic

Answer: 3

Rationale: Clients taking progestin-only drugs for birth control are instructed to wait three months to get pregnant once the drug is stopped, to avoid the risk of birth defects to the fetus. Progestin-only drugs are taken daily throughout the month. A barrier method of contraception is needed only for the first three weeks after starting the drug. Progestin-only contraceptives inhibit ovulation, but the menstrual cycle is not usually disrupted.

Nursing process: Implementation

Client need: Health Promotion and Maintenance

Cognitive level: Application

Subject area: Pharmacologic

Answer: 4

Rationale: It is not appropriate for either a licensed practical nurse or a registered nurse to inform a client on the pros and cons of hormone replacement therapy. This is the responsibility of the physician. Giving a client information or instruction on how to take a drug is a nursing task reserved for the registered nurse. Instructing a client on the purpose of a drug is the responsibility of the physician that may be reinforced by the registered nurse. A licensed practical nurse may question a client taking a nonsteroidal anti-inflammatory drug about experiencing dark tarry stools or a coffee-ground emesis. The licensed practical nurse should in turn notify the registered nurse if they are present. The registered nurse in turn notifies the physician.

Nursing process: Planning

Client need: Management of Care

Cognitive level: Analysis

Subject area: Legal and Ethical Issues

Antineoplastic Drugs

26

1. A client asks the nurse if the chemotherapy will only affect the cancer cells in the body. Which of the following is the appropriate response by the nurse?

   1. "The chemotherapy affects only the cancer cells."

   2. "The chemotherapy affects both the normal as well as the cancer cells."

   3. "It depends on the type of chemotherapy."

   4. "The effect on cells is different in every client."

2. The nurse evaluates chemotherapy to be most effective in which of the following clients?

   1. A client who is well nourished

   2. A client who has had chemotherapy before

   3. A 40-year-old male with lung cancer

   4. A 30-year-old woman with breast cancer

3. The nurse is preparing a class on chemotherapy administration for a group of student nurses. Which of the following routes of administration should the nurse include in the class?

   Select all that apply:

   [   ] **1.** Intramuscularly

   [   ] **2.** Intravenous

   [   ] **3.** Rectal

   [   ] **4.** Intrathecal

   [   ] **5.** Oral

   [   ] **6.** Directly into the tumor

Answer: 2

Rationale: Chemotherapy is a systemic treatment that affects normal as well as cancer cells. Cells of any tissue that are actively dividing will be more susceptible to its effects. While the adverse reactions experienced by any one client may vary somewhat, cancer cells and normal cells are still both affected by the treatment.

Nursing process: Analysis

Client need: Pharmacological and Parenteral Therapies

Cognitive level: Analysis

Subject area: Pharmacologic

Answer: 1

Rationale: Chemotherapy is equally effective in both men and women. The type of cancer a client has does not affect the potential of the chemotherapy. Chemotherapy may actually be somewhat less effective in those who have been exposed to chemotherapy previously, due to cancer cell resistance. Clients who are overall in better health will be able to tolerate the prescribed dose and regimen of chemotherapy better than those who are not, rendering it as effective as possible. Age does not directly affect the chemotherapy or type of cancer. Age directly relates to the client's overall condition of health.

Nursing process: Evaluation

Client need: Pharmacological and Parenteral Therapies

Cognitive level: Analysis

Subject area: Pharmacologic

Answer: 2, 4, 5, 6

Rationale: The intravenous and oral routes are the most common routes for chemotherapy administration for the majority of cancers. The intrathecal route may be used to circumvent the blood-brain barrier when cancer involves the central nervous system. Administering chemotherapy directly into the tumor is rare, and primarily used in clinical trials. The rectal route is not used for chemotherapy administration.

Nursing process: Planning

Client need: Pharmacological and Parenteral Therapies

Cognitive level: Application

Subject area: Pharmacologic

4. A client asks the nurse what was meant when the physician stated, "There has been a partial remission of the cancer." Which of the following is the appropriate response by the nurse?

  1. "The cancer has regressed 50% or more."
  2. "The cancer has progressed by 25%."
  3. "The cancer has spread to lymph nodes."
  4. "The cancer has disappeared."

5. The client asks, "Why do I need to receive all these chemotherapy medicines on the same day?" The nurse's response is based on the understanding that chemotherapy given in combination

  1. is the only way that it will be paid for by insurance.
  2. achieves the greatest tumor cell kill.
  3. shortens the length of administration.
  4. decreases the chance of allergic reaction.

6. A client asks, "Why will I lose my hair from chemotherapy?" The appropriate response by the nurse is based on which of the following?

  1. It is difficult to predict
  2. Chemotherapy affects normal cells that divide often
  3. All chemotherapy causes total alopecia
  4. Special shampoos can be used to prevent alopecia

7. The nurse is planning to care for the adverse reactions in a client receiving chemotherapy. Which adverse reaction should take priority in this plan of care?

  1. Depression
  2. Headache
  3. Fatigue
  4. Rash

Answer: 1

Rationale: A partial remission of a client's cancer indicates that it is not spreading further to lymph nodes nor growing (progressing), but rather that it has regressed (decreased) 50% or more. A complete remission would be characterized as the cancer appearing to have disappeared.

Nursing process: Analysis

Client need: Pharmacological and Parenteral Therapies

Cognitive level: Analysis

Subject area: Pharmacologic

Answer: 2

Rationale: Chemotherapy drugs are frequently used in combination because this helps to decrease cellular resistance and increase tumor cell kill. Insurance typically covers FDA-approved chemotherapy drugs given alone or in various combinations. Giving more than one chemotherapeutic drug usually increases the amount of time clients spend receiving these drugs. Combination chemotherapy is not used to decrease the incidence of allergic reaction; test dosages and premedication are used for this purpose.

Nursing process: Analysis

Client need: Pharmacological and Parenteral Therapies

Cognitive level: Analysis

Subject area: Pharmacologic

Answer: 2

Rationale: Chemotherapy drugs affect all cells of the body that divide often, such as the hair follicle cells, thus causing hair loss. Many chemotherapy drugs cause total alopecia, but some do not. There is no known, accepted method of preventing chemotherapy-related alopecia.

Nursing process: Analysis

Client need: Pharmacological and Parenteral Therapies

Cognitive level: Analysis

Subject area: Pharmacologic

Answer: 3

Rationale: Fatigue is the most common adverse reaction to chemotherapy. Clients receiving chemotherapy may experience depression and headache, but these are very individual to the client. Rash is more associated with an allergic reaction, a skin reaction to immunosuppression, or to specific types of chemotherapy, but is not common overall.

Nursing process: Planning

Client need: Management of Care

Cognitive level: Analysis

Subject area: Pharmacologic

8. A client's family asks the nurse, "Why can't the chemotherapy be given once instead of in multiple cycles?" The nurse's response is based on which of the following?

    1. Certain chemotherapy works best during certain phases of the cell cycle

    2. No one could tolerate the entire dose in one administration

    3. Chemotherapy is only covered by insurance if given in small doses

    4. Most clients prefer several doses over one dose

9. The nurse is teaching a class on the various types of chemotherapy agents. Which of the following examples of chemotherapy agents should the nurse include in the cell cycle–specific group?

    1. Cyclophosphamide (Cytoxan)

    2. Methotrexate

    3. Doxorubicin (Doxil)

    4. Nitrogen mustard

10. The nurse administers which of the following cell cycle–nonspecific chemotherapy agents to a client?

    1. Paclitaxel (Taxol)

    2. 5-fluorouracil (Adrucil)

    3. Cisplatin (Platinol)

    4. Vincristine (Oncovin)

11. Which of the following should the nurse consider before preparing to administer chemotherapy to a client?

    1. Wear disposable gown, mask, and gloves

    2. Wait for the chemotherapy to be prepared by the physician

    3. Do not assign a nurse who is pregnant to this client

    4. Prime the IV tubing with the chemotherapy agent

Answer: 1

Rationale: Chemotherapy is given in multiple cycles to allow for recuperation of normal cells between doses and to catch cancer cells in various phases of the cell cycle when the chemotherapy would have the most effect. It is true that giving too large a dose of chemotherapy could be lethal to a client, but this is not the primary reason that chemotherapy is administered in cycles. The number of cycles has been established through clinical trials and is not dependent on insurance payment.

Nursing process: Analysis

Client need: Pharmacological and Parenteral Therapies

Cognitive level: Analysis

Subject area: Pharmacologic

Answer: 2

Rationale: Methotrexate is an antimetabolite and a cell cycle–specific drug. Cyclophosphamide (Cytoxan), doxorubicin (Doxil), and nitrogen mustard are cell cycle–nonspecific.

Nursing process: Planning

Client need: Pharmacological and Parenteral Therapies

Cognitive level: Analysis

Subject area: Pharmacologic

Answer: 3

Rationale: Cisplatin (Platinol) is an alkylating agent and a cell cycle–nonspecific chemotherapy drug. Paclitaxel (Taxol), 5-fluorouracil (Adrucil), and vincristine (Oncovin) are all cell cycle–specific chemotherapy drugs.

Nursing process: Implementation

Client need: Pharmacological and Parenteral Therapies

Cognitive level: Analysis

Subject area: Pharmacologic

Answer: 1

Rationale: Nurses should always wear protective clothing such as disposable gown, mask, and gloves when administering chemotherapy. Chemotherapy drugs are usually prepared by a pharmacist or the nurse under a vented, laminar-flow cabinet. Pregnant nurses may administer chemotherapy using the usual precautions. The IV tubing should not be primed with the chemotherapy agent.

Nursing process: Analysis

Client need: Pharmacological and Parenteral Therapies

Cognitive level: Analysis

Subject area: Pharmacologic

12. The nurse should include which of the following when preparing to select the client's IV site for chemotherapy administration? Choose an IV site

    1. distal to other venipuncture sites on the extremity.

    2. on the same side as the cancer surgery.

    3. between the antecubital space and wrist.

    4. with a large-diameter vein.

13. Prior to initiating chemotherapy administration for a client, the nurse should consider which of the following principles?

    1. All chemotherapy drugs must be administered by an infusion pump

    2. Vesicant drugs should be infused before nonvesicant drugs

    3. The client's arm should be elevated throughout administration

    4. The IV line should be flushed with 20 ml of D$_5$W between drugs

14. Which of the following is the priority nursing action when a client states, "My IV site hurts!" during chemotherapy administration?

    1. Reposition the needle

    2. Notify the physician

    3. Stop the infusion

    4. Apply a cold pack to the IV site

Answer: 3

Rationale: The appropriate site for chemotherapy administration is between the antecubital space and wrist, proximal to any recent venipuncture site. Chemotherapy should be administered to a site with excellent blood return to assure the vessel is competent to receive chemotherapy without leakage. Leakage of chemotherapy through the vein can occur if it is administered distal to a recent venipuncture site. Chemotherapy is usually not administered on the arm associated with the cancer surgery, if applicable (e.g., given right mastectomy, chemotherapy will be administered to the left arm).

Nursing process: Planning

Client need: Pharmacological and Parenteral Therapies

Cognitive level: Analysis

Subject area: Pharmacologic

Answer: 2

Rationale: Vesicant chemotherapy agents should be administered before nonvesicant drugs if two such drugs are ordered in combination. This is due to the fact that the best blood flow, condition of vein, and site are desired for administration of a potentially tissue-damaging drug (vesicant). Since these factors could deteriorate during drug administration, the nurse should start with the vesicant. Some chemotherapy agents should be administered with an infusion pump, but others should not The client's arm should be in a natural, relaxed position during administration. The IV line should be flushed with approximately 10 ml of normal saline between administrations of chemotherapy drugs.

Nursing process: Analysis

Client need: Pharmacological and Parenteral Therapies

Cognitive level: Analysis

Subject area: Pharmacologic

Answer: 3

Rationale: The priority nursing action that should be taken by the nurse if the client complains of a painful IV site during chemotherapy administration is to stop the infusion. The nurse would then assess the situation to determine the cause of the pain. Caution should be used regarding repositioning of the needle so as not to damage the vein. If extravasation is suspected, the needle should be left in place, and the physician notified. Applying heat or cold to the IV site may be ordered, based on the chemotherapy being administered. All of these interventions are performed only after stopping the infusion.

Nursing process: Planning

Client need: Management of Care

Cognitive level: Application

Subject area: Pharmacologic

15. The nurse suspects that the vesicant IV chemotherapy being administered to the client has extravasated. Based on this assessment, which of the following is the priority intervention?

1. Continue administration until extravasation is confirmed by the physician
2. Stop the infusion and notify the physician
3. Remove the IV needle immediately and reinsert the needle in another area
4. Slow down the infusion and continue to observe the area

16. Which of the following client assignments is an appropriate assignment for a licensed practical nurse?

1. Administer methotrexate orally to a client with lung cancer
2. Develop a plan of care for a client receiving bleomycin (Blenoxane)
3. Administer cisplatin (Platinol) intravenously to a client with bladder cancer
4. Assist a client receiving ifosfamide (Ifex) to mark a bland diet

17. The nurse administers which of the following prescribed drugs to a client receiving chemotherapy who has developed neutropenia?

1. Leuprolide acetate (Lupron)
2. Tamoxifen (Tamofen)
3. Filgrastim (Neupogen)
4. Trastuzumab (Herceptin)

18. The nurse is caring for a 30-year-old female with ovarian cancer who is receiving cisplatin (Platinol). Which of the following is a priority to include in this client's plan of care?

1. Monitor the BUN and creatinine
2. Instruct the client to report tinnitus
3. Maintain IV hydration
4. Instruct the client to use a reliable method of birth control

Answer: 2

Rationale: The first action taken when extravasation is suspected is to stop the infusion and notify the physician. The nurse should not wait to stop the IV until confirmation of extravasation by the physician. The needle should not be removed, as it will be used to aspirate drug from the site to treat the extravasation. The drug should not be restarted until the extravasation has been properly treated and according to the physician's orders.

Nursing process: Planning

Client need: Management of Care

Cognitive level: Analysis

Subject area: Pharmacologic

Answer: 4

Rationale: Only specially trained registered nurses may administer chemotherapy drugs, regardless of the route. Developing a plan of care is a job task reserved for the registered nurse. A licensed practical nurse may assist a client receiving chemotherapy to mark a bland diet after the initial instruction has taken place.

Nursing process: Evaluation

Client need: Management of Care

Cognitive level: Analysis

Subject area: Legal and Ethical Issues

Answer: 3

Rationale: Filgrastim (Neupogen) is a colony-stimulating factor used in the treatment of neutropenia for a client receiving chemotherapy. Leuprolide acetate (Lupron) is an antineoplastic hormone used in the treatment of prostate cancer. Tamoxifen (Tamofen) is an antiestrogen used in breast cancer. Trastuzumab (Herceptin) is an antineoplastic used in the treatment of breast cancer.

Nursing process: Implementation

Client need: Pharmacological and Parenteral Therapies

Cognitive level: Analysis

Subject area: Pharmacologic

Answer: 4

Rationale: It is a priority to instruct a client who is of childbearing age and receiving cisplatin (Platinol) to take a reliable method of birth control. Monitoring the BUN and creatinine, maintaining IV hydration, and instructing the client to report tinnitus are all appropriate interventions but not the priority intervention.

Nursing process: Planning

Client need: Management of Care

Cognitive level: Analysis

Subject area: Pharmacologic

19. Which of the following is a priority for the nurse to monitor for a client receiving ifosfamide (Ifex) for testicular cancer?
    1. Hemorrhagic cystitis
    2. Alopecia
    3. Phlebitis
    4. Liver dysfunction

20. Which of the following is a priority for the nurse to monitor in a client who is receiving mitoxantrone (Novantrone) for leukemia?
    1. Congestive heart failure
    2. Amenorrhea
    3. Mucositis
    4. Pneumonia

Answer: 1

Rationale: Ifosfamide (Ifex) is an alkylating antineoplastic drug used in the treatment of testicular cancer, generally as a third-line therapy. It must always be administered with mesna (Mesnex), the antidote for ifosfamide toxicity. Ifex is metabolized to products that cause hemorrhagic cystitis. At least two liters of oral or IV fluids should be given with mesna (Mesnex) to prevent bladder toxicity. Other less serious adverse reactions include alopecia, phlebitis, and liver dysfunction.

Nursing process: Assessment

Client need: Management of Care

Cognitive level: Analysis

Subject area: Pharmacologic

Answer: 1

Rationale: Mitoxantrone (Novantrone) is an antineoplastic used in the treatment of leukemia. It can cause a potentially fatal congestive heart failure. Other less serious adverse reactions include amenorrhea, mucositis, and pneumonia.

Nursing process: Assessment

Client need: Management of Care

Cognitive level: Analysis

Subject area: Pharmacologic

Psychotropic Drugs

27

1. The nurse caring for a client diagnosed with schizophrenia administers what classification of drugs to treat hallucinations? _____

2. A client who has been taking haloperidol (Haldol) for 15 years tells the nurse of some involuntary muscle movements of the mouth, arms, and legs. The nurse reports this as what? _____

3. The nurse is admitting a client with a diagnosis of suspected schizophrenia. Which of the following clinical manifestations should the nurse assess as positive clinical manifestations of schizophrenia?

    1. Anhedonia and blunted affect

    2. Hallucinations and delusional thinking

    3. Lack of motivation

    4. Abnormal movements of the mouth

4. The nurse is caring for a client with Alzheimer's disease who is taking quetiapine (Seroquel) for paranoid ideations. Which of the following adverse reactions should the nurse assess this client for?

    Select all that apply:

    [ ] **1.** Hypertension

    [ ] **2.** Headache

    [ ] **3.** Bradycardia

    [ ] **4.** Diarrhea

    [ ] **5.** Dry mouth

    [ ] **6.** Tardive dyskinesia

Answer: Antipsychotics

Rationale: Antipsychotic drugs are the drugs of choice to treat the psychotic clinical manifestations of schizophrenia.

Nursing process: Implementation

Client need: Pharmacological and Parenteral Therapies

Cognitive level: Comprehension

Subject area: Pharmacologic

Answer: Tardive dyskinesia

Rationale: Tardive dyskinesia is a long-term adverse reaction to typical antipsychotics. It is characterized by involuntary muscle movements, particularly of the mouth and the extremities.

Nursing process: Analysis

Client need: Pharmacological and Parenteral Therapies

Cognitive level: Application

Subject area: Pharmacologic

Answer: 2

Rationale: Positive clinical manifestations of schizophrenia include hallucinations and delusional thinking. Anhedonia, blunted affect, and lack of motivation are negative clinical manifestations of schizophrenia. Abnormal movements of the mouth indicate tardive dyskinesia.

Nursing process: Assessment

Client need: Pharmacological and Parenteral Therapies

Cognitive level: Application

Subject area: Pharmacologic

Answer: 2, 5, 6

Rationale: Quetiapine (Seroquel) is an antipsychotic drug that is used for psychotic disorders. Adverse reactions include orthostatic hypotension, headache, tachycardia, constipation, dry mouth, and tardive dyskinesia.

Nursing process: Assessment

Client need: Pharmacological and Parenteral Therapies

Cognitive level: Application

Subject area: Pharmacologic

5. Which of the following should the nurse include in the plan of care for a client taking an antidepressant drug?

   1. Encourage the client to drink low-calorie beverages

   2. Instruct the client to take the drug on an empty stomach

   3. Inform the client that urinary frequency is an adverse reaction

   4. Monitor the client for bradycardia prior to administration

6. The nurse should include which of the following adverse reactions to Olanzapine (Zyprexa) in the drug instructions given to a client?

   Select all that apply:

   [ ] 1. Constipation

   [ ] 2. Weight loss

   [ ] 3. Loss of taste

   [ ] 4. Hypotonia

   [ ] 5. Insomnia

   [ ] 6. Urinary retention

7. The nurse caring for a client administers sertraline (Zoloft) for which of the following disorders?

   1. Abnormal movement disorder

   2. Brief reactive psychosis

   3. Major depressive disorder

   4. Schizophrenia

8. The client is instructed to take mirtazapine (Remeron) for depression. Which of the following would best indicate that the client is complying with the prescribed regimen? The client

   1. places the tablet on the tongue and waits 30 seconds for it to dissolve.

   2. waits two hours after administration before driving or operating dangerous equipment.

   3. avoids caffeine and irritating foods in the diet.

   4. reports adverse reactions of bloody diarrhea.

Answer: 1

Rationale: Antidepressants are used to treat depression. Adverse reactions include weight gain, gastrointestinal upset, urinary retention, and tachycardia. Clients must be cautioned to avoid high-caloric drinks to avoid weight gain.

Nursing process: Planning

Client need: Pharmacological and Parenteral Therapies

Cognitive level: Application

Subject area: Pharmacologic

Answer: 1, 5, 6

Rationale: Olanzapine (Zyprexa) is an antipsychotic drug used to treat schizophrenia and the acute mania associated with bipolar disorders. Adverse reactions include weight gain, constipation, hypertonia, insomnia, and urinary retention.

Nursing process: Planning

Client need: Pharmacological and Parenteral Therapies

Cognitive level: Application

Subject area: Pharmacologic

Answer: 3

Rationale: Sertraline (Zoloft) is a selective serotonin reuptake inhibitor (SSRI) antidepressant used in the treatment of major depression, obsessive-compulsive disorder, post-traumatic stress disorder, and panic disorders.

Nursing process: Implementation

Client need: Pharmacological and Parenteral Therapies

Cognitive level: Application

Subject area: Pharmacologic

Answer: 1

Rationale: Mirtazapine (Remeron) is a tetracyclic antidepressant used in the treatment of depression. The tablets come as oral disintegrating tablets and should be administered initially in the evening, before sleep, until the drug effects are known. The tablet should be placed on the tongue for 30 seconds until dissolved. The client should not engage in activities that require mental alertness until the drug effects are known. Although nausea and vomiting may occur, there are no food restrictions. Fluids may be encouraged for the adverse reaction to constipation.

Nursing process: Analysis

Client need: Pharmacological and Parenteral Therapies

Cognitive level: Analysis

Subject area: Pharmacologic

9. Which of the following is a priority to include in the plan of care for a client taking fluoxetine (Prozac)?
   1. Monitor the client for orthostatic hypotension
   2. Avoid giving on an empty stomach
   3. Wait 14 days after taking a monoamine oxidase inhibitor before starting Prozac
   4. Administer simultaneously with thioridazine (Mellaril)

10. A client complains of having a dry mouth. Which of the following instructions should the nurse give to the client?
    1. "Try chewing sugar-free gum and drinking cool, sugar-free sodas."
    2. "You need to drink more milk products, especially with your drugs."
    3. "Avoid drinking fluids in the evenings."
    4. "Drink more fluids early in the day."

11. The nurse should question an order for bupropion (Wellbutrin) for which of the following clients?
    1. A client with a closed head injury
    2. A client with liver failure
    3. A client with kidney failure
    4. A client with chronic gastrointestinal upset

12. The priority nursing action for the nurse administering an antidepressant drug to a client is which of the following?
    1. Check the client's mouth for possible hoarding of the drug
    2. Instruct the client that the therapeutic effects of the drug may take two weeks
    3. Administer the drug with food
    4. Monitor the blood pressure

Answer: 3

Rationale: Fluoxetine (Prozac) is a selective serotonin reuptake inhibitor antidepressant. The client should be monitored for orthostatic hypotension and instructed to change positions with caution. Prozac may be administered with food to decrease gastrointestinal upset. It is a priority to wait 14 days after discontinuing a monoamine oxidase inhibitor and administering Prozac. Five weeks should pass between stopping Prozac and starting a monoamine oxidase inhibitor. Prozac should not be administered with Mellaril.

Nursing process: Planning

Client need: Management of Care

Cognitive level: Analysis

Subject area: Pharmacologic

Answer: 1

Rationale: Clients who take antidepressants and antipsychotic drugs may experience dry mouth as an adverse reaction. The client should avoid high-calorie fluids, which may promote weight gain. Drinking low-calorie fluids and chewing sugarless gum are encouraged to avoid gaining weight.

Nursing process: Planning

Client need: Health Promotion and Maintenance

Cognitive level: Application

Subject area: Pharmacologic

Answer: 1

Rationale: Bupropion (Wellbutrin) is an antidepressant that is known to lower the seizure threshold and is contraindicated for clients with known seizure disorders or closed head injuries.

Nursing process: Analysis

Client need: Pharmacological and Parenteral Therapies

Cognitive level: Analysis

Subject area: Pharmacologic

Answer: 1

Rationale: Clients who are suicidal may attempt to hoard their drugs by "cheeking" them to be used later for a suicide attempt. Extreme caution should be used with suicidal clients.

Nursing process: Planning

Client need: Management of Care

Cognitive level: Application

Subject area: Pharmacologic

13. A nurse is instructing a client about getting blood drawn the following day for a lithium carbonate (Eskalith) level. Which of the following instructions is important?

   1. "Do not take your morning dose of lithium until your blood has been drawn."

   2. "Do not eat anything in the morning before having your blood drawn."

   3. "Do not take your evening dose of lithium tonight."

   4. "Take your morning dose of lithium carbonate with a sip of water."

14. The nurse evaluates which of the following lab results as within the normal range for a client who is receiving lithium carbonate (Eskalith)?

   1. 1.5 to 2.0 mEq/L

   2. 0.1 to 0.5 mEq/L

   3. 1.8 to 2.5 mEq/L

   4. 0.6 to 1.2 mEq/L

15. A nurse educating a client about possible signs of lithium carbonate (Eskalith) toxicity should instruct the client to report which of the following adverse reactions?

   Select all that apply:

   [   ] **1.** Weight gain

   [   ] **2.** Vomiting

   [   ] **3.** Diarrhea

   [   ] **4.** Tremor

   [   ] **5.** Salty taste

   [   ] **6.** Abdominal pain

16. The nurse is caring for a client with a psychotic disorder who is receiving thioridazine (Mellaril). The nurse should monitor this client for which of the following abnormal laboratory results?

   1. Hyperkalemia

   2. Decreased alkaline phosphatase

   3. Agranulocytosis

   4. Hypocalcemia

Answer: 2
Rationale: Lithium carbonate (Eskalith) is an antimanic drug used in the treatment of bipolar disorders (manic phase) and in the prevention of bipolar manic-depressive psychosis. The lithium blood level is most accurate if the blood is drawn 12 hours after the last dose of drug. The client should avoid eating prior to having a lithium level drawn to avoid a food-lithium interaction and an inaccurate result.
Nursing process: Planning
Client need: Reduction of Risk Potential
Cognitive level: Application
Subject area: Pharmacologic

Answer: 4
Rationale: Lithium carbonate (Eskalith) is an antimanic drug. The client's lithium carbonate level should be monitored. The normal range is 0.6 to 1.2 mEq/L.
Nursing process: Evaluation
Client need: Reduction of Risk Potential
Cognitive level: Application
Subject area: Pharmacologic

Answer: 2, 3, 4, 6
Rationale: Lithium carbonate (Eskalith) is an antimanic drug. Usual adverse reactions include headache, drowsiness, dizziness, hypotension, dry mouth, salty taste, and fatigue. Toxic adverse reactions include vomiting, diarrhea, tremors, abdominal pain, muscle weakness, lassitude, severe thirst, tinnitus, and dilute urine.
Nursing process: Planning
Client need: Health Promotion and Maintenance
Cognitive level: Analysis
Subject area: Pharmacologic

Answer: 3
Rationale: Thioridazine (Mellaril) is an antipsychotic and atypical neuroleptic used in the treatment of psychotic disorders, schizophrenia, major depressive disorders, and organic brain syndrome. Mellaril may cause agranulocytosis (reduction in the number of white blood cells).
Nursing process: Assessment
Client need: Reduction of Risk Potential
Cognitive level: Analysis
Subject area: Pharmacologic

17. The nurse is conducting a class on the adverse reactions to a variety of drugs such as lithium carbonate (Eskalith), carbamazepine (Tegretol), gabapentin (Neurontin), and valproic acid (Depakene). Which of the following common adverse reactions should the nurse include in the class?

Select all that apply:

[　] 1. Nausea

[　] 2. Restlessness

[　] 3. Diarrhea

[　] 4. Insomnia

[　] 5. Dyspepsia

[　] 6. Irritability

18. The nurse reads on the initial history and physical that anticonvulsant drugs are prescribed, but there is no diagnosis of a seizure disorder, and no report of treatment in a mental health clinic. The nurse concludes that the client is taking the anticonvulsant drugs to treat which of the following?

Select all that apply:

[　] 1. Major depression

[　] 2. Bipolar disorders

[　] 3. Anxiety disorders

[　] 4. Aggression

[　] 5. Cognitive disorders

[　] 6. Brief reactive psychosis

19. A client has been treated for depression with phenelzine (Nardil). The nurse recognizes that the drug was difficult to take for which of the following reasons?

1. It requires dosing several times a day, thus decreasing compliance

2. It has the potential for serious interactions with other medications

3. It requires adherence to a strict diet

4. It has been found to be ineffective in treating psychiatric disorders

Answer: 1, 3, 5

Rationale: Lithium carbonate (Eskalith) is an antimanic and antipsychotic drug used in the treatment of bipolar disorders. Carbamazepine (Tegretol) is an anticonvulsant used to treat absence seizures. It is also used investigationally in the treatment of bipolar disorders, schizophrenia, and psychotic behavior with dementia. Gabapentin (Neurontin) is an anticonvulsant used in the adjunct treatment of partial seizures. It also is used investigationally for bipolar disorders. Valproic acid (Depakene) is an anticonvulsant used in the treatment of seizures. Common adverse reactions for all of these drugs include nausea, diarrhea, and dyspepsia.

Nursing process: Analysis

Client need: Health Promotion and Maintenance

Cognitive level: Application

Subject area: Pharmacologic

Answer: 2, 3, 4

Rationale: Anticonvulsant drugs are being used investigationally in the treatment of bipolar disorders, anxiety disorders, and aggression.

Nursing process: Analysis

Client need: Pharmacological and Parenteral Therapies

Cognitive level: Analysis

Subject area: Pharmacologic

Answer: 3

Rationale: Monoamine oxidase inhibitors (MAOIs), such as phenelzine (Nardil), interact with tyramine found in many foods, thus requiring the individuals using these drugs to follow a strict diet. Compliance becomes an issue. Foods high in tyramine include aged cheese, salami, sauerkraut, avocados, chocolate, coffee, fava beans, and beer and wine containing yeast.

Nursing process: Analysis

Client need: Pharmacological and Parenteral Therapies

Cognitive level: Analysis

Subject area: Pharmacologic

20. The nurse is caring for a client who is taking phenelzine (Nardil). Which of the following should the nurse include in the medication instructions?

    1. "Common adverse reactions include sleepiness and agitation."

    2. "You may experience a decrease in appetite."

    3. "Tell your physician all of the other drugs you are taking."

    4. "If you have a history of low blood sugar, you should not take this drug."

21. The nurse is discharging a client taking flurazepam (Dalmane). Which of the following instructions should be given?

    1. Drink a small glass of wine at bedtime to enhance sleep

    2. Drive cautiously after taking the drug

    3. Drink low-calorie fluids for a dry mouth

    4. A "hangover effect" may be experienced in the morning

22. The nurse is instructing an older adult client who has been prescribed a hypnotic for insomnia. Which of the following instructions should be given?

    1. "Ask for help getting out of bed."

    2. "You may feel more hungry when you are taking this drug."

    3. "You may notice that you're feeling more irritable and moody when you take this drug."

    4. "This drug may cause movements of your mouth that you can't control."

Answer: 3

Rationale: Monoamine oxidase inhibitors (MAOIs), such as phenelzine (Nardil), have interactions with many different drugs, including over-the-counter drugs.

Nursing process: Planning

Client need: Health Promotion and Maintenance

Cognitive level: Application

Subject area: Pharmacologic

Answer: 4

Rationale: Flurazepam (Dalmane) is a sedative and hypnotic that is used for insomnia. Clients are advised to avoid alcohol because alcohol taken in combination with hypnotics can have a lethal effect. Clients should not drive after taking hypnotics for safety reasons. Their reflexes would be dulled. Low-calorie fluids are not necessary because dry mouth is not an adverse reaction and Dalmane has no effect on appetite.

Nursing process: Planning

Client need: Health Promotion and Maintenance

Cognitive level: Application

Subject area: Pharmacologic

Answer: 1

Rationale: Hypnotics may cause ataxia and confusion, increasing the risk of falls and fractures. Hypnotics will not increase the appetite, result in irritability, or cause extrapyramidal adverse reactions.

Nursing process: Planning

Client need: Health Promotion and Maintenance

Cognitive level: Application

Subject area: Pharmacologic

23. The nurse administers which of the following drugs to a client who is severely ill with schizophrenia, does not respond to conventional antipsychotic drugs, and has suicidal ideations?

    1. Haloperidol (Haldol)

    2. Chlorpromazine (Thorazine)

    3. Risperidone (Risperdal)

    4. Clozapine (Clozaril)

24. Which of the following interventions is a priority and will help the older adult client comply with the drug regimen?

    1. Educate the family members about drug administration

    2. Contact the client frequently as a reminder to take drugs

    3. Educate the client on ways to manage adverse reactions

    4. Count the number of pills left in the bottle at each visit

25. The nurse reads in the record that the client is receiving a stimulant drug. The nurse reviews the medical record and administers which of the following drugs?

    1. Buspirone (BuSpar)

    2. Alprazolam (Xanax)

    3. Modafinil (Provigil)

    4. Amitriptyline (Elavil)

Answer: 4

Rationale: Haloperidol (Haldol) is an antipsychotic used to treat manic states, drug-induced psychoses, and schizophrenia. Chlorpromazine (Thorazine) is an antipsychotic used to treat acute and chronic psychoses, schizophrenia, and the manic phase of manic-depression. Risperidone (Risperdal) is an antipsychotic used in the treatment of schizophrenia. Clozapine (Clozaril) is an antipsychotic used to treat severely ill schizophrenic clients who do not respond to conventional antipsychotic therapy and have suicidal ideations. It carries a risk of life-threatening agranulocytosis.

Nursing process: Implementation

Client need: Pharmacological and Parenteral Therapies

Cognitive level: Analysis

Subject area: Pharmacologic

Answer: 3

Rationale: The priority intervention is to educate the client on how to manage the adverse reactions of the drugs. Unpleasant adverse reactions are often the reason for noncompliance with drugs. Educating the family members reinforces the education given the client. It should not be the priority intervention because it takes away the control from the client. Counting the number of pills left in the bottle at each appointment with the physician and calling the client as a reminder to take the pills as prescribed also take away the control from the client and display a sense of distrust.

Nursing process: Planning

Client need: Management of Care

Cognitive level: Analysis

Subject area: Pharmacologic

Answer: 3

Rationale: Modafinil (Provigil) is an analeptic drug administered to improve wakefulness in clients with excessive daytime sleepiness associated with narcolepsy. Buspirone (BuSpar) and alprazolam (Xanax) are antianxiety drugs. Amitriptyline (Elavil) is an antidepressant drug.

Nursing process: Implementation

Client need: Pharmacological and Parenteral Therapies

Cognitive level: Analysis

Subject area: Pharmacologic

26. The nurse is preparing to delegate nursing tasks to a licensed practical nurse. Which of the following may be delegated to a licensed practical nurse?

1. Assist a client taking a monoamine oxidase inhibitor to select a menu low in tyramine foods

2. Inform a client taking a hypnotic about the risk of falls and fractures

3. Assess for abuse the parents of a child taking a stimulant

4. Instruct the client and the family on the adverse reactions to an antipsychotic drug

Answer: 1

Rationale: A licensed practical nurse may assist a client taking a monoamine oxidase inhibitor to select a low-tyramine diet. The instructional teaching that must be performed by a registered nurse has already taken place and now the focus changes to assisting a client to select appropriate foods. It would not be appropriate to assess the parents of a child taking a stimulant for abuse unless there is an indication of potential abuse. Providing the family and client information on the adverse reactions to a drug and informing the client of potential complications should be performed by a registered nurse.

Nursing process: Planning

Client need: Management of Care

Cognitive level: Analysis

Subject area: Legal and Ethical Issues

Growth and Development

28

1. Based on an understanding of Erikson's stages of psychosocial development, which of the following is a priority to communicate to the parents of an infant to assist them in meeting the basic needs of infancy?

   1. Provide the infant with entertainment and stimulation for psychological growth
   2. Talk with the infant during the times when the infant is awake
   3. Hold the infant in a way the infant prefers
   4. Attend to the infant's need for comfort, security, predictability, food, and warmth

2. The nurse is assessing a toddler's psychosocial developmental level using Erikson's eight stages. Which of the following behaviors would the nurse most likely find if the child were demonstrating being in shame and doubt instead of having mastered autonomy?

   1. Dependency and constantly looking to others for approval
   2. Sleep disturbance, crying, and vomiting
   3. Always imitating others rather than using imagination
   4. Frequent crying, emotional outbursts, and whining

3. A nurse is assessing the play of a 4-year-old child. Which of the following best describes what the nurse would observe in the play of this age preschooler?

   1. Plays alongside but not with playmates, taking toys away from others, using a pounding bench, and playing with a musical toy
   2. Interactive play, obeying limits, creating an imaginary friend, and engaging in fantasy play
   3. Engaging in group sports and games and playing with puppets
   4. Playing alone in the corner, engaged in putting a puzzle together

4. A preschooler knows ramming a tricycle into the garage door at home is not an acceptable behavior but does this at a friend's house. Which of the following statements by the nurse is the most appropriate reason for this difference in behavior at home and at the friend's house?

   1. "Preschoolers value their own house more than they value the house of a playmate."
   2. "The child's mother is much stricter and supervises children much more closely than does the playmate's mother."
   3. "A young preschool child may have difficulty applying known rules to a different situation."
   4. "There is a higher level of frustration when outside their own home and play territory."

Answer: 4

Rationale: During infancy, trust is developing, which means that the infant's basic needs must consistently be met by reliable, nurturing caregivers, usually the parents. If these needs are not met, there is a danger that mistrust will occur.

Nursing process: Analysis

Client need: Management of Care

Cognitive level: Analysis

Subject area: Pediatric

Answer: 1

Rationale: Autonomy versus shame and doubt is Erikson's stage for toddlers. Autonomy develops as children discover their new mental and physical abilities while improving language and motor skills and learning competencies related to independence (bathing, eating, toileting). Doubt occurs if children learn to mistrust not only themselves but also the immediate environment. Children demonstrating dependency and constantly needing approval for their actions have not resolved this conflict.

Nursing process: Assessment

Client need: Health Promotion and Maintenance

Cognitive level: Analysis

Subject area: Pediatric

Answer: 2

Rationale: Preschooler is an age group that follows toddlerhood and includes children between 3 and 6 years of age. Preschoolers enjoy group play and engage in imitative, dramatic, and imaginative play. They are becoming more tolerant of playmates, may have an imaginary friend, and enjoy activities that include memory games, construction toys, puzzles, books, art, and fantasy play.

Nursing process: Assessment

Client need: Health Promotion and Maintenance

Cognitive level: Application

Subject area: Pediatric

Answer: 3

Rationale: Preschool children are in the preconventional level of moral development. They are learning to conform their behavior to the expectations of others, but are not able to transfer reasons for their behavior to a different situation or environment, especially when the person rewarding them for good behavior is always around.

Nursing process: Analysis

Client need: Health Promotion and Maintenance

Cognitive level: Analysis

Subject area: Pediatric

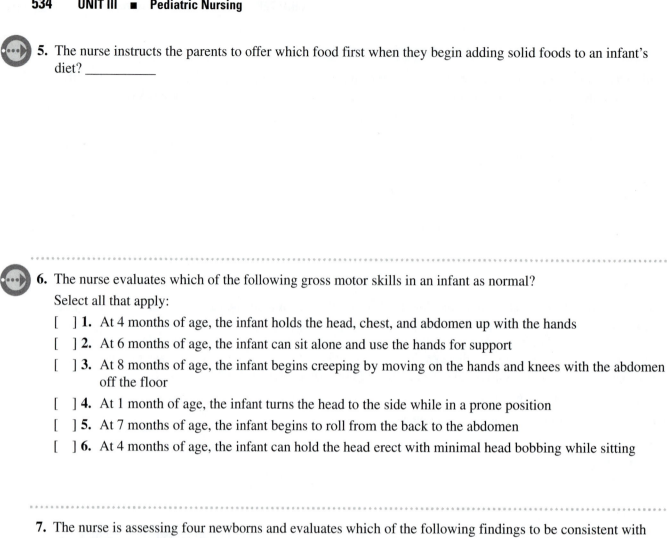

5. The nurse instructs the parents to offer which food first when they begin adding solid foods to an infant's diet? _____

6. The nurse evaluates which of the following gross motor skills in an infant as normal?

Select all that apply:

[ ] **1.** At 4 months of age, the infant holds the head, chest, and abdomen up with the hands

[ ] **2.** At 6 months of age, the infant can sit alone and use the hands for support

[ ] **3.** At 8 months of age, the infant begins creeping by moving on the hands and knees with the abdomen off the floor

[ ] **4.** At 1 month of age, the infant turns the head to the side while in a prone position

[ ] **5.** At 7 months of age, the infant begins to roll from the back to the abdomen

[ ] **6.** At 4 months of age, the infant can hold the head erect with minimal head bobbing while sitting

7. The nurse is assessing four newborns and evaluates which of the following findings to be consistent with physiologic or normal jaundice?

1. A gradual rise in bilirubin to 8 mg/dl on day 3 to 5 after birth

2. A sudden elevation of unconjugated bilirubin within the first 24 hours

3. Unconjugated bilirubin of 14 mg/dl in the breast-feeding baby

4. Jaundice in a 2-week-old, small-weight infant

Answer: Rice cereal

Rationale: Because there is less chance that an infant will have an allergic reaction to rice cereal, it is the first food to be added to an infant's diet when solid foods are added.

Nursing process: Implementation

Client need: Health Promotion and Maintenance

Cognitive level: Analysis

Subject area: Pediatric

Answer: 2, 3, 4

Rationale: It is normal for an infant at 6 months of age to sit alone and use the hands for support. It is also normal for an 8-month-old infant to begin creeping, and a 1-month-old infant in the prone position to turn the head from side to side. It is not until 5 or 6 months of age that the infant begins to hold the head, chest, and abdomen up by bearing weight with the hands. It is also abnormal for an infant 7 months of age to just start to roll from the back to the abdomen. This is a skill that starts at 2 to 3 months. A 2-month-old infant begins to hold the head with minimal head bobbing.

Nursing process: Evaluation

Client need: Health Promotion and Maintenance

Cognitive level: Application

Subject area: Pediatric

Answer: 1

Rationale: Physiologic or normal jaundice shows a gradual rise in bilirubin of 8 mg/dl at 3 to 5 days after birth. The level falls to normal the second week of life. If the unconjugated level is greater than 12 mg/dl when the baby is formula-fed, greater than 14 mg/dl if the baby is breast-fed, or if the jaundice is persistent past 2 weeks of age, further evaluation is warranted.

Nursing process: Evaluation

Client need: Health Promotion and Maintenance

Cognitive level: Analysis

Subject area: Pediatric

8. Which of the following should the nurse include in the immediate care instructions given to the parents of a newborn circumcised with a plastic bell?

    1. Gently lift the ring and squeeze warm water from a cotton ball on to the tip of the penis when changing the diaper

    2. Remove the bell when the baby is awake and active and likely to pull on the bell and dislodge it

    3. Remove the ring in five to seven days when the circumcision is nearly or completely healed

    4. Wash the bell and the penis with hydrogen peroxide several times a day

9. The mother of a breast-fed newborn tells the nurse that the baby's stool is golden yellow, pasty instead of firm, and has a sour milk odor. Which of the following would be the best response by the nurse?

    1. "You probably need to feed this baby some cereal to firm up the stool."

    2. "Cut back on your fluid intake and be careful what you eat, as you pass this on to the baby."

    3. "I need to check your temperature and your breasts to determine if you have a breast abscess."

    4. "This is a normal stool for a newborn who is breast-fed."

10. A mother tells the nurse that her 6-month-old child is grasping things such as a spoon in the palms and asks when the child will be able to grasp a spoon between the thumb and fingers. The appropriate response by the nurse would be

    1. "This is normal for this age. The pincer grasp isn't mastered until 8 months."

    2. "Encourage your child to play with an older child who uses the pincer grasp and your child will pick up the skill from the other child."

    3. "Begin teaching your baby to use the pincer grasp. It will take time."

    4. "I will ask your physician about doing developmental testing to evaluate your baby's level of development."

Answer: 1

Rationale: The immediate care of the circumcised newborn is dependent on the procedure performed. If the plastic bell was utilized, it is left on the penis. Gently lift the ring and squeeze warm water from a cotton ball onto the tip of the penis when changing the diaper. The ring will fall off in 7 to 10 days when the circumcision has healed.

Nursing process: Planning

Client need: Health Promotion and Maintenance

Cognitive level: Application

Subject area: Pediatric

Answer: 4

Rationale: Transition stools of the newborn are green-brown to yellow-brown in color. They occur by the third day. Breast-fed infants' stool is yellow to golden, pasty, and has a sour milk odor. Formula-fed newborns' stool is pale to light yellow, firmer than the stool of a breast-fed infant, and has a strong odor.

Nursing process: Analysis

Client need: Health Promotion and Maintenance

Cognitive level: Analysis

Subject area: Pediatric

Answer: 1

Rationale: During the first month of life, a primitive grasp reflex enables the infant to hold objects with a tightly clenched fist. By the end of 2 months, this primitive reflex fades and the infant begins to actively grasp and momentarily hold an object before dropping it. At 3 months of age, the infant has the ability to hold the hand open, look at the fingers, and place them in the mouth. By 5 months, the infant can voluntarily grasp an object with the whole hand (palmar grasp) and can actively manipulate all grasped objects and place them in the mouth. Between 6 and 7 months, the infant can hold a bottle securely and willingly drop any grasped object. The palmar grasp is replaced with a thumb and finger pincer grasp at approximately 8 months.

Nursing process: Analysis

Client need: Health Promotion and Maintenance

Cognitive level: Analysis

Subject area: Pediatric

11. A mother expresses concern because her infant is walking sideways while holding onto furniture. Which of the following is the appropriate statement the nurse should make to this mother?

   1. "You may want to consider a neurological evaluation to rule out a pathological cause for this behavior."
   2. "If you will hold the baby's hands while the baby walks, you can break the baby of this habit."
   3. "Infants start walking sideways while holding onto furniture before walking or standing alone."
   4. "You need to make an appointment with your pediatrician and have this problem checked out."

12. Which of the following should the nurse include when preparing to teach a class on the introduction of new foods during the first year of life?

   1. Place up to three foods on the spoon at one time with an old favorite on the front of the spoon
   2. Introduce fruits first, introduce one new fruit per day until all fruits are introduced
   3. Alternate between offering one spoonful of fruits and one spoonful of vegetables
   4. Introduce one new food at a time at seven-day intervals

13. The nurse evaluates which of the following four infants to have an abnormal language development?

   1. A 9-month-old who uses two-syllable sounds such as dada
   2. A 7-month-old who is beginning to vocalize during play and pleasure
   3. A 2-month-old who begins vocalizing in the presence of familiar sounds
   4. An 11-month-old who uses intentional gestures

14. The nurse is instructing the parents of a toddler on the development of depth perception. Which of the following should the nurse instruct the parents to watch for?

   1. An increased fear of heights and of falling out of bed at night
   2. An unusual sense of dizziness will be experienced at times
   3. A difficulty in learning to swim
   4. An increased fall risk when the toddler is learning to walk, run, and climb stairs

Answer: 3

Rationale: From 10 to 12 months, infant locomotion progresses rapidly. During this time, infants will take deliberate steps while holding onto something and will walk sideways while holding onto furniture before walking or standing alone. Once infants can stand alone, they will attempt to take a few steps alone.

Nursing process: Analysis

Client need: Health Promotion and Maintenance

Cognitive level: Analysis

Subject area: Pediatric

Answer: 4

Rationale: Due to the potential for an allergic reaction during the infant's first year of life, new foods should be introduced one at a time at seven-day intervals between each new food, so if the infant is allergic to the new food, it will be apparent. Generally, rice cereal is introduced first because it is least likely to cause allergies. Vegetables are offered next, followed by fruits. Vegetables are started before fruits to avoid getting the infant accustomed to the sweet taste.

Nursing process: Planning

Client need: Health Promotion and Maintenance

Cognitive level: Application

Subject area: Pediatric

Answer: 2

Rationale: It is abnormal for a 7-month-old infant to start vocalizing during play and pleasure. This is a language skill that normally develops between 3 and 6 months.

Nursing process: Evaluation

Client need: Health Promotion and Maintenance

Cognitive level: Analysis

Subject area: Pediatric

Answer: 4

Rationale: Before depth perception is fully developed, toddlers will have no sense of distance and may not realize how far away the floor is when learning to walk, run, and climb.

Nursing process: Planning

Client need: Health Promotion and Maintenance

Cognitive level: Analysis

Subject area: Pediatric

15. Which of the following is the most age-appropriate explanation the nurse should give a toddler who is to take medication every morning for seven days?

   1. "Your mommy will give you the medicine between 8:00 and 9:00 a.m. each morning until it is gone."

   2. "You will be taking your medicine every morning after breakfast until it is gone."

   3. "For a week you will be taking your medicine in the early morning."

   4. "Your mommy will give you your medicine every day by 9:00 a.m. until it is gone."

16. A mother tells the nurse about being frustrated by the toddler saying "no" to everything said. Which of the following statements by the nurse would be most helpful to the mother?

   1. "Reword every question so your child will eventually say 'yes.' "

   2. "This is an expression of your child's search for autonomy that will disappear at 30 months of age."

   3. "Walk away from your child when 'no' is said and pay attention when 'yes' is said so the behavior can be modified."

   4. "Start telling your child 'no' whenever something is asked for so your child will understand that negativity is not rewarding."

17. A couple is expecting their new baby any day and are concerned their 2-year-old will have problems accepting a new sister or brother. Which of the following statements by the parents would indicate they have acted on the teaching the nurse offered to help the toddler to deal with the birth of the sibling?

   1. "We started toilet training this week and, hopefully, will have our 2-year-old trained by the time the baby is born."

   2. "We told the 2-year-old that a brother or sister will be a new playmate."

   3. "The grandparents have been keeping our 2-year-old frequently."

   4. "The 2-year-old was moved out of the nursery this week so we could prepare for the baby."

18. A mother is expressing concern to the nurse that her 5-year-old occasionally is urinating in the underwear instead of going to the bathroom. Which of the following questions is the priority for the nurse to ask to determine if this is a normal occurrence?

   1. "Do you remind your child to go to the bathroom every two hours?"

   2. "Is this your firstborn child?"

   3. "Has your child started school already?"

   4. "Does this behavior occur when your child is engaged in some activity?"

Answer: 2

Rationale: Children of this age do not have the cognitive ability to understand explanations and are better able to understand time when it is associated with a familiar activity.

Nursing process: Evaluation

Client need: Health Promotion and Maintenance

Cognitive level: Analysis

Subject area: Pediatric

Answer: 2

Rationale: Toddlers often resent being given directions or not being allowed to explore what they desire in an expanding environment. Often toddlers will delight in doing the opposite of what is asked and respond "no" to frequent requests.

Nursing process: Analysis

Client need: Health Promotion and Maintenance

Cognitive level: Analysis

Subject area: Pediatric

Answer: 3

Rationale: Sibling rivalry often arises when an infant is born into a family with a toddler. The arrival of the new baby can be devastating to toddlers since they now must compete for a caregiver's attention. One way to help toddlers is to have them stay with other family members who will be caring for them when the mother is in the hospital having the new baby. Grandparents are often these family members.

Nursing process: Evaluation

Client need: Health Promotion and Maintenance

Cognitive level: Analysis

Subject area: Pediatric

Answer: 4

Rationale: It is not uncommon for preschoolers to become so engaged in their play or other interesting activities that they do not realize they need to go to the bathroom.

Nursing process: Assessment

Client need: Management of Care

Cognitive level: Analysis

Subject area: Pediatric

19. A mother is concerned about the preschool child running into the street without looking. Which of the following instructions would be the priority for the nurse to give this mother?

  1. Offer verbal reminders to look before crossing the street

  2. Punishment is essential to prevent this behavior

  3. Prevent the child from crossing the street without the parent

  4. Children this age seldom run into the street without looking, unless distracted

20. Which of the following should the nurse include when instructing a mother to administer vitamins to a preschooler?

  1. Give the vitamins with sips of milk

  2. Give preschoolers half a vitamin

  3. Store the vitamins in a locked cabinet that the child cannot access

  4. Allow the child to be independent by self-administering the vitamins

21. Which of the following statements by the parents of a preschooler would indicate that the parents had implemented the nurse's instructions on dental hygiene practices?

  1. "Our child brushes his or her teeth without any help from us."

  2. "We give our child a pea-sized amount of fluoride toothpaste."

  3. "When our child is 6 years old, we will make an appointment to see the dentist."

  4. "When our child does a good job brushing we offer a lollipop."

22. The nurse caring for preschoolers in a day care center will find which of the following problems to be more common at this age than at any other?

  1. Appendicitis and tonsillitis requiring day surgeries or one-day hospitalization

  2. Accidents, cuts, bruises, and major traumas requiring emergency room care

  3. Poisoning with lead, plants, household chemicals, and other sources

  4. Minor illnesses such as colds, otitis media, and GI disturbances

Answer: 1
Rationale: Preschoolers have the cognitive ability to understand directions and consequences of their behavior. However, to help them remember to behave in a certain way, they often need to be reminded.
Nursing process: Implementation
Client need: Management of Care
Cognitive level: Analysis
Subject area: Pediatric

Answer: 3
Rationale: Multivitamins for children often taste like candy. Because preschoolers like the taste of these vitamins, they may be tempted to take more pills than needed unless the pills are stored in a locked cabinet the child has difficulty accessing.
Nursing process: Planning
Client need: Health Promotion and Maintenance
Cognitive level: Application
Subject area: Pediatric

Answer: 2
Rationale: Toothpaste often contains fluoride, and young children are in danger of receiving too much fluoride if the amount used in tooth brushing is larger than a pea.
Nursing process: Evaluation
Client need: Health Promotion and Maintenance
Cognitive level: Analysis
Subject area: Pediatric

Answer: 4
Rationale: Common illnesses of the preschool years include mostly minor illnesses, such as otitis media, colds, or gastrointestinal disturbances. In fact, minor illnesses are more common during this time than at any other time in life because this is the age at which children start playing together more frequently, attend childcare, or start preschool activities and thus have greater exposure to illness.
Nursing process: Analysis
Client need: Health Promotion and Maintenance
Cognitive level: Analysis
Subject area: Pediatric

23. Based on the growth and development of adolescent girls, the school nurse understands which of the following is the priority regarding body image?

1. Most girls are satisfied with their physical appearance

2. Few girls are satisfied with their physical appearance

3. The majority of girls think they are too thin

4. Girls are only concerned with their abdomen and hips

24. An adolescent tells the parents that refusing to go to school on a particular day doesn't have anything to do with not having anything appropriate to wear and having a "zit" (skin eruption) on the face. The nurse explains to the parents that this behavior exemplifies which of the following concepts?

1. Imaginary audience

2. Extreme and diagnosable narcissism

3. Adolescent instability of emotions

4. Disrespect for the school system

25. The nurse is teaching a class of adolescents to improve their diets. Which of the following approaches would be most helpful in achieving this goal?

1. Send dietary information to the parents of the adolescents

2. Have the adolescents get involved in meal planning after receiving information on dietary needs

3. Show a film on dietary needs and what happens to the body if those needs are not met

4. Conduct a series of lectures by a variety of health specialists on dietary needs of the adolescent

Answer: 2

Rationale: Body image, or the mental conception of one's physical appearance, varies with maturation and changes across time, situations, and experiences one has with others. Adolescent females are more dissatisfied with their appearance and more likely to be concerned about particular parts of their bodies than are their male counterparts.

Nursing process: Analysis

Client need: Management of Care

Cognitive level: Analysis

Subject area: Pediatric

Answer: 1

Rationale: The imaginary audience refers to the adolescent's belief of always being on stage and that others are always aware of the adolescent's physical appearance.

Nursing process: Implementation

Client need: Health Promotion and Maintenance

Cognitive level: Analysis

Subject area: Pediatric

Answer: 2

Rationale: Adolescents always seem hungry but often do not eat appropriately. Instead they prefer snack foods that are easy to prepare, faddish, and full of empty calories. Adolescent food habits are influenced by concerns about their body image, peer pressure, emotional problems, busy schedules, or unsupervised meal preparation or purchase. They also may skip meals, eat fast foods, or snack frequently. The best way to help adolescents improve their nutrition is to explain the importance of a good diet and encourage adolescents to become involved in meal planning.

Nursing process: Analysis

Client need: Health Promotion and Maintenance

Cognitive level: Analysis

Subject area: Pediatric

26. The registered nurse is preparing the clinical assignments for a pediatric unit. Which of the following assignments may the nurse delegate to a licensed practical nurse?

   1. Evaluate the growth and development of a preschooler

   2. Monitor the play activity of a toddler

   3. Assist a toddler in walking

   4. Instruct the parents on the dietary requirements of a school-age child

27. The nurse identifies which of the following as a characteristic of defecation in toddlers?

   1. Control of defecation normally begins after 3 years of age

   2. Toddlers frequently delay defecation because of play

   3. Constipation is a common problem among toddlers

   4. Control of defecation starts between 1 and 2 years of age

Answer: 3

Rationale: Clinical assignments such as skills that involve evaluation, monitoring, and instructing belong to the registered nurse. A licensed practical nurse may assist a toddler in walking.

Nursing process: Planning

Client need: Management of Care

Cognitive level: Analysis

Subject area: Legal and Ethical Issues

Answer: 4

Rationale: Control of defecation generally starts in toddlers between 1 and 2 years of age. Preschoolers, between 3 and 6 years of age, frequently delay defecation because of play and may experience constipation.

Nursing process: Implementation

Client need: Health Promotion and Maintenance

Cognitive level: Application

Subject area: Pediatric

Eye, Ear, Nose, and Throat Disorders

29

1. A mother brings her infant to the clinic for a 9-month well-baby exam. She expresses concern to the nurse that her infant's "soft spot" in the front is still palpable. The nurse's response would be based on the understanding that the anterior fontanel closes

   1. by 6 months of age.

   2. before 18 months of age.

   3. shortly after birth.

   4. before 12 months of age.

2. A 5-year-old girl presents for a vision screen. A screening using an HOTV chart is completed with the following results: 10/15 right eye, 10/12.5 left eye. Which of the following interpretations by the nurse is correct?

   1. The results indicate that this is a failing response and the child requires immediate referral to an ophthalmologist

   2. The eyes should be retested at 20 feet for more accurate results

   3. These results are considered passing and no referral is required

   4. These results are inconclusive and the child should be rescreened using the Snellen alphabet chart

3. At a well-child exam, a 3-year-old boy is diagnosed with strabismus. Which of the following clinical manifestations does the nurse interpret as indicative of this disorder?

   Select all that apply:

   [   ] **1.** Excessive eye rubbing

   [   ] **2.** Squinting

   [   ] **3.** Difficulty doing close work

   [   ] **4.** Positioning self close to TV

   [   ] **5.** Closing one eye to see

   [   ] **6.** Tilting head to one side to see

4. On testing, a 3-year-old boy is found to have left esotropia. The physician directs the nurse to instruct the parent on "patching" to treat the strabismus. The nurse instructs the parent to place

   1. the patch on the right eye.

   2. the patch on the left eye.

   3. patches on both eyes for a short time each day.

   4. the patch on the right and left alternately throughout the day.

Answer: 2

Rationale: The anterior fontanel closes between 12 and 18 months of age, with average closure at 14 months. The parent of a 9-month-old should be reassured that the anterior fontanel is still palpable. The nurse should measure its size and plot it on the occipital frontal circumference chart.

Nursing process: Analysis

Client need: Health Promotion and Maintenance

Cognitive level: Analysis

Subject area: Pediatric

Answer: 3

Rationale: A 5-year-old child screened using the HOTV chart should achieve at least a 10/15 in both eyes without a two-line difference, so this is considered a passing test. An HOTV test is the preferred test for children ages 3 to 5, because most children at these ages are unable to read the letters on a Snellen chart. The recommended testing distance is 10 feet.

Nursing process: Analysis

Client need: Reduction of Risk Potential

Cognitive level: Analysis

Subject area: Pediatric

Answer: 2, 5, 6

Rationale: The child tilts the head to one side in an effort to improve visual alignment. In strabismus, the eyes are misaligned, so the child makes efforts to improve focus. Other clinical manifestations include squinting, appearing cross-eyed, or closing one eye to see. Excessive eye rubbing, difficulty doing close work, and sitting close to the television are all manifestations of myopia.

Nursing process: Assessment

Client need: Health Promotion and Maintenance

Cognitive level: Application

Subject area: Pediatric

Answer: 1

Rationale: For a client with esotropia, the stronger eye should be patched to increase visual stimulation in the weaker eye, thus strengthening the eye muscles. Patching the weaker eye would worsen the problem. Patching both eyes is impractical, unnecessary, and counter to the goals of treatment. Esotropia (convergent) occurs when the eye turns toward the midline.

Nursing process: Implementation

Client need: Health Promotion and Maintenance

Cognitive level: Application

Subject area: Pediatric

5. In addition to instructing the mother on patching, the nurse informs her that it is important that the strabismus was recognized before the age of 6 years. This reflects the nurse's understanding that untreated strabismus may result in

   1. myopia.

   2. astigmatism.

   3. amblyopia.

   4. hyperopia.

6. To pass pure tone audiometry testing, the nurse understands that a child should be able to hear a frequency of 500 Hz at how many decibels (db)?

   1. 30 db

   2. 25 db

   3. 20 db

   4. 15 db

7. An 18-month-old child is to have a tympanogram. The mother asks what that is. Which of the following statements by the nurse best describes the purpose of tympanometry?

   1. "It is a diagnostic test that measures tympanic membrane compliance (mobility)."

   2. "It is a diagnostic test that is used most effectively in infants under age 6 months."

   3. "It is a diagnostic test that indicates the degree of hearing loss in a child."

   4. "It is a diagnostic test that measures external auditory canal air pressure."

8. A 2-year-old boy is sent home from day care because of red, itchy eyes. The nurse notes mucopurulent discharge from both eyes, and the physician treats the boy with antibiotic eyedrops. The nurse providing discharge education recognizes a need to repeat instruction when the mother states

   1. "He cannot return to day care for 24 hours after starting the eyedrops."

   2. "He needs to have the eyedrops regularly, so I will have to bring them to day care."

   3. "We should wash our hands frequently."

   4. "I need to clean his eyes from the outer corner inward."

Answer: 3

Rationale: Strabismus is a condition where the visual lines of the two eyes do not focus simultaneously on the same object in space because of a lack of muscle coordination, resulting in a cross-eyed appearance. If left untreated, it leads to eventual loss of vision in the weaker eye and may lead to blindness. Astigmatism, myopia, and hyperopia are disorders that, while significant, are refractory errors and can be corrected with special lenses.

Nursing process: Analysis

Client need: Health Promotion and Maintenance

Cognitive level: Analysis

Subject area: Pediatric

Answer: 2

Rationale: Inability to hear any frequency at 25 db is considered a failure. Most children are able to hear frequencies higher than 500 Hz at 20 db.

Nursing process: Analysis

Client need: Reduction of Risk Potential

Cognitive level: Analysis

Subject area: Pediatric

Answer: 1

Rationale: Tympanometry is used to measure tympanic membrane compliance. It also estimates middle ear pressure. It does not indicate the degree of hearing loss. It is not useful in infants under age 6 months, because of hypercompliance of the tympanic membrane. It does not measure external auditory canal air pressure.

Nursing process: Evaluation

Client need: Reduction of Risk Potential

Cognitive level: Application

Subject area: Pediatric

Answer: 4

Rationale: The eye should be cleaned from the inner canthus of the eye downward and outward. This will lessen the potential of infecting the other eye. It would be appropriate to prevent the child from returning to day care for 24 hours after starting antibiotics to prevent spreading the infection. It is also necessary to administer the antibiotic on a regular basis and to wash the hands frequently.

Nursing process: Evaluation

Client need: Health Promotion and Maintenance

Cognitive level: Analysis

Subject area: Pediatric

9. The nurse evaluates which of the following laboratory tests and pathogens that cause acute otitis media in children?

   1. Group A beta-hemolytic *streptococcus*
   2. *Escherichia coli*
   3. *Haemophilus influenzae* and *Streptococcus pneumoniae*
   4. *Staphylococcus aureus* and *Pasteurella*

10. The mother of a 9-month-old infant calls the triage nurse with a concern that her child, who has a bad cold, might have an ear infection. The triage nurse elicits additional history. Which of the following can be identified from the health history as a risk factor for the development of otitis media in children?

    1. Day care attendance
    2. Breastfeeding
    3. Female gender in infants
    4. Introduction of a new solid food

11. A 3-year-old boy is accompanied by his mother for follow-up of fluid in his middle ears. He had a bilateral ear infection three months ago and the fluid in his middle ears has persisted at all of his subsequent appointments. The nurse, based on an understanding of bilateral middle ear effusion, recognizes that this child should be

    1. reassured that this is a normal complication of otitis media.
    2. screened for hearing loss.
    3. rescheduled for follow-up at 6 months because not enough time has elapsed to reevaluate the ears.
    4. avoiding milk products because they thicken upper respiratory tract secretions.

Answer: 3

Rationale: *H. influenzae* and *Str. pneumoniae* are upper respiratory pathogens. These most often cause otitis media. Group A beta-hemolytic *streptococcus* is also an upper respiratory pathogen, but is not implicated in acute otitis media. *S. aureus* is commonly found on skin and *E. coli* is a bowel organism. *Pasteurella* is an infection associated with animal bites.

Nursing process: Evaluation

Client need: Reduction of Risk Potential

Cognitive level: Application

Subject area: Pediatric

Answer: 1

Rationale: Day care attendance is recognized as a risk factor in otitis media because of increased exposure to bacterial pathogens and the likelihood that some of these pathogens may have developed resistance to antimicrobial therapy. Breastfeeding has been shown to decrease the incidence of otitis media in infants compared to bottle-feeding. Males less than school age are more at risk than females for the development of otitis media. There is currently no substantial evidence to support the link between the introduction of new foods and the development of otitis media, although some theories propose that allergies may play a role in the development of otitis media.

Nursing process: Assessment

Client need: Health Promotion and Maintenance

Cognitive level: Analysis

Subject area: Pediatric

Answer: 2

Rationale: A child who has had fluid in both middle ears for three months should have a hearing screen because there is increased potential for conductive hearing loss. Over time, conductive hearing loss could negatively affect the development of speech, language, and cognition. Otitis media with effusion can be a normal consequence of otitis media but should resolve by three months. There is no evidence to support limiting milk products to treat otitis media effusion.

Nursing process: Analysis

Client need: Health Promotion and Maintenance

Cognitive level: Analysis

Subject area: Pediatric

12. A 5-year-old female has received tympanostomy tubes. The discharge nurse instructs the parent and child regarding tympanostomy tubes and their care. Which of the following would be included in the education plan?

    1. The child should never be allowed to go swimming

    2. The tympanostomy (PE) tubes will remain in place for five years

    3. The child with tympanostomy tubes in place will not experience any further episodes of otitis media

    4. Earplugs are recommended for activities such as diving, submerging, bathing, and shampooing

13. A 12-year-old child has experienced repeated otitis externa. The child swims daily on a swim team and is unwilling to give that up. The nurse instructs the child and parents on methods to prevent further episodes. Which of the following is included in the plan?

    1. Instruct parent and child to remove water from within the ear with a cotton-tipped swab

    2. Instruct the parent and child to instill rubbing alcohol into the ears after swimming

    3. Instruct the parent and child to instill a 50% solution of vinegar and water into the ears after swimming

    4. Instruct the parent and child to stay in the water for no more than two hours at a time

14. A 6-year-old child is scheduled for a tonsillectomy. The nurse is obtaining the preoperative history. Because of risks associated with this surgery, the nurse should report which of the following to the surgeon?

    1. There is a family history of bleeding tendencies

    2. Current upper respiratory infection is denied

    3. The child recently visited the dentist

    4. The child does not have a cleft palate

Answer: 4

Rationale: While swimming does not increase the risk of infection, diving, jumping, and submerging may. Bath water carries a higher risk of infection because it is contaminated, as is lake water. The use of earplugs is recommended for these activities. Soap reduces the surface tension of water, facilitating its entry into the tube, so earplugs are also recommended when shampooing. Most tympanostomy (PE) tubes fall out by 12 months and should be removed after 2 years. Children with tympanostomy tubes in place most often experience otitis when there is otorrhea from the PE tube.

Nursing process: Planning

Client need: Health Promotion and Maintenance

Cognitive level: Application

Subject area: Pediatric

Answer: 3

Rationale: Instilling dilute vinegar and water into the ear of a child with otitis externa establishes an acidic environment, which is less conducive to bacterial growth. A cotton-tipped swab is not recommended for removal of water, because it may further damage the sensitive ear canal. Similarly, undiluted rubbing alcohol would be too harsh for the sensitive ear canal and may further damage tissue. The usual recommendation for water exposure is less than one hour at a time with a one- to two-hour interval between repeated exposures.

Nursing process: Planning

Client need: Health Promotion and Maintenance

Cognitive level: Application

Subject area: Pediatric

Answer: 1

Rationale: The operative site in a tonsillectomy is highly vascular, so family bleeding tendencies would require additional alertness for this potential problem in this client. It is ideal that the child does not have a concurrent upper respiratory infection, but this would not require notification of the surgeon. The child's mouth should be assessed for loose teeth prior to surgery, so this notation is of little significance. Cleft palate is a contraindication to tonsillectomy.

Nursing process: Analysis

Client need: Health Promotion and Maintenance

Cognitive level: Analysis

Subject area: Pediatric

15. The nurse is caring for a child following tonsillectomy. Which of the following observations should the nurse immediately report?

   1. The presence of dark brown blood on the teeth

   2. The presence of blood trickling down the throat

   3. An episode of vomiting

   4. A complaint of a sore throat

16. A 7-year-old child who has undergone tonsillectomy is alert, and the nurse is reviewing postoperative instructions. Which of the following should be included in the instructions?

   1. A soft diet will be ordered once the child is alert

   2. Coughing, clearing of throat, and blowing of the nose is discouraged

   3. The client should continue to be positioned prone or in a side-lying position for 24 hours

   4. Milk is the choice of fluid following the tonsillectomy to provide nutrients

17. The mother of a child asks the nurse when the frontal sinuses in children develop. Which of the following is the appropriate response by the nurse? "The frontal sinuses are fully developed

   1. at birth."

   2. by age 3 months."

   3. by age 7 years."

   4. in puberty."

Answer: 2

Rationale: The presence of blood trickling down the throat following a tonsillectomy is a sign of bleeding and should be communicated to the surgeon immediately. The dark brown blood is old and is commonly found on the teeth, in the nose, and in the emesis following tonsillectomy. It does not signify hemorrhage. Vomiting may be a normal sequela following surgery and does not need to be communicated to the surgeon. If, however, the vomitus contains bright red blood, then the surgeon should be notified immediately, as this is an indication of bleeding. A client complaint of a sore throat is an anticipated finding posttonsillectomy.

Nursing process: Analysis

Client need: Reduction of Risk Potential

Cognitive level: Analysis

Subject area: Pediatric

Answer: 2

Rationale: Coughing, clearing of the throat, and blowing the nose should be discouraged following a tonsillectomy. A soft diet, an oral intake of milk, and positioning the client prone or side-lying once alert may all stress the operative site and cause bleeding or hemorrhage. Typically, a cold, clear liquid diet is begun and advanced slowly as tolerated. The client may prefer an upright position once alert. The prone and side-lying positions are recommended until the client is alert. Milk products can be given later in the course, but should be avoided if they cause excessive clearing of the throat.

Nursing process: Planning

Client need: Health Promotion and Maintenance

Cognitive level: Application

Subject area: Pediatric

Answer: 3

Rationale: The frontal sinuses develop by age 7 years. The maxillary and ethmoid sinuses are present at birth, but they are very small. The sphenoid sinus does not develop fully until puberty.

Nursing process: Analysis

Client need: Health Promotion and Maintenance

Cognitive level: Analysis

Subject area: Pediatric

18. A 9-year-old girl was diagnosed with strep throat and an antibiotic was prescribed. The mother asks the nurse when the child can return to school. Which of the following is the priority response by the nurse?

    1. "She may return immediately if she is afebrile."
    2. "She may return after 1 week if she is feeling better."
    3. "She may return after the 10-day course of antibiotic."
    4. "She may return after taking the antibiotic for a 24-hour period."

19. An adolescent experiences recurrent aphthous stomatitis. Which of the following should the nurse include in the instructions for a client with aphthous ulcers?

    1. Encourage fluids through a straw and soft diet while the ulcers are present
    2. Recommend the use of a hard-bristle toothbrush to remove affected tissue
    3. Administer antiviral drugs such as acyclovir (Zovirax) to shorten course
    4. Inform the client that the ulcers will last one to two days

20. The nurse understands that viscous lidocaine is sometimes prescribed for clients with aphthous ulcers. The nurse should question a physician's prescription for viscous lidocaine in which of the following clients?

    1. An adolescent male with stomatitis
    2. An adult female with stomatitis
    3. A toddler male with stomatitis
    4. An alert 60-year-old female with stomatitis

21. The nurse should assess for what related condition in a 4-month-old infant who has oral candidiasis?

    1. Eczema
    2. Diaper rash
    3. *Herpes simplex* infection
    4. Aphthous ulcers

Answer: 4

Rationale: Twenty-four hours of antibiotic therapy decreases the number of colonies in respiratory secretions, thus lessening the infectious nature of strep throat. The child can return to school after 24 hours of antibiotic therapy when she is feeling better and is afebrile. This will likely be sooner than one week. The antibiotic is typically prescribed for 10 days, but this does not necessitate missing school for that period of time.

Nursing process: Analysis

Client need: Health Promotion and Maintenance

Cognitive level: Analysis

Subject area: Pediatric

Answer: 1

Rationale: Aphthous stomatitis is canker sores. Eating a soft diet and using a straw will help avoid additional trauma and contact with painful lesions allowing the child to eat. A soft-bristle toothbrush is recommended to avoid further trauma and irritation of the ulcers. Antiviral drugs such as acyclovir (Zovirax) are helpful to treat herpetic lesions but are not used in the treatment of aphthous ulcers. Aphthous ulcers typically last 4 to 12 days.

Nursing process: Planning

Client need: Health Promotion and Maintenance

Cognitive level: Application

Subject area: Pediatric

Answer: 3

Rationale: Viscous lidocaine can be prescribed for a client with aphthous ulcers. The client must be able to keep one teaspoon of the solution in the mouth for two to three minutes and then expectorate. The toddler patient would be unlikely to be able to do this. Adolescents and adults would likely be able to do this.

Nursing process: Analysis

Client need: Health Promotion and Maintenance

Cognitive level: Analysis

Subject area: Pediatric

Answer: 2

Rationale: Oral candidial lesions can spread to other body systems including the gastrointestinal tract and via poor hand washing by the caregiver. Concomitant monilial diaper rash is common. Although eczema, *herpes simplex* infection, and aphthous ulcers may be present, they are not directly related to the oral candidiasis.

Nursing process: Assessment

Client need: Health Promotion and Maintenance

Cognitive level: Analysis

Subject area: Pediatric

22. A 2-month-old breast-fed infant has oral thrush. Which of the following is the most appropriate intervention to be included in the nurse's plan of care?

    1. The oral lesions should be treated with an over-the-counter topical anesthetic such as Anbesol

    2. Administer oral nystatin before feedings as prescribed

    3. Instruct the mother on treatment of her nipples if she continues breastfeeding

    4. Add cereal to the diet to decrease the need for sucking

23. The nurse is teaching a class on allergic rhinitis. The nurse should include which of the following in the class?

    1. Unlike asthma, there is no familial predisposition to allergic rhinitis

    2. Allergic rhinitis is a disorder that occurs seasonally

    3. A nasal smear for eosinophils is the hallmark diagnostic test of allergic rhinitis

    4. Peak incidence of allergic rhinitis occurs in the adolescent and postadolescent population

24. An 8-year-old boy will be undergoing skin allergy testing. The nurse should include which of the following precautions in the preparations?

    1. Evaluate for dermographism before beginning the testing

    2. Notify the physician if not on site that testing has begun

    3. Reassure the parent and child that no allergic reactions generally occur with this method

    4. Inject the allergen solution to a depth to elicit bleeding

Answer: 3

Rationale: The nipples of a mother who is breastfeeding an infant with oral thrush should be treated with a topical antifungal to avoid reinfection of the infant. Anbesol is not recommended in the treatment of oral candidiasis. Oral nystatin is the treatment of choice, but should be administered after feeding. Current guidelines recommend introduction of cereal at 6 months; adding cereal to the diet of a 2-month-old is inappropriate.

Nursing process: Planning

Client need: Health Promotion and Maintenance

Cognitive level: Application

Subject area: Pediatric

Answer: 4

Rationale: Allergic rhinitis can occur in any age group, but the peak incidence occurs in the adolescent and postadolescent population. Allergic rhinitis does have a familial component. It may occur seasonally or perennially. Perennial allergic rhinitis to common household allergens is more common. A nasal smear for eosinophils is a nonspecific, nonuniversal finding and is not considered a hallmark diagnostic test.

Nursing process: Planning

Client need: Health Promotion and Maintenance

Cognitive level: Application

Subject area: Pediatric

Answer: 1

Rationale: The client should be tested for dermographism before beginning skin allergy testing because dermographism may result in false-positive test results. Clients undergoing skin testing for allergies are at risk for an allergic reaction; those undergoing blood testing are unlikely to suffer allergic reactions. The physician should be on site for testing as there is potential for anaphylactic response and certainly for allergic reaction. Bleeding should be avoided during injection because this would create the potential for systemic allergen exposure and resultant anaphylaxis.

Nursing process: Planning

Client need: Health Promotion and Maintenance

Cognitive level: Application

Subject area: Pediatric

25. A 13-year-old female has been prescribed allergy injections every three to four weeks. The nurse instructs the child that following the injection, she

   1. must remain for observation for at least five minutes.

   2. must remain for observation for at least 20 minutes.

   3. must remain for observation for at least one hour.

   4. does not need to remain for observation.

26. The registered nurse is preparing the nursing tasks for a pediatric eye, ear, nose, and throat disorder unit. Which of the following nursing tasks may be delegated to a licensed practical nurse?

   1. Perform a nasopharyngeal culture

   2. Refer the parent of a child with strabismus to an ophthalmologist

   3. Instruct a client scheduled for a myringotomy on the procedure

   4. Monitor the neurological status on a child with craniosynostosis

Answer: 2

Rationale: It is recommended that the client receiving allergy injections should remain for observation for 20 to 30 minutes following the injection to ensure that no delayed reaction occurs.

Nursing process: Implementation

Client need: Reduction of Risk Potential

Cognitive level: Analysis

Subject area: Pediatric

Answer: 1

Rationale: A licensed practical nurse may perform a nasopharyngeal culture. Referring a child with strabismus to an ophthalmologist, instructing the parents of a child scheduled for a myringotomy, and monitoring the neurological status on a child with craniosynostosis are all nursing skills reserved for the registered nurse.

Nursing process: Planning

Client need: Management of Care

Cognitive level: Analysis

Subject area: Legal and Ethical Issues

Respiratory Disorders

1. The nurse informs the parents of an infant that the primary difference between the chest of an infant and that of an adult is that the chest of an infant
   1. has a more flattened front-to-back diameter.
   2. is a cone-shaped structure.
   3. is rounded in shape.
   4. consists of cartilage, bone, and muscle.

2. A mother accompanies her 6-month-old male infant to the emergency room. She is concerned because the infant has not been feeding well. The infant has had a bad cold and cough, although the cough has subsided today. The nurse assessing the infant notes that the infant is very irritable and displays nasal flaring and intercostal retractions. Which of the following is the priority intervention for the nurse to take?
   1. Offer formula because the infant appears hungry
   2. Suction the infant's nose
   3. Acknowledge the mother's concern regarding the infant's diminished feeding
   4. Notify the physician that the infant needs to be seen quickly

3. During an examination of the breath sounds in a child, the nurse assesses continuous, high-pitched musical sounds. The nurse documents this as _____.

Answer: 3

Rationale: An infant's chest is almost circular in shape; in adults, the anterior-posterior diameter is less than the lateral diameter. The thoracic cavity for both infants and adults is cone-shaped and consists of bone, cartilage, and muscle.

Nursing process: Implementation

Client need: Health Promotion and Maintenance

Cognitive level: Application

Subject area: Pediatric

Answer: 4

Rationale: Poor feeding, irritability, nasal flaring, and intercostal retractions are signs of altered respiratory function and respiratory distress in infants. It is important for the nurse to recognize these clinical manifestations in order to triage the infant, so that the physician sees this child before less ill clients. Infant feeding is likely decreased because the infant has air hunger and does not have the energy to feed. Suctioning the infant's nose would likely increase hypoxia. While it is important to acknowledge the mother's concern regarding infant feeding, a more appropriate response is to have the physician see the infant as soon as possible.

Nursing process: Planning

Client need: Management of Care

Cognitive level: Analysis

Subject area: Pediatric

Answer: wheezing

Rationale: Wheezing consists of continuous, high-pitched musical sounds.

Nursing process: Implementation

Client need: Health Promotion and Maintenance

Cognitive level: Comprehension

Subject area: Pediatric

4. While assessing a 13-year-old male following a motor vehicle accident, the nurse notes crepitus over the left lateral rib cage. Based on an understanding of crepitus, the nurse evaluates which of the following to cause the crepitus?
   1. Palpable vibrations over the chest wall that are produced by voice sounds
   2. The transmission of a pleural friction rub through the chest wall
   3. Remodeling of lung tissue secondary to asthma
   4. Air escaped from the lungs and trapped in the subcutaneous tissue

5. The parents of a 10-year-old child ask the nurse what pulmonary function testing is. Which of the following is the most appropriate response by the nurse? "Pulmonary function testing
   1. is an invasive test of pulmonary mechanics."
   2. is used to evaluate the severity of a respiratory disease."
   3. is used to diagnose specific respiratory diseases."
   4. does not differentiate between restrictive and obstructive pulmonary disease."

6. A 15-month-old infant is seen in a well-child exam. Because the infant's family has recently emigrated from East Africa where tuberculosis (TB) is endemic, a Mantoux test is performed. No one in the infant's family has currently or has in the past had tuberculosis. The mother brings the infant back to the clinic in 48 hours to have the Mantoux test read. According to this infant's risk status and age, which is the smallest amount of induration that the nurse should consider a positive finding? An area of
   1. 5 mm induration.
   2. 10 mm induration.
   3. 15 mm induration.
   4. 20 mm induration.

7. The nurse is caring for a 5-year-old child suspected of having tuberculosis. Which of the following is the preferred method of obtaining a sputum specimen for culture and smear from this child?
   1. Endotracheal suctioning
   2. Sputum collected by elicited cough
   3. Sputum collected by early morning gastric washings
   4. Thoracentesis

Answer: 4

Rationale: Tactile fremitus is a palpable vibration over the chest wall that is produced by voice sounds. A pleural friction rub is auscultated as a grating sound. Remodeling in asthma does not cause crepitus.

Nursing process: Evaluation

Client need: Health Promotion and Maintenance

Cognitive level: Comprehension

Subject area: Pediatric

Answer: 2

Rationale: Pulmonary function testing (PFT) is used to evaluate the severity of the disease. It is a noninvasive test. PFT cannot diagnose specific diseases because different diseases may have the same functional abnormalities. It is used to differentiate between restrictive and obstructive disease.

Nursing process: Analysis

Client need: Reduction of Risk Potential

Cognitive level: Comprehension

Subject area: Pediatric

Answer: 2

Rationale: For a child under the age of 4 years and born in an area of the world where tuberculosis is prevalent, a reading of 10 mm induration would be the lowest value that would be considered a positive finding in accordance with current clinical standards. While 15 mm and 20 mm induration would also be considered positive findings, given the younger age of 15 months, a positive reading would occur at 10 mm.

Nursing process: Analysis

Client need: Reduction of Risk Potential

Cognitive level: Application

Subject area: Pediatric

Answer: 3

Rationale: Because young children are likely to swallow any sputum that is produced by cough, gastric lavage is a more effective method of collecting a sputum sample. It is the preferred method of collecting sputum for culture and smear from a child who is suspected of having tuberculosis. Endotracheal suctioning, unless intubated, would not be well tolerated, and thoracentesis is both invasive and impractical on a routine basis.

Nursing process: Analysis

Client need: Reduction of Risk Potential

Cognitive level: Application

Subject area: Pediatric

8. A mother reports that her 15-month-old child has had three colds in three months during the winter while attending day care. The mother inquires whether she should use an over-the-counter antihistamine for this child, because she suspects allergies must be the cause of the frequent colds. Which of the following is the nurse's most appropriate intervention?

1. Reassure the parent that frequent episodes of nasopharyngitis are common given the child's risk factors

2. Notify the physician immediately because this information may be indicative of an immunodeficiency

3. Inform the parent that the child might have asthma because of the frequency of upper respiratory infections

4. Instruct the parent to use an over-the-counter antihistamine

9. A mother reports that her 4-month-old has a cold, but no fever. She reports noisy breathing at night and that the child's nose is very congested. The nurse advises the mother to promote maximum ventilation during sleep. Which of the following instructions about positioning would be appropriate for the nurse to include in the instructions?

1. Elevate the infant's head on a pillow to open the airway

2. Place infant in an upright (90 degrees) position

3. Elevate the head of the crib 30 degrees

4. Place the infant prone to promote drainage of secretions

10. A 3-year-old child is brought to the emergency room at night with a harsh cough, hoarseness, and noisy breathing. Although the nurse's initial assessment reveals a child who appears comfortable and whose respiratory status is within normal limits, a diagnosis of acute spasmodic laryngitis is made. Which of these instructions should the nurse include in the teaching plan?

1. This is an isolated episode and will not recur

2. This illness is usually accompanied by fever

3. Stimulating the child may help terminate the episode

4. Clinical manifestations may resolve on exposure to cool night air

Answer: 1

Rationale: Nasopharyngitis occurs more frequently in infants and young children, especially in settings like a day care center where many children interact in a small space. The most frequent transmission is by human hands, so good handwashing is essential to help prevent continuous colds. The fall and winter months are also prime times for colds. It is unlikely the child is immunosuppressed based on the circumstances and clinical manifestations. The nurse should not suggest that the child has asthma, because it is not in the scope of practice and the diagnosis is not supported by the data collected. It would not be appropriate to make a recommendation concerning over-the-counter antihistamine therapy for a child this young. Antihistamines have also been found to be ineffective in treating nasopharyngitis.

Nursing process: Planning

Client need: Health Promotion and Maintenance

Cognitive level: Application

Subject area: Pediatric

Answer: 3

Rationale: Appropriate positioning is a significant means of easing respiratory efforts in infants and small children. Elevation of the head of the crib or maintaining the infant's head at 30 degrees will promote maximum lung expansion. Resting an infant's head on a pillow is not recommended, because of the risk of sudden infant death syndrome. Positioning an infant at 90 degrees would actually compress the diaphragm and diminish respiratory function. Prone positioning of infants is generally not recommended, because of its correlation with sudden infant death syndrome. It should be noted that in the rare case that the infant is experiencing gastroesophageal reflux, positioning the infant prone may be permitted.

Nursing process: Planning

Client need: Health Promotion and Maintenance

Cognitive level: Application

Subject area: Pediatric

Answer: 4

Rationale: Exposure to cool night air or humidity may help relieve the spasm in acute spasmodic laryngitis. The parent should be advised that these attacks may be recurrent. The illness is usually not accompanied by fever. Stimulation may aggravate the dyspnea.

Nursing process: Planning

Client need: Health Promotion and Maintenance

Cognitive level: Application

Subject area: Pediatric

11. Which of the following should the nurse include in a plan of care for a 5-year-old child admitted to the hospital with the diagnosis of epiglottitis?

   1. Perform a throat culture to identify the pathogen

   2. Administer cough syrup to the child

   3. Encourage the child to assume a tripod position

   4. Restrict fluids

12. A mother calls the medical information line and reports that her 6-year-old child has awakened with a complaint of sore throat and pain on swallowing. She reports that the child was fine when going to bed. The child has a fever of 39.2°C, or 102.5°F, orally and is restless and appears quite sick. Which of the following questions is a priority for the nurse to ask to triage this client?

   1. "Has the child been drooling?"

   2. "Has the child been exposed to strep throat?"

   3. "Did you give the child an antipyretic?"

   4. "Is the child up to date on immunizations?"

13. A child in the emergency room is suspected of having epiglottitis. Which of the following is the priority to include in this client's plan of care?

   1. Explain the course of the disease to the parents

   2. Ensure that the child has a patent airway

   3. Establish IV access

   4. Accompany the child to radiology for lateral neck x-ray

Answer: 3

Rationale: Epiglottitis, also referred to as croup syndrome, is a life-threatening bacterial infection that can lead to a complete airway obstruction. Because of difficulty breathing and swallowing, the child is likely to assume a tripod position. This is characterized by the child sitting upright and leaning forward with chin thrust out, tongue protruding, and mouth open to facilitate breathing and swallowing. A throat culture should not be done, as this could cause additional or complete obstruction. Examination of the throat should only occur when emergency tracheostomy or intubation is possible. The onset of epiglottitis is usually abrupt and is more likely preceded by a sore throat than by cold manifestations. It is most common in children between the ages of 2 and 7 years. Fluids, antibiotics, and supportive care are included in the treatment plan.

Nursing process: Planning

Client need: Health Promotion and Maintenance

Cognitive level: Analysis

Subject area: Pediatric

Answer: 1

Rationale: Clinical manifestations of a sore throat, difficulty swallowing, restlessness, and temperature of 39.2°C, or 102.5°F, orally is suggestive of epiglottitis, which is a medical emergency. Confirming that the child is drooling would be additional data to support the nurse's suspicions and assist to direct the parent and child to an emergency department for evaluation and treatment. Although asking about strep throat, administration of an antipyretic, and immunizations may be appropriate questions for any parent of a child, the priority question would be to inquire about drooling.

Nursing process: Assessment

Client need: Health Promotion and Maintenance

Cognitive level: Analysis

Subject area: Pediatric

Answer: 2

Rationale: Epiglottitis, or croup syndrome, is a bacterial infection that may lead to a complete airway obstruction. It should be managed in the same way as acute respiratory distress, with maintenance of the airway being the priority. Establishing IV access and assisting with x-ray will also be done, but only after the airway has been ensured and trained personnel are available. The nurse should not perform any procedures without additional medical team support. Communicating to the parents is important, but only after the client is stabilized.

Nursing process: Planning

Client need: Management of Care

Cognitive level: Analysis

Subject area: Pediatric

14. A 4-year-old child with epiglottitis is being transferred via ambulance to the hospital. The parents and child are very fearful. The mother asks if her child can sit in her lap for transport. What is the nurse's best response?

1. "Your anxiousness is making your child upset. It is best to leave the child."

2. "Riding on your lap would be a dangerous practice and is not recommended."

3. "Letting your child ride on your lap may reduce your child's stress."

4. "Your child is very anxious so a sedative will be given so your child can sleep."

15. The father of a child with laryngotracheobronchitis asks the nurse what it is. Which of the following statements by the nurse best describes laryngotracheobronchitis?

1. "It is a reactive airway disease characterized by wheezing and cough."

2. "It is a viral illness that results in inflammation of the small airways and production of thick mucus."

3. "It is a bacterial illness that results in serious supraglottic inflammation."

4. "It is a viral illness that results in swelling around the level of the larynx characterized by a barking cough and hoarseness."

16. A child with a brassy cough, mild fever, and hoarseness is seen in the emergency department and diagnosed with croup. The physician orders discharge to home with management to include cool-temperature therapy. The nurse preparing discharge teaching notices that the child has developed continuous respiratory stridor. Which of the following is the priority nursing intervention?

1. Complete discharge instructions, including a review of the clinical manifestations of respiratory distress

2. Instruct the parent on how to perform cool-temperature therapy

3. Notify the physician of the child's status immediately

4. Request that the child follow up with the primary care provider in one week

17. The nurse administers which of the following vaccines to help prevent the development of epiglottitis?

1. Diphtheria/tetanus/acellular pertussis (DTaP) combination vaccine

2. Varicella vaccine (Varivax)

3. *Haemophilus influenzae* vaccine (HIB)

4. Pneumococcal polysaccharide vaccine (Prevnar)

Answer: 3

Rationale: Being allowed to sit on a parent's lap may actually decrease the child's (and parent's) stress and facilitate easier breathing. Such a request would need to be approved by the physician and the ambulance personnel. Isolating the child from the parents would very likely increase the child's stress and consequently the respiratory dysfunction. This would be counterproductive. Sedation would be inappropriate in this situation, as it would further compromise respiratory effort.

Nursing process: Analysis

Client need: Health Promotion and Maintenance

Cognitive level: Analysis

Subject area: Pediatric

Answer: 4

Rationale: Laryngotracheobronchitis (croup) is a viral illness that results in swelling around the level of the larynx characterized by a barking cough and hoarseness. A reactive airway disease characterized by wheezing and cough is a description of asthma. A viral illness that results in inflammation of the small airways and production of thick mucus is a description of bronchiolitis. A bacterial illness that results in serious supraglottic inflammation is a description of epiglottitis.

Nursing process: Evaluation

Client need: Health Promotion and Maintenance

Cognitive level: Comprehension

Subject area: Pediatric

Answer: 3

Rationale: Stridor is a high-pitched sound produced by an obstruction of the trachea or larynx that can be heard during inspiration or expiration. Stridor even at rest signifies progression of the croup and requires medical management. The physician should be notified immediately. It would be inappropriate to discharge the client in view of the change in status without notifying the physician. Instructing the parents on cool-temperature therapy is an appropriate intervention but not the priority.

Nursing process: Implementation

Client need: Management of Care

Cognitive level: Analysis

Subject area: Legal and Ethical Issues

Answer: 3

Rationale: *Haemophilus influenzae* is the most common causative organism of epiglottitis. The *Haemophilus influenzae* vaccine may help prevent it. Diphtheria/tetanus/acellular pertussis (DTaP) immunizes against diphtheria, tetanus, and pertussis. Varivax immunizes against varicella (chickenpox), and Prevnar immunizes against streptococcal pneumonia and to a lesser degree ear infections caused by *Streptococcus pneumoniae*.

Nursing process: Implementation

Client need: Reduction of Risk Potential

Cognitive level: Analysis

Subject area: Pediatric

18. The nurse is caring for a 5-year-old child diagnosed with bronchitis who is otherwise in good health. The child's mother verbalizes to the nurse that she is very upset that the physician did not prescribe antibiotics. The nurse's response would be based on the understanding that bronchitis is

   1. treated by antihistamines, not antibiotics.

   2. usually viral in a child under 5 years and not affected by antibiotic therapy.

   3. a minor bacterial illness and antibiotics are not recommended because of the risk of developing bacterial resistance.

   4. most appropriately controlled by cough syrup administered every four hours.

19. Which of the following infection control measures is the priority for the nurse to implement in the care provided to a 5-month-old infant admitted to the hospital with respiratory syncytial virus (RSV) bronchiolitis?

   1. Hand washing is required by all personnel and visitors having contact with the infant

   2. Gowns and masks must be worn by all personnel in the infant's room

   3. Place the infant in a private room

   4. Visitors are restricted to only the parents of the infant

20. The parents of a 5-month-old infant who has bronchiolitis ask the nurse what changes occur to the lung during the illness. The nurse informs these parents that which of the following lung changes occur?

   1. Asthma

   2. Emphysema

   3. Atelectasis

   4. Crepitus

Answer: 2

Rationale: Laryngotracheobronchitis (croup) is usually caused by a virus, especially in young children. Antibiotics are ineffective against viral illnesses. It would be appropriate for the nurse to explain this rationale to the parent as part of client-family education. Bronchitis is not treated with antihistamines. Cough suppressants should be used with caution as they may make the child drowsy and may also impede the clearance of secretions. The issue in antibiotic resistance is to treat with an adequate dose of an antibiotic that is active against the offending pathogen, not whether or not to treat.

Nursing process: Analysis

Client need: Health Promotion and Maintenance

Cognitive level: Analysis

Subject area: Pediatric

Answer: 1

Rationale: Bronchiolitis is a viral infection causing inflammation of the bronchioles and production of thick mucus that occludes the bronchiole tubes and small airways, impeding expiration. Of the infection control measures implemented, consistent hand washing and not touching the nasal mucosa or conjunctivae have been shown to be most important. Wearing masks and gowns has not been shown to be of added benefit, although the gowns may help reduce the risk of fomite spread. Infants with RSV may be in rooms with children with similar diagnosis or isolated in private rooms, dependent on hospital policy. The advisability of limiting visitors and staff in an effort to lessen the spread of infection is being studied.

Nursing process: Planning

Client need: Safety and Infection Control

Cognitive level: Analysis

Subject area: Legal and Ethical Issues

Answer: 2

Rationale: In bronchiolitis, the bronchioles and small airways become occluded due to inflammation and thick mucus. Air becomes trapped behind the occlusions, where it leads to progressive overinflation of the lungs called emphysema. While some infants may manifest asthmalike manifestations, this does not reflect the usual progression of bronchiolitis. Atelectasis is a collapse of the lung and is not a normal development in bronchiolitis. Crepitus is a crackling sound on palpation caused by the escape of air into the subcutaneous tissue and is also not common in bronchiolitis.

Nursing process: Implementation

Client need: Health Promotion and Maintenance

Cognitive level: Analysis

Subject area: Pediatric

21. The mother of a 4-month-old diagnosed with respiratory syncytial virus and bronchiolitis tells the nurse the infant has not been feeding well. Which of the following physical clinical manifestations indicates to the nurse that the client's condition is deteriorating and the client has become dehydrated?

    Select all that apply:

    [   ] **1.** Bradycardia

    [   ] **2.** Oliguria

    [   ] **3.** Decreased respirations

    [   ] **4.** Decreased skin turgor

    [   ] **5.** Sunken anterior fontanel

    [   ] **6.** Dry mucous membranes

22. Which of the following methods should the nurse use to collect a respiratory syncytial virus (RSV) culture that has been ordered on a 6-month-old infant?

    1. Use a nasopharyngeal swab

    2. Perform a nasal washing

    3. Venipuncture

    4. Gastric lavage

23. The nurse screens which of the following pediatric age groups for atypical pneumonia caused by mycoplasma?

    1. Infancy

    2. Toddlerhood

    3. School age

    4. Adolescence

24. The nurse is teaching a class on sudden infant death syndrome to parents. Which of the following should the nurse include in the class?

    1. The peak incidence is between 6 and 8 months of age

    2. Occurrence is most frequent during the summer months

    3. Being a low-birth-weight male infant increases the risk

    4. Every infant under 1 year of age should be tested

Answer: 2, 4, 5, 6

Rationale: The sunken fontanel is the most specific clinical manifestation indicating that the infant is dehydrated. Other clinical manifestations include decreased skin turgor, oliguria, dry mucous membranes, and skin color changes. The infant may also become tachypneic and tachycardic.

Nursing process: Analysis

Client need: Health Promotion and Maintenance

Cognitive level: Application

Subject area: Pediatric

Answer: 2

Rationale: The nasal washing is identified as the method of choice for collecting the nasal specimen for respiratory syncytial virus (RSV). Although sometimes used, a nasopharyngeal swab is not as effective a collection technique. Venipuncture and gastric lavage are not used to obtain specimens for RSV determination.

Nursing process: Implementation

Client need: Reduction of Risk Potential

Cognitive level: Application

Subject area: Pediatric

Answer: 3

Rationale: *Mycoplasma pneumoniae* is the most common causative agent of pneumonia in school-age children between the ages of 5 and 12 years. Viral pneumonia is the most common pneumonia overall and is seen in all age groups. Bacterial pneumonias are more prevalent in children under age 5 years.

Nursing process: Implementation

Client need: Health Promotion and Maintenance

Cognitive level: Application

Subject area: Pediatric

Answer: 3

Rationale: Sudden infant death syndrome is the unexpected death of an apparently healthy infant under the age of 1 year. Peak incidence is between 2 and 4 months. It occurs more frequently between the ages of 2 and 4 months and in the winter months. Low-birth-weight male infants are at a greater risk than are females. There is no diagnostic test for sudden infant death syndrome.

Nursing process: Planning

Client need: Health Promotion and Maintenance

Cognitive level: Application

Subject area: Pediatric

25. Which of the following clinical manifestations does the nurse assess to be present in a child in the paroxysmal stage of pertussis?

Select all that apply:

[   ] **1.** Sneezing

[   ] **2.** Low-grade fever

[   ] **3.** Flushed cheeks

[   ] **4.** Waning of paroxysmal coughing

[   ] **5.** High-pitched crowing

[   ] **6.** Protruding tongue

26. The clinical assignments on a pediatric respiratory unit have been made for the day. Which of the following assignments should be questioned?

1. Unlicensed assistive personnel are assigned to walk children with croup

2. A licensed practical nurse is assigned to teach a class to parents on sudden infant death syndrome

3. Unlicensed assistive personnel are assigned to help children who have cystic fibrosis to eat

4. A licensed practical nurse is assigned to administer a prescribed bronchodilator to a child with asthma

27. The nurse took respiratory rates on the following four pediatric clients. Which of the following clients should the nurse report as having an abnormal respiratory rate?

1. A 6-month-old infant who has respirations of 45 breaths per minute

2. A 2-year-old child who has respirations of 30 breaths per minute

3. A 10-year-old who has respirations of 28 breaths per minute

4. An 18-year-old who has respirations of 25 breaths per minute

Answer: 3, 5, 6

Rationale: The classic clinical manifestation of pertussis (whooping cough) is the "whoop" or high-pitched crowing sound that is heard at the end of the cough during the paroxysmal stage of the disease. Other clinical manifestations found in the paroxysmal stage include flushed cheeks, bulging eyes, and a protruding tongue. Sneezing and a low-grade fever are found during the catarrhal stage, when manifestations of an upper respiratory infection occur. A waning of the paroxysmal coughing is characteristic during the convalescent stage.

Nursing process: Assessment

Client need: Health Promotion and Maintenance

Cognitive level: Analysis

Subject area: Pediatric

Answer: 2

Rationale: Unlicensed assistive personnel may help a child walk and eat. A licensed practical nurse may administer a bronchodilator to a child with asthma. It is inappropriate to assign a licensed practical nurse to teach a class on sudden infant death syndrome. A registered nurse should be given responsibility for teaching such a class.

Nursing process: Analysis

Client need: Management of Care

Cognitive level: Analysis

Subject area: Legal and Ethical Issues

Answer: 4

Rationale: The respiratory rate of an infant from birth to 6 months is 30 to 50 breaths per minute. Children between 6 months and 2 years of age would have respirations from 20 to 30 breaths per minute. Children between 3 and 10 years of age have respirations between 20 and 28 breaths per minute. The respiratory rate of children between 10 and 14 years of age is between 16 and 20 breaths per minute. The respiratory rate of children between 16 and 18 years of age would be between 12 and 20 breaths per minute. An 18-year-old who has respirations of 25 breaths per minute is experiencing some degree of respiratory distress and that finding should be reported.

Nursing process: Evaluation

Client need: Health Promotion and Maintenance

Cognitive level: Analysis

Subject area: Pediatric

28. Which of the following should the nurse include in the instructions given to parents of a child with an allergy on methods to reduce allergen exposure?

Select all that apply:

[   ] 1. Trim household plants of dead leaves daily

[   ] 2. Exercise in cool, dry areas

[   ] 3. Clean moldy areas with 1:10 bleach solution

[   ] 4. Keep pets in uncarpeted areas

[   ] 5. Avoid strong odors

[   ] 6. Maintain laundry water at 37.8°C, or 100°F

29. Which of the following nursing interventions should the nurse include in the plan of care for a child with acute spasmodic laryngitis?

1. Administer antipyretic

2. Provide cold steam in the bedroom from a humidifier

3. Avoid exposure to the night air

4. Administer corticosteroids

30. The nurse is caring for a child suspected of having bacterial tracheitis. Which of the following is the primary clinical manifestation that the nurse assesses supporting this diagnosis?

1. Fever

2. Brassy cough

3. Thick purulent tracheal secretions

4. Inspiratory stridor

Answer: 3, 4, 5

Rationale: Household plants, strong odors, and exercising in cool, dry areas should be avoided in the plan of care for a child with an allergy. Moldy surfaces should be cleaned with a 1:10 bleach solution. Pets should be kept in uncarpeted areas that are easy to clean. Laundry water should be maintained at 54.4°C, or 130°F.

Nursing process: Planning

Client need: Health Promotion and Maintenance

Cognitive level: Application

Subject area: Pediatric

Answer: 2

Rationale: Acute spasmodic laryngitis is characterized by sudden, brief laryngeal obstructions that occur primarily at night. There is no fever, so antipyretics are not administered. Corticosteroids are also not administered. Exposure to the night air may terminate the laryngeal spasm. It is appropriate to provide steam from a hot bath or shower or cold steam from a humidifier to relieve mild clinical manifestations.

Nursing process: Planning

Client need: Health Promotion and Maintenance

Cognitive level: Application

Subject area: Pediatric

Answer: 3

Rationale: Bacterial tracheitis is a bacterial infection involving the mucosa of the upper trachea. Although fever, brassy cough, and inspiratory stridor are all clinical manifestations of bacterial tracheitis, the hallmark manifestation diagnostic of the condition is thick, purulent tracheal secretions. If left untreated, these secretions may result in airway obstruction or even respiratory arrest.

Nursing process: Assessment

Client need: Health Promotion and Maintenance

Cognitive level: Analysis

Subject area: Pediatric

CHAPTER

Cardiovascular Disorders

31

1. When caring for a child with a ventricular septal defect (VSD), the nurse should monitor for which clinical manifestations of hemodynamic alterations?

    Select all that apply:

    [   ] **1.** Pulmonic murmur

    [   ] **2.** Bradycardia

    [   ] **3.** Tachypnea

    [   ] **4.** Fatigue

    [   ] **5.** Dyspnea

    [   ] **6.** Anxiety

2. The nurse is reviewing the chart of a child with coarctation of the aorta. Which of the following findings would the nurse anticipate?

    1. Congestive heart failure

    2. Cerebral hypertension

    3. Hypoxemia

    4. Femoral artery hypertension

3. The nurse is planning care for a 2-year-old child immediately following cardiac catheterization. Which of these activities should have the highest priority?

    1. Change the dressing at the puncture site

    2. Apply direct pressure to the catheterization site for at least 15 minutes

    3. Monitor the heart rate for at least one minute during vital signs

    4. Start oral fluids

4. The nurse includes which of the following in a discharge teaching plan for parents of a child who has just undergone a cardiac catheterization for a cardiac defect?

    1. Monitor the dressing and stitches until the return appointment

    2. Maintain the postsurgical clear liquid diet for 48 hours

    3. Use a home cardiac monitoring system

    4. Administer antibiotics for two weeks

Answer: 3, 4, 5

Rationale: Ventricular septal defect is an abnormal connection between the right and left ventricles. Tachypnea, dyspnea, and fatigue are clinical manifestations that may indicate worsening hemodynamics and possible congestive heart failure. Pulmonic murmur, bradycardia, and anxiety are not manifestations of hemodynamic changes in ventricular septal defects.

Nursing process: Assessment

Client need: Health Promotion and Maintenance

Cognitive level: Application

Subject area: Pediatric

Answer: 2

Rationale: Coarctation of the aorta is a stenosis most commonly located within the thoracic aorta that increases systemic resistance at the site of the coarctation. This causes an increase in pressure proximal to the coarctation, causing hypertension in the cerebral arteries. Arteries distal to the coarctation have reduced pressure, causing lower extremity hypotension.

Nursing process: Analysis

Client need: Health Promotion and Maintenance

Cognitive level: Analysis

Subject area: Pediatric

Answer: 2

Rationale: Direct pressure on the site for 15 minutes and frequent monitoring of the occlusive pressure dressing will decrease the risk of complications from hematoma or hemorrhage following cardiac catheterization. The dressing should not be changed immediately postprocedure, as disruption of the clot may cause life-threatening hemorrhage. Monitoring the heart rate for one minute during vital signs and starting oral fluids are appropriate actions in postoperative care, but are of lower priority in the assessment and care of the child immediately post-op.

Nursing process: Planning

Client need: Management of Care

Cognitive level: Analysis

Subject area: Legal and Ethical Issues

Answer: 4

Rationale: After a cardiac catheterization, the dressing will be removed before discharge and stitches are not necessary for this procedure. The postprocedure diet is the child's usual diet, and home cardiac monitors are not used after cardiac catheterization. Antibiotics are used for children with heart defects prophylactically to minimize the risk of infection.

Nursing process: Implementation

Client need: Reduction of Risk Potential

Cognitive level: Application

Subject area: Pediatric

5. The nurse asks the mother of a child suspected of having a congenital heart defect about eating patterns and activities. Based on an understanding of this child's condition, which of the following should the nurse consider before recommending a plan of care?

   1. Poor feeding and activity intolerance are common in children with congenital heart disease

   2. The child's favorite foods and playtime activities are essential to compliance with therapy

   3. The parenting techniques should be assessed

   4. Mealtimes should be coordinated to the child's activity schedule

6. The nurse is evaluating heart sounds in four children. Which of the following heart sounds found in a 4-year-old child does the nurse report as pathologic?

   1. S_1

   2. S_2

   3. S_3

   4. S_4

7. A 5-year-old child is scheduled for an echocardiogram. She asks the nurse if the test will hurt. Which of the following is the nurse's best response?

   1. "It is different for everyone."

   2. "I'm not sure. You should ask your physician."

   3. "There will be a jelly that will feel cool, but it won't hurt."

   4. "The various positions you will have to assume may cause a little discomfort."

8. The nurse is caring for a child with tetralogy of Fallot who experiences an episode of acute cyanosis. Which of the following is the primary clinical manifestation the nurse will assess?

   1. Decreased respiratory rate

   2. Decreased pulse rate and blood pressure

   3. Loss of consciousness

   4. Anxiousness and irritability

Answer: 1

Rationale: Poor appetite and feeding patterns and activity intolerance are common to many congenital heart diseases. This is the primary consideration for the nurse before recommending the child's plan of care.

Nursing process: Analysis

Client need: Health Promotion and Maintenance

Cognitive level: Application

Subject area: Pediatric

Answer: 4

Rationale: The S_1 and S_2 are normal heart sounds at the beginning (closure of A-V valves) and end (closure of semilunar valves) of ventricular systole. The S_3 sound occurs early in diastole and is considered normal in children and young adults, but is a sound of cardiac disease in older adults. S_4 is a rare sound and not heard in a normal heart.

Nursing process: Implementation

Client need: Health Promotion and Maintenance

Cognitive level: Analysis

Subject area: Pediatric

Answer: 3

Rationale: An echocardiogram is noninvasive and painless. The child needs to be reassured.

Nursing process: Analysis

Client need: Reduction of Risk Potential

Cognitive level: Analysis

Subject area: Pediatric

Answer: 4

Rationale: Tetralogy of Fallot is comprised of a ventral septal defect, pulmonary stenosis, right ventricular hypertrophy, and an overriding aorta. During a cyanotic spell, pulse and respiratory rates increase to compensate for decreased oxygen levels. Anxiety and irritability are the most common manifestation in children with hypoxic spells. Loss of consciousness is more likely to be seen in states of severe heart failure.

Nursing process: Assessment

Client need: Management of Care

Cognitive level: Analysis

Subject area: Pediatric

9. Which of the following should be included in the discharge teaching the nurse is preparing for the parents of a child with tetralogy of Fallot?

   1. A demonstration of suctioning procedures

   2. The signs of infection

   3. Use of the knee-chest position for cyanotic spells

   4. Complete bed rest

10. The nurse is caring for a child with Kawasaki disease. Which of the following would indicate to the nurse that the client's condition is deteriorating?

    1. Bradycardia

    2. Strep throat

    3. Arrhythmias

    4. Hypotension

11. The nurse would expect which of the following clinical manifestations to be present in a 9-month-old infant with hypoplastic left heart?

    Select all that apply:

    [ ] **1.** Heart murmur

    [ ] **2.** Cyanosis

    [ ] **3.** Hypertension

    [ ] **4.** Heart rate of 130 beats per minute

    [ ] **5.** Tachypnea

    [ ] **6.** Syncope

12. The nurse is administering digoxin (Lanoxin) to a child with cardiac disease. The nurse should report which of the following manifestations indicative of digoxin toxicity?

    Select all that apply:

    [ ] **1.** Hypertension

    [ ] **2.** Cyanosis

    [ ] **3.** Visual disturbances

    [ ] **4.** Inconsolability

    [ ] **5.** Weakness

    [ ] **6.** Headache

Answer: 3

Rationale: Tetralogy of Fallot is comprised of a ventral septal defect, pulmonary stenosis, right ventricular hypertrophy, and an overriding aorta. The use of the knee-chest position is effective in decreasing cardiac workload. Complete bed rest is inappropriate; as much normal activity as can be tolerated is encouraged. Signs of infection and suctioning are not a part of the care for a child with a tetralogy of Fallot.

Nursing process: Planning

Client need: Health Promotion and Maintenance

Cognitive level: Application

Subject area: Pediatric

Answer: 3

Rationale: Kawasaki disease is a multisystem vasculitis that affects the coronary arteries. Hypotension and strep throat are not manifestations seen in Kawasaki disease. Cardiac complications are the most serious and contribute to morbidity and mortality. Tachycardia, a gallop rhythm, and congestive heart failure may occur.

Nursing process: Analysis

Client need: Health Promotion and Maintenance

Cognitive level: Analysis

Subject area: Pediatric

Answer: 1, 2, 5

Rationale: Heart murmur and cyanosis would be characteristic of hypoplastic left heart. Heart rate of 130 at rest is within normal range for an infant. Increasing respiratory crackles could indicate an increased load on the right ventricle and increased potential for heart failure. Hypotension is also a manifestation.

Nursing process: Evaluation

Client need: Health Promotion and Maintenance

Cognitive level: Application

Subject area: Pediatric

Answer: 3, 5, 6

Rationale: Clinical manifestations of digoxin toxicity are visual disturbances, weakness, headache, apathy, and psychosis.

Nursing process: Analysis

Client need: Pharmacological and Parenteral Therapies

Cognitive level: Application

Subject area: Pharmacologic

13. The nurse is caring for a child with a possible diagnosis of rheumatic fever. Which of the following assessment findings does the nurse evaluate as a diagnostic criterion?

1. Decreased erythrocyte sedimentation rate

2. Bradycardia

3. Elevation of antistreptolysin (ASO) levels

4. Desquamation of the fingertips

14. When preparing discharge teaching for a family of a child recovering from rheumatic fever, the nurse's priority instruction is

1. the child needs to take prophylactic antibiotics to prevent endocarditis.

2. the child should resume school activities as soon as tolerated.

3. parents should inform the school nurse of the child's illness.

4. parents should monitor the child for poor appetite and growth.

15. Which of the following should the nurse include in the discharge instructions for an infant with an atrial septal defect?

1. A discussion of speech development

2. Cardiopulmonary resuscitation

3. The necessity of monitoring for obesity

4. Home oxygen saturation monitoring

16. A child's mother asks the nurse how her child got hypertension and what it means. In explaining hypertension in children, the nurse would most appropriately respond that in children hypertension "is

1. generally related to another disease process."

2. generally not treated."

3. usually nothing to worry about."

4. related to cholesterol levels."

Answer: 3

Rationale: Streptococcal infection precedes the development of rheumatic fever by approximately two weeks. Elevation of antistreptolysin (ASO) levels indicates a recent strep infection.

Nursing process: Evaluation

Client need: Reduction of Risk Potential

Cognitive level: Analysis

Subject area: Pediatric

Answer: 1

Rationale: Rheumatic fever is thought to be an autoimmune disorder related to group A streptococcal infection. Future streptococcal infection and the risk for endocarditis can be prevented with prophylactic antibiotic administration. Resuming school activities and informing the school nurse about the illness may be appropriate interventions, but they are of lower priority. Poor appetite and growth do not generally occur with rheumatic fever unless the child already has experienced significant heart damage.

Nursing process: Planning

Client need: Management of Care

Cognitive level: Application

Subject area: Legal and Ethical Issues

Answer: 2

Rationale: An atrial septal defect is an abnormal connection between the right and left atria. Children with any heart defect are at a higher risk for heart failure. Instruction in CPR increases parental confidence and prepares them to handle an emergency.

Nursing process: Planning

Client need: Health Promotion and Maintenance

Cognitive level: Application

Subject area: Pediatric

Answer: 1

Rationale: Secondary hypertension is much more common in children than primary hypertension. It is usually a manifestation of another disease process. Hypertension in children is of concern and treatable. The association with cholesterol is not applicable.

Nursing process: Analysis

Client need: Health Promotion and Maintenance

Cognitive level: Application

Subject area: Pediatric

17. Which of the following should the nurse include in the preoperative teaching for the parents of a child scheduled for cardiac surgery?

    1. A warning to avoid bringing toys from home to the hospital

    2. A warning that siblings should not visit

    3. Concepts of pain management

    4. A tour of the general pediatric care unit

18. A nurse caring for a young child with a newly diagnosed atrial septal defect would

    1. prepare the child for echocardiogram.

    2. discuss life expectancy with the parents.

    3. assess for signs of liver damage.

    4. monitor the child for cyanotic spells.

19. To reduce cardiac workload, the nurse should implement which of the following nursing interventions for a child in heart failure?

    1. Place the child in Trendelenburg position

    2. Encourage fluids

    3. Schedule regular meals three times a day

    4. Provide a quiet environment

20. The parents of a 3-year-old child with tetralogy of Fallot tell the nurse that their child frequently squats during play. Based on an understanding of tetralogy of Fallot, the nurse recognizes that this is

    1. normal for the child's developmental age.

    2. a sign of constipation.

    3. a compensatory mechanism.

    4. a disinterest in engaging in play.

Answer: 3

Rationale: It is appropriate to instruct the parents of a child scheduled for cardiac surgery in the concepts of pain management. Toys from home can be comforting to a hospitalized child as can sibling visits. Siblings are also comforted by seeing the child in person. While a tour of the intensive care unit is appropriate, the tour of general pediatrics can come later as necessary.

Nursing process: Planning

Client need: Health Promotion and Maintenance

Cognitive level: Application

Subject area: Pediatric

Answer: 1

Rationale: An atrial septal defect is an abnormality between the left and right atria. A chest x-ray and an echocardiogram are generally performed to demonstrate the increase in the heart size and location and size of the defect. Cyanotic spells are generally not seen in atrial septal defects. Cyanosis itself is rare unless the defect in the septum is large enough to allow significant mixing of oxygenated and unoxygenated blood.

Nursing process: Implementation

Client need: Health Promotion and Maintenance

Cognitive level: Application

Subject area: Pediatric

Answer: 4

Rationale: Placing a child with a cardiac condition in a Trendelenburg position and encouraging fluids would actually increase cardiac workload. The preferred method of feeding to reduce cardiac workload is to feed five to six small meals a day. A quiet environment reduces stress and anxiety, resulting in a reduced cardiac workload.

Nursing process: Implementation

Client need: Health Promotion and Maintenance

Cognitive level: Analysis

Subject area: Pediatric

Answer: 3

Rationale: Tetralogy of Fallot is comprised of a ventral septal defect, pulmonary stenosis, right ventricular hypertrophy, and an overriding aorta. Squatting helps the child's circulatory system compensate for episodes of hypoxemia, especially during active periods.

Nursing process: Analysis

Client need: Health Promotion and Maintenance

Cognitive level: Analysis

Subject area: Pediatric

21. Which of the following should the nurse include in the plan of care for a child diagnosed with secondary hypertension?

   1. Weight control

   2. Managing cholesterol levels

   3. Use of diuretics

   4. Treatment of the underlying condition

22. The nurse caring for an infant with patent ductus arteriosus informs the parents that corrective surgery will prevent

   1. pulmonary vascular congestion.

   2. increased systemic venous pressure.

   3. cerebral vascular hemorrhage.

   4. hepatomegaly.

23. Which of the following is the nurse's priority intervention in a child with pulmonary stenosis?

   1. Monitor for indications of congestive heart failure

   2. Educate the parents regarding home medications

   3. Provide sensory preparation for a chest x-ray

   4. Discuss the child's nutritional and developmental needs

Answer: 4

Rationale: Secondary hypertension in a child is related to an underlying disease process. Treatment of that condition will most commonly significantly improve the hypertension. Weight control, use of diuretics, and managing the cholesterol level are common treatments for primary hypertension, which is rare in children.

Nursing process: Planning

Client need: Health Promotion and Maintenance

Cognitive level: Application

Subject area: Pediatric

Answer: 1

Rationale: The ductus arteriosus is a direct connection between the main pulmonary artery and the aorta. When the connection remains open several weeks after birth in a full-term infant, it is a patent ductus arteriosus. Patent ductus arteriosus causes an increase in blood flow in the reverse of what it was in fetal life as systemic pressure increases relative to pulmonary pressures. This causes an increase in pulmonary flow through the pulmonary artery. Pulmonary vascular congestion is the risk in this case.

Nursing process: Implementation

Client need: Health Promotion and Maintenance

Cognitive level: Analysis

Subject area: Pediatric

Answer: 1

Rationale: Pulmonary stenosis is a narrowing of the pulmonary valve and obstruction of the blood flow from the right ventricle to the lungs. Monitoring the child for congestive heart failure is the priority as it is potentially life threatening. Provision of sensory preparation for the x-ray is also important but not as significant as monitoring for CHF. Educating the parents about home medications and discussing the child's nutritional and developmental needs are appropriate interventions later in the hospitalization.

Nursing process: Implementation

Client need: Management of Care

Cognitive level: Analysis

Subject area: Legal and Ethical Issues

24. A child with an atrioventricular canal has been experiencing difficulty breathing and productive cough for three days. On admission, the nurse notes nasal flaring and retractions. At this point, the nurse's priority action is to

1. inform the physician of the client's worsening condition.

2. administer oxygen via mask.

3. reassure the parents.

4. obtain the child's weight.

25. The nurse is assessing an infant who has been transferred from another facility for examination of possible cardiac anomalies. The child has congestive heart failure, is severely cyanotic, and is on mechanical ventilation. The chest x-ray shows an abnormally large right ventricle and a very small left ventricle. The nurse recognizes that this is most likely

1. coarctation of the aorta.

2. atrioventricular canal defect.

3. truncus arteriosus.

4. hypoplastic left heart syndrome.

26. The registered nurse is preparing clinical assignments for a pediatric unit. Which of the following nursing assignments may be delegated to a licensed practical nurse?

1. Instruct the parents of a child with septal defect in cardiopulmonary resuscitation

2. Inform the parents of a child with an atrioventricular canal of the clinical manifestations of congestive heart failure

3. Assist a child with tetralogy of Fallot to a knee-chest position during an acute hypoxic spell

4. Assess a child with tricuspid atresia for growth retardation and failure to thrive

Answer: 2

Rationale: An atrioventricular canal is a defect that allows blood to flow among all four chambers. An atrial septal defect is continuous with a ventricular septal defect along the septum, also affecting both A-V valves (mitral and tricuspid), creating essentially one large chamber. Blood flow direction depends on the child's peripheral resistance and pulmonary resistance as well as ventricular pressures. This defect is seen in Down syndrome. This client is experiencing labored breathing and requires oxygen immediately. This can be applied quickly before calling the physician. Reassuring the parents and obtaining a weight are also important interventions, but immediate oxygen could reduce the difficulty of breathing for this child and help stabilize the condition.

Nursing process: Implementation

Client need: Management of Care

Cognitive level: Analysis

Subject area: Legal and Ethical Issues

Answer: 4

Rationale: Hypoplastic left heart syndrome is characterized by a lack of development of the left ventricle secondary to mitral valve atresia or aortic atresia. The result is a small hypoplastic left ventricle not capable of cardiac function.

Nursing process: Analysis

Client need: Health Promotion and Maintenance

Cognitive level: Analysis

Subject area: Pediatric

Answer: 3

Rationale: Nursing assignments involving skills such as instructing, informing, or assessing should be performed only by a registered nurse. A licensed practical nurse may assist a child with tetralogy of Fallot to a knee-chest position during an acute hypoxic spell because the initial instruction has taken place.

Nursing process: Planning

Client need: Management of Care

Cognitive level: Analysis

Subject area: Legal and Ethical Issues

Gastrointestinal Disorders

32

1. A mother brings an 8-month-old infant into the health clinic. An examination reveals that the infant's height and weight are below the fifth percentile, skin is dry and wrinkled, abdomen protrudes, and muscle wasting is evident. The most appropriate nursing diagnosis for this child at this time would be

   1. risk for injury related to parental abuse.

   2. failure to thrive related to unknown causes.

   3. diarrhea related to deficiency in essential nutrients.

   4. social isolation related to lack of maternal-infant bonding.

2. Which assessment provides the nurse with the most accurate information regarding a 6-month-old child admitted with a tentative diagnosis of nonorganic failure to thrive (NFTT)?

   Select all that apply:

   [ ] **1.** Irritable

   [ ] **2.** Periorbital edema

   [ ] **3.** Taut skin

   [ ] **4.** Muscle wasting

   [ ] **5.** Uninterested in the environment

   [ ] **6.** Responds to stimulation

3. An infant, who has had a cleft palate repair, is positioned side-lying or on the back. The rationale for this positioning is that it

   1. allows observation of the suture line.

   2. decreases anxiety.

   3. promotes drainage.

   4. facilitates oral intake.

4. The mother of an infant who has had a cleft lip repair tells the nurse that the physician said it was very important not to let the baby cry and wants to know why. Which of the following is the appropriate response by the nurse? "Crying

   1. impairs breathing."

   2. stresses the sutures."

   3. may result in gagging."

   4. leads to crusting."

Answer: 2

Rationale: A diagnosis of failure to thrive is an appropriate nursing diagnosis for an 8-month-old infant that falls below the fifth percentile, has dry, wrinkled skin, protruding abdomen, and muscle wasting. Although a child with diarrhea may have the clinical manifestations of failure to thrive, diarrhea is not a presenting manifestation. Diarrhea is a diagnosis in itself, but may be a defining characteristic of imbalanced nutrition.

Nursing process: Analysis

Client need: Health Promotion and Maintenance

Cognitive level: Analysis

Subject area: Pediatric

Answer: 4, 5

Rationale: In cases of nonorganic failure to thrive, the cause may be a variety of psychosocial factors such as lack of interest in the environment. Muscle wasting results from the disinterest in food. These children may be below normal in intellectual development, language skills, and social interactions, and their weight falls below the third to fifth percentiles. Irritability is found in a variety of gastrointestinal disorders such as colic. Periorbital edema and taut skin are typical manifestations of dehydration.

Nursing process: Assessment

Client need: Health Promotion and Maintenance

Cognitive level: Application

Subject area: Pediatric

Answer: 3

Rationale: After surgery for a cleft lip and palate repair, increased salivation is expected and aspiration is a potential complication. Positioning the child in a side-lying position maintains an open airway and facilitates drainage. The suture line is usually not observed unless bleeding is suspected. The rationale for the side-lying is to maintain a patent airway and promote drainage, which in turn will relieve anxiety. Prone position is not suggested as a means to facilitate feeding unless the medical condition prevents any other positioning.

Nursing process: Evaluation

Client need: Basic Care and Comfort

Cognitive level: Analysis

Subject area: Pediatric

Answer: 2

Rationale: Crying stretches the facial muscles, especially those around the lips, which stresses the suture line and leads to potential separation of the incision site following a cleft lip and repair. Impairment of breathing and gagging are more of an issue with cleft palate. Scarring occurs as a result of suture line crusting and tissue trauma from rubbing.

Nursing process: Analysis

Client need: Health Promotion and Maintenance

Cognitive level: Application

Subject area: Pediatric

5. Which of the following interventions is a priority for the nurse to implement in the postoperative care of a child with a cleft lip repair?

   1. Assess for edema of the tongue, lips, and mucous membranes

   2. Place the child prone to facilitate drainage

   3. Encourage the parents to limit their visits to allow the child to rest

   4. Restrain the child's arms with blankets to prevent the child from rubbing the suture line

6. Which of the following is the first intervention to include in the initial postoperative care of an infant following a bilateral cleft lip and palate repair?

   1. Clean the suture line to prevent formation of crusts

   2. Maintain nothing by mouth until the incision is sealed

   3. Restrain all extremities to prevent rubbing of the face and lip

   4. Administer sedation to prevent picking at the incision site

7. Ongoing nursing measures for the infant with a tracheoesophageal fistula (TEF) include

   1. observing respiratory status.

   2. isolating for respiratory precautions.

   3. keeping the room lights dimmed.

   4. giving slow oral feedings.

8. When planning the care of an infant suspected of having a tracheoesophageal fistula (TEF), it is critical for the nurse to

   1. hold the infant in an upright position after feeding.

   2. feed the infant by enteral feedings.

   3. feed the infant slowly.

   4. hold all feedings.

Answer: 1

Rationale: Trauma to the mucous membranes of the mouth that occurs with a cleft lip repair causes edema, leading to the respiratory distress and potential closing of the airway. Trauma to the suture line would occur in the prone position. Family-centered care is very important; because the parents can help calm the child, their visits are not limited. Elbow restraints, not blankets, are used to keep the child's hands away from the suture line.

Nursing process: Implementation

Client need: Management of Care

Cognitive level: Application

Subject area: Pediatric

Answer: 1

Rationale: Crusting of the suture line following a bilateral cleft lip and palate repair can lead to scarring and uneven closure of the incision. The child is not kept NPO and can take oral feedings when fully awake from anesthesia. Only the elbows are restrained to protect the suture line and only analgesics are used to control the pain.

Nursing process: Evaluation

Client need: Management of Care

Cognitive level: Application

Subject area: Pediatric

Answer: 1

Rationale: Because the fistula links the trachea and esophagus, acidic substances from the gastrointestinal tract can irritate the pulmonary system. Aspiration can occur from any secretions in the oropharyngeal cavity. There is no evidence of infection. Close observation of respiratory status is critical. The child is NPO until after surgical repair, because of the risk for aspiration.

Nursing process: Planning

Client need: Health Promotion and Maintenance

Cognitive level: Application

Subject area: Pediatric

Answer: 4

Rationale: In a tracheoesophageal fistula, the fistula forms an open connection between the trachea and esophagus. Because the client can aspirate anything entering the oral cavity, the goal of treatment is to prevent aspiration.

Nursing process: Planning

Client need: Management of Care

Cognitive level: Application

Subject area: Pediatric

9. When evaluating the assessment data of a preterm infant who has bloody stools, apnea, and bradycardia, the nurse should suspect

    1. intraventricular hemorrhage (IVH).

    2. necrotizing enterocolitis (NEC).

    3. meconium aspiration syndrome.

    4. esophageal atresia.

10. An infant with short bowel syndrome will be discharged home on total parenteral nutrition (TPN) and gastrostomy feedings. The nurse should include which of the following in the discharge instructions?

    1. Maintain a strict NPO status

    2. Provide a pacifier for nonnutritive sucking

    3. Calculate the caloric needs of the infant

    4. Secure TPN and gastrostomy tubing under diaper

11. A mother who brings a 6-week-old infant into the clinic reports that the baby has been spitting up for about three weeks. The vomitus has become more frequent and projectile since yesterday. In reviewing the child's record, the nurse notes that the child has gained only one pound since birth and suspects that the child may have pyloric stenosis. Which of the following assessment findings would confirm a diagnosis of pyloric stenosis?

    1. Immediate postfeeding vomiting

    2. Bile-stained vomitus

    3. An axillary temperature of 38°C, or 101°F

    4. A refusal to eat

12. Which of the following is the nurse's priority in the plan of care for a child admitted with pyloric stenosis?

    1. Assess the respiratory status

    2. Maintain thermoregulation

    3. Evaluate fluid status

    4. Assess perfusion

Answer: 2

Rationale: In necrotizing enterocolitis (NEC), the bowel is perforated as a result of necrosis, causing blood loss. Apnea and bradycardia are secondary to the hemorrhaging. The clinical manifestations are not always specific. Apnea and a low hematocrit are consistent with bleeding in the ventricles of the brain. Central apnea without hemorrhaging is expected with meconium aspiration. Evidence is not present for esophageal atresia.

Nursing process: Analysis

Client need: Health Promotion and Maintenance

Cognitive level: Analysis

Subject area: Pediatric

Answer: 2

Rationale: To ensure adequate growth and development in the infant, it is important to maintain developmentally appropriate behaviors even though the infant is not allowed anything by mouth. Since the child will be given enteral feeds through a gastrostomy tube, the child is not considered NPO. Calculating the caloric needs of the infant and securing the TPN and gastrostomy tube under the diaper do not promote developmentally appropriate behaviors.

Nursing process: Planning

Client need: Health Promotion and Maintenance

Cognitive level: Application

Subject area: Pediatric

Answer: 1

Rationale: In pyloric stenosis, the circular muscle of the pylorus thickens, causing constriction and obstruction of the gastric outlet. Projectile vomiting immediately after feeding is a cardinal indicator of pyloric stenosis. Bile-stained vomitus is not expected since bile is passed through the pyloric valve. Fever is an indication of an infection and is not usually seen with pyloric stenosis. With pyloric stenosis, a child will usually eat immediately after vomiting if a feeding is offered.

Nursing process: Assessment

Client need: Health Promotion and Maintenance

Cognitive level: Analysis

Subject area: Pediatric

Answer: 3

Rationale: Fluid and electrolyte imbalance is a problem because of the loss of gastric secretions and poor nutrition secondary to projectile vomiting in pyloric stenosis. Respiratory status and perfusion may be affected by severe imbalance, making it a priority to evaluate fluid status. Thermoregulation is not an issue with pyloric stenosis. Altered perfusion is a result of altered fluid balance.

Nursing process: Implementation

Client need: Management of Care

Cognitive level: Analysis

Subject area: Pediatric

13. A priority nursing diagnosis in the care of a child with pyloromyotomy is
    1. trauma related to a break in skin integrity.
    2. fluid deficit related to loss of gastric secretions.
    3. imbalanced nutrition: less than body requirements related to NPO status.
    4. ineffective breathing related to tissue trauma from vomiting.

14. In which of the following positions should the nurse place an infant following a pyloromyotomy?
    1. On the right side in a low-Fowler's position at all times
    2. In a prone position while sleeping
    3. On the right side with the head elevated after feeding
    4. On the left side in a semi-Fowler's position after feeding

15. The parents of a child with Hirschsprung's disease ask the nurse what the expected treatment is. Which of the following is the most appropriate response by the nurse?
    1. "You will be taught how to do daily neomycin enemas at home."
    2. "The nutritionist will discuss a gluten-free diet with you."
    3. "Surgery will be scheduled for a permanent colostomy."
    4. "The affected bowel segment will be surgically removed."

16. When planning the postoperative care of a child with Hirschsprung's disease, which of the following interventions should the nurse include?
    Select all that apply:
    [ ] 1. Monitor vital signs
    [ ] 2. Assess gastric pH
    [ ] 3. NPO
    [ ] 4. Strict intake and output
    [ ] 5. Administer daily enemas
    [ ] 6. Colostomy care

Answer: 2

Rationale: The priority nursing diagnosis following a pyloromyotomy is fluid status, because the loss of gastric secretions can lead to more serious dysfunction of the respiratory and cardiac systems. Tissue trauma is important but is not a priority at this time. The child is not placed NPO without maintaining nutritional status by parenteral fluids until the child is able to take nutrition by mouth. Mucous membrane irritation secondary to vomiting usually does not lead to ineffective breathing.

Nursing process: Evaluation

Client need: Management of Care

Cognitive level: Analysis

Subject area: Pediatric

Answer: 3

Rationale: Placing an infant on the right side with the head elevated after feeding facilitates gastric emptying and decreases the possibility of "dumping syndrome" following a pyloromyotomy. Prior to surgery, placing the infant on the left side with the head elevated reduces the risk of severe pyloric spasm. To reduce the risk of sudden infant death syndrome (SIDS), the infant is placed supine for sleep.

Nursing process: Planning

Client need: Reduction of Risk Potential

Cognitive level: Application

Subject area: Pediatric

Answer: 4

Rationale: Hirschsprung's disease, a congenital aganglionic megacolon, is a motility disorder of the bowel caused by the absence of parasympathetic ganglion cells in the large intestine. Feces accumulate proximal to the defect. The aganglionic segment must be removed to enable peristalsis to return, producing normal evacuation of fecal material. Antibiotic enemas are only given prior to surgery to reduce the intestinal flora. The colostomy is temporary, to allow the colon to rest before resection.

Nursing process: Analysis

Client need: Health Promotion and Maintenance

Cognitive level: Analysis

Subject area: Pediatric

Answer: 1, 3, 4, 6

Rationale: After the aganglionic segment has been removed in a child with Hirschsprung's disease, the child must be NPO until peristalsis returns. Monitoring vital signs and maintaining a strict intake and output are important to evaluate the fluid and nutritional status of the child. The child will have a temporary colostomy for several months to allow the colon to rest secondary to the tissue trauma. Gastric pH checks are performed with enteral tube placement, and the child would not have an ileostomy. Enemas are done prior to surgery and not after surgery.

Nursing process: Planning

Client need: Health Promotion and Maintenance

Cognitive level: Application

Subject area: Pediatric

17. The nurse caring for a child with Hirschsprung's disease documents the stools to have what characteristic appearance?

1. Tarry and tenacious
2. Currant jellylike
3. Frothy and foul smelling
4. Ribbonlike

18. When preparing a child with probable intussusception for a hydrostatic reduction procedure, the nurse should explain which of the following aspects of the procedure? The procedure will

1. blow air into a cavity of the bowel.
2. empty the bowel of all stool.
3. relax the bowel.
4. facilitate mixing the currant jellylike stool with normal stool.

19. The nurse assists a child with celiac disease to make which of the following menu selections?
Select all that apply:

[ ] 1. Whole wheat toast
[ ] 2. Cornbread
[ ] 3. Oatmeal
[ ] 4. Green beans
[ ] 5. Reuben sandwich with rye bread
[ ] 6. Canned tomato soup

20. Which of the following should the nurse perform to minimize reflux in a 4-month-old infant who has gastroesophageal reflux without other complications?

1. Place the infant in a Trendelenburg position after eating
2. Thicken formula with rice cereal
3. Administer continuous nasogastric tube feedings
4. Offer three meals

Answer: 4

Rationale: Ribbonlike stool is characteristically seen with Hirschsprung's disease. Tarry and tenacious stools would be related to high gastrointestinal bleeding. Currant jellylike stools are related to the presence of blood and mucus seen with intussusception. Frothy and foul-smelling stool would indicate cystic fibrosis.

Nursing process: Implementation

Client need: Health Promotion and Maintenance

Cognitive level: Analysis

Subject area: Pediatric

Answer: 1

Rationale: Intussusception occurs when one segment of the bowel telescopes into the lumen of an adjacent segment of intestine. The purpose of the hydrostatic reduction procedure is to pull the invaginated bowel out from another section of bowel, allowing normal fecal material to pass. The procedure uses barium or air insufflation; air insufflation is considered to be safer than barium insufflation. The procedure will not empty the bowel completely nor relax it. The currant jelly stools will stop when the bowel is no longer irritated.

Nursing process: Planning

Client need: Reduction of Risk Potential

Cognitive level: Analysis

Subject area: Pediatric

Answer: 2, 4

Rationale: Celiac disease is called a gluten-sensitive enteropathy and is caused by an intolerance to gluten, the protein component of wheat, rye, barley, and oats. Beans and corn do not contain the protein gluten. It is important to read labels of all prepared foods because many of these products contain flour made from wheat, barley, rye, or oats, all of which contain gluten.

Nursing process: Implementation

Client need: Basic Care and Comfort

Cognitive level: Application

Subject area: Pediatric

Answer: 2

Rationale: Gastroesophageal reflux is the reflux of the gastric contents into the lower portion of the esophagus through the lower esophageal sphincter. Thickened formula decreases acid reflux and increases the emptying time of the stomach. Reflux precautions include positioning the child supine or on the right side with head elevated. Continuous NG feedings are not necessary since the child can tolerate bolus feedings. To reduce the reflux process, small, frequent feedings are more appropriate than three large meals.

Nursing process: Planning

Client need: Health Promotion and Maintenance

Cognitive level: Application

Subject area: Pediatric

21. While assisting another nurse with the postoperative care of neonate with an omphalocele repair, the nurse explains that it is a priority to monitor which of the following?

    1. Blood pressure

    2. Pulse

    3. Respiration

    4. Skin

22. The triage nurse in the emergency department is evaluating the following four clients. Which client is the priority and a surgical emergency?

    1. A child with gastroschisis

    2. A child with hypertrophic pyloric stenosis

    3. A child with celiac disease

    4. A child with malrotation/volvulus

23. Which of the following serum bilirubin levels supports a diagnosis of pathologic jaundice?

    1. Concentrations greater than 2 mg/dl in cord blood

    2. An increase of more than 1 mg/dl in 24 hours

    3. Levels greater than 10 mg/dl in a full-term newborn

    4. An increase of 5 mg/dl or greater in 24 hours

Answer: 3

Rationale: An omphalocele is a congenital malformation that results from a failure of the intestines to reenter the abdominal cavity at approximately 7 weeks of gestation. The defect, which permits the abdominal contents to herniate through the abdominal cavity, is located centrally and includes the umbilical cord. Surgical intervention is the treatment of choice. Once the abdominal contents have been replaced into the peritoneal cavity, the organs place pressure on the diaphragm, which can lead to respiratory compromise. Decreased cardiac output, altered hemodynamics, and congestive heart failure occur secondary to a respiratory compromise.

Nursing process: Analysis

Client need: Reduction of Risk Potential

Cognitive level: Analysis

Subject area: Pediatric

Answer: 4

Rationale: Malrotation is an incomplete rotation of the midgut during the period of fetal development when the gut returns from the umbilical pouch to the abdominal cavity. With this condition, the bowel fails to rotate normally as it returns to the abdominal cavity and obstructs blood flow to the mesentery organs. This leads to bowel death and necrosis, which is not compatible with life. Malrotation is considered a surgical emergency. Gastroschisis is a congenital malformation where a defect in the abdominal wall allows a segment of the abdominal contents to herniate outside the abdominal cavity. Although surgery is the recommended treatment, it is not a priority. Hypertrophic pyloric stenosis involves a hypertrophic pyloric sphincter generally with a width four times normal that results in a narrow opening and gastric outlet obstruction. A pyloromyotomy is the surgical repair but not an emergency. Celiac disease is a gluten-sensitive enteropathy in which there is a permanent intolerance to gluten. Treatment involves providing a gluten-free diet.

Nursing process: Evaluation

Client need: Management of Care

Cognitive level: Analysis

Subject area: Pediatric

Answer: 4

Rationale: Pathologic jaundice is present when serum bilirubin exceeds 15 mg/dl at any time. Jaundice appears within the first 24 hours and is diagnosed when the serum bilirubin concentration in cord blood is greater than 4 mg/dl and there is an increase of 5 mg/dl or greater in 24 hours.

Nursing process: Assessment

Client need: Reduction of Risk Potential

Cognitive level: Analysis

Subject area: Pediatric

24. Which of the following nursing actions takes priority in the plan of care for an infant receiving phototherapy?

    1. Provide opportunities for parent-infant interaction

    2. Avoid bathing the infant who is receiving treatment

    3. Remove eye patches to allow assessment

    4. Interrupt treatment for 60 minutes per shift for tactile stimulation

25. Which of the following in a newborn's assessment should be reported as a critical sign of an imperforate anus?

    1. The first rectal temperature of 36.8°C, or 98.3°F

    2. The infant has not passed a meconium stool in the first 48 hours

    3. The infant has not voided six times in 24 hours

    4. There is a family history of congenital defects

26. The registered nurse is making the day's clinical assignments for a pediatric unit. Which of the following clinical assignments would be most appropriate to delegate to a licensed practical nurse?

    1. An infant with volvulus

    2. A child with short bowel syndrome

    3. An infant with esophageal atresia and tracheoesophageal fistula

    4. A child with celiac disease

Answer: 1

Rationale: Phototherapy is the use of high-intensity fluorescent lights as a way of reducing serum bilirubin levels to prevent kernicterus. Although the infant needs to stay under phototherapy, the infant can be removed for brief periods that should not last longer than 30 minutes. Since phototherapy interrupts parent-infant attachment during the first few days of life, it is considered very stressful for the child and family. Encouraging all opportunities for parent-infant interaction is the priority.

Nursing process: Planning

Client need: Reduction of Risk Potential

Cognitive level: Analysis

Subject area: Pediatric

Answer: 2

Rationale: An imperforate anus is an anorectal condition in which there is no obvious anal opening. A meconium stool is expected to pass within 48 hours after the neonate's birth. A rectal temperature would be indicative of a patent anus. Urine output is not indicative of an imperforate anus. A family history of congenital defects is not usually associated with an imperforate anus.

Nursing process: Assessment

Client need: Managment of Care

Cognitive level: Analysis

Subject area: Pediatric

Answer: 4

Rationale: A volvulus is a complication of malrotation. It occurs when an incompletely rotated bowel twists on itself. This leads to arterial obstruction, ischemia, and necrosis and is a surgical emergency. Short bowel syndrome is a condition that results from surgical resection of the intestine in cases of volvulus, Crohn's disease, or necrotizing enterocolitis. There is an inadequate surface area of the small intestine. Treatment focuses on maintaining optimal nutrition. This usually involves administration of total parenteral nutrition by a central line and enteral feeding by a nasogastric or gastrostomy tube, which require the skills of a registered nurse. Esophageal atresia and tracheoesophageal fistula generally occur together when the esophagus is incomplete and terminates before it reaches the stomach. After preventing aspiration pneumonia, treatment generally requires surgery and neonatal intensive care, which require the skills of a registered nurse. Celiac disease is a gluten-sensitive enteropathy caused by a permanent intolerance to gluten. Control involves medical management and control through a gluten-free diet. The licensed practical nurse can assist a child and parents of a child with celiac disease to select foods free of gluten.

Nursing process: Planning

Client need: Management of Care

Cognitive level: Analysis

Subject area: Pediatric

27. The nurse is caring for a preterm neonate who has necrotizing enterocolitis. Which of the following is a clinical manifestation that this infant's condition is deteriorating?

1. Cyanosis
2. Bloody stools
3. Decreased bowel sounds
4. Hypotension

28. Which of the following clinical manifestations should the nurse assess in a child suspected of having extrahepatic biliary atresia?

Select all that apply:

[ ] 1. Jaundice
[ ] 2. Regurgitation
[ ] 3. Light tan stools
[ ] 4. Nocturnal asthma
[ ] 5. Dark urine
[ ] 6. Failure to thrive

29. The nurse is reviewing the diagnostic criteria in a child with necrotizing enterocolitis. Which of the following findings is indicative of severe disease and perforation of the bowel?

1. Dilated bowel loops
2. Pneumatosis intestinalis
3. Pneumoperitoneum
4. Deep crypts on the intestinal mucosa

Answer: 4

Rationale: Necrotizing enterocolitis is a necrosis of the mucosa of the small and large intestine generally in preterm neonates. Classical features include abdominal tenderness and distention, bloody stools, decreased bowel sounds, increased gastric residuals, erythema of the abdominal wall, and bilious vomiting after feeding. Clinical manifestations of deterioration include bradycardia, apnea, lethargy, temperature instability, decreased urine output, and evidence of shock. A late deteriorating sign is hypotension.

Nursing process: Analysis

Client need: Reduction of Risk Potential

Cognitive level: Analysis

Subject area: Pediatric

Answer: 1, 3, 5, 6

Rationale: Extrahepatic biliary atresia is a progressive inflammatory process causing intrahepatic and extrahepatic bile duct fibrosis. Regurgitation and nocturnal asthma are clinical manifestations of gastroesophageal reflux. Jaundice, light tan stools, dark urine, and failure to thrive are clinical manifestations of extrahepatic biliary atresia.

Nursing process: Assessment

Client need: Health Promotion and Maintenance

Cognitive level: Application

Subject area: Pediatric

Answer: 3

Rationale: Necrotizing enterocolitis is a necrosis of the mucosa of the small and large intestine. Radiographic findings found in necrotizing enterocolitis include dilated bowel loops and pneumatosis intestinalis. Pneumoperitoneum or free air in the peritoneal cavity or portal circulation indicates severe disease and perforation of the bowel. Deep crypts on the intestinal mucosa are found in celiac disease.

Nursing process: Evaluation

Client need: Reduction of Risk Potential

Cognitive level: Analysis

Subject area: Pediatric

30. The nurse is caring for a child with inflammatory bowel disease. Which of the following should the nurse include in the plan of care?

1. Place the child on a gluten-free diet

2. Administer omeprazole (Prilosec)

3. Provide the child with increased calories

4. Monitor the child for melena

Answer: 3

Rationale: Inflammatory bowel disease (IBD) consists of ulcerative colitis and Crohn's disease because of an inflammation or ulceration of the small and large intestine. A gluten-free diet is the diet of choice with celiac disease. Although some children with inflammatory bowel disease poorly tolerate lactose, there is no special diet for IBD. Omeprazole (Prilosec) is a proton pump inhibitor used in the treatment of peptic ulcers. The goal of nutritional therapy is to replace nutrients and increase calories in the diet to maintain normal metabolic functions. Melena or black tarry stools occur in peptic ulcer disease.

Nursing process: Planning

Client need: Health Promotion and Maintenance

Cognitive level: Application

Subject area: Pediatric

Metabolic and Endocrine Disorders

33

1. Which of the following should the nurse include in the nursing assessment of the endocrine system in a child?
    1. The number and type of pets in the home
    2. Family health history
    3. Dietary intake of calcium
    4. History of streptococcus infection

2. A nurse is caring for a client with short stature from a growth hormone (GH) deficiency. Which of the following measures would be essential to include in the child's plan of care?
    1. Monitor linear growth
    2. Encourage at least two glasses of milk per day
    3. Assess the skin for bruising
    4. Instruct the child on weight-control issues

3. Which of the following children being cared for by the nurse is in need of treatment for precocious puberty?
    1. A 10-year-old Caucasian girl with beginning breast development
    2. An 8-year-old African-American girl with breast development
    3. An 8-year-old boy with secondary sex characteristics
    4. A 10-year-old boy with beginning pubic hair

Answer: 2

Rationale: The family health history is important, as many endocrine disorders run in families. The number of pets, calcium intake, and history of streptococcus infection are not specifically relevant to the endocrine system.

Nursing process: Assessment

Client need: Health Promotion and Maintenance

Cognitive level: Application

Subject area: Pediatric

Answer: 1

Rationale: Growth hormone deficiency is an endocrine disorder in which there is a poor growth in stature as a result of a failure of the pituitary to produce sufficient growth hormone. Linear growth is monitored to evaluate the need for medication prior to treatment and the effectiveness of medication during treatment. Bruising and weight control are not part of growth hormone deficiency. Monitoring milk intake is part of a normal healthy diet in children and not just in growth hormone deficiency.

Nursing process: Planning

Client need: Health Promotion and Maintenance

Cognitive level: Application

Subject area: Pediatric

Answer: 3

Rationale: The development of secondary sex characteristics in boys before age 9 years is abnormal and in need of treatment for precocious puberty. A 10-year-old Caucasian girl with beginning breast development, an 8-year-old African-American girl with breast development, and a 10-year-old boy with beginning pubic hair are considered within the normal range. Precocious puberty is defined as occurring in Caucasian girls with developing breasts before 7 years of age and before 6 years of age in African-American girls. Children with precocious puberty have accelerated growth rates, develop secondary sex characteristics earlier than normal, and exhibit advanced bone age, acne, body odor, and some behavioral changes. Psychosocial development is generally age-appropriate.

Nursing process: Evaluation

Client need: Health Promotion and Maintenance

Cognitive level: Analysis

Subject area: Pediatric

4. Which of the following instructions is most appropriate for the nurse to give the parents of a child with diabetes insipidus?

   1. Technique for administering desmopressin acetate (DDAVP)

   2. Directions for performing a urine dipstick

   3. Procedure for giving an insulin injection

   4. Provisions necessary for providing a safe home environment

5. The nurse is caring for a 10-year-old child who has been diagnosed with acquired hypothyroidism. The parents ask the nurse for information on the disorder. Which of the following should the nurse include in the information given to the parents?

   1. Infection is the most likely cause

   2. Weight loss is a common clinical manifestation

   3. A thyroid replacement drug will be given

   4. Fevers and diarrhea are common

6. The nurse should include which of the following in the preprocedure instruction given to the parents of a child scheduled for a thyroid function test?

   1. NPO after midnight

   2. A high-carbohydrate meal should be eaten the day before the test

   3. A concentrated glucose will be given just prior to the test

   4. It is important that the child remain still during the procedure

7. The nurse is assessing a child's thyroid status. Which of the following assessment findings should the nurse document as a subjective finding?

   1. Fatigue

   2. Weight loss

   3. Hypertension

   4. Tachycardia

Answer: 1

Rationale: Desmopressin acetate (DDAVP) is the drug of choice for the child with diabetes insipidus. It is a synthetic antidiuretic hormone that acts to increase the absorption of water in the kidney. It is important that the parents learn how to administer the drug intranasally or orally. Diabetes insipidus is a disorder of water regulation in which there is a deficiency of the antidiuretic hormone. Urine dipstick and insulin administration would be used by parents of a child with diabetes mellitus. Home safety is important for all children.

Nursing process: Planning

Client need: Pharmacological and Parenteral Therapies

Cognitive level: Application

Subject area: Pharmacologic

Answer: 3

Rationale: Acquired hypothyroidism is an endocrine disorder that generally has an autoimmune cause. It is associated with weight gain, hypothyroidism, and constipation. Thyroid replacement medication must be taken daily.

Nursing process: Planning

Client need: Health Promotion and Maintenance

Cognitive level: Application

Subject area: Pediatric

Answer: 4

Rationale: There is no special preparation for thyroid function tests except for the child to hold still during the procedure. There is no need for a child to be NPO or eat a high-carbohydrate diet or concentrated glucose before the test.

Nursing process: Planning

Client need: Reduction of Risk Potential

Cognitive level: Application

Subject area: Pediatric

Answer: 1

Rationale: A subjective finding is something the client tells the nurse. An objective finding is one the nurse detects through evaluative procedures. Fatigue, something felt and described by the child, is a subjective finding. Weight loss, hypertension, and tachycardia are all objective findings.

Nursing process: Assessment

Client need: Health Promotion and Maintenance

Cognitive level: Application

Subject area: Pediatric

8. The nurse is caring for a child with Cushing's syndrome. Which of the following should the nurse include in the plan of care?

   1. Encourage a diet high in carbohydrates

   2. Administer medication to slow growth

   3. Offer emotional support for premature puberty

   4. Encourage a diet low in sodium

9. The nurse is working with the parents of a newborn with ambiguous genitalia due to congenital adrenal hyperplasia (CAH). Which of the following instructions should the nurse provide the parents?

   1. Glucose monitoring should be performed

   2. Salt should be restricted in the daily formula

   3. Extra blankets will be used because of heat intolerance

   4. An assignment of sex may be delayed

10. When planning the education for the parents of a child with type 1 diabetes mellitus, which of the following should the nurse include?

    1. Restrict the activity of the child

    2. Rotate insulin injection sites

    3. Avoid letting the child perform the home testing of blood sugar

    4. Encourage a high-carbohydrate diet

11. The nurse is admitting a child with suspected type 1 diabetes mellitus. Which of the following questions should the nurse ask the parents?

    1. "Has the child's number and type of bowel movements changed?"

    2. "Has the child experienced nocturia or bedwetting?"

    3. "How much exercise does the child get?"

    4. "Does the child complain of headaches?"

Answer: 4

Rationale: Hypertension is common in a child with Cushing's syndrome due to sodium retention, so limiting the salt intake will help control blood pressure. Weight gain is common and a high carbohydrate intake would contribute to weight gain. Premature puberty is not part of Cushing's syndrome because growth is slowed.

Nursing process: Planning

Client need: Health Promotion and Maintenance

Cognitive level: Application

Subject area: Pediatric

Answer: 4

Rationale: Congenital adrenal hyperplasia is a group of inherited disorders characterized by a deficiency of an enzyme essential for synthesis of cortisol and occasionally aldosterone. Ambiguous genitalia are difficult for parents to adjust to and accept. The process of gender selection is controversial, which is stressful for the family, and an assignment of sex may be delayed. There is no heat intolerance with congenital adrenal hyperplasia; heat intolerance occurs with hyperthyroidism.

Nursing process: Planning

Client need: Health Promotion and Maintenance

Cognitive level: Application

Subject area: Pediatric

Answer: 2

Rationale: Rotation of injection sites is one of the most important things to do in a child with type 1 diabetes mellitus. Rotating the site allows for the best absorption and most accurate dosing of insulin. Blood sugar testing is often one of the earliest skills a child with type 1 diabetes mellitus acquires. A high-carbohydrate diet would contribute to an elevated blood sugar level. Activity is important in the treatment and management of diabetes.

Nursing process: Planning

Client need: Health Promotion and Maintenance

Cognitive level: Application

Subject area: Pediatric

Answer: 2

Rationale: Frequent urination (polyuria) is one of the classic clinical manifestations of diabetes mellitus along with increased appetite (polyphagia) and increased thirst (polydipsia). Weight loss is also common in children.

Nursing process: Assessment

Client need: Health Promotion and Maintenance

Cognitive level: Application

Subject area: Pediatric

12. Which of the following is a priority for the nurse to include in the discharge instructions for the family of a child with type 2 diabetes?
    1. How to recognize complex blood sugar patterns
    2. Changes the family will need to make
    3. Daily blood sugar and ketone testing
    4. Accurate carbohydrate counting

13. Which of the following statements by a child with type 2 diabetes mellitus indicates a lack of understanding about the disease and a need for further instructions?
    1. "I will exercise regularly."
    2. "I will count the carbohydrates I eat."
    3. "I will avoid junk food high in calories."
    4. "I will take my injections of insulin on time."

14. The parents of a child with newly diagnosed type 2 diabetes mellitus want to know more about the condition. The nurse should include which of the following?
    1. Activity is not important with type 2 diabetes.
    2. Daily insulin injections are required.
    3. Type 2 diabetes does not require intervention.
    4. Type 2 diabetes is increasing in frequency in children.

15. The nurse implements which intervention when caring for a child with hypoparathyroidism?
    1. Instruct the parents about the signs of hypocalcemia
    2. Administer a daily thyroid hormone replacement drug
    3. Instruct the parents that the child should wear a medical alert bracelet
    4. Weigh the child daily

Answer: 3

Rationale: In type 2 diabetes mellitus, the pancreas still produces some insulin. However, the body is unable to use the insulin effectively and unable to produce enough insulin to lower the glucose. Type 2 diabetes can usually be managed with an oral hypoglycemic agent, exercise, diet, and home glucose monitoring. Testing of blood sugar and ketone levels is the priority and basis for all care for children with diabetes. Recognition of complex blood sugar patterns, carbohydrate counting, and changes the family needs to make are important but not the priority.

Nursing process: Planning

Client need: Management of Care

Cognitive level: Analysis

Subject area: Pediatric

Answer: 4

Rationale: Because the pancreas still produces some insulin in type 2 diabetes mellitus, it is generally managed with oral hypoglycemic drugs, and lifestyle changes such as a healthy diet, regular exercise, carbohydrate counting, and avoidance of high-calorie junk food.

Nursing process: Evaluation

Client need: Health Promotion and Maintenance

Cognitive level: Application

Subject area: Pediatric

Answer: 4

Rationale: Type 2 diabetes is increasing in frequency, even in youth. Type 2 diabetes mellitus generally can be controlled with oral hypoglycemic drugs, diet, exercise, and home glucose monitoring.

Nursing process: Planning

Client need: Health Promotion and Maintenance

Cognitive level: Application

Subject area: Pediatric

Answer: 1

Rationale: Hypoparathyroidism is a disorder of the parathyroid hormone. The primary function of the parathyroid hormone is to maintain the serum calcium. Thyroid replacement is used with hypothyroidism. Weight is not directly affected by the parathyroid glands and daily weighing is not necessary. A medical alert bracelet is also unnecessary. A medical alert bracelet should be worn for disorders such as Addison's disease.

Nursing process: Implementation

Client need: Health Promotion and Maintenance

Cognitive level: Application

Subject area: Pediatric

16. Leuprolide acetate (Lupron) is prescribed for a child with precocious puberty. Based on an understanding of this drug, the nurse caring for this child should

    1. inform the parents that shakiness and a general malaise are common adverse reactions.

    2. administer the drug intramuscularly once every four weeks.

    3. encourage the child to increase fluids.

    4. assess blood pressure and respiration prior to giving the drug.

17. Which of the following tasks may the registered nurse delegate to unlicensed assistive personnel?

    1. Documentation of the urinary output after toileting a child with diabetes mellitus

    2. Informing a child with growth hormone deficiency that a growth hormone injection will be given

    3. Monitoring a neonate suspected of having hypoparathyroidism for jittery movements during the bath

    4. Assessing the presence of arthralgia, fatigue, and tachycardia when ambulating a child with hyperthyroidism

18. The nurse receives report on a newborn who is lethargic and exhibiting jittery movements during morning care. Which of the following is the priority nursing intervention?

    1. Administer oral calcium gluconate

    2. Evaluate the response to feeding

    3. Administer intravenous calcium

    4. Assess for the presence of bone deformities

19. The nurse should monitor a child receiving propylthiouracil (PTU) for which of the following adverse reactions indicating toxicity?

Select all that apply:

[   ] **1.** Tachycardia

[   ] **2.** Headaches

[   ] **3.** Sore throat

[   ] **4.** Loss of taste

[   ] **5.** Nausea

[   ] **6.** Fever

Answer: 2

Rationale: Leuprolide acetate (Lupron) depot injection is a GnRH analog administered once every three to four weeks by subcutaneous or intramuscular injection or intranasally two to three times a day for precocious puberty. Shakiness and a general malaise are not common adverse reactions, and assessing blood pressure or respiration prior to administration are not necessary. Fluids need not be increased with Lupron.

Nursing process: Planning

Client need: Pharmacological and Parenteral Therapies

Cognitive level: Application

Subject area: Pharmacologic

Answer: 1

Rationale: Although unlicensed assistive personnel may ambulate and bathe a child, assessing and monitoring for the presence of an abnormality are not tasks that can be delegated to them. Unlicensed assistive personnel can never inform or instruct new information. Unlicensed assistive personnel may document the urinary output after toileting a child.

Nursing process: Planning

Client need: Management of Care

Cognitive level: Analysis

Subject area: Legal and Ethical Issues

Answer: 3

Rationale: Jittery movements in a lethargic newborn indicate the presence of hypoparathyroidism and of tetany. This poses an emergency situation, and intravenous calcium is the treatment of choice and the priority. A poor feeding behavior would be assessed in any newborn but is not the priority. Oral gluconate is reserved for the nonacute treatment of transient hypocalcemia. Assessing for the presence of bone deformities would be done on a growing child and is not a priority in a newborn.

Nursing process: Implementation

Client need: Management of Care

Cognitive level: Analysis

Subject area: Legal and Ethical Issues

Answer: 3, 6

Rationale: Propylthiouracil (PTU) is an antithyroid drug used to treat hyperthyroidism. It relieves the clinical manifestations of tachycardia, restlessness, and tremors associated with hyperthyroidism. Nausea, headaches, and loss of taste are mild adverse reactions. A sore throat and high fever are adverse reactions indicating agranulocytosis, which is serious and potentially fatal.

Nursing process: Assessment

Client need: Pharmacological and Parenteral Therapies

Cognitive level: Analysis

Subject area: Pharmacologic

20. The nurse is admitting a child suspected of having hyperglycemia. Which of the following assessment findings would support a diagnosis of hyperglycemia?

Select all that apply:

[　] **1.** Hunger

[　] **2.** Pallor

[　] **3.** Tachycardia

[　] **4.** Blurred vision

[　] **5.** Polydipsia

[　] **6.** Headaches

21. The nurse is preparing discharge for a child with type 1 diabetes. Which of the following should the nurse include in the discharge instructions?

1. A physical examination should be performed every other year

2. Sugar-free products are not always carbohydrate-free

3. Conserve energy by restricting activity

4. Test the blood glucose once daily

22. A school nurse should include which of the following in the assessment of a child who has type 1 diabetes mellitus for adherence to the treatment plan?

Select all that apply:

[　] **1.** Assess the finger pads for small marks

[　] **2.** Ask the child if high-sugar foods are avoided

[　] **3.** Evaluate the injection sites for bruising

[　] **4.** Ask the child to describe the symptoms of hypoglycemia

[　] **5.** Ask the child how long it takes to use a bottle of insulin

[　] **6.** Obtain a blood glucose level

Answer: 1, 4, 5

Rationale: Hunger, polydipsia, and blurred vision are clinical manifestations of hyperglycemia. Tachycardia, pallor, and headaches are clinical manifestations of hypoglycemia.

Nursing process: Assessment

Client need: Health Promotion and Maintenance

Cognitive level: Application

Subject area: Pediatric

Answer: 2

Rationale: In type 1 diabetes mellitus, glucose accumulates in the blood, and the body cannot make efficient use of the glucose. Daily insulin doses are required. Sugar-free products are not necessarily carbohydrate-free. A physical examination should be performed annually. Activity is not restricted, but insulin should be adjusted according to exercise level. Increased insulin is necessary with increased activity. A blood glucose test should be performed before every insulin dose.

Nursing process: Planning

Client need: Health Promotion and Maintenance

Cognitive level: Application

Subject area: Pediatric

Answer: 1, 3, 5

Rationale: To evaluate a child's compliance to the type 1 diabetes mellitus treatment plan, the nurse should assess the finger pads for small stick marks and the injection sites for bruising. Asking the child how long it takes to use a bottle of insulin can serve as a way to determine whether all of the insulin was administered over the prescribed time frame. Obtaining a blood glucose level would not be an accurate evaluation of adherence to the treatment plan. It would only indicate the glucose level at the time of the test and not long-term compliance. Asking a child if high-sugar foods are avoided and what the clinical manifestations of hypoglycemia are merely evaluate the child's knowledge but not necessarily compliance.

Nursing process: Assessment

Client need: Health Promotion and Maintenance

Cognitive level: Application

Subject area: Pediatric

23. The nurse identifies which of the following adolescents with type 1 diabetes mellitus as being at greatest risk for complications? An adolescent
    1. with frequent *Candida albicans* urinary infections.
    2. who has an eating disorder.
    3. who has a fever and a sore throat.
    4. who is sexually active and taking birth control.

24. Which of the following is a priority for the nurse to include in the assessment of a child admitted with dehydration who is to begin on intravenous potassium?
    1. Obtain a weight
    2. Assess the child for edema
    3. Evaluate the output
    4. Monitor blood pressure

25. The nurse is admitting a child suspected of having acquired hypothyroidism. Which of the following assessments should the nurse evaluate as confirming the diagnosis?
    1. Goiter
    2. Exophthalmos
    3. Proptosis
    4. Hirsutism

Answer: 2

Rationale: An eating disorder poses a serious health hazard in the management of the diabetes. Not only do bulimic behaviors such as binging and vomiting pose serious complications, but starvation that occurs with anorexia nervosa also raises the potential for serious complications. The omission of insulin can lead to serious complications too. A urinary infection with *Candida albicans* is often an early sign in adolescents that type 2 diabetes may be present. Sore throat and fever do not necessarily pose serious health risks but simply may indicate that an insulin adjustment may be necessary during the illness. Sexual activity and birth control do not directly alter an adolescent's risk for complications.

Nursing process: Analysis

Client need: Reduction of Risk Potential

Cognitive level: Analysis

Subject area: Pediatric

Answer: 3

Rationale: The priority assessment in a child admitted with dehydration who is to begin on intravenous potassium is to evaluate the child's output. The child must have functioning kidneys necessary for excretion. Intravenous potassium should never be given to a child with an impaired renal output. Obtaining a blood pressure and a weight and evaluating for edema may be appropriate interventions, but not the priority.

Nursing process: Assessment

Client need: Management of Care

Cognitive level: Analysis

Subject area: Pediatric

Answer: 1

Rationale: Acquired hypothyroidism generally results from an autoimmune cause. The thyroid gland becomes inflamed, is infiltrated by the antibodies, and is progressively destroyed. Goiter is an indication found in acquired hypothyroidism. Exophthalmos and proptosis are present in hyperthyroidism. Hirsutism is a clinical manifestation in congenital adrenal hyperplasia.

Nursing process: Evaluation

Client need: Health Promotion and Maintenance

Cognitive level: Application

Subject area: Pediatric

Neurological Disorders

34

1. During hospitalization, a child experiences a tonic-clonic seizure. To provide for the client's safety, which of the following actions should the nurse take?

    1. Put a padded tongue blade between the child's teeth

    2. Perform a jaw thrust and administer oxygen

    3. Securely restrain the child in the bed

    4. Administer a benzodiazepine intramuscularly

2. Postoperatively, for placement of a shunt for hydrocephalus, the nurse should place a child in which of the following positions?

    1. Elevated 45 degrees in a supine position

    2. Flat and lying on the unoperated side

    3. Flat and lying on the operated side

    4. Elevated 30 degrees and prone

3. The parents of a 2-year-old toddler who has cerebral palsy notice the child does not sit up alone. They ask the nurse whether the child will be able to learn to walk alone or with crutches. Which of the following is the appropriate response by the nurse?

    1. "Your child will most likely not be able to walk alone or with crutches."

    2. "The chances of your child walking without crutches is good, but it is unlikely that your child will walk alone."

    3. "It is very difficult to say because every child is different."

    4. "Your child will most probably be able to walk alone and without the use of crutches."

4. The parents of a child with cerebral palsy ask the nurse what the most common cause of cerebral palsy is. The most appropriate response by the nurse is

    1. "The cord gets wrapped around the neck in the birth canal."

    2. "The result of a forceps delivery."

    3. "The result of a premature birth or very low birth weight."

    4. "Preeclampsia in the mother."

Answer: 2

Rationale: To provide for the safety of the child during a tonic-clonic seizure, the nurse should perform a jaw thrust and administer oxygen. Holding the child down, restraining the child, or putting a padded tongue blade between the child's teeth may cause injury to the child. Benzodiazepine is not used to treat a tonic-clonic seizure but is used in status epilepticus.

Nursing process: Planning

Client need: Health Promotion and Maintenance

Cognitive level: Application

Subject area: Pediatric

Answer: 2

Rationale: A child who has had a shunt revision for hydrocephalus should be placed flat in bed, lying on the unoperated side. The head-elevated position may cause the cerebrospinal fluid to drain too quickly from the ventricles. Lying on the operated side can cause injury to the shunt, and the prone position may cause interference with respiration.

Nursing process: Planning

Client need: Reduction of Risk Potential

Cognitive level: Application

Subject area: Pediatric

Answer: 1

Rationale: If a child cannot sit up by the age of 2, there is every indication that the child has cerebral palsy affecting voluntary motor control. As a result, the child will not be able to walk with or without crutches.

Nursing process: Analysis

Client need: Health Promotion and Maintenance

Cognitive level: Analysis

Subject area: Pediatric

Answer: 3

Rationale: Although the cord getting wrapped around the neck in the birth canal, a forceps delivery, and preeclampsia in the mother all place a child at risk for cerebral palsy, children born prematurely or those who have very low birth weights are the most at risk.

Nursing process: Analysis

Client need: Health Promotion and Maintenance

Cognitive level: Analysis

Subject area: Pediatric

5. When caring for a child with meningitis, it is essential that the nurse evaluate for a positive Brudzinski's sign, which would indicate

    1. increased intracranial pressure.

    2. meningeal irritation.

    3. encephalitis.

    4. intraventricular hemorrhage.

6. A nurse is providing discharge instructions to the parents of a child who suffered a head injury six hours ago. Which statement by the parents indicates additional teaching is needed?

    1. "We will call the doctor immediately if vomiting occurs."

    2. "We won't give anything stronger than Tylenol for headache."

    3. "We will provide for uninterrupted sleep when we get home."

    4. "I know continued amnesia regarding the events of the injury is expected."

7. The nurse is assigned to administer bismuth subsalicylate (Pepto-Bismol) to a 10-year-old child who has Reye's syndrome and is experiencing gastrointestinal clinical manifestations. Which of the following is the priority action for the nurse to take?

    1. Administer the prescribed dose of 1 tablet

    2. Inform the child and parents that stools will be dark in appearance

    3. Instruct the child to chew the tablet thoroughly

    4. Question the physician's order

8. The nurse is admitting an infant with setting-sun eyes with sclera above the iris, bulging fontanel, a high-pitched cry, vomiting, dilated scalp veins, and a slight alteration in consciousness. The nurse should report these findings as _____.

Answer: 2

Rationale: Brudzinski's sign, when the legs flex at both hips and knees in response to flexing the head and neck, indicates meningeal irritation.

Nursing process: Evaluation

Client need: Reduction of Risk Potential

Cognitive level: Application

Subject area: Pediatric

Answer: 3

Rationale: Waking children to check neurological status following a head injury is important, no matter the time of day. Vomiting could indicate increased intracranial pressure requiring further evaluation. Narcotics should be avoided after a head injury. Amnesia following a head injury is not uncommon.

Nursing process: Evaluation

Client need: Health Promotion and Maintenance

Cognitive level: Analysis

Subject area: Pediatric

Answer: 4

Rationale: Bismuth subsalicylate (Pepto-Bismol) contains aspirin, and there is a suspected link between aspirin and the etiology of Reye's syndrome. It is a priority to question the order for Pepto-Bismol to be given to this child. One tablet is appropriate for a child 10 years of age. Chewing the tablet and informing the child and parents that the stool will be dark in appearance are all appropriate interventions in the plan of care for a child taking Pepto-Bismol, but not for a child with Reye's syndrome.

Nursing process: Planning

Client need: Management of Care

Cognitive level: Analysis

Subject area: Legal and Ethical Issues

Answer: increased intracranial pressure

Rationale: Clinical manifestations of increased intracranial pressure include setting-sun eyes with sclera above the iris, bulging fontanel, a high-pitched cry, vomiting, dilated scalp veins, and a slight alteration in consciousness.

Nursing process: Analysis

Client need: Health Promotion and Maintenance

Cognitive level: Analysis

Subject area: Pediatric

9. The nurse assesses cranial nerve VII in a pediatric client by which of the following techniques?

   1. Gently swab the cornea with a sterile cotton-tipped applicator

   2. Hold the eyes open and turn the head from side to side

   3. Place the child's head in the midline position with the head elevated and inject ice water into the ear canal

   4. Irritate the pharynx with a tongue depressor or cotton swab

10. The nurse should monitor a child for which of the following clinical manifestations of meningeal irritation? Select all that apply:

    [   ] **1.** Nuchal rigidity

    [   ] **2.** Nausea and vomiting

    [   ] **3.** Anxiousness

    [   ] **4.** Heightened sense of environment

    [   ] **5.** Headache

    [   ] **6.** Decreased resistance to pain and extension of the leg

11. With an infant who has ancephaly, the most appropriate nursing intervention is to

    1. inform the parents that an abnormal gait with foot weakness or deformity will appear by toddlerhood.

    2. assess the infant for cerebrospinal fluid leak at the site of the defect.

    3. instruct the parents to notify the physician if difficulties in controlling bowel and bladder functions develop when toilet training is attempted.

    4. monitor the infant for respiratory failure and prepare the parents that death is imminent.

12. When planning client assignments for the day, which of the following nursing tasks would be appropriate for the registered nurse to assign to unlicensed assistive personnel?

    1. Assess a child for signs of increased intracranial pressure

    2. Explain the procedure for a skull x-ray to the parents and child

    3. Document the temperature of a child with bacterial meningitis

    4. Monitor a child for urinary retention following surgery for spina bifida

Answer: 1

Rationale: Gently swabbing the cornea with a sterile cotton-tipped applicator assesses cranial nerve VII, which evaluates the corneal reflex. Holding the eyes open and turning the head from side to side evaluates cranial nerves II, IV, and VI and the oculocephalic reflex. Placing the child's head in a midline position with the head elevated prior to injecting ice water into the ear canal evaluates cranial nerves III and VIII, or the oculovestibular reflex. Irritating the pharynx with a tongue depressor or cotton swab evaluates cranial nerves IX and X, or the gag reflex.

Nursing process: Assessment

Client need: Reduction of Risk Potential

Cognitive level: Application

Subject area: Pediatric

Answer: 1, 2, 5

Rationale: Clinical manifestations of meningeal irritation are nuchal rigidity, positive Kernig's sign (resistance to pain and extension of the leg), positive Brudzinski's sign, severe headache, loss of consciousness, photophobia, nausea, vomiting, fever, and convulsions.

Nursing process: Assessment

Client need: Health Promotion and Maintenance

Cognitive level: Application

Subject area: Pediatric

Answer: 4

Rationale: Ancephaly is the absence of the cranial vault with the cerebral hemisphere missing or reduced in size. Although the brain stem may be intact, respiratory failure and death are imminent. The abnormal gait with foot weakness or deformity appears in toddlerhood with spina bifida. Leakage of cerebrospinal fluid occurs with meningomyelocele. Difficulties in bowel and bladder functions occur at the time of toilet training with spina bifida occulta.

Nursing process: Implementation

Client need: Health Promotion and Maintenance

Cognitive level: Application

Subject area: Pediatric

Answer: 3

Rationale: It is appropriate for a registered nurse to assign only those activities that are basic cares and do not involve assessing, explaining, or teaching, or monitoring for change. Unlicensed assistive personnel are trained only to take a temperature.

Nursing process: Planning

Client need: Management of Care

Cognitive level: Analysis

Subject area: Legal and Ethical Issues

13. The nurse is caring for a child who had a seizure 15 minutes after sustaining a head injury. After assuring a patent airway, which of the following is the priority intervention?

    1. Assess fluid and electrolyte status

    2. Administer prescribed benzodiazepine

    3. Monitor for postconcussive syndrome

    4. Observe for signs of increased intracranial pressure

14. A child has received an external ventricular drainage (EVD) for treatment of an infection following shunt insertion. For which of the following clinical manifestations of overdraining ventricles should the nurse monitor the child?

    Select all that apply:

    [ ] **1.** Tachycardia

    [ ] **2.** Nausea and vomiting

    [ ] **3.** Ataxia

    [ ] **4.** Polydipsia

    [ ] **5.** Headache

    [ ] **6.** Apnea

15. The nurse receives report from an emergency room nurse that a child is being admitted with a C7 spinal cord injury. Based on this information, the nurse prepares to care for a child with which of the following deficits?

    1. Quadriplegia with total loss of respiratory function and flaccid paralysis

    2. Paraplegia with loss of leg, bowel, and bladder function

    3. Quadriplegia but with gross arm movements and diaphragmatic breathing

    4. Paraplegia, arm function intact, loss of some degree of intercostal and abdominal muscles

16. The nurse should monitor a child who has survived a submersion injury in a hot tub for pneumonia caused by which of the following organisms?

    1. *Escherichia coli*

    2. *Pseudomonas aeruginosa*

    3. *Staphylococcus aureus*

    4. *Streptococcus*

Answer: 2

Rationale: If a seizure occurs within 30 minutes of a head injury, benzodiazepine is administered intravenously to stop the seizure. If the seizure continues, phenytoin may be administered. Although the remaining interventions of assessing fluid and electrolyte status, monitoring for postconcussive syndrome, and observing for increased intracranial pressure are appropriate, the priority intervention is to stop the seizure.

Nursing process: Planning

Client need: Management of Care

Cognitive level: Analysis

Subject area: Legal and Ethical Issues

Answer: 2, 5, 6

Rationale: The clinical manifestations of overdraining ventricles following placement of an external ventricular drainage include bradycardia, apnea, severe headache, nausea, vomiting, lethargy, drowsiness, and irritability, and there is a possibility that seizures will occur.

Nursing process: Assessment

Client need: Health Promotion and Maintenance

Cognitive level: Application

Subject area: Pediatric

Answer: 3

Rationale: C1 to C2 spinal cord lesions result in quadriplegia with total loss of respiratory function and flaccid paralysis. Spinal cord lesions at C7 to C8 would result in quadriplegia with biceps intact and diaphragmatic breathing. Spinal cord lesions at T1 to T2 would result in paraplegia with loss of leg, bowel, bladder, and sexual function. Spinal cord lesions C5 to C6 would result in paraplegia with loss of varying degrees of intercostals and abdominal muscles, but gross arm movements would be present.

Nursing process: Planning

Client need: Health Promotion and Maintenance

Cognitive level: Analysis

Subject area: Pediatric

Answer: 2

Rationale: Because *Pseudomonas aeruginosa* is an organism commonly found in hot tubs, a child who suffers a submersion injury in a hot tub is at risk for pneumonia caused by this organism.

Nursing process: Assessment

Client need: Health Promotion and Maintenance

Cognitive level: Analysis

Subject area: Pediatric

17. The nurse is preparing to teach a class to educate parents about common neurological injuries in children. Which of the following should the nurse include in the class?

Select all that apply:

[   ] **1.** Most drownings occur between 1200 and 1400.

[   ] **2.** Improperly placed seat belts are the second most common cause of spinal injuries

[   ] **3.** Fifty percent of drownings occur in lakes and oceans

[   ] **4.** A lap belt in an automobile is the best way to prevent spinal cord trauma in children under the age of 13 years

[   ] **5.** Seventy-five percent of spinal injuries in children under the age of 8 years occur at the C3 level

[   ] **6.** Most spinal cord injuries in young children are the result of pedestrian-vehicle, bike-vehicle, or passenger-vehicle injuries

18. The nurse assesses a child who cries, withdraws from painful stimuli, and opens the eyes to pain to have a Glasgow Coma Scale of

1. 3.

2. 6.

3. 9.

4. 12.

19. The nurse observes a child having a seizure that begins with tonic contractions of the fingers in the left hand and progresses into tonic-clonic movements that proceed up the muscles of the left side of the body. The nurse should report these seizures as

1. Jacksonian.

2. Rolandic.

3. general.

4. complex.

Answer: 2, 5, 6

Rationale: Most drownings occur between 4 p.m. and 6 p.m. when the caregiver is busy preparing dinner and not closely supervising the child. Over 90% of drownings occur in fresh water, with 50% of those in swimming pools. Lap belts are dangerous because when a crash occurs, the lap belt is positioned on the abdomen of a child of this age. In a crash, the child is hyperflexed over the belt, which snaps back upright. The force of the lap belt continues posteriorly to the spinal column and cord, causing trauma.

Nursing process: Planning

Client need: Health Promotion and Maintenance

Cognitive level: Application

Subject area: Pediatric

Answer: 3

Rationale: Crying to painful stimuli is a 3, withdrawing from pain is a 4, and opening the eyes to painful stimuli is a 2 on the Glasgow Coma Scale. This gives a total score of 9. A score of 3 means there is neither a verbal nor a motor response to painful stimuli. A score of 12 indicates the child opens the eyes on command, withdraws at simple touch, and has an irritable cry to painful stimuli. A score of 6 is a minimal response to all of the categories, but still a response.

Nursing process: Assessment

Client need: Health Promotion and Maintenance

Cognitive level: Analysis

Subject area: Pediatric

Answer: 1

Rationale: Jacksonian seizures begin with tonic contractions of the fingers in the left hand and progress into tonic-clonic movements that proceed up the muscles of the left side of the body. Rolandic seizures include tonic-clonic movements of the face, with increased salivation and arrested speech; they commonly occur during sleep. Complex seizures have an aura, and consciousness may not be completely lost. Children are rarely violent, but may demonstrate confusion or purposeless behaviors. General seizures are secondary to diffuse electrical activity throughout the cortex and into the brain.

Nursing process: Analysis

Client need: Health Promotion and Maintenance

Cognitive level: Application

Subject area: Pediatric

20. Which of the following statements indicates the family of a child with a seizure disorder has followed the nurse's discharge instructions?

    1. "Our child has had a growth spurt, so we made an appointment to review the medication to prevent seizures."

    2. "We remind our child every day of what activities should be restricted."

    3. "Most of our time is spent with our child who has seizures, so we have little time for the other children."

    4. "Our child knows to take a dose of seizure medicine after remembering a dose that was accidentally forgotten."

21. The parents of a child suspected of having a shunt malfunction ask the nurse what caused it. The appropriate response by the nurse is which of the following?

    1. Increased flow of cerebrospinal fluid

    2. Decreased reabsorption of cerebrospinal fluid

    3. Obstructed flow of cerebrospinal fluid

    4. Decreased production of cerebrospinal fluid

22. The nurse assists the parents of a child with myoclonic seizures to make which of the following menu selections?

    1. Baked potato

    2. Creamed corn

    3. Roast beef

    4. Pecan pie with ice cream

Answer: 1

Rationale: As children gain weight, the dose of the seizure medication may need to be altered. Dosages of medications should not be missed at all. Children with seizure disorders should be allowed to participate in most activities, not be overprotected by parents, and parents should divide their time equally among all their children. Reminders of what an affected child can and cannot do should not be necessary.

Nursing process: Evaluation

Client need: Health Promotion and Maintenance

Cognitive level: Analysis

Subject area: Pediatric

Answer: 2

Rationale: Decreased reabsorption is a common cause of hydrocephalus. Increased flow of and decreased production of cerebrospinal fluid (CSF) do not relate to hydrocephalus, intracranial pressure (ICP), or shunt malfunction.

Nursing process: Analysis

Client need: Health Promotion and Maintenance

Cognitive level: Application

Subject area: Pediatric

Answer: 4

Rationale: A ketogenic diet, in which 90% of calories come from fat, and protein and carbohydrates are limited, is used in the treatment of myoclonic seizures. Roast beef is high in protein. Baked potato and creamed corn are high in carbohydrates. Pecans and ice cream are high in fat, so that menu selection is appropriate to a ketogenic diet. Why ketones affect seizures is not understood, but researchers theorize that ketones change lipid concentrations, reduce fluid and electrolyte imbalances, modify the seizure threshold, and stabilize the central nervous system.

Nursing process: Implementation

Client need: Basic Care and Comfort

Cognitive level: Application

Subject area: Pediatric

23. The nurse is planning the care for a child who has an elevated blood pressure, slow pulse, is flushed, has profuse facial perspiration, and is experiencing urinary retention and constipation four days after sustaining a C3 injury. Which of the following is the priority nursing intervention?

1. Administer the prescribed antihypertensive

2. Insert a prescribed Foley catheter

3. Remove the blankets on the bed

4. Encourage fluids

24. The nurse should monitor a client for which of the following signs of neurogenic shock after a C5 injury? Select all that apply:

[ ] **1.** Hypotension

[ ] **2.** Tachycardia

[ ] **3.** Hypothermia

[ ] **4.** Cool and pale skin

[ ] **5.** Vasoconstriction

[ ] **6.** Inability to perspire

Answer: 2

Rationale: Spinal shock occurs shortly after the injury and may persist for up to 10 days with a high cervical or thoracic injury. After the spinal shock has resolved and reflex activity has returned, high cervical or thoracic lesions may react with a potential life-threatening sympathetic nervous system response to stimuli such as a distended bladder, constipation, or fecal impaction. Spasms of the pelvic viscera and arterioles produce vasoconstriction below the lesion, resulting in hypertension, superficial vasodilatation, flushing, piloerection, and profuse perspiration above the injury. To compensate for the increased blood pressure, the heart rate is slowed via vagal stimulation. Without prompt reversal of the clinical manifestations, which is usually just removal of the stimulant, the client may have a stroke, have a seizure, or die.

Nursing process: Planning

Client need: Management of Care

Cognitive level: Analysis

Subject area: Legal and Ethical Issues

Answer: 1, 3, 6

Rationale: Neurogenic shock is a form of distributive shock that accompanies complete high spinal cord injury. It is caused by an interruption of sympathetic impulses from the spinal cord in the cervical-thoracic region. Clinical manifestations include vasodilatation, hypotension, bradycardia, warm, flushed skin, inability to perspire, and hypothermia.

Nursing process: Assessment

Client need: Health Promotion and Maintenance

Cognitive level: Application

Subject area: Pediatric

Integumentary Disorders

35

1. Which of the following instructions should the nurse include in the teaching plan for a 16-year-old client with comedonal acne being treated with topical Retin-A?

    1. Avoid sun exposure

    2. Severe headaches may be experienced

    3. Improvement will be seen in 24 hours

    4. Scrub the skin prior to application

2. Which of the following should the nurse include in the discharge instructions for a child who had a punch biopsy done on the back?

    1. Leave the site open to air

    2. Make an appointment to have the sutures removed in 5 days

    3. Keep the site clean, dry, and covered for 24 hours

    4. Avoid physical activity

3. Which of the following should the nurse include when preparing a teaching plan for a child with atopic dermatitis regarding application of steroid ointments?

    1. Apply the steroid ointment over the emollient

    2. Apply the ointment sparingly and rub into the skin

    3. Use a large amount of the ointment

    4. Apply the steroid frequently

4. The nurse should prepare an 18-year-old adolescent with acne who has not responded to antibiotic therapy for which of the following tests prior to starting treatment with isotretinoin (Accutane)?

    1. Skin biopsy

    2. Hearing test

    3. Pregnancy test

    4. Urinalysis

Answer: 1

Rationale: The main clinical manifestation of pediculosis capitis, or head lice, is intense pruritus. Nits are commonly found on the hairs of the occipital area of the scalp.

Nursing process: Planning

Client need: Management of Care

Cognitive level: Analysis

Subject area: Pediatric

Answer: 2

Rationale: Permethrin 1% (Nix) is both pediculocidal and ovicidal and generally considered the treatment of choice. Nix should be applied to clean, damp hair. It should be left on for 10 minutes followed by rinsing and combing with a fine-toothed comb to remove nits.

Nursing process: Planning

Client need: Pharmacological and Parenteral Therapies

Cognitive level: Application

Subject area: Pharmacologic

Answer: 4

Rationale: Permethrin 5% is considered the treatment of choice for scabies. The pruritus is a hypersensitivity response to the nit and its ova and feces. Following application of Elimite, the pruritus may continue for 14 to 21 days. Emollients may help to relieve the discomfort.

Nursing process: Analysis

Client need: Pharmacological and Parenteral Therapies

Cognitive level: Application

Subject area: Pharmacologic

Answer: 2

Rationale: Following the use of a pediculocide for pediculosis capitis, or head lice, the hair should not be washed for one to two days. A combination shampoo and conditioner or a cream rinse should not be used before using a pediculocide.

Nursing process: Planning

Client need: Health Promotion and Maintenance

Cognitive level: Application

Subject area: Pediatric

9. Following excision of a nevus on the arm, which of the following should the nurse include in this child's discharge instructions?

   1. Shower after 24 hours

   2. Remove the dressing after 24 hours, leaving the wound open to the air

   3. All activities may be resumed

   4. Take acetaminophen (Tylenol) for discomfort

10. The nurse informs a child with atopic dermatitis that which of the following may cause a flare?

    1. Bathing with mild soap

    2. Moisturizing the skin

    3. Wearing cotton clothing

    4. Sudden changes in temperature

11. The parent of a child infested with scabies asks the nurse how the child got scabies. Based on the nurse's knowledge of scabies, the most likely method of contracting scabies is

    1. swimming in a pool.

    2. being in close contact with an infested individual.

    3. having contact with an infected pet.

    4. airborne.

12. The client with tinea capitis asks the nurse what the condition is. The nurse should reply with what statement? _____

Answer: 4

Rationale: Following excision of a nevus, the wound should be kept dry until sutures are removed to avoid infection. Physical activity should be avoided for two to four weeks to prevent wound dehiscence.

Nursing process: Planning

Client need: Health Promotion and Maintenance

Cognitive level: Application

Subject area: Pediatric

Answer: 4

Rationale: Atopic dermatitis is a chronic inflammation of the dermis and epidermis resulting in pruritus, erythema, edema, papules, serous discharge, and crusting. Cotton clothing, daily baths, and moisturizing are all part of the plan of care for atopic dermatitis. Sudden temperature changes can cause dryness or sweating, which may contribute to a flare.

Nursing process: Implementation

Client need: Health Promotion and Maintenance

Cognitive level: Analysis

Subject area: Pediatric

Answer: 2

Rationale: Scabies is an infestation of the scabies mite with *Sarcoptes scabiei* and is dependent on a human host for survival. It is transmitted by skin-to-skin contact with an infested individual. It is less likely to contract through fomites. Animals do not carry scabies. The mite can survive for 24 to 36 hours away from the host.

Nursing process: Analysis

Client need: Health Promotion and Maintenance

Cognitive level: Analysis

Subject area: Pediatric

Answer: Tinea capitis is a fungal infection of the scalp

Rationale: Tinea capitis is a fungal infection caused by a dermatophyte (*M. canis* or *Trichophyton tonsurans*). Although often referred to as ringworm, there is no infestation by a worm.

Nursing process: Analysis

Client need: Health Promotion and Maintenance

Cognitive level: Comprehension

Subject area: Pediatric

13. The nurse should assess a child suspected of having tinea capitis for which of the following?

Select all that apply:

[   ] **1.** Scalp scaling with alopecia

[   ] **2.** Warts on the periungual regions

[   ] **3.** Orolabial lesions

[   ] **4.** Presence of kerions

[   ] **5.** Scale and black dots

[   ] **6.** Creamy-white plaques on the buccal mucosa

14. The client with tinea capitis asks the nurse what the treatment for a kerion is. Based on the treatment of tinea capitis, the nurse replies

1. "apply warm, moist soaks."

2. "apply permethrin 1% (Nix)."

3. "shave the hair."

4. "oral corticosteroids (Orapred, Prelone, Pediapred)."

15. Which of the following should the nurse include in the medication instructions for a child with tinea capitis for whom griseofulvin (Grifulvin V, Fulvicin P/G, Grisactin) has been prescribed?

1. Stop taking the drug when the scalp improves

2. Take the drug on an empty stomach

3. Take the drug with a fatty meal

4. Take the drug at bedtime only

16. The mother of a 4-week-old infant with a small hemangioma asks the nurse if the hemangioma will get any bigger. Which of the following is the most appropriate response by the nurse?

1. "Hemangiomas generally grow rapidly during the first year of life, followed by a gradual spontaneous involution."

2. "The hemangioma will not grow and get any bigger."

3. "The hemangioma will fade over time, leaving just a pink scar."

4. "Hemangiomas gradually get smaller with each passing month of life, until there is normal skin where the hemangioma was."

Answer: 1, 4, 5

Rationale: Scalp scaling with alopecia is a clinical manifestation of tinea capitis. Kerions are moist, boggy scalp nodules. Scale and black dots may also be present. Warts on the periungual region around the nail are seen in verrucae. Orolabial lesions occur in the herpes simplex virus type 1. Creamy-white plaques on the buccal mucosa are characteristic of candidiasis.

Nursing process: Assessment

Client need: Health Promotion and Maintenance

Cognitive level: Application

Subject area: Pediatric

Answer: 4

Rationale: Oral corticosteroids (Orapred, Prelone, Pediapred) are used to treat a kerion. It is not necessary to shave the hair or apply soaks. Topical treatment is ineffective.

Nursing process: Analysis

Client need: Health Promotion and Maintenance

Cognitive level: Application

Subject area: Pediatric

Answer: 3

Rationale: Griseofulvin (Grifulvin V, Fulvicin P/G, Grisactin) is the standard treatment for tinea capitis. It is best absorbed when taken with fatty foods. Treatment generally lasts for a minimum of eight weeks.

Nursing process: Planning

Client need: Pharmacological and Parenteral Therapies

Cognitive level: Analysis

Subject area: Pharmacologic

Answer: 1

Rationale: Hemangiomas are benign proliferations of the blood vessels of the skin. Although rarely present at birth, most appear by 1 to 4 weeks of life. They grow rapidly during the first year of life and then have a spontaneous involution that may begin as early as 6 to 10 months. They become soft and gray. About 50% of hemangiomas are gone by age 5 years and 90% are gone by age 12 years.

Nursing process: Analysis

Client need: Health Promotion and Maintenance

Cognitive level: Analysis

Subject area: Pediatric

17. Which of the following nursing interventions should the nurse include in the plan of care for a child with tinea pedis?

 1. Apply warm soaks to the feet

 2. Keep the feet dry

 3. Wear wool socks

 4. Administer oral steroids

18. Which of the following should the nurse include in the information given to the parents of an infant born with a port-wine stain?

 1. The port-wine stain does not grow bigger with age

 2. Most port-wine stains are the result of a medical condition

 3. Port-wine stains generally become darker and thicker with age

 4. The port-wine stain becomes raised over time

19. The nurse prepares to include which of the following in the plan of care of a child with molluscum contagiosum?

 1. Instruct the child to scratch with the knuckles instead of the fingers

 2. Instruct the parents to keep the child out of school as long as the child is contagious

 3. Administer cantharidin directly to the lesion

 4. Administer oral Prelone

20. A client with molluscum contagiosum has read on the Internet that no treatment is required and asks why the molluscum should be treated. The nurse's most appropriate response is

 1. "It will not clear spontaneously."

 2. "It is contagious, and your child cannot attend school until the molluscum is treated."

 3. "The lesions may resolve spontaneously, but they may continue to spread."

 4. "If the lesions are not treated, they grow larger."

Answer: 2
Rationale: Tinea pedis is a dermatophyte infection of the feet. Because it is generally acquired from shower room floors, the feet should be kept dry. It must be treated for four to six weeks with topical antifungals. Clients should avoid tight-fitting shoes and wear cotton socks.
Nursing process: Planning
Client need: Health Promotion and Maintenance
Cognitive level: Application
Subject area: Pediatric

Answer: 3
Rationale: A port-wine stain is a capillary malformation present at birth. It generally is not associated with any medical condition. Port-wine stains usually grow with the child, but do not become raised.
Nursing process: Planning
Client need: Health Promotion and Maintenance
Cognitive level: Analysis
Subject area: Pediatric

Answer: 3
Rationale: Molluscum contagiosum is a viral infection of the skin caused by a DNA pox virus. The main feature is a flesh-colored, dome-shaped papule with central umbilication. Cantharidin is applied with a wooden applicator directly to the lesion. Although contagious, the child does not have to be kept out of school. Corticosteroids, such as Prelone, are used in the treatment of tinea capitis.
Nursing process: Planning
Client need: Health Promotion and Maintenance
Cognitive level: Application
Subject area: Pediatric

Answer: 3
Rationale: Molluscum contagiosum is a viral infection of the skin characterized by flesh-colored, dome-shaped papules with central umbilication. Although molluscum will eventually resolve, lesions spread easily, may become infected, may be itchy or irritated, and are sometimes cosmetically objectionable. For these reasons, they are usually treated with cantharidin applied directly to the lesion.
Nursing process: Analysis
Client need: Health Promotion and Maintenance
Cognitive level: Analysis
Subject area: Pediatric

21. The child with molluscum contagiosum is going to be treated with cantharidin. The parents of the child ask the nurse how the cantharidin is given. The nurse's response would be

   1. "It is injected into each lesion."

   2. "An oral tablet is given twice a day."

   3. "A wooden applicator is used to apply the cantharidin directly to each lesion."

   4. "You will receive a prescription for the topical ointment to rub on twice a day."

22. The nurse prepares a 10-year-old child who presents with a single wart on the hand for which of the following treatments?

   1. Liquid nitrogen

   2. Tagamet

   3. Aldara

   4. Retin-A

23. The parents of a 3-month-old infant who has a hemangioma on the nasal tip asks the nurse what the treatment is. Based on an understanding of hemangiomas, which of the following is the nurse's response?

   1. "Hemangiomas are generally not treated because they are never life threatening."

   2. "Liquid nitrogen is usually applied to nasal tip hemangiomas."

   3. "Surgical excision is generally performed within the first year of life."

   4. "Nasal tip hemangiomas are treated with oral corticosteroids."

24. The nurse is admitting a 4-month-old infant with an irregularly shaped reddish-purple macular vascular lesion on the face. The mother states it was present at birth. The nurse documents this as which of the following?

   1. Hemangioma

   2. Port-wine stain

   3. Congenital melanocytic nevus

   4. Pyogenic granuloma

Answer: 3

Rationale: Molluscum contagiosum is a viral infection of the skin that causes flesh-colored, dome-shaped papules with central umbilication. Cantharidin is very potent and can cause significant burns if not used properly. It must be applied carefully to each lesion with a wooden applicator. This treatment is only done in the doctor's office. A prescription is never given and the drug is never administered in the home by the client.

Nursing process: Analysis

Client need: Pharmacological and Parenteral Therapies

Cognitive level: Analysis

Subject area: Pharmacologic

Answer: 1

Rationale: Verrucae, or cutaneous warts, are benign tumors of the epidermis caused by a human papillomavirus. For a 10-year-old child with a single wart, the most likely treatment would be liquid nitrogen. Cryotherapy with liquid nitrogen is reserved for children over the age of 8 years. Tagamet is given for multiple warts and is often used in younger children who cannot tolerate liquid nitrogen. Aldara and Retin-A are used to treat flat warts on the face. In addition, Aldara is used to treat genital warts.

Nursing process: Implementation

Client need: Health Promotion and Maintenance

Cognitive level: Analysis

Subject area: Pediatric

Answer: 4

Rationale: Hemangiomas are benign proliferations of the blood vessels in the skin. They are rarely present at birth. Most of them develop within one to four weeks after birth. To prevent excessive tissue growth on the nasal tip (Cyrano nose deformity) in a nasal tip hemangioma, oral corticosteroids (Prelone, Pediapred, Orapred) are given. Surgical intervention is recommended only after the hemangioma has involuted. It will continue to grow for up to 1 year of age. Some hemangiomas can be life threatening.

Nursing process: Analysis

Client need: Health Promotion and Maintenance

Cognitive level: Analysis

Subject area: Pediatric

Answer: 2

Rationale: Port-wine stains are capillary malformations present at birth. They are generally irregularly shaped reddish-purple macular vascular lesions. Hemangiomas are not usually present at birth and grow rapidly during the first year of life. Congenital nevi are brown. Pyogenic granulomas are raised reddish-purple papules that bleed profusely with trauma.

Nursing process: Implementation

Client need: Health Promotion and Maintenance

Cognitive level: Comprehension

Subject area: Pediatric

25. The nurse prepares a child with a pyogenic granuloma on the chin that has been bleeding for which of the following treatments?

    1. Elliptical excision
    2. Punch biopsy
    3. Shave lesion and electrodessication
    4. Pulsed dye laser

26. The registered nurse is delegating nursing tasks for the day. Which of the following tasks should the nurse delegate to a licensed practical nurse?

    1. Instruct the parents of a child with a wart to wash off the podophyllin used in the treatment in four to six hours
    2. Inform the parents of a child with a hemangioma that generally no treatment is required
    3. Administer Prelone to a child with tinea capitis who has a kerion
    4. Assess and report the characteristics of a child's port-wine stain

Answer: 3

Rationale: Pyogenic granulomas are benign growths of blood vessels that can bleed profusely with trauma. Treatment is to shave the lesion and cauterize the base to prevent recurrence. A pulsed dye laser is used to destroy wart tissue.

Nursing process: Implementation

Client need: Health Promotion and Maintenance

Cognitive level: Application

Subject area: Pediatric

Answer: 3

Rationale: Instructing, informing, and assessing are all nursing skills that are most appropriately performed by the registered nurse. A licensed practical nurse may administer a prescribed drug.

Nursing process: Planning

Client need: Management of Care

Cognitive level: Analysis

Subject area: Legal and Ethical Issues

CHAPTER

Musculoskeletal Disorders

36

1. The parents of a 4-year-old child whose femur is fractured at the growth plate ask the nurse what type of fracture this is. Based on an understanding of the growth plate, the nurse should respond, "The growth plates
   1. serve no function after birth."
   2. are found in every bone in the body."
   3. serve to produce red blood cells."
   4. control the growth of long bones."

2. The nurse completes an orthopedic assessment of a 6-year-old child who has a new cast applied for a fractured radius. Which of the following clinical manifestations is a priority for the nurse to report immediately to the physician?
   1. Skin around the cast is warm
   2. The child states that hand feels "asleep"
   3. Edema in fingers that lessens with elevation
   4. Capillary refill of 3 seconds in affected hand

3. The nurse is told in report that an infant has talipes equinovarus. In doing the physical assessment of this infant, the nurse would expect to find which of the following?
   1. Asymmetry of gluteal and thigh skin folds
   2. One foot is rotated upward slightly, but the foot is easily moved to a normal position
   3. One foot is rotated in and down and is fixed and difficult to move
   4. One knee is lower when flexing both legs

4. While assessing a newborn infant for developmental hip dysplasia (DDH), the nurse evaluates which of the following signs as indicating the presence of DDH?
   1. One knee is lower when both legs are flexed
   2. Thigh and gluteal skin folds are symmetrical
   3. Hip adduction of affected side is limited
   4. Negative Ortolani sign when hips are abducted

Answer: 4

Rationale: Growth plates are located in the metaphysis of long bones. They control bone growth until about 21 years of age. Fractures of the growth plate retard the growth of the affected long bone. Red blood cells are produced in the marrow of the bone and not the growth plate.

Nursing process: Analysis

Client need: Health Promotion and Maintenance

Cognitive level: Application

Subject area: Pediatric

Answer: 2

Rationale: The sensation of numbness or tingling indicates neurovascular impairment. If not reported immediately, the impairment can lead to permanent tissue or nerve damage. The skin around the cast often feels warm. Capillary refill of 3 seconds is acceptable. As long as edema is decreasing, this is not an adverse sign.

Nursing process: Analysis

Client need: Management of Care

Cognitive level: Analysis

Subject area: Pediatric

Answer: 3

Rationale: Talipes equinovarus, referred to as clubfoot, is a congenital abnormality characterized by the affected foot being rotated in and down while in a fixed position. Clinical manifestations of developmental hip dysplasia include asymmetry of gluteal and thigh skin folds and one knee being lower when both legs are flexed. An upward rotation of the foot is known as talipes calcaneus.

Nursing process: Assessment

Client need: Health Promotion and Maintenance

Cognitive level: Analysis

Subject area: Pediatric

Answer: 1

Rationale: Developmental hip dysplasia (DDH) is characterized by one knee being lower when both knees are flexed, asymmetrical gluteal and thigh skin folds, limited abduction of hip on affected side, and a positive Ortolani sign when the hips are abducted.

Nursing process: Evaluation

Client need: Health Promotion and Maintenance

Cognitive level: Analysis

Subject area: Pediatric

5. The nurse evaluates the musculoskeletal systems of children to be different from adults in which of the following ways?

   1. Tendons and ligaments are weaker in children until puberty

   2. Periosteum is not as strong in children

   3. Bones of children are less porous and dense than adult bones

   4. Skull bones are not rigid or fused at birth

6. While caring for a 4-year-old child with a fractured femur in skeletal traction, the nurse notes that the child is crying with pain and the foot of the affected leg is pale and pulseless. Which of the following nursing actions is a priority?

   1. Remove the weight from the traction

   2. Notify the physician of the changes noted

   3. Give the child a prescribed analgesic

   4. Document the observations and check the extremity in 15 minutes

7. The nurse is caring for a child with a new full-leg cast. Which of the following is an appropriate nursing intervention for this client?

   1. Avoid changing the child's position for 24 hours after application of the cast

   2. Handle the cast with the tips of the fingers

   3. Avoid elevating the casted extremity until the cast is completely dry

   4. Make sure that all cast edges are smooth and free of irritating projections

8. When providing information about osteogenesis imperfecta (OI) to the parents of a newly diagnosed child, the nurse should include which of the following information about the disorder?

   1. It is an inherited disease of the connective tissue

   2. When treated early, it is easily controlled

   3. With later onset, the disease usually runs a more difficult course than with early onset

   4. Braces and splints are not of therapeutic value for this condition

Answer: 4

Rationale: In the musculoskeletal systems of children, the tendons, ligaments, and periosteum are stronger than those of adults. Bones of children are more porous and less dense than bones of adults. The skull bones of children are not rigid or fused at birth to allow for ease of delivery and growth of the brain.

Nursing process: Evaluation

Client need: Health Promotion and Maintenance

Cognitive level: Analysis

Subject area: Pediatric

Answer: 2

Rationale: It is a priority to notify the physician when a child with a fractured femur in skeletal traction complains of pain in the affected foot and the foot is pale and pulseless. This may be an indication of neurovascular damage. Traction weights are not removed unless there is a doctor's order to do so. The nurse should administer an analgesic and chart the observations after notifying the physician.

Nursing process: Planning

Client need: Management of Care

Cognitive level: Analysis

Subject area: Legal and Ethical Issues

Answer: 4

Rationale: The child's position can be changed carefully using the palms of hands to allow cast to dry on all sides. The casted extremity should be elevated above the level of the heart to encourage venous return while the cast is drying. To prevent skin irritation and breakdown, the cast edges should always be smooth and free of projections.

Nursing process: Planning

Client need: Health Promotion and Maintenance

Cognitive level: Application

Subject area: Pediatric

Answer: 1

Rationale: Osteogenesis imperfecta (OI) is an inherited disease of the connective tissue that is very difficult to treat and control. Earlier onset usually means a more difficult course of the disease. Braces and splints may be of therapeutic value to treat fractures and prevent deformity.

Nursing process: Planning

Client need: Health Promotion and Maintenance

Cognitive level: Application

Subject area: Pediatric

9. While teaching 9- and 10-year-old children about safety measures to prevent injuries, the school nurse considers which of the following as the priority influence in the risk-taking behavior in this age group?

   1. Concrete thinking patterns

   2. The lack of a well-developed identity

   3. Inadequate rule enforcement

   4. Pressure from peers

10. When caring for a 4-year-old child whose left leg is in traction, the nurse notices that the traction weights are resting on the floor at the foot of the bed. What is the best action that the nurse should take in this situation?

    1. Elevate the foot of the bed

    2. Lower the head of the bed

    3. Cut the ropes to make them shorter

    4. Pull the child up in the bed

11. A mother of an infant asks the nurse when the anterior fontanel usually closes. The most appropriate response by the nurse is

    1. 6 months.

    2. 12 months.

    3. 18 months.

    4. 24 months.

12. Based on an understanding of Legg-Calvé-Perthes disease, the nurse provides the parents with what description of the disorder? _____

Answer: 4

Rationale: Although 9- and 10-year-olds have concrete thinking patterns and lack well-developed identities, peer pressure is the most likely cause of risk-taking behavior in this age group. Inadequate rule enforcement is less likely to cause risk-taking behavior.

Nursing process: Analysis

Client need: Management of Care

Cognitive level: Analysis

Subject area: Pediatric

Answer: 4

Rationale: When the traction weights are resting on the floor, the child needs to be pulled up in bed so that the weights can hang freely and the proper traction can be applied to the leg. Elevating the foot of the bed or lowering the head of the bed would not allow the proper traction to be applied to the child's leg. Cutting the ropes would not improve the traction if the child remains down at the foot of the bed.

Nursing process: Planning

Client need: Health Promotion and Maintenance

Cognitive level: Application

Subject area: Pediatric

Answer: 3

Rationale: An infant's anterior fontanel normally closes at 18 months.

Nursing process: Analysis

Client need: Health Promotion and Maintenance

Cognitive level: Application

Subject area: Pediatric

Answer: Avascular necrosis of the femoral head

Rationale: Legg-Calvé-Perthes disease can best be described as avascular necrosis of the head of the femur.

Nursing process: Implementation

Client need: Health Promotion and Maintenance

Cognitive level: Comprehension

Subject area: Pediatric

13. The nurse should assess a child admitted with a diagnosis of slipped capital femoral epiphysis for which of the following additional health problems?

1. Emaciated appearance

2. Nutritional anemia

3. Developmental delays

4. Obesity

14. The nurse should assess a teenage child suspected of having early stage scoliosis for which of the following clinical manifestations?

Select all that apply:

[   ] **1.** Unequal shoulder level

[   ] **2.** Curved spinal column

[   ] **3.** Altered gait with a limp

[   ] **4.** Truncal asymmetry

[   ] **5.** Prominence of one scapula

[   ] **6.** Limited use of one arm

15. Based on an understanding of the treatment for moderate scoliosis, which of the following is a priority?

1. Assess for more severe clinical manifestations

2. The use of a Boston or TLSO brace

3. Stretching and exercising

4. Surgery to place rods or wires

16. A school nurse is conducting a screening program for scoliosis. At which grade level should the school nurse begin testing for scoliosis?

1. Third grade

2. Fifth grade

3. Seventh grade

4. Ninth grade

Answer: 4

Rationale: The upper femoral epiphysis slips from its functional position in slipped capital femoral epiphysis. The incidence of slipped capital femoral epiphysis is greatest in African-American obese males. An emaciated appearance, anemia, and developmental delays are not usually associated with this diagnosis.

Nursing process: Assessment

Client need: Health Promotion and Maintenance

Cognitive level: Analysis

Subject area: Pediatric

Answer: 1, 2, 4, 5

Rationale: Scoliosis is a lateral curvature of the spine with vertebral body rotation. Clinical manifestations in the early stages include an unequal shoulder level, curved spinal column, truncal asymmetry, and prominence of one scapula. Severe back pain does not usually occur in the early stages. Neither a limp nor limited use of an arm is usually apparent at this time.

Nursing process: Assessment

Client need: Health Promotion and Maintenance

Cognitive level: Application

Subject area: Pediatric

Answer: 2

Rationale: When moderate scoliosis is found, the priority treatment is usually to fit the child with a brace to limit progression of the disease. The Boston brace is a prefabricated plastic shell that fits under the arm and is used for curves of the low thoracolumbar and lumbar spine. The TLSO brace is a molded custom jacket used for thoracolumbar curves. Stretching and exercising may be done in mild forms of the disease, and surgery may be performed for more severe forms of scoliosis.

Nursing process: Analysis

Client need: Management of Care

Cognitive level: Analysis

Subject area: Legal and Ethical Issues

Answer: 2

Rationale: In order to detect scoliosis in the early stage, the school nurse should begin testing for scoliosis in the fifth grade and continue testing until midadolescence. The third grade is too early to begin testing.

Nursing process: Planning

Client need: Health Promotion and Maintenance

Cognitive level: Application

Subject area: Pediatric

17. A 3-year-old child is admitted with a fractured femur and a diagnosis of osteogenesis imperfecta. On physical examination of this child, the nurse also assesses this child to have which of the following clinical manifestations?

    Select all that apply:

    [   ] 1. Blue sclerae

    [   ] 2. Chronic anemia

    [   ] 3. Dental deformities

    [   ] 4. Open posterior fontanel

    [   ] 5. Hyperlaxity of ligaments

    [   ] 6. Bowed legs

18. The mother of an 8-year-old with osteogenesis imperfecta asks the nurse if there is a sport in which her child could safely participate. Which of the following sports should the nurse suggest?

    1. Soccer

    2. Track

    3. Baseball

    4. Swimming

19. The nurse correctly assesses which of the following children for the onset of Duchenne's muscular dystrophy?

    1. An infant at birth

    2. A preschool child

    3. A school-age child

    4. An adolescent

20. The nurse caring for a child with muscular dystrophy observes the child use the Gower maneuver while trying to

    1. sit.

    2. walk.

    3. stand.

    4. bend over.

Answer: 1, 3, 5

Rationale: Osteogenesis imperfecta, also called brittle bone disease, is a connective tissue disease characterized by a disturbance of the formation of the periosteal bone. Along with fragile bones and frequent fractures, an affected child may also have blue sclerae, dental deformities, and hyperlaxity of the ligaments.

Nursing process: Assessment

Client need: Health Promotion and Maintenance

Cognitive level: Application

Subject area: Pediatric

Answer: 4

Rationale: Participating in sports is a problem for children with osteogenesis imperfecta, or brittle bone disease. Swimming is a sport that would not place stress on the child's bones. Soccer, track, and baseball are all sports that would be too dangerous for a child with osteogenesis imperfecta.

Nursing process: Planning

Client need: Health Promotion and Maintenance

Cognitive level: Analysis

Subject area: Pediatric

Answer: 2

Rationale: Duchenne's muscular dystrophy is a group of progressive degenerative inherited diseases that cause muscle wasting. It has an onset between the ages of 3 and 6 years.

Nursing process: Assessment

Client need: Health Promotion and Maintenance

Cognitive level: Application

Subject area: Pediatric

Answer: 3

Rationale: At about 5 or 6 years of age, children with muscular dystrophy must use their hands to walk up their legs to achieve the standing position. This is called the Gower maneuver.

Nursing process: Assessment

Client need: Health Promotion and Maintenance

Cognitive level: Application

Subject area: Pediatric

21. A nurse is teaching a class to parents of children with spinal deformities. Which of the following should the nurse include in the class?

    1. Lordosis is an increased posterior convex angle in the curvature of the thoracic spine.

    2. The child should be evaluated annually for progress during growth spurts.

    3. Scoliosis occurs most often during infancy and childhood.

    4. Spinal deformities may be painless and have a slow progression in the early stages.

22. The nurse is assessing four infants for fine and gross motor development. The nurse should report which of the following infants as having a problem with motor development?

    1. A 7-month-old infant who cannot sit without support

    2. A 3-month-old infant whose tonic neck and Moro reflexes are disappearing

    3. A 5-month-old infant who uses the whole hand to grasp an object

    4. A 6-month-old infant who does not have a pincer grasp

23. Which of the following should the nurse include in the home care instructions given to the parents of a child with a cast?

Select all that apply:

    [   ] **1.** With time, the cast may give off a foul-smelling odor

    [   ] **2.** Instruct the child to use a small object such as a pencil to scratch under the top of the cast

    [   ] **3.** Elevate the cast on a pillow above the level of the heart

    [   ] **4.** Avoid "petaling" the edges of the cast around the groin or perineum

    [   ] **5.** For itching, blow air into the cast with a hair dryer set on the cool setting

    [   ] **6.** Cover the cast with plastic wrap before bathing

24. The nurse is caring for a child in balanced suspension following a fracture of the femur. The child is complaining of severe, unrelenting pain distal to the break that is unrelieved by analgesics. The nurse should report this as a critical sign of _____.

Answer: 4

Rationale: Spinal deformities are generally painless and have a slow progression in the early stages. Lordosis is an increased anterior curvature of the lumbar spine. The child and family should be taught that periodic evaluation (every three to six months) during rapid growth spurts is indicated. Scoliosis most often occurs during the growth spurt of adolescence.

Nursing process: Planning

Client need: Health Promotion and Maintenance

Cognitive level: Application

Subject area: Pediatric

Answer: 1

Rationale: A 6-month-old infant should be able to sit without support. The tonic neck and Moro reflexes begin to disappear between 2 and 3 months. Using the whole hand to grasp an object occurs between 4 and 5 months. The pincer grasp begins to develop between 8 and 9 months.

Nursing process: Analysis

Client need: Health Promotion and Maintenance

Cognitive level: Analysis

Subject area: Pediatric

Answer: 3, 5, 6

Rationale: At no time should a foul-smelling odor from the cast be ignored; an odor indicates the presence of infection. Using objects to scratch under the cast can cause injuries to the skin. "Petaling"—covering the edges with moleskin or adhesive tape to protect the child's skin from rough, irritating edges—should be done in the groin and perineum to protect the cast from urine and stool.

Nursing process: Planning

Client need: Health Promotion and Maintenance

Cognitive level: Application

Subject area: Pediatric

Answer: compartment syndrome

Rationale: Compartment syndrome is a serious condition in which there is an increased pressure within one or more compartments leading to massive impairment of circulation to the area. The characteristic manifestation is unrelenting pain distal to the break, which is unrelieved by analgesics.

Nursing process: Analysis

Client need: Reduction of Risk Potential

Cognitive level: Analysis

Subject area: Pediatric

25. Which of the following pictures of traction should the nurse include in the preparation given to the parents of a child to be placed in Bryant's traction? _____

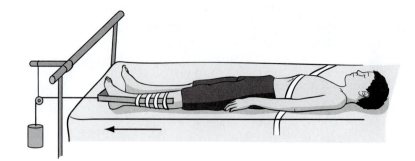

1.

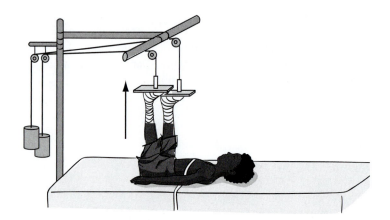

2.

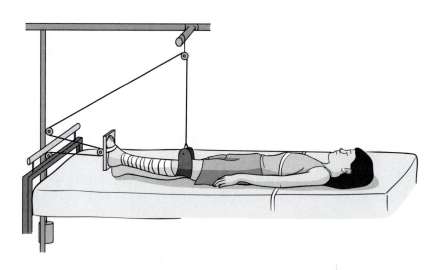

3.

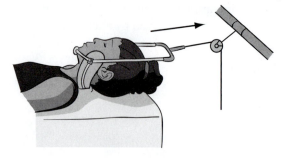

4.

Answer: 2

Rationale: Choice 1 is Buck's extension. Choice 3 is Russell's traction. Both of these are types of skin traction, as is Bryant's traction. Choice 4 is balanced suspension and a form of skeletal traction.

Nursing process: Planning

Client need: Health Promotion and Maintenance

Cognitive level: Application

Subject area: Pediatric

26. The registered nurse is preparing the clinical assignments for a pediatric musculoskeletal unit. Which of the following nursing tasks should the nurse delegate?

  1. Assess a child for juvenile rheumatoid arthritis

  2. Bathe a client with a hip spica cast

  3. Prepare a child with slipped femoral capital epiphysis for surgery including a pinning and external fixation of the femoral head

  4. Monitor a child with Bryant's traction following a fracture of the femur for compartment syndrome

27. The nurse should report which of the following pediatric musculoskeletal assessment findings as abnormal?

  1. An increased muscle tone in a 2-year-old child

  2. An 18-month-old infant who is bowlegged

  3. A 1-year-old toddler who has a wide-based gait

  4. An infant with a lumbar curvature of the spine and protuberant abdomen

Answer: 2

Rationale: Assessing, monitoring, and preparing a child for surgery are nursing tasks that require the skills of a registered nurse. A licensed practical nurse may bathe a client with a cast.

Nursing process: Planning

Client need: Management of Care

Cognitive level: Analysis

Subject area: Legal and Ethical Issues

Answer: 1

Rationale: An increased muscle tone in a 2-year-old child is abnormal. It may indicate cerebral palsy. It is normal for an 18-month-old child to be bowlegged. A wide-based gait is normal in a 1-year-old toddler. Infants normally have lumbar curvatures of the spine and protuberant abdomens.

Nursing process: Analysis

Client need: Health Promotion and Maintenance

Cognitive level: Analysis

Subject area: Pediatric

Genitourinary Disorders

37

1. The parents of a newborn with bladder exstrophy ask the nurse why a suprapubic catheter is being inserted. Which of the following is the most appropriate response by the nurse? "Suprapubic catheterization

   1. is a less painful procedure on a newborn than bladder catheterization."

   2. does not require restraining the newborn like bladder catheterization."

   3. is performed to aspirate urine when the newborn has not voided for more than one hour."

   4. is the only procedure that allows a small catheter to be used on a newborn."

2. The nurse assesses a 6-year-old child suspected of a urinary tract infection for which of the following clinical manifestations?

   Select all that apply:

   [　] 1. Enuresis

   [　] 2. Straining at urination

   [　] 3. Dribbling

   [　] 4. Urinary retention

   [　] 5. Jaundice

   [　] 6. Dysuria

3. Which of the following should the nurse include in the postoperative management of a child who had surgery for vesicoureteral reflux?

   1. Cover the bladder with a thin, clear, nonadhesive dressing

   2. Encourage the parents to have the child wear loose clothing

   3. Inform the parents that a renal ultrasound should be done at 6 months and again at 1 year

   4. Administer prescribed oxybutynin chloride (Ditropan) and desmopressin acetate (DDAVP)

Answer: 3

Rationale: Suprapubic catheterization allows the aspiration of urine when a child cannot void because of a congenital abnormality such as bladder exstrophy. Generally, suprapubic catheterization is performed when a child hasn't voided for more than an hour. It is a less desirable procedure than bladder catheterization because it is painful and the child must be restrained. It is performed less frequently now than in the past because small catheters are now available for bladder catheterization.

Nursing process: Analysis

Client need: Health Promotion and Maintenance

Cognitive level: Application

Subject area: Pediatric

Answer: 1, 2, 3, 6

Rationale: Clinical manifestations of a urinary tract infection in a child 2 years of age or older include enuresis, dysuria, frequency, urgency, fever, dribbling, foul-smelling urine, flank pain, and straining at urination.

Nursing process: Assessment

Client need: Health Promotion and Maintenance

Cognitive level: Application

Subject area: Pediatric

Answer: 3

Rationale: Postoperative care of a child who has had surgery for a vesicoureteral reflux should include a renal ultrasound at 6 months and again at 1 year to evaluate renal growth. Covering the bladder with a thin, nonadhesive dressing is an appropriate intervention before surgery for a bladder exstrophy. Encouraging the parents to have the child wear loose clothing is an appropriate intervention for cryptorchidism. Oxybutynin chloride (Ditropan) is an anticholinergic used in the treatment of enuresis. Desmopressin acetate (DDAVP), a synthetic analog of vasopressin that acts by increasing water retention and urine concentration, is also used for enuresis.

Nursing process: Planning

Client need: Health Promotion and Maintenance

Cognitive level: Application

Subject area: Pediatric

4. When working with a child with postinfectious glomerulonephritis, which of the following is most appropriate to consider when planning the goals of care?

   1. Most children fully recover from this illness

   2. Visible blood in the urine may persist for one to two years

   3. Blood pressure medications will need to be taken permanently

   4. There is a high incidence of recurrent urinary tract infections

5. When providing care for a child who is on oxybutynin chloride (Ditropan) for enuresis, the nurse should monitor the child for which of the following?

   Select all that apply:

   [   ] **1.** Facial flushing

   [   ] **2.** Nasal congestion

   [   ] **3.** Diarrhea

   [   ] **4.** Blurred vision

   [   ] **5.** Dry mouth

   [   ] **6.** Nosebleeds

6. The parents of a child in end-stage renal disease have received dietary instructions. Which of the following statements by the parents would indicate that they understood which foods to avoid in end-stage renal disease?

   Select all that apply:

   [   ] **1.** "We will avoid foods high in calcium."

   [   ] **2.** "We will avoid foods high in sodium."

   [   ] **3.** "We will avoid foods high in phosphorus."

   [   ] **4.** "We will avoid foods high in magnesium."

   [   ] **5.** "We will avoid foods high in potassium."

   [   ] **6.** "We will avoid foods high in cholesterol."

7. The nurse is admitting a child suspected of having nephrotic syndrome. After performing a physical assessment and reviewing laboratory data, the nurse notifies the physician that what three classic features are present in nephrotic syndrome? _____

Answer: 1

Rationale: Glomerulonephritis is a primary disorder or a manifestation of a systemic disorder that may range from mild to severe. The most common form is a postinfectious inflammation of the glomeruli caused by a streptococcal, pneumococcal, or viral infection. A full recovery generally occurs. Although hypertension and hematuria are clinical manifestations, they generally resolve with recovery. Recurrent urinary infections do not occur in glomerulonephritis but in vesicoureteral reflux.

Nursing process: Planning

Client need: Health Promotion and Maintenance

Cognitive level: Analysis

Subject area: Pediatric

Answer: 1, 4, 5

Rationale: Oxybutynin chloride (Ditropan) is an anticholinergic used in the treatment of enuresis by inhibiting voiding and enhancing voluntary urethral control. Common adverse reactions include facial flushing, dry mouth, constipation, heat intolerance, drowsiness, insomnia, and blurred vision. Nasal congestion and nosebleeds are adverse reactions to desmopressin acetate (DDAVP).

Nursing process: Assessment

Client need: Pharmacological and Parenteral Therapies

Cognitive level: Application

Subject area: Pharmacologic

Answer: 2, 3, 5

Rationale: Chronic renal failure is a progressive disease with the gradual destruction of over 50% of kidney function. Potassium, sodium, and phosphorus are to be avoided. Potassium and phosphorus are not well excreted, and sodium is restricted because it is associated with edema and blood pressure.

Nursing process: Evaluation

Client need: Basic Care and Comfort

Cognitive level: Application

Subject area: Pediatric

Answer: Hypoalbuminemia, hyperalbuminuria, and periorbital edema

Rationale: Nephrotic syndrome results from a glomerular injury and is manifested by periorbital edema that is generally worse in the morning. Significant laboratory data includes hypoalbuminemia and hyperalbuminuria.

Nursing process: Analysis

Client need: Health Promotion and Maintenance

Cognitive level: Analysis

Subject area: Pediatric

8. In planning the post-op care for a child who has had surgery for cryptorchidism, the nurse should perform which of the following priority nursing interventions?

   1. Encourage protein in the diet

   2. Assess the cremasteric reflex

   3. Change the diapers frequently

   4. Encourage activity

 9. Because a 3-year-old child has diurnal enuresis, plans for nursing interventions should include which of the following?

   Select all that apply:

   [   ] **1.** Restrict citrus fruits and foods high in sugar.

   [   ] **2.** Implement a bed-wetting alarm on the child's pajamas.

   [   ] **3.** Implement a behavior motivational star chart.

   [   ] **4.** Restrict fluids in the diet.

   [   ] **5.** Encourage a diet high in fiber.

   [   ] **6.** Administer prescribed luteinizing hormone-releasing hormone nasal spray.

10. A mother of a 4-year-old child asks the nurse whether control of urine or stool comes first. Which of the following responses is appropriate?

   1. "Control of urine at night occurs first."

   2. "Control of stool during the day occurs first."

   3. "Control of stool at night occurs first."

   4. "Control of urine during the day occurs first."

Answer: 3

Rationale: Cryptorchidism is failure of one or both testes to descend normally into the scrotum. Surgery is necessary to avoid exposure of the undescended testis to the body temperature, increased incidence of infertility, tumors, and physical or psychological trauma as a result of an empty scrotum. The priority nursing intervention is frequent diaper changes to prevent infection. There are no dietary restrictions, although protein will promote wound healing. Assessing the cremasteric reflex is the application of firm pressure on the external ring before palpating the abdomen or genitalia. The reflex is active in an infant and child up to 5 years of age and may result in withdrawal of the testes above the scrotum. Activity is not encouraged, and engaging in strenuous activity and playing on riding toys are to be avoided.

Nursing process: Planning

Client need: Mangement of Care

Cognitive level: Application

Subject area: Pediatric

Answer: 1, 3, 5

Rationale: Diurnal enuresis is enuresis that occurs only during the day, so a bed-wetting alarm is not necessary. Citrus fruits and heavily sugared foods are to be avoided because they are irritants to the bladder mucosa. Fiber and fluids should be increased to avoid constipation. A behavior motivational star chart is implemented to reward the child when progress is made and serves as a visual chart of successes. Luteinizing hormone-releasing hormone nasal spray is used in the treatment of cryptorchidism.

Nursing process: Planning

Client need: Health Promotion and Maintenance

Cognitive level: Application

Subject area: Pediatric

Answer: 3

Rationale: Control of the bowel occurs first at night followed by control of the bowel during the day. Subsequently, urine is controlled during the day; control of urine at night occurs last.

Nursing process: Analysis

Client need: Health Promotion and Maintenance

Cognitive level: Analysis

Subject area: Pediatric

11. When planning the care for a child with bladder exstrophy-epispadias complex, the nurse identifies a priority goal as _____.

....

12. Which of the following nursing interventions is a priority for the nurse to implement in the plan of care for a child with hemolytic uremic syndrome?

    1. Administer prescribed sodium polystyrene sulfonate (Kayexalate) rectally

    2. Restrict glucose foods

    3. Administer prescribed trimethoprim-sulfamethoxazole (Bactrim)

    4. Encourage phosphorus-rich foods

....

13. The nurse evaluates which of the following children with end-stage renal failure to be the most appropriate candidate for a renal transplant?

    1. A 12-year-old child with osteosarcoma

    2. A 2-year-old child born with the HIV virus

    3. A 3-year-old child with hemolytic uremic syndrome

    4. An 18-year-old adolescent with Hodgkin's disease

....

14. Which of the following is the priority for the nurse to monitor in a child who has had hypospadias surgery?

    1. Urethral fistula

    2. Urinary tract infections

    3. Dysuria

    4. Bladder spasms

Answer: preservation of the bladder and abdominal wall

Rationale: The priority goal in the treatment of bladder exstrophy-epispadias complex is to perform surgery within two days of birth first to preserve the bladder and abdominal wall, then to create a successful urethral sphincter, and lastly to correct genital anomalies.

Nursing process: Planning

Client need: Management of Care

Cognitive level: Analysis

Subject area: Pediatric

Answer: 1

Rationale: A priority nursing intervention for hemolytic uremic syndrome is the administration of rectal sodium polystyrene sulfonate (Kayexalate) to bind potassium in the body and remove it through the rectum. Glucose may be administered if hypoglycemia is present. Trimethoprim-sulfamethoxazole (Bactrim) is a sulfonamide that is nephrotoxic. Aluminum hydroxide gel may be given to bind with phosphorus.

Nursing process: Implementation

Client need: Management of Care

Cognitive level: Application

Subject area: Pediatric

Answer: 3

Rationale: Renal transplantation for children with end-stage renal disease is the only treatment that offers these children a chance at a normal life. The child must be free of cancer for a period of no less than two years and have no indications of an infection.

Nursing process: Evaluation

Client need: Health Promotion and Maintenance

Cognitive level: Analysis

Subject area: Pediatric

Answer: 1

Rationale: Hypospadias is a congenital defect in which the urethral meatus appears on the ventral surface of the penis. A urethral fistula results in urine leaking from the urethra and may necessitate surgery if it does not spontaneously resolve. Although dysuria, bladder spasms, and urinary tract infections may occur following urinary surgery, the priority is the leakage of urine that may occur from the urethra with a urethral fistula.

Nursing process: Assessment

Client need: Reduction of Risk Potential

Cognitive level: Analysis

Subject area: Pediatric

15. Which of the following changes in a child's assessment should the nurse report as a critical indication of a toxic reaction to oxybutynin chloride (Ditropan)?

   1. Constipation and urinary retention

   2. Dry mouth and blurred vision

   3. Tachycardia and hypertension

   4. Heat intolerance and insomnia

16. In planning the post-op care for a child following reimplantation of the ureters, the nurse should include which of the following in the plan of care to prevent urinary tract infections?

   1. Assess the tubing and ureteral stents for breaks in their integrity

   2. Monitor the intake and output

   3. Perform frequent bladder irrigations

   4. Maintain a diet high in protein and fiber

17. The nurse evaluates which of the following laboratory tests and assessment findings in a 6-month-old infant to support a diagnosis of hemolytic uremic syndrome?

   Select all that apply:

   [ ] **1.** Blood pressure of 110/70 mm Hg

   [ ] **2.** Blood urea nitrogen (BUN) of 20 mg/dl

   [ ] **3.** A platelet count of 95,000/μl

   [ ] **4.** Serum calcium of 11.0 mg/dl

   [ ] **5.** Serum potassium of 6.1 mEq/L

   [ ] **6.** Serum sodium of 131 mEq/L

Answer: 3

Rationale: Oxybutynin chloride (Ditropan) is an anticholinergic used in the treatment of enuresis. Common adverse reactions include constipation, urinary retention, dry mouth, blurred vision, heat intolerance, and insomnia. Tachycardia and hypertension are serious adverse reactions that are indications of toxicity.

Nursing process: Analysis

Client need: Pharmacological and Parenteral Therapies

Cognitive level: Analysis

Subject area: Pharmacologic

Answer: 1

Rationale: Assessing the ureteral stents and tubing for breaks in their integrity is a priority nursing intervention to prevent urinary tract infections following implantation of the ureters.

Nursing process: Planning

Client need: Health Promotion and Maintenance

Cognitive level: Application

Subject area: Pediatric

Answer: 1, 2, 3

Rationale: Hypertension, thrombocytopenia, and an elevated blood urea nitrogen are laboratory findings in hemolytic uremic syndrome. In a 6-month-old infant, normal blood pressure is approximately 90/61 mm Hg; normal blood urea nitrogen should be between 4 mg/dl and 16 mg/dl; a normal platelet count is between 84,000 and 478,000 (a platelet count less than 75,000 indicates thrombocytopenia); normal serum calcium is 9.0 mg/dl to 10.6 mg/dl; normal serum sodium is 136 mEq/l to 146 mEq/L; and a normal serum potassium is 3.9 mEq/L to 5.9 mEq/L.

Nursing process: Analysis

Client need: Reduction of Risk Potential

Cognitive level: Analysis

Subject area: Pediatric

18. The registered nurse in charge of a busy genitourinary unit should most appropriately delegate which of the following nursing tasks to the appropriate unit personnel considering budget, time, and qualifications of the employee?

    1. Assign unlicensed assistive personnel (UAP) to take the vital signs on a child suspected of being hypertensive and in renal failure

    2. Assign a registered nurse (RN) to assess an infant with hemolytic syndrome for signs of intracranial pressure

    3. Assign a licensed practical nurse (LPN) to teach the parents of a child with a urinary obstruction about an intravenous pyelography scheduled for their child and obtain an informed consent

    4. Assign unlicensed assistive personnel (UAP) to evaluate the laboratory tests of a child with acute glomerulonephritis for hematuria and elevated serum sodium and potassium levels

19. The nurse is preparing the client assignments for the day on a genitourinary unit. Which of the following assignments would be appropriate to delegate to a licensed practical nurse (LPN)?

    1. Develop the plan of care for a client with vesicoureteral reflux

    2. Instruct the parents about the surgery scheduled for an infant with hypospadias

    3. Administer the prescribed prednisolone (Prelone) to a child with nephrotic syndrome

    4. Monitor the central venous pressure of a child with hemolytic uremic syndrome

20. The nurse should assess a child suspected of being in acute renal failure for which of the following?
    Select all that apply:

    [ ] 1. Urine output of less than 1 ml/kg/hr

    [ ] 2. Hematuria

    [ ] 3. Listlessness

    [ ] 4. Anorexia

    [ ] 5. Pain

    [ ] 6. White blood cell count of greater than 100,000 CFU/ml

Answer: 2

Rationale: Only a registered nurse can perform assessments. Also, a child suspected of having signs of intracranial pressure may not be stable. It is not appropriate to delegate to unlicensed assistive personnel the task of taking the vital signs of a child suspected of being hypertensive and in renal failure. Taking the vital signs of this client would be an assessment and evaluation of the client's status, which can only be performed by a registered nurse. A licensed practical nurse cannot provide education or evaluate; such tasks must be performed by the registered nurse.

Nursing process: Planning

Client need: Management of Care

Cognitive level: Analysis

Subject area: Legal and Ethical Issues

Answer: 3

Rationale: Prednisolone (Prelone) may be administered by a licensed practical nurse (LPN). An LPN cannot plan nursing care, perform education, or perform a central venous pressure reading. These assignments may only be performed by a registered nurse.

Nursing process: Planning

Client need: Management of Care

Cognitive level: Analysis

Subject area: Legal and Ethical Issues

Answer: 1, 3, 4

Rationale: Clinical manifestations of acute renal failure include anuria or a urine output of less than 1 ml/kg/hr, listlessness, and anorexia. Other clinical manifestations associated with acute renal failure include pallor, vomiting, lethargy, and signs of dehydration. Hematuria is a clinical manifestation of acute glomerulonephritis, not renal failure. Pain and an elevated white blood cell count are not features associated with acute renal failure.

Nursing process: Assessment

Client need: Health Promotion and Maintenance

Cognitive level: Application

Subject area: Pediatric

21. The nurse is discharging a 2-month-old infant after a recurrent urinary tract infection. Which of the following are common signs of a urinary tract infection that the nurse should instruct the parents to monitor the infant for at home?

Select all that apply:

[   ] 1. Urinary frequency

[   ] 2. Failure to thrive

[   ] 3. Nausea and vomiting

[   ] 4. Enuresis

[   ] 5. Chills

[   ] 6. Abdominal distention

22. The nurse assists a 4-year-old child experiencing primary enuresis to make which of the following menu selections?

1. Hamburger, orange, and cola

2. Hot dog and a chocolate milk shake

3. Pizza, vanilla ice cream, and tea

4. Fried chicken and mashed potatoes

23. The nurse is caring for a child who is having peritoneal dialysis. The nurse should monitor this child for what complication that is the priority risk for this child? _____

24. The nurse is assessing the following four children for the risk of developing an inguinal hernia. The nurse should recognize that which of the following children has the highest risk of developing this condition?

1. A 3-week-old male who was premature and has a low birth weight

2. A 7-year-old male who has been exposed to an infectious agent

3. A 2-year-old female who has a history of urinary tract infections

4. A 1-year-old female who lives in an underdeveloped country and is known to have eaten beef contaminated with *Escherichia coli*

Answer: 1, 2, 3, 6
Rationale: Clinical manifestations of a urinary tract infection in a 2-month-old infant include urinary frequency, failure to thrive, feeding problems, nausea, vomiting, abdominal distention, diarrhea, and jaundice.
Nursing process: Planning
Client need: Health Promotion and Maintenance
Cognitive level: Application
Subject area: Pediatric

Answer: 4
Rationale: Foods such as dairy products, citrus fruits, heavily sugared foods, and beverages with artificial coloring, carbonation, and caffeine can be irritants to the bladder and increase the child's enuresis.
Nursing process: Implementation
Client need: Basic Care and Comfort
Cognitive level: Application
Subject area: Pediatric

Answer: Infection
Rationale: Contracting an infection (peritonitis) is a major risk for clients undergoing peritoneal dialysis.
Nursing process: Assessment
Client need: Reduction of Risk Potential
Cognitive level: Analysis
Subject area: Pediatric

Answer: 1
Rationale: Infantile inguinal hernias are more common within the first month of life in males. The incidence is greatly increased in males born prematurely and with a low birth weight. A 7-year-old male exposed to an infectious agent may have acute glomerulonephritis. A 2-year-old female with a history of urinary tract infections may have vesicoureteral reflux. A 2-year-old female living in an undeveloped country who ate *E. coli*-contaminated beef may have hemolytic uremic anemia, a disorder that is distributed equally between the sexes.
Nursing process: Evaluation
Client need: Health Promotion and Maintenance
Cognitive level: Analysis
Subject area: Pediatric

Oncology Disorders

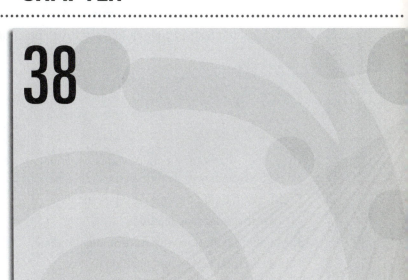

38

1. The nurse should include which of the following statements when providing education to the parents of a child who has had a bone marrow aspirate procedure?

    1. "Your child can take a shower, if desired."

    2. "You should not give your child a tub bath for 24 hours."

    3. "Your child should not sit for prolonged periods of time."

    4. "You should restrict your child's activity to quiet play for the next 12 hours."

2. The nurse is caring for a child who is experiencing severe mucositis. Which of the following measures would be essential to include in the child's plan of care?

    1. Offer oral liquid nutritional supplements

    2. Provide nasogastric feedings

    3. Maintain hydration with intravenous fluids

    4. Provide total parenteral nutrition (TPN)

3. A child is admitted to the day infusion area for two units of packed red blood cells. Which of the following clinical manifestations indicates to the nurse that the child is experiencing anemia?

    Select all that apply:

    [   ] 1. Gingival bleeding

    [   ] 2. Petechiae

    [   ] 3. Tachycardia

    [   ] 4. Pale mucous membranes

    [   ] 5. Dry mucous membranes

    [   ] 6. Headache

4. The father of a child newly diagnosed with acute lymphocytic leukemia (ALL) asks the nurse why trimethoprim-sulfamethoxazole (Bactrim) has been prescribed. The nurse would best describe the purpose of trimethoprim-sulfamethoxazole (Bactrim) therapy as a means to prevent which of the following?

    1. A certain type of pneumonia

    2. Diarrhea caused by a certain type of bacteria

    3. Upper respiratory infections caused by a certain type of virus

    4. A certain type of fungal infection in the mouth

Answer: 2

Rationale: Tub bathing and showering will compromise the integrity of the pressure dressing applied to the bone marrow aspirate site; the dressing needs to be in place for 24 hours postprocedure. Sitting for prolonged periods of time has no ill effect on the site of injury or the iliac crest. Activity restriction is regulated by the child's comfort level, since there are no activity restrictions associated with a bone marrow aspiration procedure.

Nursing process: Planning

Client need: Reduction of Risk Potential

Cognitive level: Analysis

Subject area: Pediatric

Answer: 4

Rationale: The most appropriate intervention for a child with mucositis is to provide total parenteral nutrition. Because mucositis severely alters oral cavity mucosa, oral feeding would be painful. Nasogastric feedings would not be an option, because intubation could potentially cause mechanical damage to the already injured oral and esophageal mucosa. Maintaining hydration does not allow for nutrition needs, only fluid needs.

Nursing process: Planning

Client need: Health Promotion and Maintenance

Cognitive level: Application

Subject area: Pediatric

Answer: 3, 4, 6

Rationale: Anemia, or a decrease in the number of red blood cells with oxygen-carrying hemoglobin that are circulating, produces clinical manifestations of rapid heart rate, headache, and paleness. Gingival bleeding and petechiae are manifestations of thrombocytopenia. Dry mucous membranes can indicate dehydration.

Nursing process: Analysis

Client need: Health Promotion and Maintenance

Cognitive level: Application

Subject area: Pediatric

Answer: 1

Rationale: Leukemia is a malignant disease in which normal marrow cells are replaced by abnormal, immature lymphocytes known as blast cells. It is the most common form of childhood leukemia. Trimethoprim and sulfamethoxazole (Bactrim) is prophylactic treatment for pneumonia caused by *Pneumocystis carinii*. Bactrim is ineffective against fungal and viral agents as well as ineffective in treating diarrhea.

Nursing process: Analysis

Client need: Pharmacological and Parenteral Therapies

Cognitive level: Application

Subject area: Pharmacologic

5. An adolescent with newly diagnosed osteosarcoma of the femur asks the nurse why a computerized tomography (CT) scan of the chest was ordered. The nurse should give this client which explanation of what the CT scan will show?

   1. "How well your lungs are functioning."
   2. "Your oxygenation status."
   3. "Metastatic lesions, if present."
   4. "How well your heart is pumping."

6. Before setting out for an appointment at the hematology/oncology clinic, an adolescent begins experiencing anticipatory nausea and vomiting. When informed of this situation, the nurse should instruct the adolescent to follow which of the following medication regimens?

   1. Oral lorazepam (Ativan), one hour before arriving at the clinic
   2. Intravenous lorazepam (Ativan) upon arrival at the clinic
   3. Oral dexamethasone (Decadron) half an hour before arriving at the clinic
   4. Intravenous dexamethasone (Decadron), with ondansetron (Zofran) upon arrival at the clinic

7. Which of the following assessments should the nurse perform on a child with newly diagnosed Wilms' tumor?

   1. Urine dipstick for microscopic hematuria
   2. Deep abdominal palpation
   3. Cranial nerve testing
   4. Urine electrolyte analysis

Answer: 3

Rationale: Osteosarcoma is a bone tumor that usually occurs in the growth metaphysis or the long ends of the bone. It is usually not diagnosed until there is a trauma to the bone. A chest CT scan is performed during the metastatic search. A test to determine how well the lungs are functioning would be a pulmonary function test. A test determining oxygenation would be ABG, or oxygen-saturation monitoring. A test to determine how well the heart is pumping would be an echocardiogram.

Nursing process: Analysis

Client need: Reduction of Risk Potential

Cognitive level: Application

Subject area: Pediatric

Answer: 1

Rationale: Lorazepam (Ativan) is an antianxiety medication that is effective against anticipatory nausea and vomiting. Administration of IV lorazepam (Ativan) is the incorrect route. Oral dexamethasone (Decadron) is not an antianxiety medication. Dexamethasone (Decadron) with ondansetron (Zofran) upon arrival to the clinic is not effective against anticipatory nausea and vomiting.

Nursing process: Planning

Client need: Pharmacological and Parenteral Therapies

Cognitive level: Analysis

Subject area: Pharmacologic

Answer: 1

Rationale: Wilms' tumor, or nephroblastoma, is the most common tumor of the kidney in children. Microscopic hematuria is often seen in clients diagnosed with Wilms' tumor. Deep palpation is avoided in order to keep the malignancy encapsulated. Cranial nerve testing is assessed in suspected central nervous system tumors. Urine electrolyte analysis is performed when syndrome of inappropriate antidiuretic hormone or diabetes insipidus is suspected.

Nursing process: Assessment

Client need: Health Promotion and Maintenance

Cognitive level: Analysis

Subject area: Pediatric

8. The nurse is caring for a child diagnosed with stage IV neuroblastoma. The nurse recognizes that the child may require which of the following?

   1. Total parenteral nutrition (TPN) to maintain nutritional requirements

   2. Rehabilitative services after tumor resection

   3. Placement of a ventriculoperitoneal (VP) shunt

   4. Thyroid replacement therapy after completion of chemotherapy

9. The nurse is providing postoperative care for an adolescent immediately following a limb salvage procedure of the left femur. Which of the following assessments should the nurse perform during the immediate postoperative period?

   1. Abduction of the left lower extremity

   2. Adduction of the left lower extremity

   3. Weight-bearing capacity of operative leg

   4. Circulation, movement, sensation (CMS) checks distal to operative site

10. The nurse is caring for a child receiving radiation therapy to the scapula as part of the treatment for Ewing's sarcoma. Which of the following interventions should the nurse include when performing skin care?

    1. Perform deep tissue massage of the radiation site

    2. Apply baby oil to the skin prior to daily radiation treatment

    3. Apply ice to irritated skin three times a day

    4. Apply prescribed lotion to reddened skin daily after radiation treatment

Answer: 1

Rationale: Neuroblastoma is a tumor that originates from cells that are precursors of the adrenal medulla and sympathetic nervous system. With stage IV neuroblastoma, the tumor has spread to the liver, skin, or bone marrow. Nutritional support is needed when a child is not capable of maintaining requirements. Rehabilitation services after tumor resection is needed for children undergoing limb salvage procedures. Placement of a VP shunt is needed for children experiencing hydrocephalus from a brain tumor. Thyroid replacement therapy after completion of chemotherapy is needed if the thyroid was in the radiation field and can no longer function adequately.

Nursing process: Implementation

Client need: Health Promotion and Maintenance

Cognitive level: Analysis

Subject area: Pediatric

Answer: 4

Rationale: Circulation, movement, and sensation (CMS) checks distal to the operative site are imperative perfusion assessments following a limb salvage of the left femur. Abduction and adduction of the left lower extremity would not be assessed immediately after surgery, due to tissue trauma and the potential for tissue injury. Assessment of the weight-bearing capacity of the operative leg would occur only after 24 to 48 hours of strict bed rest.

Nursing process: Assessment

Client need: Health Promotion and Maintenance

Cognitive level: Analysis

Subject area: Pediatric

Answer: 4

Rationale: Ewing's sarcoma is a highly malignant bone tumor usually present in the pelvis, tibia, fibula, and femur. It would be appropriate to apply prescribed lotion to reddened skin after radiation treatment. Massage would increase pain and mechanical cellular damage to already irritated skin. Baby oil prior to therapy would affect the efficacy of the radiation beam during therapy. Ice application would decrease circulation to the site, which needs an adequate blood supply for tissue healing.

Nursing process: Planning

Client need: Health Promotion and Maintenance

Cognitive level: Application

Subject area: Pediatric

11. The nurse is caring for a child with neutropenia secondary to chemotherapy. Which of the following measures would be essential to include in the child's discharge instructions?

    1. Call the doctor if the child has a fever greater than or equal to 38.3°C, or 101°F

    2. Do not send the child to school

    3. Discontinue granulocyte colony-stimulating factor (Neupogen)

    4. Administer acetaminophen (Tylenol) if the child complains of pain

12. The nurse is collecting a nursing history from a child with a pathological fracture of the right tibia. Which of the following questions should the nurse ask first to elicit the most accurate assessment?

    1. "Have you had any fevers recently?"

    2. "Did you experience any trauma to your right leg?"

    3. "Is there a family history of cancer?"

    4. "Are you having pain in any area other than your right leg?"

13. The nurse is collecting a nursing history from an adolescent diagnosed with Hodgkin's disease. Which of the following reported clinical manifestations are classified as B category manifestations?

    Select all that apply:

    [   ] 1. Anorexia

    [   ] 2. Productive cough

    [   ] 3. Unilateral numbness in lower extremity

    [   ] 4. Nausea and vomiting

    [   ] 5. Night sweats

    [   ] 6. Recurrent fevers

14. The nurse is caring for a child with a brain tumor. Which of the following observations should the nurse immediately report?

    Select all that apply:

    [   ] 1. Headache

    [   ] 2. Visual changes

    [   ] 3. Abdominal discomfort

    [   ] 4. Diarrhea

    [   ] 5. Decreased urine output

    [   ] 6. Vomiting

Answer: 1

Rationale: Fever is often the first sign of infection in a child with neutropenia. Not sending the child to school does not prevent infection caused by intrinsic organisms. Neupogen should be discontinued only after the neutrophil count has recovered. Administering acetaminophen (Tylenol) can mask a fever.

Nursing process: Planning

Client need: Management of Care

Cognitive level: Application

Subject area: Pediatric

Answer: 2

Rationale: Bone tumors alter the integrity of the bone, which often leads to pathological fractures. A fracture can be correlated with the onset of clinical manifestations, an important component in obtaining a health history. Recent fevers do not always give the nurse information about onset of manifestations. Family history and pains in other areas do not give the nurse information about the timing of onset of clinical manifestations.

Nursing process: Assessment

Client need: Management of Care

Cognitive level: Analysis

Subject area: Pediatric

Answer: 1, 5, 6

Rationale: Hodgkin's disease originates in the cervical lymph nodes and spreads to other lymph node regions. If treatment is not initiated, it may spread to the organs. Anorexia, night sweats, and recurrent fevers are B category clinical manifestations of Hodgkin's disease. Productive cough may be an indication of an upper respiratory infection. Altered gait and unilateral numbness in a lower extremity are clinical manifestations of a neurologic injury. Nausea, vomiting, and diarrhea are indications of a viral illness or adverse reactions to chemotherapy.

Nursing process: Assessment

Client need: Health Promotion and Maintenance

Cognitive level: Application

Subject area: Pediatric

Answer: 1, 2, 6

Rationale: Headache, visual changes, and vomiting are clinical manifestations of space-occupying intracranial lesions or ventriculoperitoneal (VP) shunt malfunction. Abdominal discomfort, diarrhea, and decreased urine output are all general clinical manifestations that a child may exhibit, but they do not necessarily require immediate attention.

Nursing process: Analysis

Client need: Reduction of Risk Potential

Cognitive level: Analysis

Subject area: Pediatric

15. The child newly diagnosed with acute lymphocytic leukemia is scheduled to have a lumbar puncture. With which of the following statements can the nurse best describe the purpose of the lumbar puncture?

    1. "It will relieve the headaches you are having."

    2. "It will allow for collection of fluid to examine for metastasis."

    3. "It will allow for collection of fluid to examine for meningitis."

    4. "It will relieve the bone pain you are having."

16. Which of the following does the nurse assess as a major presenting clinical manifestation in the child with a retinoblastoma?

    1. Icteric sclera

    2. Cat's eye reflex

    3. Chronic conjunctivitis

    4. Aniridia

17. The nurse is caring for a child with left-sided hemiparesis after a brain tumor resection. Which of the following nursing interventions is appropriate?

    1. Place the call light near the child's left hand

    2. Secure a peripheral intravenous catheter in the child's left hand

    3. Support the child's right side during transfer to a bedside commode

    4. Instill natural tears in both eyes four times a day

18. In preparing a child for a magnetic resonance image (MRI) with sedation, the nurse should include which of the following preprocedure instructions?

    1. Nothing by mouth six hours prior to exam

    2. Clear liquids until time of the test

    3. The child will need to be admitted to the hospital after the exam

    4. The child can go home immediately after the scan

Answer: 2

Rationale: The purpose of a lumbar puncture is to obtain cerebral spinal fluid to be examined for leukemic cells. Telling the client that it will relieve headaches is not appropriate, because there is a high incidence of headaches after a lumbar puncture. Examination of collected fluid for meningitis is not part of a new diagnosis evaluation of acute lymphocytic leukemia. Relieving bone pain is not correlated with accessing the intrathecal space.

Nursing process: Analysis

Client need: Reduction of Risk Potential

Cognitive level: Application

Subject area: Pediatric

Answer: 2

Rationale: Retinoblastoma tumors are tumors of the eye that create a cat's eye reflex when the light hits the eye at the right angle; the reflex is also identifiable in photographs. An icteric sclera would be associated with hepatic dysfunction. Chronic conjunctivitis is not identified as a precursor or a clinical manifestation of retinoblastoma. Aniridia is associated with Wilms' tumor.

Nursing process: Assessment

Client need: Health Promotion and Maintenance

Cognitive level: Application

Subject area: Pediatric

Answer: 2

Rationale: A peripheral intravenous catheter should be inserted in the child's left hand. The child's right hand should not be used because it would further limit the function of a compromised right side. Securing the call light near the child's left hand would not allow the child to independently call for the nurse. Supporting the child's right side does not consider safety during transfer. Instilling natural tears in both eyes four times a day suggests a bilateral intervention for a unilateral functional disability to keep the cornea protected.

Nursing process: Planning

Client need: Health Promotion and Maintenance

Cognitive level: Application

Subject area: Pediatric

Answer: 1

Rationale: Children receiving sedation for a magnetic resonance image (MRI) need to be NPO in order to prevent aspiration. Clear liquids would not be permitted. Hospital admission is not required. Postsedation monitoring is all that is required until the child is awake and alert. Immediate discharge is not allowed because the child needs to recover from sedation.

Nursing process: Planning

Client need: Reduction of Risk Potential

Cognitive level: Application

Subject area: Pediatric

19. The nurse is discharging a child with Wilms' tumor after a resection. Which of the following measures would be a priority to include in the client's discharge instructions?

    1. Low-sodium diet
    2. Restrict fluid intake
    3. Avoid contact sports
    4. Limit protein intake

20. The nurse should monitor a child with a brain stem glioma receiving vincristine sulfate (Oncovin) for which of the following adverse reactions?

    1. Constipation
    2. Diarrhea
    3. Appendicitis
    4. Typhlitis

21. The parents of a child with acute lymphocytic leukemia, positive for Philadelphia chromosome, ask the nurse to describe the treatment plan. The priority response by the nurse is "Chemotherapy

    1. until the child achieves remission."
    2. and biologic modifiers until the child achieves remission."
    3. until the child achieves remission, then radiation therapy."
    4. until the child achieves remission, then stem cell transplantation."

22. The nurse caring for a child with neuroblastoma includes which of the following assessments as a measure of tumor responsiveness?

    1. Serum copper levels
    2. Erythrocyte sedimentation rate (ESR)
    3. Urine catecholamines
    4. Urinalysis with a culture and sensitivity

Answer: 3

Rationale: Wilms' tumor is the most common childhood tumor of the kidney. Avoiding contact sports is a priority to protect the remaining kidney. A low-sodium diet is part of hypertension management. Fluid restriction and limiting protein intake are part of renal failure management.

Nursing process: Planning

Client need: Management of Care

Cognitive level: Analysis

Subject area: Legal and Ethical Issues

Answer: 1

Rationale: Vincristine sulfate (Oncovin) is an antineoplastic drug that inhibits mitosis at metaphase. It can cause neuropathy, including the gut, leading to constipation. Appendicitis and typhlitis are infectious processes that may arise during neutropenic episodes.

Nursing process: Assessment

Client need: Pharmacological and Parenteral Therapies

Cognitive level: Application

Subject area: Pharmacologic

Answer: 4

Rationale: Acute lymphocytic leukemia accounts for 80% of childhood leukemias. Children positive for Philadelphia chromosome require related or unrelated stem cell transplantation in order to eradicate the chromosomal defect. Biologic modifiers and radiation therapy will not eradicate the chromosomal defect.

Nursing process: Analysis

Client need: Pharmacological and Parenteral Therapies

Cognitive level: Analysis

Subject area: Pharmacologic

Answer: 3

Rationale: Neuroblastoma is a tumor that originates from the adrenal medulla and sympathetic nervous system. Clients with neuroblastoma produce excessive amounts of urine catecholamine metabolites (VMA, HVA, dopamine). Serum copper levels and erythrocyte sedimentation rates are tumor markers for Hodgkin's disease. Urinalysis with culture and sensitivity is an assessment conducted when urinary tract infection is suspected.

Nursing process: Assessment

Client need: Reduction of Risk Potential

Cognitive level: Analysis

Subject area: Pediatric

23. When planning the discharge of a child newly diagnosed with a malignancy, which of the following instructions should be included regarding infection prevention?

    1. Isolation is the most effective method of infection prevention

    2. Hand washing is the most effective method of infection prevention

    3. Restrict the intake of fresh fruits and vegetables

    4. Remove the carpet from the child's bedroom and play area

24. When caring for a child who has a ventriculoperitoneal (VP) shunt secondary to hydrocephalus from medulloblastoma, the nurse should include which of the following interventions?

    1. Darken the room to decrease photosensitivity

    2. Administer platelets when the platelet count drops below 50,000/mm^3

    3. Instruct the child to wear a hat instead of a wig for alopecia

    4. Restrict dietary sodium intake to 2 g/day

25. An adolescent with Ewing's sarcoma asks why radiation therapy will be needed since the entire tumor was surgically removed. In describing the purpose of multimodal therapy, the nurse should give this client which explanation of why radiation is needed?

    1. "It destroys remaining microscopic tumor cells."

    2. "It eliminates the cells damaged by chemotherapy."

    3. "It assists the injured tissue in the healing process."

    4. "It maintains function of the operative site."

Answer: 2

Rationale: Hand washing has been identified as the most effective method for preventing infection. Isolation, restricting the intake of fresh fruits and vegetables, and removing the carpet from the child's bedroom are measures instituted when a child is discharged to home after a stem cell transplant.

Nursing process: Planning

Client need: Health Promotion and Maintenance

Cognitive level: Application

Subject area: Pediatric

Answer: 2

Rationale: Platelets should be administered when the platelet count drops below 50,000/mm^3 in children with brain tumors to decrease the incidence of intracranial hemorrhage. Darkening the room to decrease photosensitivity is an intervention for migraine headaches or dilated eyes. A VP shunt has no impact on the type of head covering a child can wear. Restricting dietary sodium intake is an intervention for a child experiencing hypernatremia.

Nursing process: Planning

Client need: Health Promotion and Maintenance

Cognitive level: Application

Subject area: Pediatric

Answer: 1

Rationale: Radiation therapy is often used with radiosensitive tumors to eradicate microscopic disease in the tumor beds if surgical margins are close in cancers such as Ewing's sarcoma, a highly malignant bone tumor.

Nursing process: Analysis

Client need: Health Promotion and Maintenance

Cognitive level: Analysis

Subject area: Pediatric

26. The registered nurse is delegating the clinical assignments for a pediatric oncology unit. Which of the following clinical assignments is most appropriate for the nurse to delegate to unlicensed assistive personnel?

1. Bathe and position a child with a Wilms' tumor

2. Provide the care to a child who is neutropenic and has a temperature of 39°C, or 102.2°F

3. Dispose of the bodily fluids from a child receiving radioactive fluids

4. Bathe a child with acute lymphocytic leukemia

Answer: 4

Rationale: Great care is to be used in the bathing and handling of a child with a Wilms' tumor. It is essential to limit manipulation of the abdomen to prevent spread of the malignancy should the encapsulated mass rupture. It would not be appropriate to delegate bathing this child to unlicensed assistive personnel. A child who is neutropenic and has a fever of 39°C, or 102.2°F, would most appropriately be cared for by a nurse because of the risk of infection. Because precautions should be taken when handling bodily fluids of a client receiving radioactive fluids, this would not be the most appropriate clinical assignment for unlicensed assistive personnel. It would be appropriate to permit unlicensed assistive personnel to bathe a child with acute lymphocytic leukemia.

Nursing process: Planning

Client need: Management of Care

Cognitive level: Analysis

Subject area: Legal and Ethical Issues

Hematological Disorders

39

1. In examining a child with suspected anemia, the nurse would recognize which of the following as a significant objective finding?
   1. History of pica
   2. Daily aspirin therapy
   3. Cheilosis and glossitis
   4. Tonsillectomy three days ago

2. A child is being admitted to the hematology unit of the hospital with physician orders to obtain a complete blood count (CBC). The parent inquires about the purpose of this test. The nurse's best response would be
   1. "It provides a basic description of the types of cells present and measures the quantity of all the cells in the blood."
   2. "It provides the physician with an opportunity to view the red blood cells under a microscope."
   3. "It measures the body's stores of iron and its ability to bind iron and create hemoglobin."
   4. "It allows for the evaluation of the presence of abnormal hemoglobins and can detect hemoglobinopathies."

3. In preparing the client and family for bone marrow aspiration, the nurse should explain the procedure thoroughly. Which of the following statements represents appropriate family preparation?
   1. "The child will be required to lie perfectly still while the physician obtains the specimen from the sternum."
   2. "This procedure is virtually painless and well-tolerated by all children so anesthesia is not necessary."
   3. "The test measures with a stopwatch the length of time it takes the child to stop bleeding once the procedure is completed."
   4. "The physician will use sterile technique while obtaining a small sample of bone marrow through a needle inserted into the child's hip bone."

Answer: 3

Rationale: Cheilosis (fissures in the angles of the lips) and glossitis (inflammation of the tongue) are observable physical abnormalities that tend to occur in clients experiencing significant anemia. A history of pica, daily aspirin therapy, and tonsillectomy three days ago are all examples of subjective findings that may be associated with anemia.

Nursing process: Analysis

Client need: Health Promotion and Maintenance

Cognitive level: Application

Subject area: Pediatric

Answer: 1

Rationale: The CBC (complete blood count) is a basic diagnostic exam that measures the number, quality, variety, concentrations, and percentages of the blood cells. A peripheral smear allows the clinician to view blood cells under a microscope. Serum iron and TIBC (total iron-binding capacity) measure iron stores and the capacity of the body to bind with iron and form hemoglobin. Hemoglobin electrophoresis measures both normal and abnormal hemoglobins and is the diagnostic test required to identify hemoglobinopathies.

Nursing process: Analysis

Client need: Reduction of Risk Potential

Cognitive level: Comprehension

Subject area: Pediatric

Answer: 4

Rationale: Children will be positioned on the abdomen for the procedure since the posterior iliac crest is the preferred site for bone marrow aspiration in children. Sterile technique is used during the procedure to minimize the risk for infection. The sternum is an acceptable site for bone marrow aspiration in adults, but not in children. Bone marrow aspiration is associated with discomfort during needle insertion and specimen aspiration. The length of time it takes a client to form a clot is a measure of bleeding time.

Nursing process: Planning

Client need: Reduction of Risk Potential

Cognitive level: Application

Subject area: Pediatric

4. Which of the following should be included in the discharge instructions for a child with iron deficiency anemia?

   1. Take two iron supplements after missing a dose

   2. Iron supplements should be taken between meals with orange juice and monitor for black, tarry stools

   3. Increase vitamin D milk consumption in infants less than 12 months of age to increase dietary iron

   4. Avoid foods high in vitamin C, since they decrease the absorption of iron supplements

5. After assessing four clients with sickle cell anemia, which of the following clients is the priority for the nurse to administer care to first?

   1. A client whose speech is slurred and has hemiparesis

   2. A client complaining of painful swelling of the hands or feet

   3. A client who is experiencing pallor, icteric sclera, and fatigue

   4. A client complaining of abdominal pain after eating a high-fat meal

6. A nurse is caring for a child with sickle cell anemia. Which of the following measures would be a priority to include in the plan of care to prevent infection?

   1. Increase oral fluid intake and administer prescribed analgesics

   2. Administer penicillin twice daily and immunize with Pneumovax

   3. Infuse packed red blood cells monthly as prescribed

   4. Administer prescribed antipyretics for temperatures greater than 38.3°C, or 101°F

Answer: 2

Rationale: Iron supplements should be given on an empty stomach with a source of vitamin C to increase absorption and may be given between meals to decrease stomach upset. Black, tarry stool is a common side effect of iron therapy. Making up for missed doses of iron supplements is never recommended. Whole milk consumption by young infants is responsible for a large number of cases of iron deficiency anemia. The immature GI tract in infants cannot process whole milk, and this can lead to GI bleeding, blood loss, and anemia. Vitamin C increases the absorption of iron from the GI tract.

Nursing process: Planning

Client need: Health Promotion and Maintenance

Cognitive level: Application

Subject area: Pediatric

Answer: 1

Rationale: Hemiparesis and slurred speech may be indicative of stroke. Stroke requires immediate admission to the hospital for an exchange transfusion to prevent permanent motor damage. Painful swelling of the hands or feet is called dactylitis and can be managed at home with fluids and analgesics, unless fever is present. Pallor, icteric sclera, and fatigue are continuously present in a large number of clients with sickle cell disease due to underlying anemia. Abdominal pain, which occurs after eating greasy foods, is associated with gallstones and is not a medical emergency.

Nursing process: Analysis

Client need: Management of Care

Cognitive level: Analysis

Subject area: Pediatric

Answer: 2

Rationale: All children with sickle cell anemia who are less than 6 years of age should be on penicillin twice daily to prevent pneumococcal sepsis. In addition to regular immunizations, these children should receive Pneumovax, to further protect them from infection. Increasing fluids and administering analgesics are measures aimed at treating painful episodes. Monthly blood transfusions increase a client's hematocrit and decrease the risk for stroke, but do not prevent infection in sickle cell clients. Antipyretics are not effective in preventing infection.

Nursing process: Planning

Client need: Management of Care

Cognitive level: Analysis

Subject area: Pediatric

7. The nurse is admitting a child suspected of having beta thalassemia major. Which of the following findings should be reported?

Select all that apply:

[   ] 1. Excessive bruising

[   ] 2. Hematuria

[   ] 3. Severe anemia

[   ] 4. Pallor

[   ] 5. Maxillary hyperplasia

[   ] 6. Joint pain

8. In caring for a child with aplastic anemia, the nurse should immediately report which of the following assessment findings?

1. Fever of 39°C, or 102°F

2. Splenomegaly

3. Pallor and fatigue

4. Amenorrhea

9. The nurse should include which of the following instructions for the parents of a child with hemophilia A (factor XIII deficiency)?

1. Participation in contact sports is permitted with supervision and protective equipment

2. All forms of physical activity should be avoided in order to prevent bleeding episodes

3. Apply warm packs to hemarthroses to decrease associated discomfort

4. Encourage age-appropriate immunizations

10. The nurse is caring for a child suspected to have idiopathic thrombocytopenic purpura (ITP). Which of the following questions would be most important to ask while obtaining the history?

1. "Has your child been sick recently?"

2. "What blood type does your child have?"

3. "What medications have you given your child?"

4. "Are there any pets in the home?"

Answer: 3, 4, 5

Rationale: Maxillary hypertrophy results from bone marrow hyperplasia in response to the severe anemia that occurs in beta thalassemia major. Pallor is also a result of the severe anemia. Excessive bruising and hematuria are common manifestations of hemophilia, not beta thalassemia major. Joint pain is not a common manifestation of beta thalassemia major; however, it is experienced in clients with sickle cell anemia and hemophilia.

Nursing process: Analysis

Client need: Health Promotion and Maintenance

Cognitive level: Application

Subject area: Pediatric

Answer: 1

Rationale: Children with aplastic anemia are at increased risk for overwhelming sepsis due to neutropenia. Any fever greater than 38.3°C, or 101°F, is considered a medical emergency and requires immediate treatment. Splenomegaly is not commonly associated with aplastic anemia. Pallor and fatigue are common in clients with aplastic anemia, but do not usually require immediate evaluation. Amenorrhea is actually induced in many clients with aplastic anemia to prevent further blood loss and increasing anemia.

Nursing process: Analysis

Client need: Management of Care

Cognitive level: Analysis

Subject area: Pediatric

Answer: 4

Rationale: Immunizations should be administered in children with hemophilia, but should be given s.q. In addition, pressure should be applied to the site of injection for 15 minutes. Children with hemophilia are allowed participation in noncontact sports only. Exercise is important for children with hemophilia to build flexibility, strength, and cardiovascular endurance. Ice should be applied to areas of bleeding to constrict blood vessels and decrease bleeding.

Nursing process: Planning

Client need: Health Promotion and Maintenance

Cognitive level: Application

Subject area: Pediatric

Answer: 3

Rationale: Drugs such as aspirin products and nonsteroidal anti-inflammatory drugs can adversely affect children and cause bleeding. This needs to be ruled out before making a diagnosis of idiopathic thrombocytopenic purpura (ITP). Many children with ITP have a history of preceding viral illness, although it is not a definitive indication that the child will develop ITP. The child's blood type does not play a role in the diagnosis of ITP, although it might be necessary to know this if initial treatment options are unsuccessful. Pets in the home are insignificant for ITP.

Nursing process: Assessment

Client need: Health Promotion and Maintenance

Cognitive level: Analysis

Subject area: Pediatric

11. The nurse is caring for a child suspected of having von Willebrand's disease. The nurse should prepare the client for which of the following laboratory tests?

Select all that apply:

[　] **1.** Complete blood count (CBC) with differential

[　] **2.** Platelet count

[　] **3.** Bone marrow aspiration

[　] **4.** Hemoglobin electrophoresis

[　] **5.** Bleeding time

[　] **6.** Ristocetin cofactor

12. The nurse preparing a child for a bone marrow aspiration assists the physician to cleanse and prepare which site for the aspiration? _____

13. Which of the following should the nurse include in the plan of care for a child with disseminated intravascular coagulation (DIC)?

1. Administer blood thinners

2. Monitor the child for signs of bleeding

3. Administer intravenous analgesics

4. Monitor the child's respiratory status

Answer: 2, 5, 6

Rationale: Platelet count, bleeding time, and ristocetin cofactor are all essential to confirm a diagnosis of von Willebrand's disease. A complete blood count (CBC) and hemoglobin electrophoresis are instrumental in the diagnosis of hemoglobinopathies. Bone marrow aspiration looks at the cellular components of the bone marrow and is utilized in the diagnosis of many hematological conditions, but not von Willebrand's disease.

Nursing process: Planning

Client need: Reduction of Risk Potential

Cognitive level: Analysis

Subject area: Pediatric

Answer: Posterior iliac crest and sternum

Rationale: The preferred site for a bone marrow aspiration on a child is the posterior iliac crest and sternum.

Nursing process: Implementation

Client need: Reduction of Risk Potential

Cognitive level: Application

Subject area: Pediatric

Answer: 2

Rationale: The nurse should be acutely aware of any bleeding that occurs, since hypovolemic shock can be a complication of disseminated intravascular coagulation (DIC). Blood thinners, such as heparin, are usually administered only in severe cases because they create a risk for bleeding. IV analgesics are not routinely utilized in clients with disseminated intravascular coagulation. The child's respiratory status is not usually compromised in DIC.

Nursing process: Planning

Client need: Health Promotion and Maintenance

Cognitive level: Application

Subject area: Pediatric

14. Which of the following laboratory findings would the nurse expect to be ordered for a child with disseminated intravascular coagulation (DIC)?

Select all that apply:

[   ] 1. Prolonged partial thromboplastin time (PTT)

[   ] 2. Decreased white blood cell count (WBC)

[   ] 3. Increased red blood cell count (RBC)

[   ] 4. Decreased platelet count

[   ] 5. Increased reticulocyte count

[   ] 6. Decreased fibrinogen

15. Which of the following drugs should the nurse administer to a child with sickle cell anemia to decrease painful episodes and prevent hospitalizations?

1. Morphine sulfate (MS Contin)

2. Meperidine (Demerol)

3. Acetaminophen with codeine (Tylenol #3)

4. Hydroxyurea (Hydrea)

16. The parent of a child with a hematological disorder inquires about the purpose of the red blood cells in the body. The nurse should respond, "Red blood cells

1. serve as the body's defense against infection."

2. assist in the formation of blood clots."

3. carry oxygen to the tissues."

4. are primarily responsible for removing debris from the bloodstream."

Answer: 1, 4, 6

Rationale: Prolonged partial thromboplastin time is common in clients with disseminated intravascular coagulation (DIC), due to the body's attempt to dissolve the clots formed as a result of the increased activity of coagulation factors. The platelet count and fibrinogen may drop, due to the fibrinolysis which may occur. The white blood cell count (WBC) does not play a role in the pathophysiology of disseminated intravascular coagulation (DIC) and is unrelated to this condition. The red blood cell count (RBC) is usually decreased from bleeding. Increased reticulocyte count is associated with certain types of anemia.

Nursing process: Analysis

Client need: Reduction of Risk Potential

Cognitive level: Analysis

Subject area: Pediatric

Answer: 4

Rationale: Hydroxyurea (Hydrea) is a daily drug prescribed to decrease painful crises and prevent hospitalization of a child with sickle cell anemia. Morphine sulfate, meperidine (Demerol), and acetaminophen with codeine are all drugs utilized during acute pain episodes.

Nursing process: Planning

Client need: Pharmacological and Parenteral Therapies

Cognitive level: Analysis

Subject area: Pediatric

Answer: 3

Rationale: Red blood cells are responsible for carrying oxygen to the tissues and removing carbon dioxide from them. White blood cells are the body's primary defense against infection. Platelets are the cellular components of blood that assist in the formation of blood clots. Phagocytosis is the process of removing debris from the bloodstream and is carried out by white blood cells.

Nursing process: Analysis

Client need: Health Promotion and Maintenance

Cognitive level: Comprehension

Subject area: Pediatric

17. The nurse is caring for a child with anemia. Which of the following would indicate to the nurse that the client's condition is deteriorating?

    1. Circumoral pallor
    2. Fatigue with exertion
    3. Cardiac murmur
    4. Irritability

18. The nurse is instructing the family of a child with iron deficiency anemia about the importance of increasing iron in the diet. Which of the following foods should the nurse include?

    Select all that apply:

    [   ] 1. Fortified cereals
    [   ] 2. Green leafy vegetables
    [   ] 3. Vitamin D milk
    [   ] 4. Pasta
    [   ] 5. Dried fruits
    [   ] 6. Tea

19. The nurse is caring for a child with sickle cell disease who is experiencing hematuria. Which of the following actions is an appropriate intervention?

    1. Restrict activity
    2. Administer ibuprofen (Motrin)
    3. Push fluids
    4. Check the child's temperature

20. The nurse is discharging an infant who was recently diagnosed with sickle cell anemia, or hemoglobin SS disease. It is a priority to provide these parents information on which of the following complications?

    1. Avascular necrosis
    2. Retinopathy
    3. Gallstones
    4. Dactylitis

Answer: 3
Rationale: Cardiac murmurs are only present in children with significant anemia and indicate their condition is deteriorating. Pallor, fatigue with exertion, and irritability are findings that may be present with all levels of anemia.
Nursing process: Analysis
Client need: Health Promotion and Maintenance
Cognitive level: Analysis
Subject area: Pediatric

Answer: 1, 2, 5
Rationale: Fortified cereals, green leafy vegetables, and dried fruits are all excellent sources of iron and should be included in this child's diet. Vitamin D milk is high in calcium. Tea blocks the absorption of iron and should be excluded from the child's diet. Pasta is not a significant source of dietary iron.
Nursing process: Planning
Client need: Basic Care and Comfort
Cognitive level: Application
Subject area: Pediatric

Answer: 3
Rationale: Increasing fluid intake will dilute the urine and reduce further kidney damage and may possibly correct the hematuria. Restricting activity is not specific to hematuria. Ibuprofen has no indication in the treatment of hematuria. Evaluation of temperature is not indicated in the treatment of sickle cell anemia and hematuria.
Nursing process: Planning
Client need: Health Promotion and Maintenance
Cognitive level: Application
Subject area: Pediatric

Answer: 4
Rationale: Dactylitis is the first painful episode a sickle cell client may experience and usually occurs between 6 months and 3 years of age. This information would be most relevant for the parents of an infant who was just diagnosed. Avascular necrosis and retinopathy tend to be complications experienced in adolescence and adulthood. Gallstones are not common in infancy.
Nursing process: Planning
Client need: Reduction of Risk Potential
Cognitive level: Analysis
Subject area: Pediatric

21. Which of the following drugs should the nurse administer to a child with beta thalassemia major who has been on chronic transfusion therapy for several years?

    1. Acetaminophen with codeine (Tylenol #3)

    2. Deferoxamine (Desferal)

    3. Hydroxyurea (Hydrea)

    4. Cyclosporine (Sandimmune, Neoral)

22. The nurse is caring for a child with aplastic anemia. Which of the following measures should be included in the child's plan of care?

    1. Recommendation of genetic counseling

    2. Education on the proper administration of iron supplements

    3. Administration of antithymocyte globulin (ATG)

    4. Encourage interaction with other children at day care

23. The nurse is caring for a child with severe hemophilia A (factor XIII deficiency). Which of the following measures is most appropriate for the nurse to implement in this child's plan of care?

    1. Pad the bed rails

    2. Force fluids

    3. Administer intravenous immune globulin (IVIG)

    4. Monitor temperature

24. After a health interview with an adolescent child, which of the following findings should the nurse report as significant?

    1. Heavy menstrual flow

    2. Accelerated growth curve

    3. Delayed puberty

    4. Spinal curvature

Answer: 2

Rationale: Children who are receiving chronic transfusion therapy are at risk for iron overload and subsequent organ damage. Deferoxamine (Desferal) is a chelation agent that binds with iron and helps the body remove the excess. Tylenol with codeine and hydroxyurea (Hydrea) are drugs used in the treatment and prevention of sickle cell pain. Cyclosporine (Sandimmune, Neoral) is an immunosuppressive agent used in the treatment of aplastic anemia.

Nursing process: Planning

Client need: Pharmacological and Parenteral Therapies

Cognitive level: Application

Subject area: Pediatric

Answer: 3

Rationale: Antithymocyte globulin (ATG) is routinely used to treat clients with aplastic anemia. Genetic counseling is not indicated for families experiencing aplastic anemia, since it is not a hereditary condition. Iron supplementation is not usually indicated for clients with aplastic anemia. Because children with this disease should avoid exposure to sources of infection, they should not be encouraged to interact in day care. Day care centers and schools are common sources of infection.

Nursing process: Planning

Client need: Health Promotion and Maintenance

Cognitive level: Application

Subject area: Pediatric

Answer: 1

Rationale: Padding the bed rails may help to decrease the chances of injury in a child with hemophilia. Forcing fluids is not part of routine care for hemophilia clients. Intravenous immune globulin (IVIG) is utilized in clients with idiopathic thrombocytopenic purpura (ITP). Monitoring temperatures is necessary in all clients, but is not the most appropriate intervention for this child.

Nursing process: Implementation

Client need: Health Promotion and Maintenance

Cognitive level: Application

Subject area: Pediatric

Answer: 3

Rationale: Delayed puberty is common in adolescents with sickle cell disease. Heavy menstrual flow is more commonly associated with bleeding disorders, such as von Willebrand's disease. Children with sickle cell anemia have a strong tendency to be smaller and weigh less than their peers and often do not follow a normal growth curve. Spinal curvature is not associated with having sickle cell disease.

Nursing process: Analysis

Client need: Health Promotion and Maintenance

Cognitive level: Application

Subject area: Pediatric

25. Parents who are both carriers of the beta thalassemia gene have one child with the disease and want to have another child. They ask the nurse what the chances are of having another child with this disorder. The appropriate response by the nurse is

    1. "There is a 25% chance."

    2. "There is approximately a 50% chance."

    3. "There is no chance for the next child to be affected."

    4. "The second child will be born with the disorder."

26. The registered nurse is delegating the nursing tasks for a pediatric hematology unit. Which of the following tasks should the nurse delegate to a licensed practical nurse?

    1. Administer deferoxamine (Desferal) IV to a child with beta thalassemia major

    2. Monitor the platelet count in a child with aplastic anemia

    3. Assess a child with immune thrombocytopenia purpura for indications of bleeding

    4. Administer desmopressin (DDAVP) intranasally to a child with mild hemophilia A

Answer: 1

Rationale: If both parents are carriers of the disease gene of beta thalassemia major, there will be a 25% chance of having a child with the condition with each pregnancy. The parents are both carriers of a recessive gene that has a 25% chance of being expressed with each pregnancy.

Nursing process: Analysis

Client need: Health Promotion and Maintenance

Cognitive level: Analysis

Subject area: Pediatric

Answer: 4

Rationale: Administering a drug IV, monitoring a platelet count, and assessing a child for indications of bleeding are all tasks that require the skills of a registered nurse. A licensed practical nurse may administer a drug intranasally.

Nursing process: Planning

Client need: Management of Care

Cognitive level: Analysis

Subject area: Legal and Ethical Issues

Infectious and Communicable Disorders

40

1. The nurse instructs a group of nurses about the impact of infectious diseases in the childhood population of the world. The nurse should include which of the following statements in the discussion?

   1. Since the development of vaccines, infectious diseases are no longer a worldwide concern

   2. Severe infectious diseases have been eliminated

   3. Most infectious diseases are minor childhood ailments

   4. Despite improved methods of treatment, infectious diseases continue to be a health concern

2. The nurse is educating a group of health care providers on the great strides toward eradicating infectious diseases in the world that were made during the twentieth century. Which of the following events should the nurse include as having played a major role?

   1. Decreased fertility and birth rates

   2. Steroid-enhanced dairy products

   3. Modern sanitation

   4. The Immunization Act of 1986

3. When instructing a client, which of the following statements should the nurse include in explaining communicable diseases? They

   1. commonly occur in infancy, childhood, and adolescence.

   2. are transmitted by direct or indirect contact.

   3. are limited in physiologic involvement.

   4. are insidious and develop rapidly.

4. The parent of a child asks the nurse what the term "local infection" means. The nurse's appropriate response is, "A local infection

   1. occurs in many individuals in a common geographic area."

   2. is minor and easily treated."

   3. can be spread to others in close contact with the infected individual."

   4. is limited to one area of the body."

Answer: 4

Rationale: Infectious diseases continue to account for many serious illnesses, and prevention of infection is a major goal of the World Health Organization.

Nursing process: Planning

Client need: Safety and Infection Control

Cognitive level: Analysis

Subject area: Pediatric

Answer: 3

Rationale: Modern sanitation and our ability to sanitize surfaces and instruments used in daily activities have had a huge impact on reducing the spread of infectious diseases. Infections such as sexually transmitted diseases have played a part in reducing fertility and birth rates. Steroid-enhanced protein sources have no direct role in the spread of infectious or communicable diseases. The Immunization Act of 1986 is a legal act of Congress protecting individuals harmed by vaccines.

Nursing process: Planning

Client need: Safety and Infection Control

Cognitive level: Analysis

Subject area: Pediatric

Answer: 2

Rationale: Infectious or communicable diseases occur in humans of all ages. Certain infectious illnesses occur in specific age or developmental groups. Most infectious diseases are transmitted by direct or indirect contact, and isolation categories are assigned accordingly. Many infectious diseases have total systemic involvement or sequelae. Many infectious diseases develop slowly after a prolonged incubation period.

Nursing process: Planning

Client need: Safety and Infection Control

Cognitive level: Application

Subject area: Pediatric

Answer: 4

Rationale: A local infection is limited to one locality of the body but may have some systemic repercussions, such as fever and malaise. An infection occurring in a geographic area is an endemic outbreak. Local infections are not always treated easily; treatment is dependent on the causative agent. Local infections can become severe. Local infections are not usually contagious.

Nursing process: Analysis

Client need: Safety and Infection Control

Cognitive level: Comprehension

Subject area: Pediatric

5. A client hospitalized with a systemic infection asks the nurse what is meant by a systemic infection. The appropriate response by the nurse is that a systemic infection is _____.

6. A child is hospitalized with an infection that develops rapidly and resolves in a short period of time. The nurse informs the parents that the diagnosis is which of the following?

1. A local infection

2. A childhood illness

3. Varicella

4. An acute infection

7. The nurse instructs the parents of a child that the greatest weapon and priority available to reduce the spread of disease is which of the following?

1. Antibiotics

2. Isolation techniques

3. Ethyl alcohol wipes before injections

4. Hand washing

Answer: an infection that is spread throughout the body

Rationale: Systemic defines the degree of involvement and virulence of an organism that invades the body.

Nursing process: Analysis

Client need: Safety and Infection Control

Cognitive level: Comprehension

Subject area: Pediatric

Answer: 4

Rationale: An acute infection develops rapidly and resolves in a short period of time, but if not treated completely or with the appropriate pharmaceuticals, an acute infection could become chronic.

Nursing process: Implementation

Client need: Safety and Infection Control

Cognitive level: Comprehension

Subject area: Pediatric

Answer: 4

Rationale: Antibiotics, isolation, and ethyl alcohol have places in preventing the spread of disease, but the simplest and most effective weapon against the spread of disease is hand washing.

Nursing process: Implementation

Client need: Safety and Infection Control

Cognitive level: Application

Subject area: Pediatric

8. The nurse instructs student nurses that the Centers for Disease Control (CDC) recommends that isolation be based on which of the following?
    1. Method of disease transmission
    2. Severity of client illness
    3. Availability of personal protective equipment
    4. The client's health care coverage and ability to pay for private room

9. The mother of a child whose chickenpox rash first appeared eight days ago asks the nurse when her child may return to school without being contagious. Which of the following is the nurse's most appropriate response?
    1. "Your child cannot return to school until all the lesions disappear."
    2. "Your child is contagious as long as your child is itching."
    3. "The contagious state of chickenpox is generally 2 weeks."
    4. "Your child is not contagious and may return to school now."

10. When planning the care of a client diagnosed with asymptomatic herpes simplex virus type 2 (HSV-2), which of the following should the nurse consider?
    1. There is no risk of transmitting the condition to anyone else
    2. After prescribed treatment, herpes simplex virus type 2 is cured
    3. An antibiotic is used successfully in the treatment
    4. The client is a carrier, and still able to transmit the disease

Answer: 1

Rationale: In 2002, the CDC guidelines for isolation of clients with infectious or communicable diseases were revised to align according to methods of transmission. The extent of illness is not a useful indication of communicability. Many infectious diseases are spread because the infected individual feels well enough to be out and about. Appropriate personal protective equipment should be readily available to all health care workers in America, so lack of such equipment is not a justifiable reason to employ isolation. A client's ability to pay should never define the appropriate treatment course.

Nursing process: Implementation

Client need: Safety and Infection Control

Cognitive level: Application

Subject area: Pediatric

Answer: 4

Rationale: The chickenpox infection begins one to two days before the eruption of the rash and the contagious state ends six days after the onset of the lesions, when crusts have formed.

Nursing process: Analysis

Client need: Safety and Infection Control

Cognitive level: Analysis

Subject area: Pediatric

Answer: 4

Rationale: The herpes simplex virus type 2 (HSV-2) is characterized by periods of latency between outbreaks and recurrence. The virus can be shed, and is contagious when the client is asymptomatic. There are effective treatments available, but no known cure, for HSV-2. Antibiotics are not effective against viruses.

Nursing process: Planning

Client need: Safety and Infection Control

Cognitive level: Analysis

Subject area: Pediatric

11. Which of the following interventions should the nurse include in the plan of care of a child with mumps?

   1. Initiate respiratory isolation with the appearance of a rash

   2. Administer ganciclovir (Cytovene)

   3. Provide a high-calorie diet

   4. Monitor the white blood cell count

12. The nurse is teaching a class on how to prevent infectious diseases. Which of the following are priorities for the nurse to include in the class?

   Select all that apply:

   [ ] **1.** Hand washing

   [ ] **2.** Rest

   [ ] **3.** Immunization

   [ ] **4.** Nutrition

   [ ] **5.** Drug prophylaxis

   [ ] **6.** Herbal therapy

13. A mother asks the nurse how her child became infected with rotavirus. The most appropriate response by the nurse is, "Rotavirus is primarily spread by

   1. the fecal-oral route."

   2. inhalation of infected droplets."

   3. infected blood."

   4. sexual contact."

14. The nurse should consider which of the following when planning the care of a child infected with hepatitis B?

   1. Treatment is aimed at symptom management

   2. Administer oral acyclovir (Zovirax)

   3. Administer doxycycline (Vibramycin) and azithromycin (Zithromax)

   4. Treatment is directed by the results of the white blood cell test

Answer: 3

Rationale: It would be appropriate to provide children with mumps with high-calorie diets because they frequently have nutritional problems. Spicy and irritating foods that require a lot of chewing may cause discomfort for the child. Respiratory isolation should be initiated for four days after the appearance of a rash with rubeola (measles). Ganciclovir (Cytovene) is an antiviral used to treat life-threatening cytomegalovirus in immunocompromised hosts. The white blood cell count is monitored in infectious mononucleosis.

Nursing process: Planning

Client need: Safety and Infection Control

Cognitive level: Application

Subject area: Pediatric

Answer: 1, 3, 5

Rationale: The most effective methods of controlling infectious disease are drug prophylaxis, immunization, and hand washing. There is no evidence that herbal therapies are effective against infection. A general state of wellness, including good nutrition and rest, is important to general health, but is not the most effective approach to reducing the spread of infectious diseases.

Nursing process: Planning

Client need: Management of Care

Cognitive level: Application

Subject area: Pediatric

Answer: 1

Rationale: Rotavirus is the most common cause of severe diarrhea in children. It is primarily spread by the fecal-oral route.

Nursing process: Analysis

Client need: Safety and Infection Control

Cognitive level: Application

Subject area: Pediatric

Answer: 1

Rationale: There is no specific treatment for hepatitis B. Treatment focuses on symptom management. Oral acyclovir (Zovirax) is an antiviral used in the treatment of herpes genitalis (HSV-2). Doxycycline (Vibramycin) and azithromycin (Zithromax) are antibiotics used in the treatment of chlamydia. Monitoring the white blood cell is important in the treatment of infectious mononucleosis.

Nursing process: Planning

Client need: Safety and Infection Control

Cognitive level: Application

Subject area: Pediatric

15. The nurse assesses which of the following to be present in an infant born prematurely with congenital syphilis?

Select all that apply:

[   ] **1.** Hepatosplenomegaly

[   ] **2.** Pain in the chest

[   ] **3.** Weight loss

[   ] **4.** Mucocutaneous lesions

[   ] **5.** Lymphadenopathy

[   ] **6.** Generalized pruritic rash

16. The nurse is caring for a child with varicella (chickenpox). Which of the following assessments are priorities to report and indicate a secondary infection requiring prompt medical attention?

1. Generalized pruritic rash and mild fever

2. Skin pain and purulent discharge

3. Body rash and Koplik's spots

4. Red facial (slapped cheek) rash and circumoral pallor

17. A mother of a child diagnosed with erythema infectiosum (Fifth's disease) asks the nurse when the child may return to school without being contagious. The nurse should tell the mother that her child may return to school after

1. the appearance of the rash.

2. the appearance of a generalized pruritic rash.

3. being immunized.

4. the diarrhea disappears.

Answer: 1, 4, 5

Rationale: Clinical manifestations for congenital syphilis include hepatosplenomegaly, mucocutaneous lesions, and lymphadenopathy. Pain in the chest and weight loss are clinical features of tuberculosis. A generalized rash is characteristically present in varicella (chickenpox).

Nursing process: Assessment

Client need: Safety and Infection Control

Cognitive level: Application

Subject area: Pediatric

Answer: 2

Rationale: Varicella (chickenpox) is a varicella zoster virus that is highly contagious through direct contact or may be airborne-spread from respiratory secretions. Severe skin pain, burning, or purulent discharge may indicate a secondary infection, and prompt medical attention is required. Clinical manifestations that are anticipated in chickenpox include a generalized pruritic rash and mild fever. A body rash that begins on the upper body and head and progresses to the lower body and Koplik's spots are clinical manifestations of rubeola (measles). A red facial (slapped cheek) rash and circumoral pallor are characteristically found in erythema infectiosum (Fifth's disease).

Nursing process: Assessment

Client need: Management of Care

Cognitive level: Analysis

Subject area: Pediatric

Answer: 1

Rationale: Erythema infectiosum (Fifth's disease) is an infectious disorder spread through contact with respiratory secretions. The child is highly contagious before the onset of the illness. Children may return to school after the appearance of the rash because they are no longer contagious. There is no immunization for Fifth's disease. A generalized pruritic rash is characteristic of chickenpox; a child with such a rash is highly contagious. Diarrhea is not a clinical manifestation of Fifth's disease.

Nursing process: Analysis

Client need: Safety and Infection Control

Cognitive level: Analysis

Subject area: Pediatric

18. The nurse is instructing the adolescent client about birth control and sexually transmitted diseases. Which of the following methods of birth control should the nurse include that is 100% effective in protecting against sexually transmitted disease?

1. Birth control pills

2. Abstinence from sexual behavior

3. Withdrawal method

4. Latex condoms and spermicidal foam

19. The nurse assesses what clinical manifestation to be the priority manifestation in a child with *Enterobius* (pinworm)? _____

20. Which of the following is a priority nursing intervention when caring for an adolescent client to lessen the client's risk of infection?

1. Assess for high-risk behaviors, such as unprotected sex, drug use, and gang relationships

2. Encourage continuity of health care providers

3. Provide personal privacy and avoid discussing embarrassing issues

4. Include the adolescent's parent in all discussions

Answer: 2

Rationale: Birth control pills, withdrawal method, and latex condoms and spermicidal foam are not 100% effective in preventing the spread of sexually transmitted diseases. Each method contains some risk of infection. Birth control pills simply protect individuals from pregnancy. The withdrawal method is ineffective in every way. Latex condoms and spermicidal foam are ineffective barriers in the event of tears or breakage of the device or incorrect application. Only abstinence from sexual behavior is 100% effective in protecting against sexually transmitted disease.

Nursing process: Planning

Client need: Safety and Infection Control

Cognitive level: Application

Subject area: Pediatric

Answer: Nocturnal anal itching

Rationale: *Enterobius* (pinworm) is the most common helminth infection in the United States. It frequently occurs in preschoolers and school-age children, in crowded conditions, institutions, and families. The classic feature is nocturnal anal itching.

Nursing process: Assessment

Client need: Management of Care

Cognitive level: Analysis

Subject area: Pediatric

Answer: 1

Rationale: Adolescents frequently participate in behaviors that put them at risk for infection, and they falsely believe themselves not at risk. Unprotected sex, drug use, and gang relationships are behaviors that put them at risk for infection. Continuity of health care is important with all clients and not just adolescents. All clients require personal privacy, and, although embarrassing, they are encouraged to discuss personal physical concerns. Making the parents a part of a discussion of personal issues with an adolescent will actually make the adolescent uncomfortable and reluctant to discuss pertinent issues.

Nursing process: Planning

Client need: Management of Care

Cognitive level: Analysis

Subject area: Pediatric

21. The nurse is working with a group of parents getting ready to send their children to day care for the first time. The nurse instructs the parents that immunizations are

 1. improved and stronger, so "booster" shots are no longer required.

 2. safe and without risks.

 3. an improved part of health promotion.

 4. available in oral form if the client does not like injections.

22. A child is receiving an immunization before starting preschool. Which of the following assessments is a priority for the nurse to make at this time?

 1. The child's general state of health

 2. Preexisting diseases the client has

 3. The child's immunization history

 4. Recent exposure to infectious diseases

23. Which of the following drugs should the nurse use in the treatment of a child with *Giardia*?

 1. Penicillin G

 2. Furazolidone (Furoxone)

 3. Mebendazole (Vermox)

 4. Ceftriaxone (Rocephin)

24. The nurse assesses which of the following to be a clinical manifestation of human papillomavirus (HPV)?

 1. Soft papules in the anogenital area

 2. Nocturnal anal itching

 3. Erythematous and macular rash on the ankles and wrists

 4. Painful raised vesicles

Answer: 3

Rationale: Immunizations are an important part of health promotion and disease prevention. Improvements have been made, but booster shots are still required. Although a small percentage of the population, some clients have an adverse reaction to immunizations. Some immunizations are available in oral forms, but not every required immunization can be taken orally.

Nursing process: Implementation

Client need: Safety and Infection Control

Cognitive level: Analysis

Subject area: Pediatric

Answer: 3

Rationale: The child's general state of health, preexisting diseases, and any recent exposure to infectious diseases are important considerations in the general assessment of any child. The failure to collect this information may cause a delay in administration of the vaccine. It is a priority to obtain the child's immunization history. This is most important in deciding which vaccines are required and determining the appropriate schedule for immunization.

Nursing process: Assessment

Client need: Management of Care

Cognitive level: Analysis

Subject area: Pediatric

Answer: 2

Rationale: Penicillin G is used in the treatment of tetanus. *Giardia* is a protozoan disorder transmitted by hand-to-mouth transfer of cysts from feces of an infected individual. Furazolidone (Furoxone) is the drug of choice in treatment. Mebendazole (Vermox) is used in the treatment of *Enterobius* (pinworm). Ceftriaxone (Rocephin) is used in the treatment of gonorrhea.

Nursing process: Planning

Client need: Pharmacological and Parenteral Therapies

Cognitive level: Analysis

Subject area: Pharmacologic

Answer: 1

Rationale: Soft, fleshy single or multiple papules occur in the anogenital area (genital warts) in human papillomavirus (HPV). Nocturnal anal itching is a manifestation in *Enterobius* (pinworm). Erythematous and macular rash on the ankles and wrists is found in *Rickettsia rickettsii* (Rocky Mountain spotted fever). Painful raised vesicles are the initial lesions in herpes genitalis (HSV-2).

Nursing process: Assessment

Client need: Safety and Infection Control

Cognitive level: Application

Subject area: Pediatric

25. Which of the following drugs should the nurse administer to a child with tetanus who is experiencing muscle spasms and seizures?

    1. Methocarbamol (Robaxin)

    2. Cyclobenzaprine (Flexeril)

    3. Tizanidine (Zanaflex)

    4. Diazepam (Valium)

26. The registered nurse is preparing the clinical assignments for an infectious and communicable disease unit. Which of the following assignments should the nurse delegate to a licensed practical nurse?

    1. Teach an immunization class to a group of parents

    2. Provide comfort measures for a child with mumps

    3. Counsel the parents of a child with herpes genitalis (HSV-2) about the potential for recurrent outbreaks

    4. Monitor a child with hepatitis B for progressive liver disease

27. Which of the following is the priority nursing intervention for the nurse to include in the plan of care for a child with rotavirus presenting with severe stomach cramps and explosive diarrhea?

    1. Provide a high-calorie diet

    2. Encourage the child to rest

    3. Monitor the serum electrolytes

    4. Administer normal saline bolus at a rate of 50 ml/kg

28. The nurse is admitting a child with a cough, shortness of breath, difficulty breathing, hypoxia, fever of 38.9°C, or 102°F, and radiographic evidence of pneumonia. The nurse should report which of the following disorders? _____

Answer: 4

Rationale: Although methocarbamol (Robaxin), cyclobenzaprine (Flexeril), tizanidine (Zanaflex), and diazepam (Valium) are all skeletal muscle relaxants, Valium is the drug of choice in the treatment of tetanus to control muscle spasms and seizures.

Nursing process: Planning

Client need: Pharmacological and Parenteral Therapies

Cognitive level: Analysis

Subject area: Pharmacologic

Answer: 2

Rationale: A licensed practical nurse may provide comfort measures to a child with mumps. Teaching, counseling, and monitoring are all nursing assignments that require the skills of a registered nurse.

Nursing process: Planning

Client need: Management of Care

Cognitive level: Analysis

Subject area: Legal and Ethical Issues

Answer: 4

Rationale: Although providing a high-calorie diet, encouraging the child to rest, and monitoring the serum electrolytes are appropriate interventions, the priority is to replace the fluid lost with the explosive diarrhea. A rate of 50 ml/kg is an appropriate fluid replacement for this child.

Nursing process: Planning

Client need: Management of Care

Cognitive level: Application

Subject area: Legal and Ethical Issues

Answer: Severe acute respiratory syndrome

Rationale: Clinical manifestations of a mild to moderate respiratory disorder and a temperature greater than 38°C, or 100.4°F, and radiographic evidence of pneumonia are significant and must be immediately reported as a possible case of SARS (severe acute respiratory syndrome).

Nursing process: Analysis

Client need: Safety and Infection Control

Cognitive level: Analysis

Subject area: Pediatric

29. A parent asks the nurse how human immune deficiency virus (HIV) is contracted. What is the appropriate response by the nurse? _____

30. Parents of a child with Rocky Mountain spotted fever ask the nurse how their child contracted this disease. What is the appropriate response by the nurse? _____

31. Which of the following is the appropriate nursing intervention when a child develops a reactive purified protein derivative (PPD)?

  1. Refer the child to the physician for immediate treatment

  2. Obtain a full health and immunization history

  3. Reassess the site in five days

  4. Don personal protective equipment

Answer: It is transmitted by contact with infected blood or body fluids, sexual contact, and perinatally.

Rationale: Human immune deficiency virus (HIV) may be transmitted through transfer of blood or body fluids and through the placenta.

Nursing process: Analysis

Client need: Safety and Infection Control

Cognitive level: Application

Subject area: Pediatric

Answer: The disease is vector-borne.

Rationale: Rocky Mountain spotted fever is transmitted through the bite of an infected tick. Disease transmission through an intermediate carrier occurs when a tick or mosquito transfers the organism from another animal to the human host. This mode of transmission is termed vector-borne.

Nursing process: Analysis

Client need: Safety and Infection Control

Cognitive level: Application

Subject area: Pediatric

Answer: 2

Rationale: The nurse should investigate whether the child has had contact with an individual who has tuberculosis. The nurse also should assess whether the child has received any treatment for TB, what clinical manifestations the child has, and whether the child received the immunization BCG, which creates a positive skin test response to the PPD injection. A positive reaction to the skin test does not indicate a need for immediate treatment. Retesting the PPD skin test is most reactive within 72 hours, and the response will begin to subside after that. A positive reaction to PPD is not a positive indication that the client is infectious.

Nursing process: Planning

Client need: Safety and Infection Control

Cognitive level: Application

Subject area: Pediatric

UNIT IV

Maternity and Women's Health Nursing

The Antepartal Period

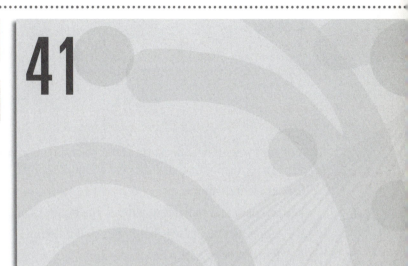

41

1. During a prenatal visit, the nurse evaluates the fundal height of the uterus to be at the umbilicus. The nurse should estimate the gestation at
   1. 16 weeks.
   2. 20 weeks.
   3. 24 weeks.
   4. 28 weeks.

2. A client is receiving education about preterm labor during a prenatal visit. Which of the following is a priority for the nurse to instruct the client to report?
   1. Nausea and vomiting
   2. Back pain that radiates down into the buttocks and legs
   3. Feeling that the baby is balling up and relaxing
   4. Vaginal spotting after a vaginal exam

3. A client asks the nurse what is the purpose of the placenta. Based on the understanding of the metabolic functions of the placenta, which of the following would be the most appropriate response by the nurse? The purposes of the placenta for the baby include which of the following?

   Select all that apply:
   [ ] 1. Cushion
   [ ] 2. Protects the skin
   [ ] 3. Respiration
   [ ] 4. Excretion
   [ ] 5. Pancreatic function
   [ ] 6. Nutrition

4. The client is 32 weeks pregnant, hospitalized for pre-eclampsia, and asks why the drug magnesium sulfate is infusing. What is the appropriate response by the nurse? _____

Answer: 2
Rationale: The fundal height rises 1 cm/week until the 36th week of gestation and is at the umbilicus (20 cm) at 20 weeks of gestation.
Nursing process: Evaluation
Client need: Health Promotion and Maintenance
Cognitive level: Analysis
Subject area: Maternity and Women's Health

Answer: 3
Rationale: A feeling that the baby is balling up and relaxing is a classic clinical manifestation of preterm labor. Nausea, vomiting, and back pain that radiates down the buttocks and legs should be reported if they continue, but are not indications of preterm labor. Vaginal spotting after a vaginal exam is a normal finding.
Nursing process: Planning
Client need: Management of Care
Cognitive level: Analysis
Subject area: Maternity and Women's Health

Answer: 3, 4, 6
Rationale: The placenta is responsible for the gas exchange (respiration), for nutrients that actively and passively cross the placental membrane for the fetus (nutrition), and for removal of metabolic waste for the fetus (excretion).
Nursing process: Analysis
Client need: Health Promotion and Maintenance
Cognitive level: Comprehension
Subject area: Maternity and Women's Health

Answer: "Magnesium sulfate prevents seizures."
Rationale: Magnesium sulfate is an anticonvulsant given to the client in pre-eclampsia to prevent seizures caused by neurologic irritability associated with hypertension.
Nursing process: Analysis
Client need: Pharmacological and Parenteral Therapies
Cognitive level: Application
Subject area: Pharmacologic

5. A client is 24 weeks pregnant and has just been told at her prenatal visit that her amniotic fluid volume has decreased. She is confused and asks the nurse, "What does that mean for my baby?" Which of the following is the appropriate response by the nurse?

   1. "The amniotic fluid is important for the baby. You should ask your doctor about that."

   2. "The less amniotic fluid, the more your baby is at risk for complications. The fluid protects the baby from trauma and helps the baby develop."

   3. "Your membranes may have ruptured, which heralds the beginning of labor. I think it would be a good idea to notify your labor support person."

   4. "You need to ask the doctor that question. In the meantime, I will notify the hospital you will be coming."

6. A pregnant client is admitted to the hospital for preterm labor. The nurse's first intervention is to

   1. obtain a complete history and update the physician.

   2. initiate IV hydration and begin tocolytic medication.

   3. obtain a fetal fibronectin and a CBC.

   4. monitor for contractions and fetal well-being.

7. After a routine screening ultrasound, a pregnant client in her third trimester asks the nurse to explain where all the fluid comes from that surrounds her baby. The nurse's response should be based on the understanding that the amniotic fluid is

   1. fluid from the maternal serum that diffuses passively across the membranes.

   2. primarily fetal urine maintained by a balance of production and reabsorption.

   3. produced primarily by the placenta and remains static unless ROM has occurred.

   4. fluid from the fetal serum that diffuses actively across the membranes.

Answer: 2

Rationale: Telling the client that less amniotic fluid places the baby at risk for complications, and that the fluid protects the baby from trauma and helps the baby develop, answers the client's question using as much information as the nurse has at the time, without assuming the fluid is low from ruptured membranes. Although telling the client that the amniotic fluid is good for the baby is true, it does not answer the client's question. Telling the client that the membranes may have ruptured and labor has started informs the client that she will be hospitalized for labor and delivery of a 24-week infant; there is no information in the question to indicate that. Telling the client that she will need to ask the doctor her question puts the client off, and there may be no need for the client to go to the hospital.

Nursing process: Analysis

Client need: Health Promotion and Maintenance

Cognitive level: Analysis

Subject area: Maternity and Women's Health

Answer: 4

Rationale: The first information the nurse should assess in a case of suspected preterm labor is to determine the labor pattern and if the fetus is evidencing any distress. This information will drive the rest of the plan of care.

Nursing process: Implementation

Client need: Management of Care

Cognitive level: Application

Subject area: Maternity and Women's Health

Answer: 2

Rationale: After the first trimester, the amniotic fluid is almost entirely fetal urine and is continually recycled via fetal swallowing and urinating.

Nursing process: Analysis

Client need: Health Promotion and Maintenance

Cognitive level: Analysis

Subject area: Maternity and Women's Health

8. A pregnant client who is 28 weeks pregnant and is taking an exercise class calls the prenatal clinic to ask if there are any maneuvers that should be avoided. Which of the following should the nurse instruct the client to avoid?

1. Lifting the arms over the head

2. Pelvic rocking

3. Sitting with the knees tucked up against the chest

4. Lying supine

9. Admitting a pregnant client to the hospital from the prenatal clinic for preterm premature rupture of membranes, the nurse includes in the client teaching which of the following treatment expectations?

1. Drugs will include antibiotic coverage

2. Activity will be restricted to ambulating in the hospital room

3. Blood pressure will need to be continuously monitored

4. Amniotic fluid volume will need to be continuously monitored

10. The nurse working in a triage clinic should return which one of the following clients' telephone messages first? A woman who is at

1. 37 weeks of gestation with shortness of breath.

2. 10 weeks of gestation with breast tenderness.

3. 35 weeks of gestation with feet that swell at the end of the day.

4. 12 weeks of gestation with darkening blotches of skin over her cheekbones.

Answer: 4

Rationale: Lifting the arms over the head, pelvic rocking, and sitting with the knees tucked up against the chest do not need to be avoided because of pregnancy. Lying supine should be avoided because it will cause compression of the vena cava by the gravid uterus and result in supine hypotension, which will impair uterine blood flow and possibly cause the pregnant woman to faint.

Nursing process: Planning

Client need: Health Promotion and Maintenance

Cognitive level: Application

Subject area: Maternity and Women's Health

Answer: 1

Rationale: The client is at risk for an intrauterine infection and infection of the membranes called chorioamnionitis once there has been a rupture of membranes. Antibiotic coverage is the standard of care. Ambulation is restricted to prevent further loss of fluid. Blood pressure is not affected by loss of amniotic fluid. Amniotic fluid will need to be regularly monitored, but not continuously.

Nursing process: Planning

Client need: Health Promotion and Maintenance

Cognitive level: Application

Subject area: Maternity and Women's Health

Answer: 1

Rationale: Darkening blotches of skin over the cheekbone describes chloasma and is a normal finding called the mask of pregnancy. Breast tenderness from early pregnancy and hormonal changes are common. The swelling of feet at the end of the day is benign, as long as the swelling is resolved by morning. This can also indicate pre-eclampsia, a concern that should be investigated further. However, the first call should be made to the woman who is complaining of dyspnea. A woman who is in her 37th week can have dyspnea from the term gravid uterus pushing up on her diaphragm, but she may also be experiencing a respiratory emergency such as pulmonary embolus.

Nursing process: Analysis

Client need: Management of Care

Cognitive level: Analysis

Subject area: Maternity and Women's Health

11. A pregnant client asks the nurse about gestational diabetes mellitus. The nurse responds based on the understanding that gestational diabetes in pregnancy is

    1. an impaired glucose tolerance.

    2. beta cell failure in pregnancy.

    3. type 1 DM undetected prior to pregnancy.

    4. type 2 DM undetected prior to pregnancy.

12. A client of Mediterranean descent tells the nurse that her mother told her she was at greater risk for which of the following blood disorders?

    1. Sickle-cell disease

    2. Tay-Sachs disease

    3. Thalassemia

    4. Phenylketonuria

13. Which of the following is the appropriate pregnancy classification for a client pregnant for the third time, whose first pregnancy ended in a miscarriage at 9 weeks and second pregnancy was a vaginal delivery at 39 weeks of gestation and the child is 3 years old now?

    1. Gravida 3 para 1-0-1-1

    2. Gravida 2 para 2-1-1-0

    3. Gravida 3 para 3-2-0-1-0

    4. Gravida 2 para 2-1-0-0

14. Which of the following health indicators for a client does the nurse evaluate as a risk factor for diabetes mellitus in pregnancy?

Select all that apply:

    [   ] **1.** History of ovarian tumors

    [   ] **2.** Caucasian

    [   ] **3.** Prior stillbirth

    [   ] **4.** Polyhydramnios

    [   ] **5.** History of DES exposure

    [   ] **6.** Overweight

Answer: 1

Rationale: Impaired glucose tolerance in pregnancy is the definition of gestational diabetes mellitus. Beta cell failure is the hallmark of type 1 diabetes mellitus.

Nursing process: Analysis

Client need: Health Promotion and Maintenance

Cognitive level: Analysis

Subject area: Maternity and Women's Health

Answer: 3

Rationale: Thalassemia is an autosomal recessive genetic condition that causes an inadequate production of normal hemoglobin. It occurs in clients of Mediterranean descent. Sickle-cell disease is genetically linked to clients of African descent. Tay-Sachs disease is linked to Ashkenazi Jews. Phenylketonuria is an inborn error of metabolism.

Nursing process: Evaluation

Client need: Health Promotion and Maintenance

Cognitive level: Analysis

Subject area: Maternity and Women's Health

Answer: 1

Rationale: This client has conceived three times and has delivered a term infant and has one living child. A nine-week miscarriage is a spontaneous abortion.

Nursing process: Evaluation

Client need: Health Promotion and Maintenance

Cognitive level: Analysis

Subject area: Maternity and Women's Health

Answer: 3, 4, 6

Rationale: Risk factors include overweight, family history of diabetes mellitus, previous gestational diabetes mellitus, ethnic predisposition (African American, Native American, Hispanic), prior birth of infant over 9 lb, polyhydramnios, and stillbirth.

Nursing process: Evaluation

Client need: Reduction of Risk Potential

Cognitive level: Analysis

Subject area: Maternity and Women's Health

15. The nurse has implemented education about HIV in pregnancy. Which statement illustrates that the pregnant HIV-positive client understood the nurse's teaching about HIV and pregnancy?

1. "My baby will not have AIDS."

2. "I will need to take a drug throughout my pregnancy."

3. "They will start giving me a drug for HIV when I come in to deliver."

4. "I will need to continue taking the HIV drug the entire time I breast-feed."

16. A pregnant client is African American and had a 10 lb 2 oz baby with her last pregnancy. Based on this information, the nurse expects that the oral glucose tolerance test should be done

1. at the first prenatal appointment.

2. at 28 weeks of gestation.

3. at the end of the first trimester.

4. when the client evidences glucose in the urine.

17. During a prenatal visit, a client approaching term asks many questions about labor and delivery. The nurse's response should be based on the understanding of normal adaptation to pregnancy because

1. anger and confusion often follow initial ambivalence as the client nears term.

2. a client has fears for safe laboring and delivery as the end of pregnancy approaches.

3. it is typical for a client to only have questions as the end of the pregnancy approaches.

4. pregnant clients will enter a phase of trust at term and ask questions only as they near term.

18. During pregnancy, the client's cervix softens. The nurse documents this as _____.

Answer: 2
Rationale: Drugs (antiretrovirals) should be taken throughout pregnancy and not started at the onset of labor. The newborn will be considered infected with maternal antibodies and will be medicated until 18 months of age, when the infant can seroconvert to negative status. It is unknown if the infant will develop AIDS. Breastfeeding is prohibited to lower the risk of transmission to the newborn.
Nursing process: Evaluation
Client need: Health Promotion and Maintenance
Cognitive level: Analysis
Subject area: Maternity and Women's Health

Answer: 1
Rationale: A history of macrosomia is a positive finding in the client's medical history indicating early screening for gestational diabetes mellitus with this pregnancy. Macrosomia is a cause of cephalopelvic disproportion.
Nursing process: Analysis
Client need: Health Promotion and Maintenance
Cognitive level: Analysis
Subject area: Maternity and Women's Health

Answer: 2
Rationale: Expressing fears of a safe delivery for the infant and self is a normal part of adaptation to pregnancy.
Nursing process: Analysis
Client need: Health Promotion and Maintenance
Cognitive level: Analysis
Subject area: Maternity and Women's Health

Answer: Goodell's sign
Rationale: Cervical softening is a positive Goodell's sign.
Nursing process: Assessment
Client need: Health Promotion and Maintenance
Cognitive level: Application
Subject area: Maternity and Women's Health

19. The nurse emphasizes the importance of good glycemic control during pregnancy to a client. Which of the following potential fetal complications does the nurse include in the education?

Select all that apply:

[   ] **1.** Intraventricular hemorrhage (IVH)

[   ] **2.** Organ malformations

[   ] **3.** Placenta previa

[   ] **4.** Pre-eclampsia

[   ] **5.** Pancreatic tumors

[   ] **6.** Macrosomia

20. During pregnancy, the client experiences infrequent, nonpainful, uterine contractions. The nurse documents this as _____.

21. After delivering a newborn infant, a client asks about the appearance of the umbilical cord. Based on an understanding of anatomy and physiology, which of the following responses by the nurse would be appropriate?

1. "There is protective tissue called chorionic villi, which surround the vessels in the cord."

2. "The umbilical cord is normally coiled with three vessels evident from any side of the cord."

3. "The umbilical cord normally develops one to two knots during pregnancy from fetal movement."

4. "The vessels in the cord are surrounded by a connective tissue called Wharton's jelly."

22. Based on the understanding of the physiologic adaptations of pregnancy, the nurse understands the client may have complications because of which of the following?

1. Blood volume increases 30 to 50% during pregnancy

2. Thyroid function decreases 10 to 25% during pregnancy

3. Respiratory rate increases by one-third during pregnancy

4. FSH and LH production is stimulated and overproduced during pregnancy

Answer: 2, 4, 6

Rationale: Fetal complications from diabetes mellitus in pregnancy include macrosomia, stillbirth, organ malformations, pre-eclampsia, and increased chance of operative delivery.

Nursing process: Planning

Client need: Reduction of Risk Potential

Cognitive level: Analysis

Subject area: Maternity and Women's Health

Answer: Braxton-Hicks

Rationale: Braxton-Hicks contractions are ineffectual uterine contractions from uterine stretching during pregnancy.

Nursing process: Assessment

Client need: Health Promotion and Maintenance

Cognitive level: Comprehension

Subject area: Maternity and Women's Health

Answer: 4

Rationale: The umbilical cord is usually straight and the vessels are surrounded by a protective connective tissue called Wharton's jelly.

Nursing process: Analysis

Client need: Health Promotion and Maintenance

Cognitive level: Analysis

Subject area: Maternity and Women's Health

Answer: 1

Rationale: Blood volume increases to perfuse the placenta and can cause complications for clients with cardiac disease or hypertension. Thyroid function increases to meet the demands of pregnancy. Other compensatory mechanisms in the respiratory system negate the need for tachypnea during pregnancy. FSH and LH are suppressed once their role in fertilization is completed.

Nursing process: Analysis

Client need: Reduction of Risk Potential

Cognitive level: Analysis

Subject area: Maternity and Women's Health

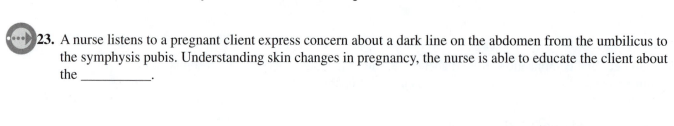

23. A nurse listens to a pregnant client express concern about a dark line on the abdomen from the umbilicus to the symphysis pubis. Understanding skin changes in pregnancy, the nurse is able to educate the client about the _____.

24. A pregnant client is hospitalized for vaginal bleeding from suspected abruptio placentae. The nurse bases the appropriate interventions on which understanding of the pathology?

1. Placenta tears away from the cervical os during dilation and results in fetal hemorrhage

2. Placental abruption is umbilical cord hemorrhage from trauma

3. Placental abruption is premature separation of the normally implanted placenta from the uterine wall

4. Abruptio placentae is the rupturing of membranes along the uterine wall and the resulting loss of fetal blood and amniotic fluid

25. The registered nurse is delegating client assignments on a maternity unit. Which of the following assignments should the nurse delegate to a licensed practical nurse?

1. Provide the care to a client suspected of having abruptio placentae

2. Provide the care to a woman in her 37th week of gestation experiencing dyspnea

3. Teach a pregnancy class to a group of women

4. Document the characteristics of a woman's lochia

26. The nurse assesses a blotchy irregular pigmentation on the face of a pregnant client. The nurse documents this finding as _____.

Answer: linea nigra

Rationale: The dark line on the abdomen from the umbilicus to the symphysis pubis is the linea nigra.

Nursing process: Analysis

Client need: Health Promotion and Maintenance

Cognitive level: Application

Subject area: Maternity and Women's Health

Answer: 3

Rationale: Abruptio placentae incorporates a premature separation of the normally implanted placenta from the uterine wall.

Nursing process: Planning

Client need: Health Promotion and Maintenance

Cognitive level: Application

Subject area: Maternity and Women's Health

Answer: 4

Rationale: Providing the care to a woman suspected of abruptio placentae and a woman in her 37th week of gestation experiencing dyspnea both require the skills of a registered nurse. A woman in her 37th week of gestation experiencing dyspnea may have a pulmonary embolus and requires the critical thinking skills of the registered nurse. Teaching a pregnancy class should be done by a registered nurse. A licensed practical nurse may document a woman's lochia.

Nursing process: Planning

Client need: Management of Care

Cognitive level: Analysis

Subject area: Legal and Ethical Issues

Answer: melasma

Rationale: Melasma is a blotchy irregular pigmentation on the face of a pregnant client. It is also known as chloasma.

Nursing process: Implementation

Client need: Health Promotion and Maintenance

Cognitive level: Comprehension

Subject area: Maternity and Women's Health

27. A pregnant client asks the nurse when the stretch marks will disappear. The most appropriate response by the nurse is

    1. "They will disappear with the birth of the infant."

    2. "They will take up to six months to disappear."

    3. "They will fade but do not totally disappear."

    4. "They will disappear with a nutritionally balanced diet and exercise."

Answer: 3

Rationale: The stretch marks a pregnant woman experiences will fade after the birth of the infant, but will not totally disappear.

Nursing process: Analysis

Client need: Health Promotion and Maintenance

Cognitive level: Application

Subject area: Maternity and Women's Health

The Intrapartal Period

42

1. When caring for the mother with premature rupture of the membranes, the nurse monitors the mother and fetus for indications of
   1. chorioamnionitis.
   2. placenta previa.
   3. hemorrhage.
   4. arrest of descent.

2. The nurse should monitor for which of the following fetal life-threatening emergencies when the fetal head is not engaged and the membranes rupture?
   1. Uterine hyperstimulation
   2. Placenta previa
   3. Cord prolapse
   4. Abruptio placentae

3. When observing a mother receiving oxytocin (Pitocin) for induction of labor, which of the following should the nurse assess for?
   1. Maternal hypotension
   2. Uterine hyperstimulation
   3. Maternal hyperthermia
   4. Placenta previa

4. After observing variable decelerations of the fetal heart rate on the fetal monitor tracing, the nurse should plan to care for a possible
   1. head compression.
   2. uteroplacental insufficiency.
   3. cord compression.
   4. cardiac conduction defect.

Answer: 1

Rationale: Loss of the protective barrier provided by the membranes increases the risk of infection (chorioamnionitis). The likelihood of placenta previa, hemorrhage, and arrest of descent are not increased by rupture of the membranes.

Nursing process: Assessment

Client need: Health Promotion and Maintenance

Cognitive level: Analysis

Subject area: Maternity and Women's Health

Answer: 3

Rationale: While uterine hyperstimulation, placenta previa, and abruptio placentae all pose a threat to the fetus, only cord prolapse is the direct result of rupture of membranes. While the other conditions pose a threat to mother as well as fetus, cord prolapse threatens only fetal well-being.

Nursing process: Assessment

Client need: Reduction of Risk Potential

Cognitive level: Analysis

Subject area: Maternity and Women's Health

Answer: 2

Rationale: Oxytocin (Pitocin) is an oxytocic drug used in the treatment of induction or stimulation of labor at term. Excessive use of oxytocin is associated with uterine hyperstimulation.

Nursing process: Assessment

Client need: Pharmacological and Parenteral Therapies

Cognitive level: Analysis

Subject area: Pharmacologic

Answer: 3

Rationale: Variable decelerations are caused by cord compression. Head compression, uteroplacental insufficiency, and cardiac conduction defect are associated with other types of periodic changes in fetal heart rate.

Nursing process: Planning

Client need: Health Promotion and Maintenance

Cognitive level: Analysis

Subject area: Maternity and Women's Health

5. The nurse notes late decelerations of the fetal heart rate on the fetal monitor tracing and suspects the cause to be _____.

6. The nurse observes early decelerations of the fetal heart rate on the fetal monitor tracing of a mother who has an epidural anesthesia and denies pain with the contractions. Which of the following is the intervention the nurse should take?

1. Perform a sterile vaginal examination

2. Assist the mother to change positions from side to side

3. Anticipate starting an amnioinfusion

4. Administer oxygen

7. The nurse should monitor for complications of disseminated intravascular coagulation (DIC) after observing which of the following decelerations of the fetal heart rate on the fetal monitor tracing? Decelerations that are

1. uniform in shape and timing.

2. variable in shape and timing.

3. uniform in shape and variable in timing.

4. variable in shape and uniform in timing.

Answer: uteroplacental insufficiency

Rationale: Late decelerations are caused by uteroplacental insufficiency, which is a compromised blood flow from the placenta to the fetus.

Nursing process: Analysis

Client need: Health Promotion and Maintenance

Cognitive level: Analysis

Subject area: Maternity and Women's Health

Answer: 1

Rationale: Early decelerations of the fetal heart rate may indicate the cervix is dilated and the labor may have progressed to the second stage. Changing the position of the mother from side to side is the intervention if umbilical cord compression is suspected. An amnioinfusion is the instillation of an isotonic glucose-free solution into the uterus to form a cushion for the umbilical cord or to thin out the meconium. It is also used when cord compression is present. Administration of oxygen is also performed when cord compression is suspected, because the oxygen will saturate the mother's blood, with the goal of supplying an adequate oxygen source to the fetus when the cord compression is relieved.

Nursing process: Implementation

Client need: Health Promotion and Maintenance

Cognitive level: Application

Subject area: Maternity and Women's Health

Answer: 2

Rationale: Variable decelerations most frequently occur after rupture of the membranes. They are variable in shape and timing.

Nursing process: Assessment

Client need: Reduction of Risk Potential

Cognitive level: Analysis

Subject area: Maternity and Women's Health

8. The nurse should document decelerations that are uniform in shape and timing and occur 15 seconds after the onset of a contraction as what type of deceleration? _____

9. Which of the following fetal heart rate patterns would the nurse anticipate seeing from a fetus who has anencephaly?

1. Early onset decelerations

2. Absent long-term variability

3. Accelerations

4. Late onset decelerations

10. After noting early decelerations on the fetal monitor tracing, the nurse should

1. prepare for emergency cesarean section.

2. administer an IV fluid bolus.

3. administer oxygen to the mother.

4. continue to observe the tracing.

11. In planning the care for the following four clients, which of the clients is a priority for the nurse to begin preoperative instructions and preparation for cesarean section?

1. A client with a complete placenta previa

2. A client who has a placenta abruptio

3. A client experiencing variable decelerations on the fetal monitor

4. A client with a fever

Answer: Late deceleration

Rationale: Late decelerations are uniform in both shape and timing.

Nursing process: Implementation

Client need: Health Promotion and Maintenance

Cognitive level: Application

Subject area: Maternity and Women's Health

Answer: 2

Rationale: Absent long-term variability seen on the fetal heart monitor is seen in congenital brain anomalies such as anencephaly. Anencephaly is a fatal condition in which the infant is born with a severely underdeveloped brain and skull. The infant most certainly dies shortly after birth.

Nursing process: Analysis

Client need: Health Promotion and Maintenance

Cognitive level: Analysis

Subject area: Maternity and Women's Health

Answer: 4

Rationale: Early decelerations do not reflect fetal jeopardy. Observation for the source of head compression (e.g., possible descent of fetal head) is all that is indicated.

Nursing process: Planning

Client need: Health Promotion and Maintenance

Cognitive level: Application

Subject area: Maternity and Women's Health

Answer: 1

Rationale: While a client with a complete placenta abruptio, a client experiencing variable decelerations, or a client with a fever may require a cesarean birth, complete placenta previa always mandates a cesarean birth.

Nursing process: Planning

Client need: Management of Care

Cognitive level: Analysis

Subject area: Maternity and Women's Health

12. A mother in labor is admitted with profuse, bright red vaginal bleeding and late decelerations on the fetal monitor. Which of the following questions is a priority for the nurse to ask the client to determine whether the source of the bleeding is placenta previa or abruptio placentae?

   1. "Are you having pain?"

   2. "Do you have a fever?"

   3. "Is this your first baby?"

   4. "Do you have a headache or blurred vision?"

13. The nurse is caring for a mother at 32 weeks of gestation who thinks her "water broke" about one hour prior to arrival at the hospital. The nurse prepares the client for which procedure to evaluate the status of the membranes?

   1. Digital vaginal exam

   2. Ultrasound

   3. Fern test

   4. Group B beta strep culture

14. The nurse is reviewing the laboratory results of a mother in labor. Which of the following nursing actions should the nurse implement with a white blood cell count of 14,000?

   1. Notify the physician

   2. Repeat the test in two hours

   3. Continue to monitor the client

   4. Prepare the client for a cesarean delivery

Answer: 1

Rationale: Both placenta previa and abruptio placentae can lead to uteroplacental insufficiency and threaten fetal well-being. The bleeding of placenta previa is usually painless and different from that for abruptio placentae. Questions regarding fever and gravida or para can be asked later. Headache and blurred vision are clinical manifestations of pre-eclampsia.

Nursing process: Assessment

Client need: Management of Care

Cognitive level: Analysis

Subject area: Maternity and Women's Health

Answer: 3

Rationale: A sterile speculum exam is performed to obtain a sample of vaginal fluid for a fern test to evaluate the status of the membranes. In the fern test, a sample of fluid is obtained from the vagina with a cotton-tipped applicator during a speculum exam. Swab the fluid-soaked applicator over a glass slide and examine it under the microscope. A frondlike pattern indicates the presence of amniotic fluid. A digital exam should be deferred until the status of the membranes is determined. Ultrasound would not detect the leakage of a small amount of fluid. The nurse might obtain a vaginal group B beta strep culture after rupture of the membranes is confirmed by the fern test.

Nursing process: Implementation

Client need: Reduction of Risk Potential

Cognitive level: Analysis

Subject area: Maternity and Women's Health

Answer: 3

Rationale: During labor, a white blood cell count of 14,000 is normal, due to the physical stress of labor. No further action is necessary.

Nursing process: Implementation

Client need: Reduction of Risk Potential

Cognitive level: Application

Subject area: Maternity and Women's Health

15. Which of the following nursing interventions should the nurse take after assessing slight respiratory alkalosis on the arterial blood gas analysis of a pregnant client?

    1. Notify the physician

    2. Repeat the test in one hour

    3. No action needed

    4. Consult respiratory therapy

16. The nurse is admitting a mother in labor who reports a small amount of dark red, mucoid vaginal discharge. The nurse should

    1. prepare for immediate cesarean delivery.

    2. proceed with the admission.

    3. obtain a specimen for coagulation studies.

    4. notify the physician.

17. The nurse is caring for a mother in labor whose membranes spontaneously rupture. The amniotic fluid is wine-colored. The appropriate action is to

    1. continue to observe the mother and fetus.

    2. test the fluid with Nitrazine paper to determine the pH.

    3. notify the physician and review the fetal monitor tracing.

    4. obtain a group B beta strep culture.

Answer: 3

Rationale: During pregnancy, a slight respiratory alkalosis occurs, resulting from the 30 to 40% increase in tidal volume. The increased PaO_2 and the decreased PCO_2 of the maternal circulation facilitate the removal of the carbon dioxide from the fetal circulation. The decreased PCO_2 of the mother is compensated by the increased renal excretion of the bicarbonate permitting the arterial pH to remain in the normal range. No action is necessary.

Nursing process: Planning

Client need: Reduction of Risk Potential

Cognitive level: Analysis

Subject area: Maternity and Women's Health

Answer: 2

Rationale: The mother is describing "bloody show," a normal finding in a mother in labor. This does not reflect coagulopathy, so no laboratory studies are indicated. Notifying the physician, obtaining coagulation studies, and preparing for a cesarean section apply to bright red vaginal bleeding, which is an abnormal finding.

Nursing process: Planning

Client need: Health Promotion and Maintenance

Cognitive level: Analysis

Subject area: Maternity and Women's Health

Answer: 3

Rationale: The "port wine" staining of the fluid is associated with abruptio placentae. Continuing to observe could place the mother and fetus in jeopardy. Obtaining culture or testing with Nitrazine paper is not indicated. The nurse should notify the physician and monitor the fetus for evidence of abruptio placentae.

Nursing process: Implementation

Client need: Reduction of Risk Potential

Cognitive level: Application

Subject area: Maternity and Women's Health

18. After a mother received an epidural anesthesia for labor and vaginal delivery, the nurse should evaluate the expected outcome of

    1. a decrease in sensation and motor control of lower extremities, bladder, and vasomotor tone.

    2. a heaviness in the legs and numb feet bilaterally.

    3. a postdural epidural headache and a decrease in blood pressure.

    4. sedation and a decrease in the mother's ability to push.

19. The nurse is caring for a newly delivered Asian mother and notes the family has piled blankets on the mother and brought her hot water and soup. The nurse understands this behavior is

    1. to prevent the mother from experiencing fever and chills.

    2. an indication of the cultural beliefs about birth.

    3. to compensate for a cool room temperature.

    4. to prevent exposure and preserve the modesty of the mother.

20. The nurse should prepare for a forceps and vacuum delivery after determining which of the following pelvis types to be present?

Select all that apply:

    [   ] **1.** Gynecoid

    [   ] **2.** Android

    [   ] **3.** Platypelloid

    [   ] **4.** Anthropoid

Answer: 1

Rationale: Epidural anesthesia for labor and delivery produces anesthesia from T10 caudal to block both first- and second-stage pain. The block is usually higher for cesarean delivery. Correctly administered, regional anesthesia does not produce sedation or loss of consciousness. A postdural epidural headache results from an accidental puncture of the dura, which creates a larger hole and increases the incidence of postdural epidural headache. An epidural may lengthen the second stage of labor, resulting in a decreased ability of the mother to push. A heaviness in the legs and numb feet indicate the epidural catheter has gone into the subarachnoid space and should be withdrawn.

Nursing process: Evaluation

Client need: Health Promotion and Maintenance

Cognitive level: Analysis

Subject area: Maternity and Women's Health

Answer: 2

Rationale: Many cultures consider the postpartum mother to be in a "cold" state, and keep the mother warm to help regain the heat lost in childbirth. While the family may have concerns about room temperature or modesty, drinking warm liquids is a cultural practice. To prevent fever is not correct because the practice of drinking hot liquids is cultural, not medical.

Nursing process: Analysis

Client need: Health Promotion and Maintenance

Cognitive level: Application

Subject area: Maternity and Women's Health

Answer: 2, 4

Rationale: The narrow dimensions of the android pelvis and the anthropoid pelvis cause slow descent of the fetal head, making the likelihood of forceps and vacuum delivery greater. The gynecoid pelvis has wider suprapubic arches and is favorable for a vaginal delivery. A platypelloid pelvis is present in only 3% of women, but a vaginal delivery may be performed.

Nursing process: Planning

Client need: Health Promotion and Maintenance

Cognitive level: Analysis

Subject area: Maternity and Women's Health

21. The nurse prepares a client with dystonia for which type of delivery? _____

22. The nurse should perform which of the following hourly assessments when a pregnant woman is receiving magnesium sulfate for pre-eclampsia and eclampsia?

1. Romberg sign

2. Deep tendon reflexes

3. Temperature

4. Maternal heart rate

23. Which of the following is a priority for the nurse to assess in a mother receiving magnesium sulfate?

1. Loss of patellar reflex

2. Diaphoresis

3. Respiratory rate less than 16

4. Flushing

24. When the nurse notes an absent patellar reflex in a client receiving magnesium sulfate, the correct action is

1. increase the rate of infusion per protocol.

2. discontinue the infusion per protocol.

3. administer an IV fluid bolus without medication.

4. administer oxygen.

Answer: Cesarean delivery

Rationale: Dystonia, or a failure of the labor to progress, would necessitate a cesarean section to be performed.

Nursing process: Implementation

Client need: Health Promotion and Maintenance

Cognitive level: Application

Subject area: Maternity and Women's Health

Answer: 2

Rationale: Magnesium sulfate decreases neuromuscular transmission of impulses; thus, reflexes would be affected. Also, loss of patellar reflex is the first sign of magnesium sulfate toxicity. Urine output and respiratory status are also assessed hourly or more often.

Nursing process: Assessment

Client need: Pharmacological and Parenteral Therapies

Cognitive level: Application

Subject area: Pharmacologic

Answer: 1

Rationale: Adverse reactions to magnesium sulfate include diaphoresis, flushing, and decreased respirations. Loss of deep tendon reflexes, including the patellar reflex, is a sign of impending toxicity and the priority assessment.

Nursing process: Assessment

Client need: Management of Care

Cognitive level: Analysis

Subject area: Pharmacologic

Answer: 2

Rationale: Since an absent patellar reflex is an early sign of toxicity, the magnesium sulfate infusion should be discontinued and the physician notified. Administering IV fluids or oxygen would not treat the toxicity. Increasing the rate would increase toxicity.

Nursing process: Planning

Client need: Pharmacological and Parenteral Therapies

Cognitive level: Application

Subject area: Pharmacologic

25. A client who is pre-eclamptic complains of blurred vision and scotomata to the nurse. The nurse should report this as indicating which of the following?

1. Glaucoma

2. Cerebral edema

3. Spinal cord injury

4. Hydrocephalus

26. The registered nurse is preparing clinical assignments for a maternity unit. Which of the following assignments should the nurse delegate to a licensed practical nurse?

1. Administer oxytocin (Pitocin) IV to a woman in labor

2. Instruct a mother on the clinical manifestations of eclampsia

3. Initiate prescribed magnesium sulfate to a mother experiencing toxemia

4. Walk a woman in labor to the delivery room

Answer: 2
Rationale: Visual disturbances may reflect cerebral edema in the pre-eclamptic client.
Nursing process: Analysis
Client need: Health Promotion and Maintenance
Cognitive level: Analysis
Subject area: Maternity and Women's Health

Answer: 4
Rationale: Administering oxytocin (Pitocin), instructing a mother on the clinical manifestations of eclampsia, and initiating magnesium sulfate to a mother experiencing toxemia should all be performed by a registered nurse. A licensed practical nurse may walk a woman in labor to the delivery room.
Nursing process: Planning
Client need: Management of Care
Cognitive level: Analysis
Subject area: Legal and Ethical Issues

The Postpartal Period

43

1. Twelve hours after delivery, the nurse assesses a client's vital signs. Which of the following findings should be reported?

   1. Temperature of 37.8°C, or 100.2°F

   2. Respiratory rate of 18 bpm

   3. Blood pressure of 120/80

   4. Pulse of 96

2. The nurse documents a client's lochia that is normal 24 hours after giving birth as _____.

3. After assessing a postpartum client's breast, diagnosed with mastitis, the nurse notices a red streak and tenderness around the right areola. Which of the following is the most important nursing intervention?

   1. Apply cold soaks to the area

   2. Avoid administering pain medication

   3. Instruct the client to empty the breasts frequently

   4. Instruct the client to avoid breastfeeding due to pain

4. During the 24-hour postpartum assessment, the nurse anticipates the uterine fundus to be in which of the following positions?

   1. U/3

   2. U/4

   3. Unable to palpate, too low in the pelvic cavity

   4. U/U

Answer: 4

Rationale: Relative bradycardia is normal after delivery due to an increased maternal blood volume. The presence of tachycardia warrants exploration. Temperature of 37.8°C, or 100.2°F, respiratory rate of 18 bpm, and blood pressure of 120/80 are all normal variants of vital signs.

Nursing process: Analysis

Client need: Health Promotion and Maintenance

Cognitive level: Application

Subject area: Maternity and Women's Health

Answer: lochia rubra

Rationale: Lochia rubra is normally present for the first three to four days postpartum.

Nursing process: Implementation

Client need: Health Promotion and Maintenance

Cognitive level: Comprehension

Subject area: Maternity and Women's Health

Answer: 3

Rationale: It is important to empty the breasts frequently to prevent milk stasis. Warm soaks would be warranted for an infection. Pain medication is appropriate and will help during breastfeeding. The milk stasis allows the infection a warm medium to continue to grow and proliferate.

Nursing process: Planning

Client need: Health Promotion and Maintenance

Cognitive level: Application

Subject area: Maternity and Women's Health

Answer: 4

Rationale: U/U is a normal involution of the uterus and indicates a normal process of healing. U/3, U/4, and a uterus that is unable to palpate because it is too low in the pelvic cavity all indicate that the uterus is further along in the involution process.

Nursing process: Analysis

Client need: Health Promotion and Maintenance

Cognitive level: Analysis

Subject area: Maternity and Women's Health

5. The nurse is giving a client who is postpartum the discharge instructions from the hospital. The nurse should instruct the client to return immediately for evaluation if which of the following occurs?

    1. Temperature of 37.2°C, or 99°F

    2. Slight swelling in the lower legs without pain or redness

    3. Bleeding becomes heavier than a heavy period

    4. Small hemorrhoids

6. A client phones the nurse to express concern about having intercourse six weeks after delivery. She is breastfeeding and reports that intercourse is uncomfortable. Which of the following is the appropriate response by the nurse?

    1. "Excess abdominal fat after delivery leads to painful intercourse."

    2. "Your estrogen levels are low and there is decreased mucous production and dryness."

    3. "Your vaginal walls are smooth and have not redeveloped rugae, making intercourse uncomfortable."

    4. "Intercourse is uncomfortable because of the distention of the vaginal canal."

7. A client who had a vaginal delivery the previous day asks the nurse what it meant when she was informed that she had a third-degree laceration. The nurse's response should be based on the understanding that a third-degree laceration is characterized by a tear

    1. through the skin and into the muscle.

    2. that extends through the anal sphincter.

    3. that involves the anterior rectal wall.

    4. that extends through the perineal muscle layer.

8. A client who had breast augmentation one year ago asks the nurse after delivery if she will be able to breast-feed. Based on a knowledge of breastfeeding, the nurse responds

    1. "Yes, you will be able to breast-feed without any problems."

    2. "No, you will be unable to breast-feed because the milk ducts were severed."

    3. "No, you will be unable to breast-feed because the implants will chemically alter the milk."

    4. "No, you will be unable to breast-feed due to the risk of infection."

Answer: 3

Rationale: Bleeding heavier than a period after discharge indicates hemorrhage and warrants evaluation. A temperature under 38°C, or 100.4°F, is insignificant. Slight swelling in the lower legs without redness or pain is a normal variant after delivery, due to excess fluids. The development of small hemorrhoids is a normal finding during the postpartum period.

Nursing process: Planning

Client need: Health Promotion and Maintenance

Cognitive level: Application

Subject area: Maternity and Women's Health

Answer: 2

Rationale: Estrogen allows for the production of mucus in the vaginal area. The estrogen levels return at a slower pace if a woman is breastfeeding exclusively. Abdominal fat has no effect on intercourse. Vaginal rugae reappear three weeks after delivery. Distention would not lead to discomfort.

Nursing process: Analysis

Client need: Health Promotion and Maintenance

Cognitive level: Analysis

Subject area: Maternity and Women's Health

Answer: 2

Rationale: A third-degree laceration goes through the perineal muscle layer with involvement of the anal sphincter. A tear through the skin and into the muscles defines a first-degree laceration. A tear that involves the anterior rectal wall defines a fourth-degree laceration. A tear that extends through the perineal muscle layer defines a second-degree laceration.

Nursing process: Analysis

Client need: Health Promotion and Maintenance

Cognitive level: Application

Subject area: Maternity and Women's Health

Answer: 2

Rationale: If milk ducts were severed during breast augmentation surgery, breastfeeding will not be possible due to the lack of a functioning ductal system. Surgery alters the breast's collection system. Implants have not been found to alter milk composition. Breast surgery does not lead to an increased risk of infection.

Nursing process: Analysis

Client need: Health Promotion and Maintenance

Cognitive level: Analysis

Subject area: Maternity and Women's Health

9. The nurse caring for a client who delivered one hour ago assesses the uterine fundus to be displaced to the right. Which of the following is the priority intervention the nurse should implement?

    1. Take the client's vital signs

    2. Check the client's perineal area

    3. Reevaluate the client after assisting to the bathroom to void

    4. Check the client's legs for swelling

10. The nurse informs a graduate nurse on a postpartum unit that the human chorionic gonadotropin (HCG) would no longer be detected in the client's blood at

    1. one week postpartum.

    2. two days postpartum.

    3. four weeks postpartum.

    4. one hour postpartum.

11. A postpartum client delivered a baby 24 hours ago. The client's blood type is O−. The baby's blood type has come back O+. The nurse evaluates the need for RhoGam and concludes that RhoGam is

    1. not needed because they both have type O blood.

    2. needed because the baby has a positive antibody.

    3. not needed until the infant is three months old.

    4. given to all infants to prevent an antibody reaction.

12. A client who is HIV positive has just given birth to her first child by cesarean section. The client received an antiviral medication during pregnancy and received the same medication through an IV during the delivery process. The client asks the nurse what is the risk of giving the baby HIV. Which of the following is the appropriate response by the nurse?

    1. "10%."

    2. "35%."

    3. "50%."

    4. "1%."

Answer: 3

Rationale: Excessive bleeding can occur with bladder distention because the uterus cannot fully contract. Frequent voiding is therefore important to prevent this from happening and putting the postpartum client at risk for hemorrhage. Although taking the client's vitals, checking the client's perineal area, and checking the client's legs for swelling are all important to assess, they are not the priority with the findings observed.

Nursing process: Planning

Client need: Management of Care

Cognitive level: Analysis

Subject area: Legal and Ethical Issues

Answer: 1

Rationale: HCG is produced by the placenta and is nonexistent by the first week postpartum.

Nursing process: Implementation

Client need: Health Promotion and Maintenance

Cognitive level: Application

Subject area: Maternity and Women's Health

Answer: 2

Rationale: The Rh-negative client who delivers an Rh-positive infant receives RhoGam to prevent the formation of antibodies that might complicate future pregnancies. The nurse should look at Rh factor, not blood type. RhoGam must be given within 72 hours of delivery. The only clients who need RhoGam are those with an Rh-negative blood type who have an Rh-positive infant.

Nursing process: Evaluation

Client need: Health Promotion and Maintenance

Cognitive level: Analysis

Subject area: Maternity and Women's Health

Answer: 4

Rationale: Current treatment with antiviral medications has greatly reduced the transmission to 1% after a surgical delivery through this prophylactic treatment plan.

Nursing process: Analysis

Client need: Health Promotion and Maintenance

Cognitive level: Analysis

Subject area: Maternity and Women's Health

13. A client who is postpartum is complaining of perineal pain. The nurse implements which of the following interventions?

Select all that apply:

[   ] 1. Apply an ice pack to the perineal area

[   ] 2. Administer a pain medication

[   ] 3. Change position

[   ] 4. Apply a warm pack to the perineal area

[   ] 5. Administer a smooth muscle relaxant

[   ] 6. Increase fluids

14. Which of the following is the most appropriate consideration to include in the plan of care for an Asian postpartum client who delivered three days ago and refuses to drink ice water or use ice packs on her perineum?

1. The client does not like water.

2. It is an important cultural belief.

3. The ice feels uncomfortable.

4. The client is in too much pain.

15. A client delivered an infant 12 hours ago and has lots of questions regarding care, but shows little initiative in caring for the newborn. According to Rubin's theory, the client is exhibiting which stage?

1. Taking-in stage

2. Taking-hold stage

3. Letting-go stage

4. Good bonding behavior

16. A postpartum client's complete blood count reflects a white blood cell count immediately after delivery to be 14,000 per cubic mm. The nurse reports this as

1. abnormal and indicating an infection is present.

2. an atypically low level.

3. elevated but normal following delivery.

4. within the normal range.

Answer: 1, 2, 3

Rationale: Administering an ice pack to the perineal area, administering a pain medication, and changing the client's position are comfort measures that should help decrease pain. Warm packs cause vasodilation and increase inflammation.

Nursing process: Implementation

Client need: Health Promotion and Maintenance

Cognitive level: Application

Subject area: Maternity and Women's Health

Answer: 2

Rationale: Cultural values influence personal self-care. The Asian culture believes that exposure to cool air leads to infection; therefore, Asian mothers will not put themselves at risk for this through oral fluids or ice packs.

Nursing process: Analysis

Client need: Health Promotion and Maintenance

Cognitive level: Application

Subject area: Maternity and Women's Health

Answer: 1

Rationale: The taking-in stage usually occurs during the first 24 hours postpartum. This is a time when the client is concerned about her own needs and illustrates little initiative in performing infant care.

Nursing process: Implementation

Client need: Health Promotion and Maintenance

Cognitive level: Application

Subject area: Maternity and Women's Health

Answer: 3

Rationale: An increase in the white blood count is a protective mechanism after delivery. It helps to protect the client from infection and is in response to the stress associated with the labor process.

Nursing process: Analysis

Client need: Reduction of Risk Potential

Cognitive level: Application

Subject area: Maternity and Women's Health

17. The nurse is reviewing physician orders for a client in the postpartum period in the hospital who is exhibiting clinical manifestations of pulmonary emboli (PE). Which of the following procedures should the nurse ensure is done first?

    1. Pulmonary angiogram

    2. Spiral CT scan

    3. V/Q scan

    4. Duplex ultrasonogram

18. When preparing a client who is not pregnant for an oral glucose tolerance test (OGTT or GTT), it is essential for the nurse to explain that the client must drink what amount of glucose?

    1. 25 grams

    2. 50 grams

    3. 75 grams

    4. 100 grams

19. A client after a vaginal delivery is at risk for postpartum hemorrhage. Nursing education to prevent postpartum hemorrhage is based on the knowledge that priority explanation for the cause is

    1. laceration of the perineal area.

    2. uterine rupture.

    3. high parity.

    4. uterine atony.

20. While assessing a client who just delivered a 9 lb 6 oz baby, the nurse assesses a firm fundus that is midline at U/U. There is also a constant trickle of blood from the vaginal area. Which of the following is the priority nursing intervention?

    1. Suspect postpartum hemorrhage and massage the uterus

    2. Question the client regarding a history of hemorrhoids

    3. Notify the physician of a possible laceration

    4. Document this as a normal finding

Answer: 1

Rationale: Pulmonary angiogram is considered the definitive test because x-rays can visualize the emboli after catheterization and contrast dye is injected. A spiral CT scan is the test used if the V/Q scan is not diagnostic. The V/Q scan is only suggestive and not a definitive test for PE. A duplex ultrasonogram is a test that shows a disruption of blood flow in the lower legs.

Nursing process: Planning

Client need: Reduction of Risk Potential

Cognitive level: Analysis

Subject area: Maternity and Women's Health

Answer: 3

Rationale: Drinking 25 or 50 grams of glucose is not enough to challenge the pancreas when evaluating for diabetes mellitus. 100 grams is widely used to screen for gestational diabetes mellitus. 75 grams of glucose is the recommended glucose load to screen the nonpregnant pancreas for diabetes mellitus or impaired glucose tolerance.

Nursing process: Planning

Client need: Reduction of Risk Potential

Cognitive level: Application

Subject area: Maternity and Women's Health

Answer: 4

Rationale: About 75% of all hemorrhages are due to uterine atony, which is the lack of uterine tone. Laceration of the perineal area, uterine rupture, and high parity are other causes of hemorrhage, but they are not as likely.

Nursing process: Planning

Client need: Management of Care

Cognitive level: Application

Subject area: Maternity and Women's Health

Answer: 3

Rationale: The bleeding from a laceration is not due to uterine atony but to a lacerated area in the perineal, vaginal, or cervical area. It is a priority to notify the physician of a possible laceration. The uterus is firm midline and at an appropriate level.

Nursing process: Implementation

Client need: Management of Care

Cognitive level: Application

Subject area: Legal and Ethical Issues

21. A client with a history of hypertension had an oxytocin drug ordered due to increased bleeding after delivery. The nurse appropriately administers which of the following drugs?

    1. Oxytocin (Pitocin)

    2. Methylergonovine maleate (Methergine)

    3. Ergonovine (Ergotrate)

    4. Acetylsalicylic acid (aspirin)

22. Following giving birth, a client complains of excruciating pain around her labial area. Upon assessment, the nurse observes a bluish, bulging area just under the skin on the left labia majora. The nurse reports this as

    1. a hemorrhage.

    2. an indication of infection.

    3. a hematoma.

    4. a laceration.

23. A client who delivered an infant three days ago is complaining of pain and frequency of urination and nausea. The nurse takes the temperature and it is 38.9°C, or 102°F. Which of the following is the priority intervention?

    1. Call the physician to obtain an order for a urine specimen for culture

    2. Increase fluids and reassess the temperature in four hours

    3. Tell the client that this is a normal finding and not to worry

    4. Administer prescribed pain medication

24. A nurse is discharging a postpartum client who has anemia. The nurse instructs the client that which of the following food selections are iron-rich?

    Select all that apply:

    [ ] **1.** Red meats

    [ ] **2.** Milk

    [ ] **3.** Cheese

    [ ] **4.** Fish

    [ ] **5.** Poultry

    [ ] **6.** Yogurt

Answer: 1

Rationale: Oxytocin (Pitocin) may cause hypotension, but this would not be of much concern in a client who is hypertensive. Hypertension is an adverse reaction to both methylergonovine maleate (Methergine) and ergonovine (Ergotrate). These drugs would be contraindicated for the client with hypertension. Aspirin inhibits the synthesis of clotting factors and can increase the risk of bleeding.

Nursing process: Implementation

Client need: Pharmacological and Parenteral Therapies

Cognitive level: Analysis

Subject area: Pharmacologic

Answer: 3

Rationale: Extreme pain is a classic indication of a hematoma. This pain is caused by pressure from the swelling of tissues in the pelvic area from damage to a vessel wall.

Nursing process: Analysis

Client need: Reduction of Risk Potential

Cognitive level: Application

Subject area: Maternity and Women's Health

Answer: 1

Rationale: Pain and frequency of urination and nausea are all common clinical manifestations of a urinary tract infection. The postpartum client is at risk due to decreased tone and sensation of the bladder after delivery. Since the ureters are enlarged after delivery due to the effects of pregnancy, infection may travel up to the kidneys. It is therefore very important to have prompt intervention and treatment started immediately. It is important to notify the physician of any deviations.

Nursing process: Planning

Client need: Management of Care

Cognitive level: Application

Subject area: Legal and Ethical Issues

Answer: 1, 4, 5

Rationale: Foods high in iron include red meats, fish, and poultry.

Nursing process: Planning

Client need: Basic Care and Comfort

Cognitive level: Application

Subject area: Maternity and Women's Health

25. The nurse is caring for a client postoperatively following a cesarean section. It is a priority for the nurse to monitor the client for

   1. postpartum depression.

   2. infection.

   3. dehydration.

   4. blood clots.

26. The registered nurse is delegating nursing tasks on a postpartum maternity unit. Which of the following tasks should the nurse delegate to a licensed practical nurse?

   1. Assess the fundus post delivery

   2. Administer oxytocin (Pitocin) IV after delivery of the placenta

   3. Maintain an accurate intake and output

   4. Report lochia rubra ten days after delivery

Answer: 2

Rationale: The nurse should closely monitor a client postoperatively for infection, which has an incidence ranging from 4 to 12% due to increased tissue trauma. Postpartum depression, dehydration, and blood clots are possible complications, but they occur at a lower incidence.

Nursing process: Assessment

Client need: Management of Care

Cognitive level: Application

Subject area: Maternity and Women's Health

Answer: 3

Rationale: Assessing the fundus post delivery, administering oxytocin (Pitocin), and reporting abnormal lochia are all skills that should be performed by a registered nurse. Maintaining an accurate intake and output is a task that can be delegated to a licensed practical nurse. The client experiences diuresis post delivery.

Nursing process: Planning

Client need: Management of Care

Cognitive level: Analysis

Subject area: Legal and Ethical Issuess

Newborn Care

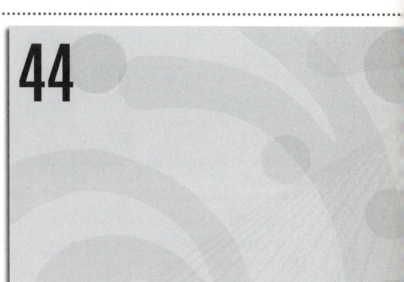

44

1. Which of the following is a priority for the nurse to monitor in an infant born to a mother who has diabetes mellitus?
   1. Hypoglycemia
   2. Rh sensitization
   3. ABO incompatibility
   4. Hypothermia

2. Based on an understanding of maternal hyperglycemia, which of the following is a priority to assess in the newborn?
   1. Cardiac anomalies
   2. Group B beta-hemolytic strep pneumonia
   3. Group B beta-hemolytic strep meningitis
   4. Inborn errors of metabolism

3. The nurse is preparing to administer vitamin K to an infant when the mother asks why her newborn is receiving a vitamin K injection. Which of the following is the most appropriate response? "Vitamin K is administered to
   1. prevent excessive bleeding from heel sticks."
   2. prevent petechiae that may occur from routine cares."
   3. prevent excessive bleeding from IM injection sites."
   4. protect against intracranial hemorrhage."

Answer: 1

Rationale: Maternal hyperglycemia causes the fetus to produce more insulin. After delivery, when maternal glucose is suddenly withdrawn, this excessive insulin produces neonatal hypoglycemia. Although Rh sensitization, ABO incompatibility, and hypothermia may be appropriate to assess in any newborn, they are not associated with maternal diabetes.

Nursing process: Assessment

Client need: Management of Care

Cognitive level: Analysis

Subject area: Maternity and Women's Health

Answer: 1

Rationale: Maternal hyperglycemia has a teratogenic effect. Infants born to mothers with insulin dependence are at greater risk for cardiac anomalies.

Nursing process: Assessment

Client need: Management of Care

Cognitive level: Analysis

Subject area: Maternity and Women's Health

Answer: 4

Rationale: An injection of prophylactic vitamin K is administered by intramuscular injection into the newborn's thigh during the first hour of life to stimulate the production of vitamin K by the bacteria in the newborn's intestine. Because the newborn's intestinal tract is considered to be sterile at birth, serious consequences, such as central nervous system hemorrhages, may result if vitamin K is not administered. Deficiencies rapidly occur within the first two to three days of life. Heel sticks and IM injections do not cause excessive bleeding in the normal newborn. Petechiae are associated with abnormalities of coagulation, not with adaptation to extrauterine life.

Nursing process: Analysis

Client need: Pharmacological and Parenteral Therapies

Cognitive level: Application

Subject area: Pharmacologic

4. When preparing the delivery room to care for the newborn, which of the following should the nurse obtain?

   1. A radiant warmer
   2. Formula
   3. Cool washcloths
   4. Clothing and blankets

5. When caring for a newborn who is small for the gestational age, the nurse understands that the newborn is at risk for hypoglycemia due to _____.

6. The nurse caring for a large-for-gestational-age newborn monitors blood glucose to detect hypoglycemia as the result of

   1. limited glycogen stores.
   2. hyperinsulinemia.
   3. large body surface-to-weight ratio.
   4. excessive brown fat stores.

7. The nurse admitting a preterm newborn to the nursery should assess the newborn for which of the following?

   1. Respiratory distress
   2. Shoulder dystocia
   3. Clavicle fracture
   4. Palsies

Answer: 1

Rationale: Due to the high ratio of a newborn's body surface to weight and the inability to shiver, newborns are at risk for hypothermia. Newborns lose heat to the environment through conduction, radiation, evaporation, and convection. A radiant warmer decreases these losses. Applying cool washcloths would increase heat loss. Clothing would prevent warmth from reaching the skin. Formula is not indicated immediately after delivery.

Nursing process: Planning

Client need: Health Promotion and Maintenance

Cognitive level: Application

Subject area: Maternity and Women's Health

Answer: limited glycogen stores

Rationale: Small-for-gestational-age newborns have limited glycogen and brown fat stores. When these are exhausted, hypoglycemia results. Hyperinsulinemia is associated with large-for-gestational-age newborns or with infants of diabetic mothers.

Nursing process: Analysis

Client need: Health Promotion and Maintenance

Cognitive level: Analysis

Subject area: Maternity and Women's Health

Answer: 2

Rationale: Large-for-gestational-age newborns are likely to develop hyperinsulinemia in order to adapt to elevated maternal blood glucose. When the delivery of maternal glucose ceases with the clamping of the cord, the newborn's blood sugar may plummet. Large-for-gestational-age newborns do not have limited glycogen stores. While they may have excessive fat stores, this does not cause hypoglycemia. A large body surface-to-weight ratio is true of all newborns.

Nursing process: Assessment

Client need: Health Promotion and Maintenance

Cognitive level: Analysis

Subject area: Maternity and Women's Health

Answer: 1

Rationale: Preterm newborns may not have adequate pulmonary surfactant. This increases the work of breathing and may cause respiratory distress and failure. Shoulder dystonia, clavicle fractures, and palsies are complications associated with larger newborns.

Nursing process: Assessment

Client need: Health Promotion and Maintenance

Cognitive level: Analysis

Subject area: Maternity and Women's Health

8. When planning the care for a newborn whose mother is positive for hepatitis B surface antigen, the nurse should prepare to administer what within 12 hours after birth? _____

9. The nurse caring for a newborn of an Rh-negative mother determines the newborn may be at risk for which of the following?

1. Hemolytic disease
2. Sepsis
3. Cardiac anomalies
4. Petechiae

10. After reviewing the medical record of a mother, the nurse evaluates a type A fetus to be at risk of ABO incompatibility from the mother because she has a blood type of

1. A.
2. B.
3. AB.
4. O.

11. The nurse reviewing a newborn's chart informs the parents that ABO incompatibility is not possible in their newborn because the mother's blood type is

1. A.
2. B.
3. AB.
4. O.

Answer: Hepatitis B vaccine and hepatitis B immune globulin

Rationale: The newborn born to a mother positive for hepatitis B should receive both hepatitis B vaccine and immune globulin for immediate, passive (immune globulin), and, later, active (vaccine) immunity. Administration of either the vaccine or immune globulin alone would not provide full immunity.

Nursing process: Planning

Client need: Reduction of Risk Potential

Cognitive level: Analysis

Subject area: Maternity and Women's Health

Answer: 1

Rationale: Rh sensitization is the most common cause of maternal immunization and hemolysis (destruction of the red blood cells) in the newborn. The sensitized Rh-negative mother produces antibodies to the Rh factor. In the Rh-positive fetus and newborn, these antibodies cause hemolysis. Petechiae, sepsis, and cardiac anomalies are not associated with hemolytic disease of the newborn.

Nursing process: Evaluation

Client need: Reduction of Risk Potential

Cognitive level: Application

Subject area: Maternity and Women's Health

Answer: 4

Rationale: Type O persons produce both anti-A and anti-B antibodies. Type AB persons produce no antibodies. Type A and type B persons produce the antibody to the opposite type. For example, a type B person would produce anti-A antibodies. ABO incompatibility occurs when a type O mother is pregnant with a type A or type B fetus. The mother may develop antibodies that may result in hemolysis in the fetus and newborn. The infants may go on to develop hyperbilirubinemia, requiring phototherapy.

Nursing process: Evaluation

Client need: Reduction of Risk Potential

Cognitive level: Analysis

Subject area: Maternity and Women's Health

Answer: 3

Rationale: Type O persons produce both anti-A and anti-B antibodies. Type AB persons produce no antibodies. Type A and type B persons produce the antibody to the opposite type. For example, a type B person would produce anti-A antibodies. No ABO incompatibility occurs with a type AB mother regardless of the fetus's blood type.

Nursing process: Implementation

Client need: Reduction of Risk Potential

Cognitive level: Analysis

Subject area: Maternity and Women's Health

12. Based on an understanding of plantar creases in the newborn, the nurse assesses plantar creases immediately after birth because

    1. after footprinting, creases will be obscured by residual ink.

    2. fluid loss may give the appearance of more plantar creases.

    3. they will fade as the skin dries in the first hours after birth.

    4. as acrocyanosis resolves, creases will be more difficult to see.

13. The parents of a newborn ask why their newborn is undergoing testing for inborn errors of metabolism, congenital adrenal hyperplasia, and hypothyroidism. The nurse informs the parents that the priority reason that all newborns are tested is to

    1. prepare them for complex medical care for life.

    2. detect conditions that require special diet and drugs.

    3. permit them to prepare advance directives.

    4. prepare them for the child's illness.

14. When admitting a newborn to the nursery, the nurse prepares to administer erythromycin ointment to the newborn's eyes to prevent blindness caused by which of the following?

Select all that apply:

[   ] **1.** Gonorrhea

[   ] **2.** Syphilis

[   ] **3.** Herpes simplex virus

[   ] **4.** Hepatitis

[   ] **5.** Chlamydia

[   ] **6.** Human immunodeficiency virus (HIV)

15. The nurse is performing a newborn assessment and evaluates a collection of blood beneath the newborn's scalp that does not cross suture lines. The nurse documents this as

    1. caput succedaneum.

    2. cephalohematoma.

    3. occiput.

    4. sinciput.

Answer: 2

Rationale: Newborns lose fluid in the first few days, which may produce the appearance of more plantar creases. The process of footprinting does not obscure the crease. Acrocyanosis and drying of the surface of the skin do not affect the creases.

Nursing process: Assessment

Client need: Health Promotion and Maintenance

Cognitive level: Analysis

Subject area: Maternity and Women's Health

Answer: 2

Rationale: Early detection and treatment of inborn errors of metabolism, congenital adrenal hyperplasia, and hypothyroidism will prevent complications and disabilities, such as mental retardation and developmental delays. These conditions are preventable.

Nursing process: Implementation

Client need: Management of Care

Cognitive level: Analysis

Subject area: Maternity and Women's Health

Answer: 1, 5

Rationale: Erythromycin prevents blindness due to gonorrhea and chlamydia. Erythromycin does not treat syphilis, herpes simplex virus, hepatitis, and human immunodeficiency virus. None of these illnesses causes blindness in the newborn.

Nursing process: Planning

Client need: Pharmacological and Parenteral Therapies

Cognitive level: Application

Subject area: Pharmacologic

Answer: 2

Rationale: Cephalohematoma is the collection of blood between a cranial bone and its periosteum. Because it is contained by the periosteum, the cephalohematoma does not cross suture lines. Caput succedaneum is a soft tissue swelling that does cross the suture line. Occiput and sinciput are anatomical points on the head.

Nursing process: Implementation

Client need: Health Promotion and Maintenance

Cognitive level: Application

Subject area: Maternity and Women's Health

16. The nurse is assessing a newborn following delivery. Which of the following assessments is abnormal and determines that further evaluation is needed?

    1. Rosy skin color

    2. Heart rate of 138 beats per minute

    3. Noisy breath sounds

    4. An axillary temperature of 36.5°C, or 97.7°F

17. The nurse is assessing the reflexes of a newborn. The nurse assesses which of the following reflexes by placing a finger in the newborn's mouth?

    1. Moro reflex

    2. Sucking reflex

    3. Rooting reflex

    4. Babinski reflex

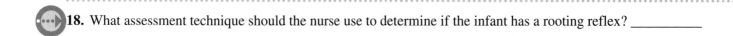

18. What assessment technique should the nurse use to determine if the infant has a rooting reflex? _____

19. The nurse assesses which of the following reflexes by lifting the newborn's body slightly above the crib, followed by suddenly lowering the body and observing for bilateral arm extension and leg flexion?

    1. Moro reflex

    2. Gallant reflex

    3. Palmar grasp

    4. Babinski reflex

Answer: 3

Rationale: A newborn's skin should be pink or rosy as circulation improves. An infant's heart rate should decrease from a high of 150 to 160 beats per minute to a rate of between 130 and 140 beats per minute. Noisy breath sounds may indicate an obstruction of the air flow through the nares and oropharynx. Suctioning with a bulb syringe may clear the nasal passage of fluid and debris. As a result, the breath sounds would become quiet. Axillary infant temperature should be between 36.5°C and 37.6°C, or 97.7°F and 99.7°F.

Nursing process: Assessment

Client need: Health Promotion and Maintenance

Cognitive level: Analysis

Subject area: Maternity and Women's Health

Answer: 2

Rationale: The sucking reflex is tested by placing something, such as a finger, in the infant's mouth and seeing if the infant begins to suck on the object. The Moro reflex is tested by suddenly lowering the newborn's body. The infant should demonstrate a bilateral arm extension and leg flexion. The rooting reflex is tested by stroking the cheek. The infant may open the mouth. The Babinski reflex is tested by firmly stroking the plantar surface. The anticipated response is the incurving of the toes as in plantar grasp with uncurling and fanning out.

Nursing process: Assessment

Client need: Health Promotion and Maintenance

Cognitive level: Application

Subject area: Maternity and Women's Health

Answer: Stroke the infant's cheek

Rationale: The assessment technique used to assess the rooting reflex is to stroke the infant's cheek. The infant should turn the head toward the stroking finger and open the mouth as if to begin sucking on an object.

Nursing process: Assessment

Client need: Health Promotion and Maintenance

Cognitive level: Application

Subject area: Maternity and Women's Health

Answer: 1

Rationale: The Moro reflex is assessed by lifting the newborn's body slightly above the crib, followed by suddenly lowering the body and observing for bilateral arm extension and leg flexion. The Babinski reflex is tested by firmly stroking the plantar surface. The palmar grasp is assessed by watching the infant wrap fingers around an object placed across the palm. The Gallant reflex is performed by holding an infant prone and stroking the lateral aspect of the leg from below the knee superiorly to the buttocks.

Nursing process: Implementation

Client need: Health Promotion and Maintenance

Cognitive level: Application

Subject area: Maternity and Women's Health

20. The nurse documents which of the following reflexes as being responsible for an infant incurving the toes with uncurling and fanning out of the toes when the lateral plantar surface is stroked?

1. Moro reflex

2. Gallant reflex

3. Rooting reflex

4. Babinski reflex

21. The parents of a newborn ask the nurse why their infant must be tested for phenylketonuria. The appropriate response by the nurse is "to

1. prevent mental retardation."

2. prevent chronic lung infections."

3. treat conductive deafness effectively."

4. treat hematuria and proteinuria before complications develop."

22. Parents of a newborn ask the nurse why the doctor said the infant must be tested for galactosemia. The nurse should inform the parents that galactosemia is an inborn error of metabolism, in which the newborn cannot metabolize which of the following?

1. Phenylalanine

2. Lactose

3. Saccharine

4. Ketones

Answer: 4

Rationale: The Babinski reflex is tested by firmly stroking the plantar surface. The anticipated outcome is the incurving of the toes with uncurling and fanning out of the toes. The Moro reflex is tested by suddenly lowering the newborn's body. The expected outcome is bilateral arm extension and leg flexion. The rooting reflex is tested by stroking the cheek. The anticipated outcome is the infant turning the head in the direction of the stroking and opening the mouth. The Gallant reflex is performed by holding an infant prone and stroking the lateral aspect of the leg from below the knee superiorly to the buttocks. The infant reacts by moving the buttocks toward the side that is stroked in a curving movement.

Nursing process: Implementation

Client need: Health Promotion and Maintenance

Cognitive level: Application

Subject area: Maternity and Women's Health

Answer: 1

Rationale: Phenylketonuria is deficiency of phenylalanine hydroxylase, which results in failure to metabolize phenylalanine. A deficiency of phenylalanine may result in mental retardation. Cystic fibrosis is a chronic lung disease in which recurrent infections occur, resulting from the inability of the ciliated epithelium to secrete mucus. Osteogenesis imperfecta type I involves osteoporosis and recurrent fractures of the long bones. It is characterized by blue sclera, conductive deafness, and discolored teeth. Polycystic kidney disease causes cysts in the kidneys, liver, pancreas, and spleen. Hematuria and proteinuria result.

Nursing process: Analysis

Client need: Health Promotion and Maintenance

Cognitive level: Application

Subject area: Maternity and Women's Health

Answer: 2

Rationale: Galactosemia is a deficiency in beta galactosidase, which results in failure to properly metabolize lactose.

Nursing process: Analysis

Client need: Health Promotion and Maintenance

Cognitive level: Application

Subject area: Maternity and Women's Health

23. The nurse evaluates a newborn to have which of the following STORCH (syphilis, toxoplasmosis, rubella, cytomegalovirus, and herpes) diseases because the newborn's mother handled cat feces and ate raw or undercooked meat during pregnancy?

1. Cytomegalovirus
2. Herpes
3. Rubella
4. Toxoplasmosis

24. The nurse informs a mother that which of the following occupations during pregnancy puts the infant at risk for developing cytomegalovirus?

1. Veterinary assistant
2. Waitress
3. Day care worker
4. Cook

25. When caring for a premature infant, the nurse will assess for neonatal respiratory distress syndrome due to an insufficient amount of what? _____

26. The registered nurse is preparing clinical assignments for a newborn care unit. Which of the following clinical assignments should the nurse delegate to a licensed practical nurse?

1. Assess an infant for cephalohematoma
2. Monitor an infant for tachypnea
3. Administer vitamin K to an infant
4. Instruct the parents of an infant on normal nutrition

Answer: 4

Rationale: Toxoplasmosis is a STORCH disease transmitted by handling cat feces or eating raw and undercooked meat. Cytomegalovirus, herpes, and rubella are diseases that are transmitted by humans.

Nursing process: Evaluation

Client need: Health Promotion and Maintenance

Cognitive level: Application

Subject area: Maternity and Women's Health

Answer: 3

Rationale: Cytomegalovirus is transmitted in the urine of infected persons. Individuals who work in day care during pregnancy put the infant at risk for developing cytomegalovirus. Toxoplasmosis is transmitted by cat feces and by raw or undercooked meat.

Nursing process: Implementation

Client need: Health Promotion and Maintenance

Cognitive level: Application

Subject area: Maternity and Women's Health

Answer: Surfactant

Rationale: Pulmonary surfactant is not produced until 32 weeks. Levels sufficient for pulmonary function after delivery are not produced until 34 weeks. It is produced later in some cases, such as in the infant of a diabetic mother. The premature infant is at risk for respiratory distress due to insufficient surfactant.

Nursing process: Assessment

Client need: Health Promotion and Maintenance

Cognitive level: Application

Subject area: Maternity and Women's Health

Answer: 3

Rationale: A licensed practical nurse may administer vitamin K to an infant. Assessing an infant for cephalohematoma, monitoring an infant for tachypnea, and instructing the parents of an infant on normal nutrition are nursing tasks that require the skills of a registered nurse.

Nursing process: Planning

Client need: Management of Care

Cognitive level: Analysis

Subject area: Legal and Ethical Issues

27. The nurse is teaching a well baby class to a group of pregnant clients on the characteristics of the feces of newborns and toddlers. Which of the following should the nurse include?

1. Infants who are breast-fed have dark yellow or tan formed feces.

2. During the first week of life, the feces of the newborn are brown, formed, and firm.

3. For the first 24 hours, the feces passed by the newborn are black, tarry, and sticky.

4. Infants who are formula-fed have bright yellow or golden colored feces.

Answer: 3

Rationale: For the first 24 hours of life, the feces of the newborn are called meconium stools and are black, tarry, and sticky. Generally by the third day of life, the stools become greenish brown to yellowish brown, thin and less sticky than the meconium stool. Infants who are breast-fed have stools that are bright yellow or golden colored and pasty. Stools of infants who are bottle-fed have stools that are pale yellow to tan and formed.

Nursing process: Planning

Client need: Health Promotion and Maintenance

Cognitive level: Analysis

Subject area: Maternity and Women's Health

Reproductive Disorders

45

1. The nurse is preparing a client for an ultrasound of her uterus. Which of the following nursing interventions should the nurse perform prior to sending the client for the examination?

   1. Ask the client if she has any allergies to iodine
   2. Have the client drink two glasses of water
   3. Ask the client to remove all metal jewelry and hair clips
   4. Have the client void before she leaves the nursing unit

2. Which of the following statements by the nurse should be included in the instructions for a client with endometriosis who is scheduled for a laparoscopy?

   1. "Do not drink carbonated beverages for 48 hours after the procedure."
   2. "The dressing should be removed the next day and the incision left open to air."
   3. "The dye that is used will color your urine blue for the first few voidings."
   4. "Notify your physician if you experience any pain in the shoulder area."

3. Which of the following should the nurse include in the instructions for a client who is to have a cervical biopsy?

   1. Food and fluids are to be restricted four hours before the procedure.
   2. A cleansing douche should be done the morning of the procedure.
   3. Sexual intercourse may be resumed the day after the procedure.
   4. The procedure must be scheduled for one week after menses begin.

4. A client beginning menopause asks the nurse, "What can I expect if I don't go on hormone replacement therapy?" The best response of the nurse should be

   1. "You will eventually be symptom-free once your body adjusts to the withdrawal of estrogen from your ovaries."
   2. "You may be more prone to fracturing a bone if you fall or injure yourself, so you will need to be very careful."
   3. "You will have occasional periods of spotting, which is normal for the first few years, and then it will stop."
   4. "You will be free of your monthly periods and won't have to worry about getting pregnant from here on."

Answer: 2

Rationale: An ultrasound uses high-frequency sound waves to provide an image of an organ. An ultrasound of the uterus requires that the bladder be full in order to visualize the uterus; thus, the client needs to drink fluids prior to the examination. An ultrasound does not use contrast media, such as iodine preparations, and metal objects, such as jewelry and hair clips, are not contraindicated for an ultrasound. Having the client void before the examination would prevent the visualization of the uterus.

Nursing process: Planning

Client need: Reduction of Risk Potential

Cognitive level: Application

Subject area: Maternity and Women's Health

Answer: 1

Rationale: Clients having a laparoscopy should refrain from drinking carbonated beverages for 48 hours after the procedure because the beverages may react with the carbon dioxide used in the procedure, causing vomiting. The laparoscope is inserted through a stab wound, thus eliminating the necessity of a surgical incision and dressing. A blue dye is not used for assessment of endometriosis. Clients having laparoscopy normally have mild pain in the shoulder area due to the insufflation of carbon dioxide during the procedure.

Nursing process: Analysis

Client need: Reduction of Risk Potential

Cognitive level: Application

Subject area: Maternity and Women's Health

Answer: 4

Rationale: A cervical biopsy must be scheduled for one week after menses begin to minimize the possibility that the client might be pregnant. The client should be NPO after midnight for the procedure. The client should not douche or have intercourse for 48 hours before the procedure. The client should not have sexual intercourse until the biopsy site has healed, which is at least 72 hours after the procedure.

Nursing process: Planning

Client need: Reduction of Risk Potential

Cognitive level: Application

Subject area: Maternity and Women's Health

Answer: 2

Rationale: Menopausal women who do not take estrogen replacement therapy are at risk for developing osteoporosis and will be more prone to fractures. Some of the manifestations of menopause do not disappear, such as vaginal and urethral atrophy. Women going through menopause will have irregular menses, not spotting. Women beginning menopause are still ovulating irregularly and may get pregnant if contraception is not used.

Nursing process: Analysis

Client need: Pharmacological and Parenteral Therapies

Cognitive level: Analysis

Subject area: Pharmacologic

5. The nurse instructs a client in menopause to eat foods that are high in calcium. The nurse includes which of the following foods that has the highest calcium content in these instructions?

   1. Low-fat plain yogurt

   2. Egg omelet

   3. Ice cream

   4. Eggnog

6. Which of the following nursing diagnoses would be most important for the nurse to include in the nursing care plan for a 55-year-old client who has had amenorrhea for one year?

   1. High risk for sexual dysfunction

   2. Self-care deficit

   3. Impaired skin integrity

   4. Risk for impaired physical mobility

7. The nurse instructs the client with premenstrual syndrome (PMS) that, prior to starting her menses when she notices fluid retention, she should eat which of the following?

   Select all that apply:

   [   ] **1.** Asparagus

   [   ] **2.** Cranberry juice

   [   ] **3.** Brussels sprouts

   [   ] **4.** Celery

   [   ] **5.** Bananas

   [   ] **6.** Parsley

8. The nurse instructs the client with premenstrual syndrome (PMS) to avoid which of the following?

   Select all that apply:

   [   ] **1.** Exercise

   [   ] **2.** Coffee

   [   ] **3.** Chocolate

   [   ] **4.** Applications of heat

   [   ] **5.** Vitamin B supplements

   [   ] **6.** Tea

Answer: 3

Rationale: Calcium is present in all of the food groups, but is highest in dairy products. Ice cream contains 1406 mg per serving. Low-fat plain yogurt contains 415 mg per serving. Egg nog contains 330 mg per serving and an egg omelet contains 47 mg per serving.

Nursing process: Implementation

Client need: Health Promotion and Maintenance

Cognitive level: Application

Subject area: Maternity and Women's Health

Answer: 4

Rationale: Menopause is considered complete after amenorrhea for one year in the older adult woman. A menopausal client is at risk for impaired mobility due to osteoporosis in the spine. Menopausal women can continue to function sexually and perform self-care measures. Although the skin becomes dryer in menopause, it is not of major consequence.

Nursing process: Planning

Client need: Management of Care

Cognitive level: Analysis

Subject area: Maternity and Women's Health

Answer: 1, 4, 6

Rationale: Asparagus, celery, and parsley are natural diuretics, which are recommended when the client experiences fluid retention. Cranberry juice, brussels sprouts, and bananas are fruits and vegetables that are high in water content and would promote fluid retention rather than alleviate it.

Nursing process: Implementation

Client need: Basic Care and Comfort

Cognitive level: Application

Subject area: Maternity and Women's Health

Answer: 2, 3, 6

Rationale: Clients with premenstrual syndrome should limit foods with caffeine, such as coffee, tea, cola, and chocolate, to decrease breast discomfort and prevent depression. Exercise should be encouraged to reduce stress. Applications of heat are effective in relieving the abdominal and pelvic cramping symptoms of PMS. Vitamin B supplements, especially B complex and vitamin B_6, are helpful in treating the depression that accompanies PMS.

Nursing process: Implementation

Client need: Basic Care and Comfort

Cognitive level: Application

Subject area: Maternity and Women's Health

9. The nurse assesses a client with a vesicovaginal fistula to have which of the following?

1. Fecal material passing into the vagina

2. Urine passing from the urethra into the vagina

3. Urine leaking continuously from the bladder into the vagina

4. Passage of urine from the ureter to the vagina

10. Which of the following diets should the nurse include in the teaching plan for a client who has a rectovaginal fistula?

1. Low fat

2. Low residue

3. Bland

4. Clear liquid

11. The nurse includes which of the following in the discharge instructions for a client with a rectovaginal fistula?

1. Do not douche until the area is healed

2. Use antifungal vaginal suppositories to prevent infection

3. Limit fluid intake until the vaginal discharge ceases

4. Avoid straining to have a bowel movement

Answer: 3

Rationale: A fistula is an abnormal opening between two organs or between an organ and the external body. The name of the fistula identifies the two areas of the body that are connected by the abnormal opening. Therefore, a vesicovaginal fistula connects the bladder with the vagina, resulting in urine from the bladder leaking continuously out the vagina. Fecal material in the vagina would be a rectovaginal fistula and urine passing from the urethra into the vagina would be a urethrovaginal fistula. The passage of urine from the ureter to the vagina is a ureterovaginal fistula.

Nursing process: Assessment

Client need: Physiological Adaptation

Cognitive level: Analysis

Subject area: Maternity and Women's Health

Answer: 2

Rationale: A low-residue diet is prescribed for the client with a rectovaginal fistula, to decrease the stool bulk and slow the transit time. A low-fat diet would be ordered for clients having gastrointestinal symptoms related to fat intolerance. A bland diet is ordered for disorders of the stomach and eliminates foods that may be irritating to the stomach mucosa. A clear liquid diet is a short-term, very restrictive diet that would not provide the necessary calories and protein needed for tissue repair.

Nursing process: Planning

Client need: Basic Care and Comfort

Cognitive level: Application

Subject area: Maternity and Women's Health

Answer: 4

Rationale: Clients with rectovaginal fistulas are advised not to strain to have a bowel movement, because the increase in pressure aggravates the fistula and usually increases the size of the opening. Clients are advised to use either cleansing or deodorizing douches during the course of treatment. Clients with rectovaginal fistulas are prone to bacterial infections rather than fungal infections. Fluid intake should not be limited as it causes constipation, which in turn puts pressure on the site of the fistula when one strains to have a bowel movement.

Nursing process: Implementation

Client need: Health Promotion and Maintenance

Cognitive level: Application

Subject area: Maternity and Women's Health

12. The client who had a rectovaginal fistula surgically repaired a year ago asks the nurse, "Why does the surgeon want to see me again in six months?" The best response of the nurse would be, "The doctor

    1. has to write a new prescription for the paregoric every six months."

    2. wants to be sure you're adhering to the diet and not gaining weight."

    3. wants to monitor the site to be sure the fistula hasn't returned."

    4. needs to be sure that the perineal area has healed completely."

13. The nurse monitors the urinary output every four hours of a postoperative client who had a cystocele and rectocele repair (anterior and posterior colporrhaphy). Which of the following measurements is the maximum amount of urine that should accumulate in the bladder?

    1. 150 ml

    2. 100 ml

    3. 200 ml

    4. 250 ml

14. Which of the following assessment findings is an anticipated finding for the client with a rectocele?

    1. Difficulty in voiding

    2. Hemorrhoids

    3. Tarry stools

    4. Stress incontinence

15. The nurse instructs a client with vaginitis to cleanse her douching equipment with what solution after each use? _____

Answer: 3

Rationale: Rectovaginal fistulas that are surgically repaired may recur within two years after the repair, necessitating follow-up care for a two-year period. Paregoric is prescribed to inhibit bowel action and would be contraindicated for a rectovaginal fistula. Weight gain would not be a consequence of this type of surgery and would not be a contributing factor for a recurrence of the fistula. A rectovaginal fistula is repaired internally and any related perineal irritation should have healed shortly after the surgery.

Nursing process: Analysis

Client need: Reduction of Risk Potential

Cognitive level: Analysis

Subject area: Maternity and Women's Health

Answer: 2

Rationale: The client who has a cystocele and rectocele repair should not have more than 100 ml of urine accumulating in the bladder to prevent tension on the suture line. Amounts of 150 ml, 200 ml, and 250 ml enlarge the bladder sufficiently to put pressure on the operative site.

Nursing process: Evaluation

Client need: Reduction of Risk Potential

Cognitive level: Analysis

Subject area: Maternity and Women's Health

Answer: 2

Rationale: A rectocele is herniation of the rectum into the vagina. As a rectocele enlarges, the client has difficulty having a bowel movement, becomes constipated, and begins to strain to have a bowel movement, resulting in hemorrhoids. A rectocele does not affect the urinary tract. Tarry stools would occur with gastrointestinal bleeding at a site remote from the rectum.

Nursing process: Assessment

Client need: Physiological Adaptation

Cognitive level: Analysis

Subject area: Maternity and Women's Health

Answer: Bleach

Rationale: Clients with reproductive system infections should soak douching equipment in bleach for 30 minutes after each use. Soap and water is not strong enough to kill the virulent organisms of vaginitis. Vinegar and bicarbonate of soda are used as douching solutions to change the pH, not as anti-infective agents.

Nursing process: Implementation

Client need: Reduction of Risk Potential

Cognitive level: Application

Subject area: Maternity and Women's Health

16. Which of the following statements by the nurse should be included in the instructions for a client receiving treatment for vaginitis?

    1. "The vagina needs to be acidic to decrease your chance of another infection."
    2. "Douching more frequently will help to rid the vagina of organisms."
    3. "Sexual intercourse is permitted as long as your partner uses protection."
    4. "A water-soluble lubricant should be used until your symptoms are gone."

17. The nurse should monitor which of the following clients for a potential vaginal infection?

    1. A menstruating client who uses sanitary napkins
    2. A menopausal client who is sexually active
    3. A client treated with Bactrim for a urinary tract infection
    4. A client given broad-spectrum antibiotics for a wound infection

18. The nurse should include which of the following in the discharge instructions for a client with herpes virus type 2?

    1. Sexual activity is permitted as long as the partner wears protection.
    2. The lesions should be covered when they break open.
    3. The antibiotic therapy should be sufficient to prevent recurrence.
    4. Abstinence from sex is necessary when the prodromal symptoms are noticed.

Answer: 1

Rationale: The normal pH of the vagina is approximately 3.5 to 5.5 and it is the acidic nature of the vaginal discharge that protects the vagina from infection by bacteria. Douching decreases the amount of normal vaginal discharge, which alters the acid nature of the vagina. Sexual intercourse, with or without protection, should not be done when a vaginal infection is present. A water-soluble lubricant has no therapeutic value in the treatment of vaginitis.

Nursing process: Planning

Client need: Health Promotion and Maintenance

Cognitive level: Analysis

Subject area: Maternity and Women's Health

Answer: 4

Rationale: Broad-spectrum antibiotics decrease the quantity of helpful bacteria as well as the harmful bacteria, so a client on broad-spectrum antibiotics for a period of time may develop vaginitis due to a decrease in the normal vaginal flora. Use of sanitary napkins has not been related to vaginal infections, but tampon use is the suspected cause of toxic shock syndrome, a bacterial infection. A sexually active menopausal client would not normally be at risk for vaginitis. Trimethoprim-sulfamethoxazole (Bactrim), an antibacterial prescribed for urinary tract infections, does not normally alter the flora in the vagina and rectum.

Nursing process: Assessment

Client need: Physiological Adaptation

Cognitive level: Analysis

Subject area: Maternity and Women's Health

Answer: 4

Rationale: The client with herpesvirus type 2 is considered infectious when the prodromal clinical manifestations occur, as the virus is being shed throughout this time. Wearing protection for sexual intercourse will not totally prevent contact with the virus, as any break in the mucous membranes or skin that comes into contact with an active lesion may become infected. Lesions should not be covered, but should be left open to the air to dry. Herpesvirus type 2 is a viral infection with no known cure. Antibiotics will not prevent a recurrence.

Nursing process: Planning

Client need: Health Promotion and Maintenance

Cognitive level: Application

Subject area: Maternity and Women's Health

19. Which of the following assessment findings would indicate to the nurse that a client with a history of gonorrhea is experiencing a complication of the disease?

    1. Inability to conceive

    2. Cottage cheese-like vaginal discharge

    3. Multiple ruptured vesicles on vagina and perineum

    4. Heavy vaginal bleeding after several missed periods

20. The nurse should include which of the following questions in a nursing history from a client admitted with pelvic inflammatory disease (PID)?

    1. "When did you first notice the heavy bleeding with clots?"

    2. "When did you start to have the sudden high fever?"

    3. "Have you ever used an intrauterine device?"

    4. "Do you have spotting after intercourse?"

21. The nurse should report which of the following client assessments as consistent with a diagnosis of toxic shock syndrome?

    Select all that apply:

    [ ] **1.** Menorrhagia

    [ ] **2.** Sudden temperature elevation of 39.2°C, or 102.6°F

    [ ] **3.** Complaints of headache and dizziness

    [ ] **4.** Muscle pain

    [ ] **5.** Red, macular rash

    [ ] **6.** Hemoglobin of 12 gm/dl

Answer: 1

Rationale: One of the complications of gonorrhea is sterility, caused by scarring of the fallopian tubes during the course of the disease and resulting in strictures. A cottage cheese-like vaginal discharge would occur with the client with candidiasis, a fungal infection. Multiple ruptured vesicles on the vagina and perineum occur when the client has herpes virus type 2. A client having heavy vaginal bleeding after several missed periods is probably experiencing a miscarriage, which indicates that the conceived ovum was transported through the fallopian tube to the uterus.

Nursing process: Evaluation

Client need: Physiological Adaptation

Cognitive level: Application

Subject area: Maternity and Women's Health

Answer: 3

Rationale: Clients who use or have used intrauterine devices are at risk for developing pelvic inflammatory disease (PID). The discharge for PID is foul smelling and purulent, not bloody with clots. Clients with PID may have fever and chills, but the temperature elevation is not sudden, and they do not normally have spotting after intercourse.

Nursing process: Assessment

Client need: Physiological Adaptation

Cognitive level: Analysis

Subject area: Maternity and Women's Health

Answer: 2, 4, 5

Rationale: One of the most pronounced clinical manifestations of toxic shock syndrome is a sudden temperature elevation above 38.9°C, or 102°F. Other clinical manifestations include chills; muscle pain; vomiting and diarrhea; red, macular rash that looks like a sunburn; and hypotension. The condition is not known to affect menses or to give rise to complaints of headache and dizziness. A hemoglobin of 12 gm/dl is within the normal range of 12 to 16 gm/dl for a female.

Nursing process: Analysis

Client need: Physiological Adaptation

Cognitive level: Application

Subject area: Maternity and Women's Health

22. The nurse develops a plan of care for the immediate postoperative period for a client who had an abdominal hysterectomy. The plan should include measures to

  1. assess intake and output every shift.

  2. clamp wound suction catheter in the morning.

  3. assess for abdominal distention.

  4. maintain bed rest until the morning, followed by assisted ambulation.

23. The nurse performs an assessment on a client diagnosed with endometriosis. Which of the following assessment findings would be indicative of this disorder?

Select all that apply:

  [   ] **1.** Spotting after intercourse

  [   ] **2.** Pain prior to menstruation

  [   ] **3.** Dyspareunia

  [   ] **4.** Menorrhagia

  [   ] **5.** Mass felt on palpation

  [   ] **6.** Yellow purulent discharge

24. The nurse is collecting a nursing history from a client admitted with an ectopic pregnancy. Which of the following questions should the nurse ask?

  1. "Has your partner's sperm been examined?"

  2. "Do you have frequent miscarriages?"

  3. "Do you have a family history of ectopic pregnancies?"

  4. "Have you ever had an infection in your pelvis?"

25. The nurse should include which of the following in the instructions to the client who has selected a barrier method of contraception?

  1. Spermicides lose effectiveness after one hour.

  2. A condom can be used a second time if washed with soap and water.

  3. Condoms are the safest form of contraception.

  4. A diaphragm should not be removed for 24 hours post coitus.

Answer: 3

Rationale: Abdominal distention in a postoperative client who had an abdominal hysterectomy could be an indication of the complication of a paralytic ileus. Intake and output should be assessed more frequently than every shift to detect postoperative complications of urinary retention and paralytic ileus. Wound suction catheters should remain open to prevent abscess formation. Clients should be ambulated the evening of surgery to prevent thrombophlebitis.

Nursing process: Planning

Client need: Physiological Adaptation

Cognitive level: Application

Subject area: Maternity and Women's Health

Answer: 2, 3, 4

Rationale: Pain in endometriosis occurs one to two days before menstruation and lasts for two to three days after menses begins. Other clinical manifestations include dyspareunia (pain during intercourse), menorrhagia (excessive bleeding with periods), feeling in the lower abdomen, irregular menstrual cycles, and infertility. Clients with endometriosis do not spot after intercourse or have an infection noted by a yellow purulent discharge. The endometrial cells, which are seeded in the pelvis, cannot be palpated.

Nursing process: Assessment

Client need: Physiological Adaptation

Cognitive level: Application

Subject area: Maternity and Women's Health

Answer: 4

Rationale: Clients who have had previous pelvic infections, such as chlamydia, gonorrhea, or pelvic inflammatory disease, are at risk for having an ectopic pregnancy, due to the strictures and adhesions created by these conditions. The cause of an ectopic pregnancy is not related to a problem with the male partner. Women at risk for an ectopic pregnancy are women who have had induced abortions, not miscarriages. Ectopic pregnancies are not genetic.

Nursing process: Assessment

Client need: Physiological Adaptation

Cognitive level: Application

Subject area: Maternity and Women's Health

Answer: 1

Rationale: Spermicides in the form of gels, foams, creams, or tablets kill sperm and should be used a few minutes before intercourse by placing them on condoms, diaphragms, or inserting them into the vagina. Their effectiveness lasts approximately one hour. Condoms should be used once and discarded, as slippage, breaks, or tears in the condom are possible. Condoms have a 10 to 15% failure rate, which is more than other forms of contraception. Diaphragms should not be left in place more than 24 hours.

Nursing process: Planning

Client need: Health Promotion and Maintenance

Cognitive level: Application

Subject area: Maternity and Women's Health

26. The registered nurse is preparing the clinical assignments on a women's health unit. Which of the following assignments would be appropriate to delegate to a licensed practical nurse?

    1. Perform an admission assessment of a woman admitted with vaginitis

    2. Conduct a health history on a woman suspected of having endometriosis

    3. Develop a plan of care on a woman following a hysterectomy

    4. Ask the woman about an allergy prior to a diagnostic test

27. A client describes an odorless, white, and cottage cheese-like vaginal discharge to the nurse. The nurse interprets this finding as indicative of what disorder? _____

Answer: 4

Rationale: A registered nurse may delegate asking a woman about an allergy prior to a diagnostic test. Performing an admission assessment, conducting a health history, and developing a plan of care involve the skills of a registered nurse.

Nursing process: Planning

Client need: Management of Care

Cognitive level: Analysis

Subject area: Legal and Ethical Issues

Answer: Candidiasis

Rationale: Candidiasis causes an odorless, white, and cottage cheese-like vaginal discharge.

Nursing process: Analysis

Client need: Physiological Adaptation

Cognitive level: Comprehension

Subject area: Maternity and Women's Health

UNIT V

Psychiatric Nursing

CHAPTER 46

Anxiety Disorders

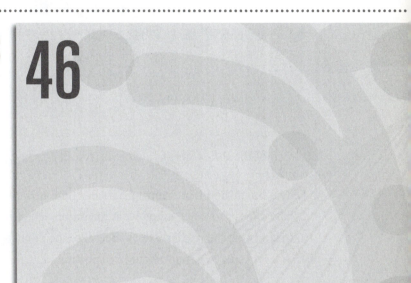

1. A client diagnosed with social phobia asks the nurse about the likelihood of children inheriting this disorder from their parents. Which of the following is the most appropriate response by the nurse?
   1. "It is only inherited if the child's father carries the trait."
   2. "There is no research supporting the heritability of social phobia."
   3. "The child of a parent with a social phobia has a 25% chance of inheriting it."
   4. "The chances of developing social phobia increase about 10% if a parent has the disorder."

2. Which of the following should be the priority consideration for the nurse caring for a client performing overt rituals?
   1. The ritual should be interrupted every time it is observed.
   2. The client should be asked what the rationale is for performing the ritual.
   3. Performing the ritual serves to decrease the client's anxiety.
   4. A less disruptive ritual should be substituted.

3. Which of the following instructions should the nurse give a client about relaxation techniques?
   1. Relaxation techniques are most effective when practiced regularly.
   2. Heart rate should be carefully monitored when relaxing.
   3. Avoid teaching these techniques to children under 12.
   4. To avoid dependence, these techniques should be used only when really needed.

4. While educating a client who has a social phobia about the use of a selective serotonin reuptake inhibitor (SSRI), the nurse assesses the client's knowledge about the drug. The client tells the nurse the physician explained that the drug will correct a "chemical imbalance" but states being unsure about what that means. Which of the following is the appropriate response by the nurse?
   1. "You should ask the physician to explain the purpose of your medication again."
   2. "Sometimes the brain produces too little of a chemical called serotonin and the SSRI corrects this."
   3. "What do you think chemical imbalance means?"
   4. "I'm also unsure what chemical imbalance means."

Answer: 4

Rationale: Although the precise mechanism of inheritance is unknown, developing a social phobia is 11% more likely if a family member has the disorder.

Nursing process: Analysis

Client need: Psychosocial Integrity

Cognitive level: Analysis

Subject area: Psychiatric and Mental Health

Answer: 3

Rationale: The purpose served by rituals is anxiety reduction. A ritual should only be interrupted as part of a carefully crafted program of exposure response prevention. The rationale the client gives for the ritual is seldom helpful in decreasing the behavior. The substitution of a less disruptive behavior only prolongs the treatment process.

Nursing process: Evaluation

Client need: Management of Care

Cognitive level: Analysis

Subject area: Psychiatric and Mental Health

Answer: 1

Rationale: The ability to effectively use relaxation techniques takes significant practice. Although heart rate often decreases during relaxation, monitoring it is unnecessary. Very young children can effectively use relaxation techniques. Relaxation can be safely and effectively used on most occasions.

Nursing process: Planning

Client need: Health Promotion and Maintenance

Cognitive level: Application

Subject area: Psychiatric and Mental Health

Answer: 2

Rationale: The nurse should tell the client that a SSRI produces the chemical serotonin in the brain of a client who naturally produces too little. This is a simple but accurate explanation of why this particular drug will help. The nurse, along with the physician, is responsible for medication education. This client already admitted to knowing about it. The nurse is responsible for knowing what a chemical imbalance means.

Nursing process: Analysis

Client need: Pharmacological and Parenteral Therapies

Cognitive level: Analysis

Subject area: Pharmacologic

5. A client with a dog phobia has undergone desensitization to this stimulus. The nurse evaluates which of the following client behaviors that indicates the treatment was successful?

1. The client recounts how the fear of dogs began, stating this fear is both unreasonable and excessive.
2. The client visits caged dogs in the pet shelter for 10 minutes three times a week.
3. The client states the fear of dogs is greatly diminished.
4. The client can pet the neighbor's dog without undue anxiety.

6. During an assessment interview, a female client explains that "Every morning I must check that my hair, makeup, and clothes are just so. I often have to redo my hair and makeup and change clothes several times before leaving the house because I worry that I just don't look quite right." The nurse documents this behavior as _____.

7. While preparing a client for surgery the next day, the nurse observes that the client is having trouble paying attention to instructions, is trembling, and has sweaty palms, a rapid heart rate, and rapid respirations. The client states, "All I can think about is this surgery tomorrow, and whether everything will go all right." The nurse notifies the physician that the client's level of anxiety is

1. mild.
2. moderate.
3. severe.
4. panic.

8. Which of the following client assessments on the use of a benzodiazepine would be a priority concern to the nurse?

1. A history of alcohol or substance abuse
2. A lack of adequate coping skills
3. A history of closed head injury
4. A diet high in tyramine-rich foods

Answer: 4

Rationale: Success in phobic desensitization is shown when the client is able to do what the average person can do without undue anxiety. Clients with phobias routinely believe their fears are unreasonable before treatment begins. A client visiting a dog shelter three times a week and stating that fears are greatly diminished are both steps in the overall desensitization process, but they are not the end result.

Nursing process: Evaluation

Client need: Psychosocial Integrity

Cognitive level: Analysis

Subject area: Psychiatric and Mental Health

Answer: obsessive-compulsive disorder

Rationale: The client's major difficulty in obsessive-compulsive disorder is in having to do and redo an activity, such as a ritual to reduce the anxiety about something's not being quite right.

Nursing process: Implementation

Client need: Psychosocial Integrity

Cognitive level: Application

Subject area: Psychiatric and Mental Health

Answer: 3

Rationale: When the client begins to display frank sympathetic arousal, clinical manifestations, and verbalize distress, the level of anxiety is severe.

Nursing process: Implementation

Client need: Psychosocial Integrity

Cognitive level: Analysis

Subject area: Psychiatric and Mental Health

Answer: 1

Rationale: Because benzodiazepines have a serious abuse potential, they are generally contraindicated for clients with a history of alcohol or substance abuse. A lack of adequate coping skills, a closed head injury, and a diet high in tyramine-rich foods are not factors in prescribing benzodiazepines.

Nursing process: Assessment

Client need: Pharmacological and Parenteral Therapies

Cognitive level: Analysis

Subject area: Pharmacologic

9. Which of the following would be the most appropriate statement for the nurse to make to a client found pacing in the hall?

   1. "The ballgame is on in the dayroom. Perhaps you'd like to watch it."

   2. "I noticed you've been pacing. Can you tell me how you're feeling?"

   3. "I think you'd be much more comfortable in your room."

   4. "I can tell something is wrong. What is it?"

10. When a client has panic-level anxiety, plans for nursing intervention should include

    1. darkening the room and offering warm blankets.

    2. having the client describe how he or she usually copes with anxiety.

    3. staying with the client.

    4. alerting security to the situation.

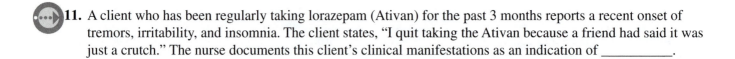

11. A client who has been regularly taking lorazepam (Ativan) for the past 3 months reports a recent onset of tremors, irritability, and insomnia. The client states, "I quit taking the Ativan because a friend had said it was just a crutch." The nurse documents this client's clinical manifestations as an indication of _____.

12. A client diagnosed with generalized anxiety disorder reports feeling increasingly ineffective at work and at home states, "I'm letting everyone down. I don't know what to do anymore." Which of the following diagnoses should the nurse select as most appropriate?

    1. Thought processes, disturbed

    2. Conflict, decisional

    3. Adjustment, impaired

    4. Role performance, ineffective

Answer: 2

Rationale: What the nurse needs to do is assess what is happening with the client. Distraction is unlikely to resolve this degree of agitation. Being alone tends to increase anxiety. It is assumed the client can explain the agitation.

Nursing process: Analysis

Client need: Psychosocial Integrity

Cognitive level: Analysis

Subject area: Psychiatric and Mental Health

Answer: 3

Rationale: Staying with the client reduces the anxiety and helps assure safety. Darkening the room may increase anxiety for a client whose perceptions may already be distorted. When in a panic level of anxiety, a client can focus only on the present and cannot think clearly enough to describe usual behaviors. Security would only be necessary if the client loses behavioral control.

Nursing process: Planning

Client need: Psychosocial Integrity

Cognitive level: Application

Subject area: Psychiatric and Mental Health

Answer: withdrawal

Rationale: Clinical manifestations of tremors, irritability, and insomnia are the classic features of withdrawal from benzodiazepines. Lorazepam (Ativan) is a benzodiazepine used in the treatment of anxiety.

Nursing process: Implementation

Client need: Pharmacological and Parenteral Therapies

Cognitive level: Analysis

Subject area: Pharmacologic

Answer: 4

Rationale: A client who has a generalized anxiety disorder expresses difficulty in performing usual roles in work and family environments. There is no evidence that the client's thinking is not reality based. There is no particular decision with which the client is wrestling. There is no indication that the client is facing any change in circumstances.

Nursing process: Planning

Client need: Psychosocial Integrity

Cognitive level: Analysis

Subject area: Psychiatric and Mental Health

13. While assessing a new client, the nurse asks the client about any fears. The client states, "Well, I've been afraid to go up and down the basement steps since my hip replacement last fall. I let my children do the laundry." The nurse should evaluate this response as

1. manipulative behavior.

2. normal anxiety.

3. a phobic reaction.

4. chronic anxiety.

14. A client being assessed for anxiety disorder relates to the nurse a concern with many physical clinical manifestations. The client states, "My heart races, my chest gets tight, and I can't breathe. I must be having a heart attack." Which of the following is the nurse's most appropriate response?

1. "Those clinical manifestations, although frightening, are very common with anxiety."

2. "Has anyone in your family had a heart attack?"

3. "Maybe we should ask the doctor to run some tests on your heart."

4. "Those are the clinical manifestations I get, too, when I am anxious."

15. The nurse is reviewing the care plan for a client diagnosed with generalized anxiety disorder. Which of the following is an appropriate client goal? The client will

1. describe the traumatic event in detail.

2. report no dissociative episodes.

3. be able to confront the phobic stimulus if accompanied.

4. report tolerating the presence of mild anxiety during activities.

Answer: 2

Rationale: It is adaptive and normal for people to be afraid to trust the reliability of a recently repaired joint. There is no indication that the client's motive is to avoid work. The client is not afraid of the stairs themselves but is afraid of getting hurt. There is no indication that this fear has persisted for a long time.

Nursing process: Evaluation

Client need: Psychosocial Integrity

Cognitive level: Analysis

Subject area: Psychiatric and Mental Health

Answer: 1

Rationale: Accurate information about the physical clinical manifestations of anxiety can be reassuring. Telling the client that the clinical manifestations are frightening and common in anxiety not only reassures the client but lets the client know the etiology of the clinical manifestations. Asking a client if anyone in the family has had a heart attack will likely increase anxiety and will not help to address the client's main concern. Telling a client that the doctor should run some tests only reinforces the concern with physical manifestations. It is inappropriate to self-disclose and will not likely comfort the client.

Nursing process: Analysis

Client need: Psychosocial Integrity

Cognitive level: Analysis

Subject area: Psychiatric and Mental Health

Answer: 4

Rationale: It is an unrealistic goal for clients with generalized anxiety disorder to be anxiety-free. Being able to tolerate mild anxiety so the client can perform activities is a realistic goal. Describing a traumatic event, reporting no dissociative episodes, or confronting a phobic stimulus are not goals for a general anxiety disorder.

Nursing process: Evaluation

Client need: Psychosocial Integrity

Cognitive level: Analysis

Subject area: Psychiatric and Mental Health

16. A new client in a mental health center program asks the nurse about the purpose of an assigned cognitive reframing group. Which of the following explanations should the nurse give?

    1. "This group will help you with your short-term memory."

    2. "This group will help you socialize more effectively with others."

    3. "All new clients are assigned to this group for assessment."

    4. "This group will help you change your faulty beliefs."

17. The nurse is assessing an obviously anxious client. Which of the following approaches should the nurse use?

    1. Avoid any questioning about the anxiety until it has subsided

    2. Ask specific, direct questions about the anxiety

    3. Don't mention the anxiety unless the client does

    4. Teach the client a relaxation exercise

18. A client reports having stopped the buspirone (BuSpar) prescribed for generalized anxiety disorder because, after taking it for a week, it did not seem to be helping. Which of the following explanations should the nurse give?

    1. Buspirone is not indicated for anxiety disorder.

    2. It is likely that the dosage is too low.

    3. Buspirone takes 2 to 3 weeks to become effective.

    4. Buspirone must be taken on an empty stomach.

19. The nurse is teaching the client how to care for a new colostomy. Although apparently attentive, the client is having difficulty repeating the sequence of actions required. The client states, "I'm sorry. Could you go over that again?" What level of anxiety would the nurse assess the client to have? _____

Answer: 4

Rationale: Cognitive reframing and restructuring helps clients change maladaptive beliefs that negatively affect their emotions and behavior. Helping a client with a short-term memory and socializing more effectively with others occur in other groups. Psychosocial assessment is not typically done in groups.

Nursing process: Analysis

Client need: Psychosocial Integrity

Cognitive level: Analysis

Subject area: Psychiatric and Mental Health

Answer: 2

Rationale: Specific, direct questions will help the client become aware of the anxiety and give pertinent information about it. Not questioning the client until the anxiety has subsided or not mentioning the anxiety unless the client does avoids assessing the client's anxiety, which must be done for the assessment to proceed. Teaching a client a relaxation exercise is an intervention, without adequate assessment.

Nursing process: Planning

Client need: Psychosocial Integrity

Cognitive level: Application

Subject area: Psychiatric and Mental Health

Answer: 3

Rationale: The full effect of buspirone (BuSpar) takes at least 2 to 3 weeks to become apparent. BuSpar is routinely used for chronic anxiety. The adequacy of the dose cannot be assessed until after the drug has been taken for at least 2 to 3 weeks. There is no evidence that food or the absence of it has any effect on absorption.

Nursing process: Analysis

Client need: Pharmacological and Parenteral Therapies

Cognitive level: Application

Subject area: Pharmacologic

Answer: Moderate

Rationale: Although at a moderate level of anxiety, individuals continue to be motivated to learn. Their functional ability decreases and thus they have difficulty learning new skills.

Nursing process: Assessment

Client need: Psychosocial Integrity

Cognitive level: Analysis

Subject area: Psychiatric and Mental Health

20. A client with agoraphobia tells the nurse in the outpatient clinic, "Now that my medication is working, I don't think I need to come here for therapy anymore." The most therapeutic response by the nurse should be which of the following?

1. "Your medicine will only work if you continue with therapy."

2. "You need to tell the doctor you want to quit therapy."

3. "You made a commitment to stay in therapy for at least six sessions."

4. "Combining medicine and therapy gives better, more lasting results."

21. The spouse of a client with a phobia of water has planned a sailing vacation to the islands and says to the nurse, "I think the best way to overcome these silly fears is to confront them head on." The nurse's most helpful response is which of the following?

1. "That kind of exposure may well do more harm than good."

2. "I agree. I think a vacation would be a good idea."

3. "For a plan like that to work, I think it would have to be a surprise."

4. "Have you discussed this plan with other family members?"

22. During an assessment interview, a client replies to the nurse's question about work relationships, "Oh no. I don't go to lunch with anyone at work. I've never been able to eat in front of other people." Which of the following disorders should the nurse consider?

1. Generalized anxiety disorder

2. Obsessive-compulsive disorder

3. Social phobia

4. Xenophobia

Answer: 4

Rationale: Research demonstrates a better outcome with combination therapy when treating a client with agoraphobia. A drug will decrease clinical manifestations on its own. Telling the client to tell the doctor about wanting to quit therapy passes off the nurse's responsibility to address this issue presently. Reminding a client about the commitment to stay in therapy for six sessions tries to keep the client in therapy by inducing guilt.

Nursing process: Analysis

Client need: Psychosocial Integrity

Cognitive level: Analysis

Subject area: Psychiatric and Mental Health

Answer: 1

Rationale: Intense exposure to feared stimuli without careful planning and the agreement of the client is likely to increase clinical manifestations and decrease trust. Affirming the spouse's comments shows the nurse's lack of understanding of the dynamics of phobia. Telling the spouse that such a plan should be a surprise demonstrates a lack of respecting the need for client involvement in the treatment planning. Asking the client's spouse if other family members' opinions have been sought is beside the point.

Nursing process: Analysis

Client need: Psychosocial Integrity

Cognitive level: Analysis

Subject area: Psychiatric and Mental Health

Answer: 3

Rationale: One of the variants of social phobia is being unable to perform some common activity, such as eating, speaking, or writing, in the presence of others. Individuals with a general anxiety disorder worry about a number of things. A client with a social phobia does not report either obsessive thoughts or compulsive behaviors. Xenophobia is a fear of strangers, and this client reports a phobic reaction with associates.

Nursing process: Assessment

Client need: Psychosocial Integrity

Cognitive level: Analysis

Subject area: Psychiatric and Mental Health

23. A client recently diagnosed with obsessive-compulsive disorder says to the nurse, "I know the doctor said this was just an anxiety problem, but I think I must really be crazy. I keep thinking that people are mad at me, and then I have to keep telling them I'm sorry." Which of the following is the most appropriate response by the nurse?

1. "Be careful. You might offend someone by using the word 'crazy.'"

2. "Very often, people's obsessive ideas seem rather bizarre to them."

3. "This is serious. We must let the doctor know."

4. "What makes you think someone is angry with you?"

24. The registered nurse is preparing to delegate clinical assignments for a psychiatric unit. Which of the following assignments should the nurse delegate to a licensed practical nurse?

1. Encourage a client with a generalized anxiety disorder to verbalize personal feelings

2. Develop a plan of care for a client with obsessive-compulsive disorder

3. Monitor the laboratory tests of a client admitted to a psychiatric unit

4. Take a detailed social history from a client admitted with a social phobia

25. A client approaches the nurse and says, "I don't know what's going on, but I have this terrible feeling that something awful is going to happen." The nurse's best response is which of the following?

1. "Don't worry, you're very safe here."

2. "Can you tell me what you think is going to happen?"

3. "It sounds like you're having some anxiety."

4. "Would you like some anxiety medication?"

Answer: 2

Rationale: Obsessive thoughts are commonly considered to be odd, foreign, and shameful to those who have them. Telling a client that using the word "crazy" may be offensive to someone may well prompt the client to feel the nurse and others will be angry. It would be inappropriate to tell a client with an obsessive-compulsive disorder that it is serious. The doctor would know that these kinds of thoughts are typical in obsessive-compulsive disorders. Clients pose no particular danger to self or others. It would be inappropriate to ask why the client thinks someone is angry, because the client has no idea why this is believed and this question will just increase the client's anxiety.

Nursing process: Analysis

Client need: Psychosocial Integrity

Cognitive level: Analysis

Subject area: Psychiatric and Mental Health

Answer: 1

Rationale: Developing a plan of care, monitoring laboratory tests, and taking a detailed social history are all assignments that should be performed by a registered nurse. It would be appropriate to delegate to a licensed practical nurse talking to a client and encouraging the verbalization of feelings.

Nursing process: Planning

Client need: Management of Care

Cognitive level: Analysis

Subject area: Legal and Ethical Issues

Answer: 3

Rationale: Saying that the client may be having some anxiety encourages the client to become aware of and explore the anxiety. Telling the client not to worry, for whatever the reason, cuts off an exploration of the client's concern. It would be inappropriate to ask a client to anticipate what might happen, because the client has already indicated having only a general sense of impending doom. Offering the client some medication is incorrect because such an intervention is premature.

Nursing process: Analysis

Client need: Psychosocial Integrity

Cognitive level: Analysis

Subject area: Psychiatric and Mental Health

26. An inpatient behavioral health unit employs some unlicensed assistive personnel. Which of the following activities may the nurse appropriately delegate to unlicensed assistive personnel?

Select all that apply:

[ ] **1.** Document the response of a client with social phobia to a cinema field trip

[ ] **2.** Evaluate the effect of a client's relaxation practice on the level of anxiety reported

[ ] **3.** Monitor a client's blood pressure after a new drug is given

[ ] **4.** Plan the weekly current events for a client discussion group

[ ] **5.** Teach the client about dietary restrictions

[ ] **6.** Inform the client on the visiting hours

Answer: 1, 3, 6

Rationale: Unlicensed assistive personnel are trained to document behavior accurately. Monitoring vital signs and informing the client about visiting hours are within the capabilities and job description of unlicensed assistive personnel. Only a registered nurse (RN) can evaluate the effect of a treatment, such as relaxation techniques. The RN is the only one who can be responsible for planning therapeutic activities or teaching clients.

Nursing process: Planning

Client need: Management of Care

Cognitive level: Analysis

Subject area: Legal and Ethical Issues

Somatoform Disorders

47

1. The nurse is assessing a client who has repeatedly complained of back pain. What is the diagnostic criterion found to be present in a client with a somatoform disorder? _____

2. The nurse informs another nurse that stress is an essential component of somatoform disorders because stress

  1. is the only feature of this disorder.

  2. exacerbates the illness.

  3. is a positive force in overcoming the illness.

  4. is not a precursor to the development of this disorder.

3. Which of the following is the most critical component leading to the client's ability to adapt to a somatoform disorder?

  1. The client's psychological makeup

  2. The etiology of the stress

  3. The nurse's ability to manipulate the environment

  4. The establishment of a medical etiology

4. When interviewing a client with a somatoform disorder, which of the following factors is important for the nurse to understand?

  1. The client is able to remember the precipitating event.

  2. Somatoform disorder is not usually within the awareness of the client.

  3. Somatoform disorders are generally within the awareness of the client.

  4. The client's behavior is an attempt to manipulate the nurse.

Answer: The presence of physical clinical manifestations without supporting laboratory findings and physiological cause

Rationale: One of the essential criteria for making a diagnosis of somatoform disorder is the absence of laboratory findings and physiological cause to support the clinical manifestations exhibited by the client.

Nursing process: Analysis

Client need: Psychosocial Integrity

Cognitive level: Application

Subject area: Psychiatric and Mental Health

Answer: 2

Rationale: Stress is one of the key components that exacerbates and intensifies the somatoform clinical manifestations. Stress is not the only feature, however, because there are psychological, neurobiological, and familial components as well. Stress does not contribute to overcoming the illness. The presence of stress actually makes the condition worse. Stress is a precursor to developing somatoform disorders.

Nursing process: Implementation

Client need: Psychosocial Integrity

Cognitive level: Application

Subject area: Psychiatric and Mental Health

Answer: 1

Rationale: A psychological makeup determines the client's ability to recognize the dysfunctional manifestations of a somatoform disorder and take corrective action. The etiology of the stress is outside the nurse's control. The ability to manipulate the environment also depends on external sources for control. The somatoform disorder does not have a medical etiology.

Nursing process: Analysis

Client need: Psychosocial Integrity

Cognitive level: Analysis

Subject area: Psychiatric and Mental Health

Answer: 2

Rationale: The cure for somatoform disorder lies in the client being able to identify the etiology of the disorder. The client may not be able to link the precipitating event to the disorder. The disorder is not within the awareness of the client. Unlike malingering, the primary goal is not manipulation.

Nursing process: Evaluation

Client need: Psychosocial Integrity

Cognitive level: Analysis

Subject area: Psychiatric and Mental Health

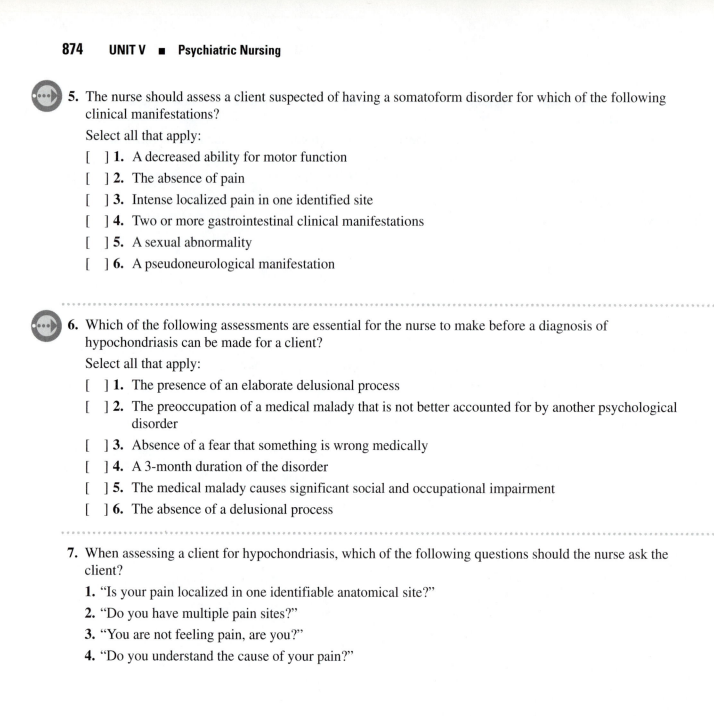

5. The nurse should assess a client suspected of having a somatoform disorder for which of the following clinical manifestations?

Select all that apply:

[   ] **1.** A decreased ability for motor function

[   ] **2.** The absence of pain

[   ] **3.** Intense localized pain in one identified site

[   ] **4.** Two or more gastrointestinal clinical manifestations

[   ] **5.** A sexual abnormality

[   ] **6.** A pseudoneurological manifestation

6. Which of the following assessments are essential for the nurse to make before a diagnosis of hypochondriasis can be made for a client?

Select all that apply:

[   ] **1.** The presence of an elaborate delusional process

[   ] **2.** The preoccupation of a medical malady that is not better accounted for by another psychological disorder

[   ] **3.** Absence of a fear that something is wrong medically

[   ] **4.** A 3-month duration of the disorder

[   ] **5.** The medical malady causes significant social and occupational impairment

[   ] **6.** The absence of a delusional process

7. When assessing a client for hypochondriasis, which of the following questions should the nurse ask the client?

1. "Is your pain localized in one identifiable anatomical site?"

2. "Do you have multiple pain sites?"

3. "You are not feeling pain, are you?"

4. "Do you understand the cause of your pain?"

8. A female client reports to the nurse that she feels she is too fat. The nurse suspects what somatoform disorder? _____

Answer: 4, 5, 6

Rationale: Clinical manifestations of a somatoform disorder include at least four pain manifestations, two gastrointestinal manifestations other than pain, one sexual, and one pseudoneurological manifestation. Somatoform disorders manifest with numerous physical complaints in multiple sites in the body, including the head, abdomen, back, joints, extremities, chest, and rectum. Motor function is not impaired by the disorder. The pain is not localized to a single site.

Nursing process: Assessment

Client need: Psychosocial Integrity

Cognitive level: Application

Subject area: Psychiatric and Mental Health

Answer: 2, 5, 6

Rationale: Hypochondriasis is the fear of having a medical malady based on the incorrect interpretation of the body's function. There is no delusional process involved. The preoccupation with a medical malady is not better accounted for by another psychological disorder. The disorder generally has at least a 6-month duration. The medical malady causes significant social and occupational impairment.

Nursing process: Assessment

Client need: Psychosocial Integrity

Cognitive level: Application

Subject area: Psychiatric and Mental Health

Answer: 2

Rationale: Hypochondriasis manifests itself in at least four sites to meet the diagnostic criteria. Pain is manifested in multiple sites. The client does not recognize the etiology of the pain.

Nursing process: Assessment

Client need: Psychosocial Integrity

Cognitive level: Analysis

Subject area: Psychiatric and Mental Health

Answer: Body dysmorphic disorder

Rationale: A body dysmorphic disorder is a preoccupation with an imagined or exaggerated defect in the body.

Nursing process: Analysis

Client need: Psychosocial Integrity

Cognitive level: Comprehension

Subject area: Psychiatric and Mental Health

9. The nurse evaluates the etiology of a conversion disorder to be _____.

10. The nurse assesses which of the following for a client with a conversion disorder?

Select all that apply:

[   ] **1.** One or more sensory or motor manifestations

[   ] **2.** Intentionally produced clinical manifestations

[   ] **3.** Minimal distress or impairment

[   ] **4.** Clinical manifestations not limited to pain or sexual dysfunction

[   ] **5.** Condition not caused by a medical problem

[   ] **6.** Absence of causative psychologic factors

11. The nurse is caring for a client who is complaining of a headache that cannot be confirmed by diagnostic tests. Which of the following factors would be critical before making a diagnosis of somatoform disorder?

1. The client has feelings of guilt.

2. There is an absence of other physical complaints.

3. The manifestations occurred at age 40 years.

4. Laboratory tests showed an abnormal EEG.

12. When planning to care for the client with hypochondriasis, the nurse should include which of the following?

1. Avoid focusing on the preoccupation with the disease

2. Attempt to identify the sources of anxiety

3. Inform the client about normal sensations

4. Discourage the client from making frequent visits to health care specialists

Answer: primarily psychological

Rationale: A conversion disorder is a psychologic disorder in which the client exhibits physical clinical manifestations not explained by a physical or neurologic disorder.

Nursing process: Evaluation

Client need: Psychosocial Integrity

Cognitive level: Application

Subject area: Psychiatric and Mental Health

Answer: 1, 4, 5

Rationale: Conversion disorder is not within the control of the client. One or more clinical manifestations affect the sensory or motor function, suggesting a medical or neurologic disorder. The clinical manifestations are not intentionally produced. There is significant distress or impairment in the client's functioning that may bring the client to the health care provider. The clinical manifestations are not limited to pain or sexual dysfunction. Conversion disorders are not caused by a medical disorder, and there are always psychologic manifestations present.

Nursing process: Assessment

Client need: Psychosocial Integrity

Cognitive level: Application

Subject area: Psychiatric and Mental Health

Answer: 1

Rationale: An unresolved guilt is a major contributor to somatoform disorder. Once the guilt is cleared up, the disorder abates. Somatoform disorder is accompanied by multiple physical complaints before the age of 30 years. Physiologic laboratory tests fail to show any physical abnormalities in somatoform disorder.

Nursing process: Evaluation

Client need: Psychosocial Integrity

Cognitive level: Analysis

Subject area: Psychiatric and Mental Health

Answer: 2

Rationale: The major treatment objective of hypochondriasis is to identify the source of anxiety and treat it. Ignoring the client's preoccupation with illness will escalate the behavior. Acknowledgment of the client's concern with a redirection toward the source of anxiety is more therapeutic. Telling the client about normal sensations does not help the client deal with personal manifestations. Health care visits should be encouraged at routine times to discourage overuse for the purpose of gaining attention.

Nursing process: Planning

Client need: Psychosocial Integrity

Cognitive level: Application

Subject area: Psychiatric and Mental Health

13. The nurse is caring for a client with somatization disorder. Which of the following nursing measures should be included in this client's plan of care?

  1. Encourage the use of pain relievers or anxiolytics

  2. Support medical intervention

  3. Discourage social interactions

  4. Identify somatic clinical manifestations as coping strategies

14. A nurse is caring for a client with body dysmorphic disorder. The client asks the nurse about the disorder. Which of the following would be an appropriate response by the nurse?

  1. "There is no medical cause for your disorder."

  2. "Because of your disorder, you will be exceptionally needy."

  3. "Significant distress in social functioning is a result of your disorder."

  4. "The defects you are experiencing are real."

15. A client is admitted to the psychiatric unit with sudden unexplained blindness. Which of the following conditions does the nurse need to establish before making a diagnosis of conversion disorder?

  1. Establish where the clinical manifestation is prominent.

  2. The client is indifferent to the condition.

  3. The clinical manifestations are produced for secondary gain.

  4. The clinical manifestations are unrelated to unresolved conflict.

16. The nurse is assessing a client with factitious disorder. Which of the following information is a priority for the nurse to understand before making a diagnosis?

  1. The clinical manifestations are real.

  2. The clinical manifestations are feigned.

  3. There is a secondary gain.

  4. The clinical manifestations are unintentionally produced.

Answer: 4
Rationale: The priority intervention for a client with a somatization disorder is that the client recognizes that the pain is a coping strategy. The use of pain relievers or anxiolytics should be discouraged to avoid dependence. The primary source of a pain disorder is psychologic, so medical interventions are not effective. The need for social interaction is important, because the consequences of diminished social interaction is social isolation.
Nursing process: Planning
Client need: Psychosocial Integrity
Cognitive level: Application
Subject area: Psychiatric and Mental Health

Answer: 3
Rationale: Social isolation is a major contributor to a body dysmorphic disorder. It is a cyclical process in which the more withdrawn the client becomes, the more the dysmorphic belief will contribute to more withdrawal. The disorder will become even more pronounced. There may be a minor problem, but the response to it is beyond reasonable. Clients tend to avoid social contact because of self-consciousness with the imagined defect. The defects the client is experiencing are not real.
Nursing process: Analysis
Client need: Psychosocial Integrity
Cognitive level: Analysis
Subject area: Psychiatric and Mental Health

Answer: 2
Rationale: One of the classic signs of conversion disorder is the client's indifference to sudden and severe impairment, "la belle indifférence." The site of the clinical manifestations is not as important as the precipitating factors. The disorder is not to achieve secondary gain and is out of the client's control. Conversion disorder is directly related to underlying conflict.
Nursing process: Analysis
Client need: Psychosocial Integrity
Cognitive level: Analysis
Subject area: Psychiatric and Mental Health

Answer: 3
Rationale: Factitious disorder is well within the awareness of the client, and clinical manifestations may be real or feigned. It is the secondary gain, for attention or financial reward, that is the priority feature for diagnosis of factitious disorder. Clinical manifestations are intentionally produced for personal gain.
Nursing process: Analysis
Client need: Management of Care
Cognitive level: Analysis
Subject area: Psychiatric and Mental Health

17. When establishing a diagnosis of malingering, the nurse should assess the client for which of the following features of the disorder?

    1. The clinical manifestations are confirmed with lab tests.

    2. The client attempts to hide the clinical manifestations.

    3. The client actively seeks attention.

    4. The client has a tendency to withdraw.

18. The registered nurse is delegating the clinical assignments on a psychiatric unit. Which of the following assignments should the nurse delegate to a licensed practical nurse?

    1. Notify the physician of a child being admitted who has a mother suspected of Munchausen's syndrome by proxy

    2. Assess a client for the diagnostic criteria of a somatization disorder

    3. Empathize with a client who has a somatoform disorder by understanding the client's pain

    4. Establish the nursing diagnoses for a client with a somatization disorder

19. Which of the following information would the nurse consider significant when assessing a client for a somatoform disorder?

    1. The clinical manifestations are under the client's voluntary control.

    2. The client fails to see the relationship between clinical manifestations and conflicts.

    3. The client's ability to perform usual tasks is unaltered.

    4. The client is unaware of the clinical manifestations.

20. Which of the following interventions should the nurse include in the plan for the client with a somatoform disorder?

    1. Assist the client to recognize somatic clinical manifestations

    2. Avoid focusing on the client's secondary gains

    3. Confront the client's defenses

    4. Administer drug therapy

Answer: 3

Rationale: Malingering is characterized by the client's deliberate attempt to gain attention. The clinical manifestations are not confirmed by lab tests. The client will bring the clinical manifestations to the attention of others for secondary gain. The client does not withdraw but becomes demanding of health care providers and others.

Nursing process: Assessment

Client need: Psychosocial Integrity

Cognitive level: Analysis

Subject area: Psychiatric and Mental Health

Answer: 3

Rationale: Notifying the physician of a client being admitted with a suspected condition, assessing the client for the diagnostic criteria, and establishing the nursing diagnoses are assignments that should be performed by a registered nurse. Any nurse working with a client with a somatization disorder should be prepared to empathize with the client by understanding the client's pain. Empathizing would be appropriate to delegate to a licensed practical nurse.

Nursing process: Planning

Client need: Management of Care

Cognitive level: Analysis

Subject area: Legal and Ethical Issues

Answer: 2

Rationale: Somatoform disorder is characterized by the client's inability to link the clinical manifestations with unresolved conflicts. This link is a key to overcoming the disorder. The client has no voluntary control over the clinical manifestations. The client's ability to perform tasks is highly diminished. The client is very aware of the clinical manifestations and only unaware of their etiology.

Nursing process: Analysis

Client need: Psychosocial Integrity

Cognitive level: Analysis

Subject area: Psychiatric and Mental Health

Answer: 1

Rationale: The key to treatment of a client with a somatoform disorder is to recognize when the clinical manifestations are somatic in nature and when they are of a medical origin. The secondary gains must be addressed so that the client can make more healthy adaptation to meet personal needs. Confrontation of defenses will increase the client's fixation. Administering a drug is not a cure but will only complicate the treatment.

Nursing process: Planning

Client need: Psychosocial Integrity

Cognitive level: Application

Subject area: Psychiatric and Mental Health

21. When teaching a client with a somatoform disorder how to deal with the clinical manifestations, the nurse should
    1. instruct the client to ignore the clinical manifestations.
    2. encourage the client to minimize the number of health care visits.
    3. instruct the client about alternative medicine.
    4. caution the client about dependence on drugs.

22. The nurse administers which of the following drugs to a client with somatoform disorder?
    1. Benzodiazepines
    2. Anxiolytics
    3. Selective serotonin reuptake inhibitor
    4. Antipsychotics

23. A client is admitted with a body dysmorphic disorder. Which of the following clinical manifestations does the nurse interpret as indicative of an exacerbation? The client will
    1. exhibit an increased preoccupation with appearance of an imagined defect.
    2. display an excessive need for social contact.
    3. exhibit a decrease in grooming behaviors.
    4. emotionally disengage.

24. The nurse is caring for a client on benzodiazepines for a pain disorder. Which of the following observations is a priority for the nurse to immediately report?
    1. Agitation
    2. An abrupt rise in temperature
    3. Restlessness
    4. Excessive sleeplessness

Answer: 4

Rationale: Somatoform disorder is characterized by the risk that the client may become addicted to either pain medications or anxiolytics. Careful client teaching is necessary to help the client avoid an overdependence on drugs. The client will need to understand the purpose of the clinical manifestations before relinquishing them. Routine health care visits are essential to not encourage anxiety or overuse. Shifting treatment to alternative medicine does not address the etiology of the disorder, but merely shifts the dependence to another substance.

Nursing process: Planning

Client need: Psychosocial Integrity

Cognitive level: Application

Subject area: Psychiatric and Mental Health

Answer: 3

Rationale: Selective serotonin reuptake inhibitors are the drugs recommended in the treatment of somatoform disorders, because they have relative few adverse effects and a good response. The benzodiazepines are addictive. There is a high potential for dependence on the anxiolytics as well. The antipsychotics are inappropriate, because the client is not psychotic.

Nursing process: Implementation

Client need: Pharmacological and Parenteral Therapies

Cognitive level: Application

Subject area: Pharmacologic

Answer: 1

Rationale: The primary clinical manifestation of a body dysmorphic disorder is an increased preoccupation with appearance of the imagined defect. Social withdrawal is common. There is an increase in grooming behaviors. The client does not disengage but becomes increasingly anxious.

Nursing process: Evaluation

Client need: Psychosocial Integrity

Cognitive level: Application

Subject area: Psychiatric and Mental Health

Answer: 2

Rationale: Neuromalignant syndrome is characterized by a high fever 39.4°C (103°F) or higher and can be fatal. The client's agitation may be from sources other than a drug. The client's restlessness may be from a drug; however, the clinical manifestations need to be observed over a period of time. The client may be sleeping due to factors other than drugs.

Nursing process: Analysis

Client need: Management of Care

Cognitive level: Analysis

Subject area: Psychiatric and Mental Health

25. When the nurse monitors the client diagnosed with hypochondriasis, it is important that the nurse assesses for which of the following behaviors?

1. The client has an increased ability to cope with anxiety.

2. The client's clinical manifestations move from the primary site to a secondary site.

3. The client asks for more medication.

4. The client reports additional clinical manifestations.

26. Which of the following instructions should the nurse include in the plan of care for a client with a body dysmorphic disorder?

1. Encourage a well-balanced diet

2. Encourage the client to achieve control over family dynamics

3. Instruct the client to avoid social interaction

4. Educate the client that binging and purging are methods to control weight

Answer: 1

Rationale: The reduction in clinical manifestations is manifested in the ability to appropriately deal with psychological anxiety. The client's clinical manifestations need to abate rather than move. The need for an additional drug is not a sign of dealing with hypochondria. The clinical manifestations should diminish rather than increase.

Nursing process: Assessment

Client need: Psychosocial Integrity

Cognitive level: Application

Subject area: Psychiatric and Mental Health

Answer: 1

Rationale: Even the client who complains about being too heavy must maintain life-sustaining nutrition. The client's core struggle is over family dynamics and it is expressed in eating disorders. Avoiding social interaction exacerbates the disorder. Binging and purging are dysfunctional means of coping.

Nursing process: Planning

Client need: Psychosocial Integrity

Cognitive level: Application

Subject area: Psychiatric and Mental Health

Dissociative Disorders

48

1. The nurse is assessing a client suspected of having a dissociative disorder. Which of the following describes a dissociative disorder? Dissociative disorders

    1. are produced by extreme anxiety.

    2. appear only in schizophrenia.

    3. are fixed and chronic.

    4. are voluntary.

2. When assessing a client who is experiencing dissociative fugue, the nurse should assess for which of the following clinical manifestations?

    Select all that apply:

    [　] **1.** Travel away from common locations

    [　] **2.** Chronic long-term state

    [　] **3.** Recollection of the fugue after an acute phase

    [　] **4.** Not preceded by a stress event

    [　] **5.** Unable to recall past identity

    [　] **6.** Assumes new identity

3. The nurse admitting a client suspected of dissociative amnesia would report which of the following manifestations?

    1. The client is unable to recall personal information.

    2. The amnesia has its etiology in a medical condition.

    3. The amnesia is the result of prolonged substance abuse.

    4. The client exhibits common forgetfulness.

4. The nurse identifies which of the following as the primary feature of dissociative identity disorder (DID)?

    1. The presence of alternating control by two or more personalities.

    2. The personalities are always unaware of each other.

    3. The condition is unique to schizophrenia.

    4. All of the personalities possess similar sexual, racial, and intellectual characteristics.

Answer: 1

Rationale: Dissociative disorders are produced by extreme anxiety, when circumstances become overwhelming and the traditional coping mechanism cannot contain the anxiety. Dissociative disorders are not confined to schizophrenia but are a diagnostic category by itself. Dissociative disorders are not fixed and chronic but change and can be temporary. Dissociative disorders are not voluntary.

Nursing process: Analysis

Client need: Psychosocial Integrity

Cognitive level: Application

Subject area: Psychiatric and Mental Health

Answer: 1, 5, 6

Rationale: Clinical manifestations of dissociative fugue include travel away from common locations, inability to recall past identity, and assuming a new identity. Dissociative fugue is not long term and can remit spontaneously. There is no recollection of the fugue state. Dissociative fugue is precipitated by stress.

Nursing process: Assessment

Client need: Psychosocial Integrity

Cognitive level: Application

Subject area: Psychiatric and Mental Health

Answer: 1

Rationale: A client with dissociative amnesia is unable to recall familiar personal information. The amnesia is not associated with a medical condition, such as brain injury, trauma, or toxicity of substances. The amnesia is beyond common forgetfulness.

Nursing process: Analysis

Client need: Psychosocial Integrity

Cognitive level: Application

Subject area: Psychiatric and Mental Health

Answer: 1

Rationale: The presence of multiple personalities is a classic feature of dissociative identity disorder. The personalities are sometimes aware of each other but often out of the awareness of the primary personality. Dissociative identity disorder is a condition in a diagnostic category by itself and is not necessarily tied to schizophrenia. The personalities may possess different sexual, racial, and intellectual characteristics.

Nursing process: Implementation

Client need: Psychosocial Integrity

Cognitive level: Application

Subject area: Psychiatric and Mental Health

5. Which of the following is the priority goal for a client with dissociative identity disorder?

 1. Meet safety and security needs

 2. Reorient the client to the true identity

 3. Assist the client to forget the stress-producing events

 4. Avoid discussing stress-producing subjects

6. When establishing a diagnosis of a dissociative disorder for a client, what information is a priority for the nurse to assess?

 1. Conduct an interview until all lost information is available

 2. Rule out the use of substances or the existence of a medical condition

 3. The client has been treated for depression

 4. The client's ability to recall the precipitating event

7. When treating a client with a dissociative disorder, which of the following is a priority intervention that the nurse should implement for early intervention?

 1. Establish a therapeutic alliance

 2. Complete the history that the client cannot recall

 3. Suggest hypnosis to uncover repressed information

 4. Try to establish the triggering events

8. Which of the following clinical manifestations should the nurse assess in a client with depersonalization disorder?

 1. Anger

 2. A loss of reality testing ability

 3. Mechanical dreamy or detached feelings

 4. Ambivalence

Answer: 1

Rationale: Ensuring the safety and security needs of the client are the priority goals for a client experiencing dissociative identity disorder, because the normal protective processes for the client are impaired. Reorientation of the client to the identity is done with a therapist at the appropriate time in the therapy. The client will need to understand the stress-producing events in the course of therapy in order to deal with the anxiety. The client will need to discuss stress-producing subjects to help develop methods of dealing appropriately with the stress.

Nursing process: Evaluation

Client need: Management of Care

Cognitive level: Application

Subject area: Psychiatric and Mental Health

Answer: 2

Rationale: It is essential that the use of substances and the existence of a medical condition are ruled out, because they may cause the same type of clinical manifestation. The client cannot recall all lost information. The client may or may not be depressed, which is not a precondition for a dissociative disorder. The client may not remember what precipitated the dissociative event.

Nursing process: Assessment

Client need: Management of Care

Cognitive level: Analysis

Subject area: Psychiatric and Mental Health

Answer: 1

Rationale: The nurse must establish a therapeutic alliance, so that trust may develop and the client may be able to reveal traumatic events with reduced anxiety. The nurse should not fill in the history for the client, because the client may find it frustrating and because mobilizing the memory is healing for the client. Hypnosis has been used with mixed success and is now being employed much less effectively than initially thought. Establishing the triggering event is the work of the client and the psychotherapist at the appropriate time in the therapy.

Nursing process: Planning

Client need: Management of Care

Cognitive level: Application

Subject area: Psychiatric and Mental Health

Answer: 3

Rationale: A client with depersonalization disorder has a mechanical dreamy or detached feeling. Client anger is not a cardinal sign. The client does not lose the ability to perform reality tests. Ambivalence is not a criterion for the diagnosis of depersonalization disorder.

Nursing process: Assessment

Client need: Psychosocial Integrity

Cognitive level: Application

Subject area: Psychiatric and Mental Health

9. The spouse of a female client brings her to the hospital after she woke up one day in an apartment building in a different city, appeared confused, and didn't know how she got there. The nurse documents this as which of the dissociative disorders? _____

10. Which of the following is the goal of therapy that is a priority when treating a client with a dissociative disorder?

1. Behavioral therapy
2. Cognitive restructuring
3. Family therapy
4. Safety

11. The nurse is recording the history of a client with a dissociative disorder. Which of the following events would most likely contribute to the diagnosis? History of

1. brain tumor.
2. substance abuse.
3. child abuse.
4. seizures.

12. Which of the following interventions is appropriate for the nurse to include in a plan of care for a client with a dissociative disorder?

1. Avoid confirming the identity of the client
2. Recall past events for the client
3. Assist the client to understand the benefits of dissociation to cope
4. Avoid letting the client make decisions

Answer: Dissociative fugue

Rationale: Dissociative fugue is a dissociative disorder characterized by travel away from the home environment. The individual does not remember getting to the new location. A person with dissociative fugue does not generally look for personal attention.

Nursing process: Implementation

Client need: Psychosocial Integrity

Cognitive level: Application

Subject area: Psychiatric and Mental Health

Answer: 4

Rationale: Safety is the priority goal when caring for a client with a dissociative disorder, because the client's natural protective instincts have been compromised. Behavioral therapy is inappropriate for a dissociative disorder, because it involves cognitive restructuring. Family therapy may be appropriate at a later date but is not usually indicated.

Nursing process: Planning

Client need: Management of Care

Cognitive level: Analysis

Subject area: Psychiatric and Mental Health

Answer: 3

Rationale: Traumatic events are often precipitating factors in dissociative disorders because they result in the individual's attempt to protect the self from remembering traumatic events. Brain tumor, substance abuse, and epilepsy have not been established as positive links to dissociative disorders.

Nursing process: Analysis

Client need: Psychosocial Integrity

Cognitive level: Application

Subject area: Psychiatric and Mental Health

Answer: 3

Rationale: The nurse should assist the client who has a dissociative disorder to understand the benefits of the dissociation to cope. The client should be reoriented to person, place, and time. The nurse should encourage and assist the client to make personal decisions.

Nursing process: Planning

Client need: Psychosocial Integrity

Cognitive level: Application

Subject area: Psychiatric and Mental Health

13. The nurse is assessing the client with dissociative amnesia. Which of the following clinical manifestations is most indicative of the disorder?

 1. The inability to recall important personal information, usually of a traumatic nature

 2. Disturbance occurs exclusively during the course of other mental disorders

 3. Existence of two or more subpersonalities

 4. Memory is retrievable at the will of the client

14. A client is admitted to the psychiatric ward of a hospital with complaints of a loss of a sense of self. The nurse treating the client anticipates which of the following clinical manifestations?

 1. The presence of a change in voice and mannerism when under stress

 2. The presence of active hallucinations

 3. The inability of the client to follow simple directions

 4. A history of substance abuse

15. When planning the care of a client with a dissociative disorder, the nurse should include which of the following interventions?

 1. Aid the client to learn to deal constructively with stress

 2. Instruct the client to suppress anxiety-producing thoughts

 3. Encourage the client to ignore the personalities

 4. Assist the client to maintain occupational pursuits

16. The nurse is working with a client who has a dissociative disorder. Which of the following would indicate to the nurse that the client's condition is deteriorating?

 1. Expressions of suicide and hopelessness

 2. Expressions of forgetfulness

 3. The presence of substance abuse

 4. The inability to take care of basic needs

Answer: 1

Rationale: The inability to recall important personal information is paramount in dissociative amnesia, because the memory does not selectively block information when attempting to suppress traumatic events. Disturbances occur outside the course of other mental disorders. The clinical manifestations create great distress. Memory is not voluntarily retrievable. The existence of two distinct subpersonalities is a feature of dissociative identity disorder.

Nursing process: Evaluation

Client need: Psychosocial Integrity

Cognitive level: Analysis

Subject area: Psychiatric and Mental Health

Answer: 1

Rationale: The presence of alternate personalities with different affective states and changes in mannerisms, voice, and gender may appear under stress in a client with a dissociative disorder. There is no presence of hallucinations as there is in schizophrenia. The client can follow directions because the ability to understand instructions is not impaired. The etiology of the disorder is not due to substance abuse or a medical condition.

Nursing process: Assessment

Client need: Psychosocial Integrity

Cognitive level: Application

Subject area: Psychiatric and Mental Health

Answer: 1

Rationale: Stress precipitates the splitting off of personalities in a client with a dissociative disorder. Constructive reintegration relies on the ability to deal with stress. The client should not suppress anxiety, because it will reemerge in the subpersonality. Clients cannot ignore the alternative personalities, even though they lie outside of the client's control. Clients are often unable to maintain occupational functioning due to the intensity of the disorder.

Nursing process: Planning

Client need: Psychosocial Integrity

Cognitive level: Application

Subject area: Psychiatric and Mental Health

Answer: 1

Rationale: Expressions of suicidal ideation and feelings of hopelessness and worthlessness are critical markers for impending suicide attempts in a client who has a dissociative disorder. They indicate that the client's condition is deteriorating and that intervention is imperative. Forgetfulness is not in itself a dangerous risk. Substance abuse may preclude the diagnosis of a dissociative disorder because the substance masks the disorder. The client with a dissociative disorder maintains the ability to conduct activities of daily living.

Nursing process: Analysis

Client need: Psychosocial Integrity

Cognitive level: Analysis

Subject area: Psychiatric and Mental Health

17. The nurse evaluating the progress of a client with a dissociative disorder should consider which of the following behaviors as significant?

   1. The client can voluntarily call up all of the subpersonalities.

   2. The client successfully suppresses feelings about events in the past.

   3. The client has difficulty recognizing the environment.

   4. The client identifies significant others.

18. The client with clinical manifestations of a dissociative disorder may develop secondary manifestations. Which of the following behaviors should be a priority for the nurse to consider?

   1. The client's confusion clears after identity is reestablished.

   2. The client decreases assaultive behavior.

   3. The client controls panic during a depersonalization experience.

   4. The client attempts self-harm from alternate personalities.

19. The nurse is caring for a client with a dissociative disorder. Which of the following is a priority to include in the client's health teaching?

   1. Prevent dissociative episodes by becoming aware of triggers

   2. Avoid outside activities that divert the focus of care from the disorder

   3. Avoid focusing on delusional processes

   4. Delegate stressful tasks away from the client and to other family members

20. The registered nurse is preparing to delegate nursing assignments to various team members in a psychiatric unit. Which of the following assignments is appropriate for the nurse to delegate?

   1. A licensed practical nurse establishes the nursing diagnoses for a client with a dissociative disorder.

   2. Unlicensed assistive personnel provide a safe environment for a client with a dissociative disorder.

   3. A licensed practical nurse assesses a client for clinical manifestations of dissociative fugue.

   4. Unlicensed assistive personnel encourage a client with a dissociative disorder to verbalize feelings of suicide.

Answer: 4

Rationale: As personality disturbances clear with a dissociative disorder, the client will regain the ability to identify and recognize significant others. There will be an absence of subpersonalities. Feelings will not be suppressed but will become available for recall. The client can identify and recognize the environment.

Nursing process: Evaluation

Client need: Psychosocial Integrity

Cognitive level: Analysis

Subject area: Psychiatric and Mental Health

Answer: 4

Rationale: The client's attempt of self-harm is a secondary manifestation in a dissociative disorder. The client's confusion and assaultive behavior may worsen. The client is likely to experience an escalation in panic.

Nursing process: Analysis

Client need: Management of Care

Cognitive level: Analysis

Subject area: Psychiatric and Mental Health

Answer: 1

Rationale: Awareness of the triggers of the dissociative process allows the client the control to reduce the occurrence of episodes. Outside activities are encouraged, such as music, physical activity, and socialization. Therapy involves the free exchange of communication, including any existence of delusions. The client's recovery depends on the ability of the client to deal with the stressors in life.

Nursing process: Planning

Client need: Management of Care

Cognitive level: Application

Subject area: Psychiatric and Mental Health

Answer: 2

Rationale: Unlicensed assistive personnel may provide a safe environment for a client with a dissociative disorder. Only a registered nurse should write nursing diagnoses to direct a plan of care. A registered nurse should assess a client for clinical manifestations. It is inappropriate for unlicensed assistive personnel to encourage a client to verbalize feelings of suicide.

Nursing process: Planning

Client need: Management of Care

Cognitive level: Analysis

Subject area: Legal and Ethical Issues

21. The nurse assesses which of the following clinical manifestations in a client suspected of depersonalization disorder?

Select all that apply:

[   ] 1. Thoughts of being someone else

[   ] 2. Sensations of not being human

[   ] 3. Intact reality testing

[   ] 4. Impaired social and occupational functioning

[   ] 5. Indifference to personal condition

[   ] 6. Onset before the age of 20 years

22. The nurse is caring for a client who has amnesia related to a traumatic event. Which of the following nursing diagnoses would be most appropriate for the client?

1. Disturbed body image

2. Ineffective coping

3. Anxiety

4. Disturbed personal identity

23. The nurse is teaching a client with dissociative identity disorder about the disorder. Which of the following interventions would be a priority?

1. Make a suicide contract with the client

2. Explain the client's behavior to other clients

3. Inform the client of the forgotten material

4. Encourage anxiety-producing activities to bring out subpersonalities

24. The nurse should include which of the following interventions in the plan of care for a client with a dissociative disorder?

1. Avoid placing the client in group therapy

2. Provide the client with complex instructions for maintenance of activities of daily living

3. Decrease the confusion and noise in the environment

4. Avoid social interaction with other clients

Answer: 2, 3, 4

Rationale: Sensations of not being human or alive are common in depersonalization disorders. The thought of being someone else is not characteristic. The incidence of depersonalization disorder decreases as the client ages. There is great distress associated with a depersonalization episode.

Nursing process: Assessment

Client need: Psychosocial Integrity

Cognitive level: Application

Subject area: Psychiatric and Mental Health

Answer: 4

Rationale: The appropriate nursing diagnosis for a client who is experiencing amnesia related to a traumatic event would be disturbed personal identity.

Nursing process: Evaluation

Client need: Psychosocial Integrity

Cognitive level: Analysis

Subject area: Psychiatric and Mental Health

Answer: 1

Rationale: One-to-one supervision and making a suicide contract with a client who has a dissociative disorder are priorities to meet the safety needs of the client under distress. Confidentiality is of the utmost importance. Never try to force recall of information the client is not prepared to know. Reduction of anxiety helps avoid the emergence of subpersonalities.

Nursing process: Planning

Client need: Management of Care

Cognitive level: Application

Subject area: Psychiatric and Mental Health

Answer: 3

Rationale: Nursing interventions appropriate for a client with a dissociative disorder include decreasing confusion and noise in the environment. This will decrease anxiety. Group therapy is recommended. Simple instructions for grooming and activities of daily living are recommended. Social interaction is encouraged to avoid withdrawal and isolation.

Nursing process: Planning

Client need: Psychosocial Integrity

Cognitive level: Application

Subject area: Psychiatric and Mental Health

25. Following a serious car accident, a client is admitted to the psychiatric unit of the hospital with memory loss. Which of the following behaviors would the nurse assess that would support a diagnosis of dissociative amnesia? The client

1. has an inability to recall important information of the event.

2. experienced a flashback while high on PCP, which resulted in the accident.

3. has a seizure disorder, which precipitated the accident.

4. is not concerned about the accident.

26. The nurse understands which of the following to be a manifestation of dissociative identity disorder?

1. The personalities are all aware of one another.

2. The disorder is never chronic.

3. The recall of traumatic events is intact.

4. The client was confronted with an intolerable terror event.

Answer: 1

Rationale: Inability to recall important personal information of the event is a diagnostic criterion for dissociative amnesia. It is not precipitated by substances or a medical condition. The amnesia causes great distress to the client.

Nursing process: Assessment

Client need: Psychosocial Integrity

Cognitive level: Analysis

Subject area: Psychiatric and Mental Health

Answer: 4

Rationale: The initial event of a dissociative disorder was an event the client confronted and found so intolerable that the client's memory split off into another personality. The personalities are often out of the awareness of the primary personality. The disorder can be episodic or chronic. Recall of the traumatic event is not available to the primary personality.

Nursing process: Evaluation

Client need: Psychosocial Integrity

Cognitive level: Application

Subject area: Psychiatric and Mental Health

Personality Disorders

49

1. At what stage of life does the nurse anticipate the clinical manifestations of personality disorders to become evident in the client's behaviors and actions? _____

2. The nurse should include which of the following interventions in the plan of care for a client with dependent personality disorder?

   1. Limit the client's opportunity to make decisions

   2. Ask the client's family to make important decisions for the client

   3. Acknowledge the client's situation with empathy while encouraging independence

   4. Withhold feedback regarding the client's situation until the client has made decisions

3. The nurse assesses a client suspected of having histrionic personality disorder for which of the following behaviors?

   Select all that apply:

   [   ] **1.** Dissatisfaction associated with being in a group

   [   ] **2.** Concerned about appearance

   [   ] **3.** Idealizes the nurse and then devalues the nurse

   [   ] **4.** Verbalizations of grand things done or planned

   [   ] **5.** Compliment-seeking behavior

   [   ] **6.** Has rapid shifts of emotion

4. Which of the following should the nurse include when planning to provide education to a client with schizoid personality disorder?

   1. Provide education in a large group setting to encourage socialization

   2. Deliver education individually in a clear and concise manner

   3. Present the information in a theoretical format

   4. Engage the client in a therapeutic relationship before providing education

Answer: Adolescence or early adulthood

Rationale: Personalities are formed during childhood. Therefore, dysfunctional pathology will not appear until the client's personalities have been tested by the trials of life. These life events begin in adolescence or early adulthood.

Nursing process: Analysis

Client need: Psychosocial Integrity

Cognitive level: Application

Subject area: Psychiatric and Mental Health

Answer: 3

Rationale: Clients with dependent personality disorder feel inadequate to make decisions for themselves. By acknowledging their difficulties, confidence is built. In turn, the confidence will facilitate independence from care providers and others they may be dependent on.

Nursing process: Planning

Client need: Psychosocial Integrity

Cognitive level: Application

Subject area: Psychiatric and Mental Health

Answer: 2, 5, 6

Rationale: Although the person with histrionic personality disorder seeks attention and craves novelty, stimulation, and excitement, the satisfaction for this person comes from attention given by others, not from within the self. The dialect of first valuing and then devaluing the nurse is indicative of borderline personality disorder. People with histrionic personality disorder seek out groups or other people to validate themselves.

Nursing process: Assessment

Client need: Psychosocial Integrity

Cognitive level: Application

Subject area: Psychiatric and Mental Health

Answer: 2

Rationale: The client with schizoid personality disorder is technically minded. Attempting to draw the client into a personal or therapeutic relationship or to participate in a group or social setting may push the client to withdraw and become isolated.

Nursing process: Planning

Client need: Psychosocial Integrity

Cognitive level: Application

Subject area: Psychiatric and Mental Health

5. When caring for a client with a personality disorder, the nurse documents that the client has difficulty maintaining what kind of relationships? _____

6. Which of the following assessments would provide the nurse with the most accurate information regarding a low serotonin level in a client with a personality disorder?

1. Psychosis and hallucinations

2. Delusions and paranoia

3. Depression and impulsiveness

4. Restlessness and agitation

7. During an initial interview with a client who has a personality disorder, the nurse evaluates which of the following to be present in the client's personality traits?

1. Changes in the personality that have come about because of a stressful event

2. Personality traits that are beyond the range found in most people

3. Personality traits that have changed with advanced age

4. Changes in personality that differ to fit the situation

8. The nurse is caring for a client with schizoid personality disorder. In determining what the plan of care should consist of, which of the following should the nurse consider? The client

1. quickly becomes attached to the group leader.

2. displays behavior lacking social tact or grace in a group.

3. becomes overly emotional in the group setting.

4. attempts to build intimate relationships with other group members.

Answer: Interpersonal

Rationale: Any relationship that an individual perceives as personal or interpersonal will also be perceived as some type of threat. Clients with personality disorders struggle to find balance in relationships; they want to be fulfilled as human beings, yet they push others away because of fear of abandonment.

Nursing process: Implementation

Client need: Psychosocial Integrity

Cognitive level: Analysis

Subject area: Psychiatric and Mental Health

Answer: 3

Rationale: Serotonin is believed to maintain mood stability and control impulsivity, rage, aggression, and depressive clinical manifestations. Delusions result from a faulty thought structure and are related to thought disturbances such as paranoia and grandiose beliefs. Restlessness and agitation are symptomatic of increased serotonin levels.

Nursing process: Assessment

Client need: Psychosocial Integrity

Cognitive level: Application

Subject area: Psychiatric and Mental Health

Answer: 2

Rationale: Personality characteristics are formed in childhood to early teens. The characteristics are set and stable over time. Events and situations may make characteristics more apparent, but these characteristics do not change. Changes in personality in advanced age are potentially related to a medical condition. The prolonged stability of the personality structure makes treating personality disorders a difficult and long process.

Nursing process: Evaluation

Client need: Psychosocial Integrity

Cognitive level: Analysis

Subject area: Psychiatric and Mental Health

Answer: 2

Rationale: Individuals with schizoid personality disorder have difficulty showing and sharing their emotions. They lack the desire to be part of a group or have intimacy in their relationships. This leads to inappropriate behaviors and a lack of social tact and grace in a group or social setting.

Nursing process: Analysis

Client need: Psychosocial Integrity

Cognitive level: Analysis

Subject area: Psychiatric and Mental Health

9. The nurse evaluates a client with schizoid personality disorder to exhibit which of the following behaviors? Select all that apply:

[   ] **1.** Irresponsibility with intentional deceit of others

[   ] **2.** Grandiosity and a lack of empathy for others

[   ] **3.** Peculiar with exaggerated social anxiety

[   ] **4.** Social isolation

[   ] **5.** Restricted range of emotion

[   ] **6.** Appears indifferent to praise

10. The nurse documents a client exhibiting suspiciousness and hypersensitivity to criticism and who expresses a feeling of being taken advantage of to have which of the following types of personality disorder? _____

11. Which of the following interventions should the nurse include in the plan of care for a client with schizoid personality disorder?

1. Empathize with the situation and avoid validating the distortions

2. Promote trust by recognizing the distortions

3. Use reality orientation whenever possible

4. Dispel the distortions by identifying their bizarre nature

Answer: 4, 5, 6

Rationale: Irresponsibility and intentional deceit are descriptive of antisocial personality disorder. Grandiosity and lack of empathy are behaviors of narcissistic personality disorder. A client with schizotypal personality disorder would have behaviors that were peculiar and show exaggerated social anxiety. Schizoid personality disorder behaviors are described as social isolation, restricted range of emotion, and indifferent to praise.

Nursing process: Evaluation

Client need: Psychosocial Integrity

Cognitive level: Application

Subject area: Psychiatric and Mental Health

Answer: Paranoid personality disorder

Rationale: A client with paranoid personality disorder will have characteristics of being highly suspicious, being hypersensitive to criticism, and have a feeling of being taken advantage of. This is contrasted to other disorders, such as borderline personality disorder, antisocial personality disorder, and schizotypal personality disorder. A client with borderline personality disorder will project discomfort with criticism by making others feel or look bad. Thus, it appears that such a client is hypersensitive to criticism. It is not common for someone with borderline personality to feel suspicious or be taken advantage of. Clients with antisocial personality disorder will internalize the criticism and are usually the ones who are taking advantage of others. Persons with schizotypal personality disorder believe they have magical powers and are preoccupied and superstitious but not paranoid.

Nursing process: Implementation

Client need: Psychosocial Integrity

Cognitive level: Application

Subject area: Psychiatric and Mental Health

Answer: 1

Rationale: Schizoid personality disorder is a personality disorder characterized by a marked detachment from people and events around them. Such clients lack close friends, spend most of their time alone, and show little emotion. Empathizing with the client and not endorsing the distortions that validate the client is the appropriate approach. This will allow the client to trust the nurse as the caregiver. Statements should be used that validate a client's response and feelings to the distortions, such as "I can see this is upsetting to you." Challenging the client's reality will push away the client and may elicit an aggressive reaction.

Nursing process: Planning

Client need: Psychosocial Integrity

Cognitive level: Application

Subject area: Psychiatric and Mental Health

12. The nurse is planning the care of a client with borderline personality disorder based on which of the following behaviors?

Select all that apply:

[   ] 1. Chronic feelings of emptiness

[   ] 2. Unstable interpersonal relationships

[   ] 3. Suicidal gestures or self-mutilation

[   ] 4. Excessive attention to appearance

[   ] 5. Holding of grudges for long periods of time

[   ] 6. Submissive behaviors

13. The nurse is caring for a client who is seeing UFOs and asks if the nurse is also afraid of the UFOs. Which of the following would be an appropriate response from the nurse?

1. "I don't know what you are talking about; I don't see any UFOs."

2. "I can tell that what you're seeing frightens you; how can I help to make you more comfortable?"

3. "I see the UFOs too, and they scare me; what are we going to do?"

4. "I don't see the UFOs; are you ready to come to group?"

14. A client comes to group provocatively dressed and is dramatic in conversation, often straying from the topic. The nurse should use which of the following approaches to maintain a therapeutic environment in the group?

1. Allow the client to express oneself and encourage independence

2. Address the client with closed-ended questions and permit only responses that are relevant

3. Avoid acknowledging the client and speak only to group members who remain on track

4. Reprimand the client for unacceptable behavior and inappropriate dress

Answer: 1, 2, 3

Rationale: Suicidal gestures, self-mutilation, chronic feelings of emptiness, and unstable interpersonal relationships are behaviors found in persons with borderline personality disorder. The client with histrionic personality disorder will pay excessive attention to appearance. A client with paranoid personality disorder will hold grudges for long periods of time. Submissive behaviors are descriptive of dependent personality disorder.

Nursing process: Evaluation

Client need: Psychosocial Integrity

Cognitive level: Analysis

Subject area: Psychiatric and Mental Health

Answer: 2

Rationale: Telling the client who complains of seeing UFOs that "I can tell that what you're seeing frightens you; how can I help to make you more comfortable?" validates the client's feelings without agreeing with or challenging the client's irrational beliefs.

Nursing process: Analysis

Client need: Psychosocial Integrity

Cognitive level: Analysis

Subject area: Psychiatric and Mental Health

Answer: 2

Rationale: Histrionic personality disorder is a personality disorder in which the client seeks attention and has excessive emotionality. The client with histrionic personality disorder needs to know from the group leader what the boundaries of the group are. This learning may need to be shown by example. Simply ignoring the client will only escalate the behavior, while allowing or endorsing the behavior will be maladaptive to the group and the individual. For clients with personality disorders, this is how they have learned to have their needs met in the past. They need to relearn appropriate behavior. Reprimanding the client may lead to the client's lack of investment in therapy.

Nursing process: Planning

Client need: Psychosocial Integrity

Cognitive level: Application

Subject area: Psychiatric and Mental Health

15. The nurse assesses which of the following behaviors to be present in a client who has antisocial personality disorder?

Select all that apply:

[　] 1. Disregards the rights of others

[　] 2. Shows a dramatic emotion to situations

[　] 3. Self-blames for situations

[　] 4. Avoids engaging in interactions with the nurse

[　] 5. Voices a lack of responsibility for situations

[　] 6. Demonstrates impulsivity

16. Which of the following should the nurse consider when planning the care of a client who has antisocial personality disorder?

1. The client's lack of ability to engage with the nurse

2. The client's attempts to manipulate the nurse

3. The client's hindered ability to justify actions

4. The client's openness and honesty about past experiences

17. In planning care for a client with borderline personality disorder, the nurse should consider which of the following?

1. The client's desire for outward perfection

2. The client's fear of abandonment

3. The client's lack of ability to show affection

4. The client's desire to be the center of attention

Answer: 1, 5, 6
Rationale: Antisocial personality is a personality disorder in which classic features include blatant disregard for others, verbalization of a lack of responsibility for situations, and impulsivity. Dramatic emotion is descriptive of histrionic personality disorder. Self-blaming would be a behavior exhibited by a client with dependent personality disorder. Avoiding interactions with the nurse would be descriptive of avoidant personality. Clients with antisocial personality disorder engage easily with others on a superficial level, often in an attempt to exploit them. They lack insight and responsibility for their behavior and are deceitful.
Nursing process: Assessment
Client need: Psychosocial Integrity
Cognitive level: Application
Subject area: Psychiatric and Mental Health

Answer: 2
Rationale: Clients with antisocial personality disorder engage in relationships easily and need to have rapport built to engage in therapeutic relationships. Clients with antisocial personality disorder misrepresent themselves in an effort to meet their needs above all else. Their behavior is manipulative. The client with this disorder also embellishes or exaggerates an experience in an effort to appear different from those around him or her.
Nursing process: Analysis
Client need: Psychosocial Integrity
Cognitive level: Analysis
Subject area: Psychiatric and Mental Health

Answer: 2
Rationale: Clients with borderline personality disorders have an extreme instability in their relationships with a great fear of being abandoned. Their behaviors are maladaptive but they attempt to keep people close to them. They have a poor sense of self, which leads to their behaviors causing problems for others so that they feel secure. Outward perfection and the desire to be the center of attention are descriptions of histrionic personality disorder. Lack of ability to show affection is found in schizoid and schizotypal personality disorders.
Nursing process: Analysis
Client need: Psychosocial Integrity
Cognitive level: Analysis
Subject area: Psychiatric and Mental Health

18. The nurse should monitor a client admitted with borderline personality disorder for what self-destructive behavior? _____

19. Which of the following is an appropriate goal for the nurse caring for a client who has a diagnosis of borderline personality disorder?
1. To identify irrational thoughts and beliefs that the client's decision making is founded on
2. To eliminate boundaries between the client and nurse so the client can more easily share problems
3. To eliminate the immediate focus on the client by encouraging the client to focus on relationships with others
4. To eliminate the client's involvement in treatment planning because of the accompanying irrational thoughts and beliefs

20. The nurse is collecting a nursing history on a client suspected of having narcissistic personality disorder. Which of the following assessments would the nurse expect to find?
1. A style of speech that lacks detail
2. An unconscious dependency on others
3. A lack of empathy for others
4. Attempts to promote self-esteem in others

21. The registered nurse is preparing to make out clinical assignments on a psychiatric unit. Which of the following assignments does the nurse appropriately delegate to a licensed practical nurse?
1. Report the empathy that a client with a narcissistic personality has
2. Assist a client with borderline personality disorder to the dayroom for group therapy
3. Develop a plan of care for a client with schizoid personality disorder
4. Assess a client suspected of having paranoid personality disorder

Answer: Self-mutilation

Rationale: Borderline personality disorder is a pattern of unstable interpersonal relationships, impulsive behavior, and negative self-image and affect. Self-mutilation and parasuicide behaviors are common in clients diagnosed with borderline personality disorder, posing a serious self-destructive behavior.

Nursing process: Assessment

Client need: Psychosocial Integrity

Cognitive level: Application

Subject area: Psychiatric and Mental Health

Answer: 1

Rationale: An appropriate goal for helping a client with borderline personality disorder is to focus on the client and the client's belief system in order to encourage an understanding of how those beliefs impact on relationships. The client with borderline personality disorder is already focused on relationships with others, which continues the chaotic relationship. The client focuses on others and fails to focus on oneself. Once the client can distinguish between rational and irrational thoughts, the client can begin to evaluate surrounding relationships.

Nursing process: Evaluation

Client need: Psychosocial Integrity

Cognitive level: Analysis

Subject area: Psychiatric and Mental Health

Answer: 3

Rationale: Lack of empathy, arrogance, and a need for admiration are key characteristics of narcissistic personality disorder. Persons with this disorder want to feel better or more important than others, so they would not promote self-esteem in another person. Their dependency is outwardly expressed in the need for admiration, so they focus on surrounding themselves with "special" people, those who are considered to be important or influential. A style of speech that lacks detail is characteristic of histrionic personality disorder.

Nursing process: Assessment

Client need: Psychosocial Integrity

Cognitive level: Application

Subject area: Psychiatric and Mental Health

Answer: 2

Rationale: Skills that involve reporting, developing a plan of care, and assessing a client are all assignments that should be performed by a registered nurse. A licensed practical nurse may assist a client to a dayroom for group therapy.

Nursing process: Planning

Client need: Management of Care

Cognitive level: Analysis

Subject area: Legal and Ethical Issues

22. Because a client has narcissistic personality disorder, plans for nursing intervention should include

    1. promoting a rapport by showing interest in personal stories.

    2. making interactions limited in time and technical in nature.

    3. decreasing the tendency for embellishment by acknowledging that the client is better than others.

    4. using reality focus, which occurs by challenging the client's misrepresentations.

23. When planning the care for a client with avoidant personality disorder, the nurse understands that the best intervention is to

    1. allow the client to stay in the room until he or she feels comfortable with people.

    2. avoid acknowledging goals achieved by the client.

    3. enable the client to set and drive the goals independent of the nurse.

    4. promote self-esteem by praising the client's success.

24. The nurse anticipates finding which of the following characteristics in a client who has a diagnosis of obsessive-compulsive personality disorder?

Select all that apply:

[   ] **1.** Is rigid and inflexible

[   ] **2.** Avoids details

[   ] **3.** Is indecisive

[   ] **4.** Delegates tasks

[   ] **5.** Is envious of others

[   ] **6.** Is excessively devoted to work and productivity

Answer: 1

Rationale: Engaging, listening, and connecting with the client will build rapport with a client who has narcissistic personality disorder. The nurse should never encourage the grandiosity but must remain nonjudgmental to what the client says. Approaching the client in a cold, technical manner will stop the grandiosity but will also impair the therapeutic relationship.

Nursing process: Planning

Client need: Psychosocial Integrity

Cognitive level: Application

Subject area: Psychiatric and Mental Health

Answer: 4

Rationale: A client with avoidant personality disorder disregards and violates the rights of others. Classic features are social inhibition and feelings of inadequacy. The client may never feel comfortable enough on one's own to join the group, so the client remains isolated and fosters avoidance behaviors. The client needs encouragement to participate along with acknowledgment of vulnerability. Any successes and accomplishments by the client should be praised. Goal setting should be a combined effort by the nurse and client. The nurse needs to drive the advancement of the goals for the client to make progress.

Nursing process: Planning

Client need: Psychosocial Integrity

Cognitive level: Application

Subject area: Psychiatric and Mental Health

Answer: 1, 3, 6

Rationale: The client with obsessive-compulsive personality disorder does not like to relinquish control for fear something may go wrong. Such clients are rigid and inflexible. Their constant drive for perfection leads to indecisiveness, because they fear making the wrong decision. They are not envious of others; in fact, they often pity others for not being more like themselves. They are reluctant to delegate tasks and are often excessively devoted to work and productivity.

Nursing process: Assessment

Client need: Psychosocial Integrity

Cognitive level: Application

Subject area: Psychiatric and Mental Health

25. Which of the following behaviors in a client suspected of obsessive-compulsive personality disorder validates the diagnosis and should be reported?

    1. Fantasies about unlimited success

    2. Looks for hidden meanings from others

    3. Task completion hampered by perfectionism

    4. Task completion hampered by lack of confidence

26. Based on an understanding of obsessive-compulsive personality disorder, which of the following should be considered before planning the care?

    1. The client is eager to become involved in a therapeutic relationship because there is a sense of attachment.

    2. The client is eager to tell personal stories and have others admire what has been accomplished in the past.

    3. The client views the therapeutic relationship as a waste of time because the client doesn't see a personal behavior problem.

    4. The client may vacillate between wanting the therapeutic relationship and pushing it away, depending on what threat is seen.

Answer: 3

Rationale: A client with obsessive-compulsive disorder likes to hoard money and finds it hard to discard worn-out possessions. Such a client is preoccupied with details, aspires to perfection, is excessively devoted to work, is overconscientious, is rigid, and is reluctant to delegate tasks. Aspirations for perfection may hamper task completion. Fantasies of unlimited success are related to narcissistic personality disorder. Clients with paranoid personality disorder look for hidden meanings in the actions of others. Task completion hampered by lack of confidence is indicative of dependent personality disorder.

Nursing process: Analysis

Client need: Psychosocial Integrity

Cognitive level: Analysis

Subject area: Psychiatric and Mental Health

Answer: 3

Rationale: A client with obsessive-compulsive personality disorder views a therapeutic relationship as a waste of time, because personal behavior is not recognized as a problem. A client with dependent personality is eager to start any kind of relationship. Such a client will go anywhere at any time for the sense of attachment and security. A client eager to be admired falls into the category of narcissistic personality disorder. The vacillation between wanting a relationship and then pushing it away is indicative of borderline personality disorder.

Nursing process: Analysis

Client need: Psychosocial Integrity

Cognitive level: Analysis

Subject area: Psychiatric and Mental Health

Mood Disorders

50

1. The nurse is assessing the client who is suicidal. Which of the following is the priority nursing intervention?

  1. Ask the client, "Do you have a plan to kill yourself?"

  2. Get the client to the hospital for further evaluation

  3. Assess the client for suicidal risk, method, and ability to carry the plan out

  4. Assess for past suicide attempts

2. The nurse should instruct a client that which of the following would be an expected clinical manifestation for up to 2 months following an electroconvulsive therapy treatment?

  1. Dizziness

  2. Heartburn

  3. Nausea and vomiting

  4. Short-term memory loss

3. When assessing a client for a bipolar disorder, the nurse should include which of the following in the mental status exam to make a positive diagnosis of a bipolar disorder? Assessment of

  1. gait.

  2. mood.

  3. emotional developmental level.

  4. nutritional status.

Answer: 3

Rationale: Assessing the client is necessary before determining if the client needs to be hospitalized or not. Assessing for past suicide attempts is very important as well as asking if the client has a plan to kill oneself. Asking if the client has a plan, assessing past suicide attempts, or taking the client to the hospital are also important interventions, but the priority is to determine if the client has a plan.

Nursing process: Planning

Client need: Management of Care

Cognitive level: Analysis

Subject area: Psychiatric and Mental Health

Answer: 4

Rationale: Short-term memory loss would be an expected clinical manifestation following electroconvulsive therapy (ECT), occurring after treatment and lasting for 1 week to 2 months or more. Unilateral placement of the electrodes may decrease the amount of short-term memory loss, because the current passes through only the nondominant side of the brain. Unilateral placement is less effective in treating depression than bilateral placement. While dizziness, heartburn, and nausea and vomiting may be experienced post ECT, they would not be expected clinical manifestations for 1 week to 2 months post ECT.

Nursing process: Planning

Client need: Psychosocial Integrity

Cognitive level: Analysis

Subject area: Psychiatric and Mental Health

Answer: 2

Rationale: While it is necessary to assess the client's gait, emotional developmental level, and nutritional status, these are not part of a mental status exam. Assessing the client's mood (either mania, hypomania, or depression) would provide the information needed to assist in verifying a diagnosis of a bipolar disorder.

Nursing process: Assessment

Client need: Psychosocial Integrity

Cognitive level: Application

Subject area: Psychiatric and Mental Health

4. The parents of a client diagnosed with major depression and who attempted suicide ask the nurse what the difference is between major depression and a bipolar disorder. The most appropriate response by the nurse is

   1. "Major depression and bipolar disorder are two different mood disorders, but the treatment is the same."

   2. "Bipolar disorder is an upswing of mood while major depression is a downward mood swing. They require very similar treatment modalities."

   3. "Major depression is a downward swing of mood with treatment, including mood stabilizers, whereas bipolar depression is an upward swing of mood with antidepressants given to bring the mood down."

   4. "Major depression is a depressed mood state that requires antidepressant medication, while a bipolar disorder is an upward swing of mood that requires mood stabilizers for treatment."

5. During an admission interview, which of the following clinical manifestations should the nurse report as indicative of hypomania?

   Select all that apply:

   [   ] **1.** Decreased delusions of grandeur

   [   ] **2.** Decreased self-esteem

   [   ] **3.** Pressured speech

   [   ] **4.** Talkativeness

   [   ] **5.** Decreased motivation

   [   ] **6.** Flight of ideas

6. A female client expresses difficulties with irritability, depressed mood, and decreased interest during the last week of luteal phase during most of her menstrual cycles in the past year. Which of the following nursing interventions are most appropriate when planning nursing care for this client with premenstrual dysphoric disorder?

   1. Instruct the client to avoid focusing on mood, sleep, and appetite during the month

   2. Administer vitamin B_6 100 mg per day for 2 weeks prior to the menstrual cycle

   3. Encourage intake of water and juice

   4. Instruct the client to consume caffeine-containing beverages and chocolate

Answer: 4

Rationale: Major depression and bipolar disorder are two different mood disorders with different treatment regimens. Major depression is a downward swing of mood, and bipolar disorder is an upward swing of mood (mania) and a downward swing of mood (hypomania). Major depression is treated with an antidepressant, while a bipolar disorder is treated with a mood stabilizer such as gabapentin (Neurontin) or divalproex sodium (Depakote).

Nursing process: Analysis

Client need: Psychosocial Integrity

Cognitive level: Analysis

Subject area: Psychiatric and Mental Health

Answer: 3, 4, 6

Rationale: Hypomania is a form of mania in which the clinical manifestations are less severe than those of mania. Clinical manifestations of hypomania include pressured speech, talkativeness, flight of ideas, delusions of grandeur, inflated self-esteem, and increased motivation.

Nursing process: Assessment

Client need: Psychosocial Integrity

Cognitive level: Application

Subject area: Psychiatric and Mental Health

Answer: 2

Rationale: Instructing a client to monitor mood, sleep, and appetite during the month is an appropriate nursing intervention to assist the nurse in knowing when the client is having difficulty with clinical manifestations. Encouraging the intake of fluids will increase water retention and will increase irritability. Administering vitamin B_6 100 mg per day for 2 weeks prior to the menstrual cycle is the most appropriate. Vitamin B_6 is a precursor to serotonin, which can assist in decreasing clinical manifestations of depressed mood and irritability. Instructing the client to consume caffeine-containing beverages and chocolate would not be appropriate because it would increase fluid retention and therefore increase clinical manifestations of irritability and depression.

Nursing process: Planning

Client need: Psychosocial Integrity

Cognitive level: Application

Subject area: Psychiatric and Mental Health

7. The nurse is planning the care of a client with cyclothymia. Currently, the client has a hypomanic mood episode. Which of the following nursing interventions would be a priority when caring for this client?

   1. Set limits with the client if the client is getting into the personal space of others
   2. Increase stimuli in the environment to prevent the client from becoming depressed
   3. Ask the client about issues related to self-esteem
   4. Encourage the client to decrease physical activity

8. The nurse is preparing to care for a client with major depression. The priority nursing intervention is to assess the client's

   1. response to medication administration.
   2. current mood and activity level.
   3. appetite and weight.
   4. risk of suicide.

9. A client has been making derogatory remarks about herself and states, "I'm not able to get a boyfriend because I am worthless." Which of the following cognitive nursing interventions would be most appropriate at this time?

   1. Encourage the client to explore feelings of worthlessness
   2. Instruct the client not to feel that way
   3. Encourage the client to explore positive thoughts about self
   4. Instruct the client to take an antidepressant drug as prescribed

Answer: 1

Rationale: Cyclothymia is a mood disorder that is generally chronic, lasting 2 years, and involves hypomanic and dysthymic mood swings. Setting limits for a client with hypomania is a priority nursing intervention, because the client is unaware of the intrusiveness and the annoyance of this behavior to other clients. The client who is hypomanic presents an inflated self-esteem or grandiosity but is using it to cover chronic feelings of low self-esteem. Asking about issues related to self-esteem would be an appropriate nursing intervention but is not the priority at this time. Encouraging the client to perform relaxation techniques during the hypomanic state is also appropriate but not a priority. Increasing stimuli in the environment will not prevent the client who is hypomanic from becoming depressed and would not be an appropriate nursing intervention, because it would further increase the irritable or elevated mood.

Nursing process: Planning

Client need: Management of Care

Cognitive level: Application

Subject area: Psychiatric and Mental Health

Answer: 4

Rationale: While it is important for the nurse to assess the client's areas of functioning, current mood, and fluid/electrolyte balance, assessing the suicide risk of the client with major depression takes priority.

Nursing process: Assessment

Client need: Management of Care

Cognitive level: Application

Subject area: Psychiatric and Mental Health

Answer: 1

Rationale: Instructing a client who is feeling worthless not to feel that way and exploring positive thoughts about herself minimizes and discourages the exploration of the client's thoughts and feelings about feeling worthless. Instructing the client to take an antidepressant drug disregards the comment made by the client. By exploring feelings of worthlessness, the client will more easily identify the source of the feelings. The client will also feel a sense of having been heard by the nurse, thus increasing trust.

Nursing process: Evaluation

Client need: Psychosocial Integrity

Cognitive level: Application

Subject area: Psychiatric and Mental Health

10. A client scheduled to receive phototherapy asks the nurse what phototherapy is. The nurse should respond with which of the following statements?

 1. "It is a camera that takes pictures of your brain to see why you are becoming depressed."

 2. "It is a bright white light that is used to help treat depression in the winter months."

 3. "It assists in decreasing stress and will help you function better at work in the winter months."

 4. "It is used to treat depression that is resistant to electroconvulsive therapy."

11. The client asks the nurse how long phototherapy should be used each day. Which of the following is the appropriate response by the nurse?

 1. "If you get a headache, then you have sat in front of the light too long."

 2. "Each individual is different. Sit in front of the light just enough so that you do not get a headache."

 3. "Sit in front of the light while reading, preferably in the evening."

 4. "You may sit in front of the light as long as you are comfortable doing so."

12. Which of the following is the priority intervention to encourage a client who is depressed to discuss any suicidal thoughts, plan, or intent?

 1. Instruct the client about the consequences of hidden anger

 2. Focus on the need to keep the client safe

 3. Avoid discussion of depressing topics

 4. Encourage the client to verbalize feelings

Answer: 2

Rationale: Phototherapy is a bright white light that is used to treat seasonal affective depression in the winter months, generally between September and March. The light (approximately 2500 to 10,000 lux) can be used from 30 minutes to 2 hours each day during the winter months. It does not decrease stress and most likely would be used prior to or after electroconvulsive therapy treatments.

Nursing process: Analysis

Client need: Psychosocial Integrity

Cognitive level: Application

Subject area: Psychiatric and Mental Health

Answer: 2

Rationale: If a client sits in front of the phototherapy light for too long, the client will develop a headache. The length of time is different for each individual. Some individuals may experience a headache within 30 minutes. Sitting in front of the light while reading or comfortable are statements of when, not how long, the client should use phototherapy each day. During the first one or two treatments, the client may get a headache because the period of treatment has not yet been established nor does the client know yet what reaction there will be to the treatment.

Nursing process: Analysis

Client need: Psychosocial Integrity

Cognitive level: Application

Subject area: Psychiatric and Mental Health

Answer: 4

Rationale: The best plan for a nursing intervention for the client who may be contemplating suicide is to encourage the client to discuss feelings, because this will allow the nurse to understand the client's emotional state and the client's mood. While instructing the client about the consequences for hidden anger and talking to the client about the need to keep safe, neither of these is a priority nursing intervention. Avoiding depressing topics is not the priority nursing intervention, because there may be depressing topics or situations that may be contributing to the depression.

Nursing process: Planning

Client need: Management of Care

Cognitive level: Application

Subject area: Psychiatric and Mental Health

13. While assessing a client in the emergency room after an attempted suicide, the priority question the nurse should ask the client is
    1. "What is happening in your life that would cause you to attempt to kill yourself?"
    2. "How are you feeling since you have awakened after your overdose?"
    3. "Where is the pill bottle of the medications that you had taken?"
    4. "What can be done to make your life better?"

14. The priority intervention for an outpatient nurse to perform for a client who is depressed and has told the nurse that "I am worthless and there is nothing to live for" would be
    1. immediately seek a psychiatric hospitalization for the client.
    2. explore feelings of worthlessness and hopelessness.
    3. encourage the client to identify self-deprecating thoughts.
    4. remove all potentially dangerous objects from the immediate area.

15. The nurse who is caring for a client who is manic and exhibiting psychomotor agitation implements which of the following interventions as the priority?
    1. Explore alternative behaviors with the client for use when feeling anxious or hyperactive
    2. Provide limits for the client while allowing the client space
    3. Explore stressors that precipitate manic behavior
    4. Assist the client in identifying negative consequences of behavior

Answer: 1

Rationale: Although asking a client how he or she is feeling after an overdose, where the pill bottle is, and what can be done to make life better are appropriate interventions, the priority is to ask the client what has led to the attempted suicide. This gets at the heart of the matter of a suicide attempt and encourages the building of the nurse-client relationship. This encouragement will allow the client to further express personal thoughts and feelings.

Nursing process: Assessment

Client need: Management of Care

Cognitive level: Analysis

Subject area: Psychiatric and Mental Health

Answer: 2

Rationale: While it is important to encourage the client to identify self-defeating thoughts, it is not the most appropriate intervention in the outpatient setting. While exploring the client's feelings of worthlessness and hopelessness, the nurse can assist the client in exploring a sense of worth, value, and hope. There are numerous clients living in the community who are chronically suicidal and can be managed on an outpatient basis. Removing all potentially dangerous objects from the immediate area or seeking immediate psychiatric hospitalization are premature.

Nursing process: Planning

Client need: Management of Care

Cognitive level: Analysis

Subject area: Psychiatric and Mental Health

Answer: 2

Rationale: A client who is manic and exhibiting the clinical manifestation of psychomotor agitation is only minimally able to have insight into those behaviors or ways to change the behavior. This client requires limits within provided structure and space.

Nursing process: Implementation

Client need: Management of Care

Cognitive level: Application

Subject area: Psychiatric and Mental Health

16. When completing an admissions assessment of a client with schizoaffective disorder, the nurse should assess for the presence of which of the following clinical manifestations?

    Select all that apply:

    [   ] 1. Increased use of substances

    [   ] 2. Decreased libido

    [   ] 3. Hallucinations

    [   ] 4. Feelings of entitlement

    [   ] 5. Decreased energy

    [   ] 6. Anhedonia

17. A client diagnosed with a bipolar disorder and who has a superimposed seasonal affective depression is using phototherapy as a treatment to lift the depression. The client calls the nurse at the outpatient mental health clinic, reporting, "My mood, libido, and interest in shopping have improved dramatically." Based on this information, which of the following is the priority to assess first?

    1. Explore energy level and level of appetite

    2. Ascertain how much money the client is spending

    3. Identify the time of day the client is utilizing the phototherapy treatment

    4. Encourage the client to explore thoughts of improved self-worth

18. Discharge plans are being made for a client hospitalized for depression. Which of the following is the priority outcome for a diagnosis of depression?

    1. Share more realistic expectations of the client and the situation

    2. Identify negative, unrealistic thoughts about oneself and ways to counteract those thoughts

    3. Discuss reasons why the client has turned the anger inward

    4. Openly express thoughts and feelings of depression

Answer: 3, 5, 6

Rationale: Schizoaffective disorder is characterized by elements of schizophrenia and manic-depressive disorder. Clinical manifestations include hallucinations, decreased energy, and anhedonia (lack of interest in pleasure or daily activities).

Nursing process: Assessment

Client need: Psychosocial Integrity

Cognitive level: Application

Subject area: Psychiatric and Mental Health

Answer: 3

Rationale: A client with a bipolar disorder and a superimposed seasonal affective depression needs to be careful about the time of day that the phototherapy is utilized. Because of circadian rhythms, it has been found that bipolar clients with seasonal depression do best if they utilize the phototherapy treatment in the later afternoon. If the phototherapy is used in the morning, manic manifestations may result. Exploring appetite, energy level, feelings of self-worth, and how much money the client is spending may all be important interventions, but determining the time of day the client is using the phototherapy allows the nurse to obtain the information that may be causing the dramatic change and elevation in mood.

Nursing process: Assessment

Client need: Management of Care

Cognitive level: Analysis

Subject area: Psychiatric and Mental Health

Answer: 4

Rationale: The priority outcome for a client with depression would be to openly express thoughts and feelings of depression. Although not the priority, it may prove beneficial to share a more realistic expectation of the client, to help the client identify negative and unrealistic thoughts about oneself, and discuss reasons why the client has turned the anger inward.

Nursing process: Evaluation

Client need: Management of Care

Cognitive level: Analysis

Subject area: Psychiatric and Mental Health

19. A nurse is caring for a client with a major depressive disorder who is undergoing electroconvulsive treatments. While planning the postprocedure care, the priority nursing intervention is _____.

20. The nurse receives a report on a client with dysthymia. It would be most important for the client to make which of the following assessments?

Select all that apply:

[   ] **1.** Chronic feelings of low self-esteem

[   ] **2.** Poor concentration

[   ] **3.** Flight of ideas

[   ] **4.** Hallucinations

[   ] **5.** Depressed mood

[   ] **6.** Increased libido

21. A night-shift nurse is planning the preprocedural care for a depressed client who is scheduled to have electroconvulsive therapy at 0800. The priority nursing intervention for this client is _____.

22. The nurse is preparing the nursing care for a client with major depression who is to have electroconvulsive therapy. What is the priority for the nurse to assess from the client's medical record? _____

Answer: to ensure an open airway and prevent aspiration

Rationale: Following electroconvulsive therapy (ECT), the priority is to ensure a patent airway and prevent aspiration. As with any condition, it is always the priority to remember the A (airway), B (breathing), and C (circulation) first. After ensuring a patent airway, the client should be reassured, oriented to the surroundings, and the response to ECT should be evaluated.

Nursing process: Planning

Client need: Management of Care

Cognitive level: Analysis

Subject area: Psychiatric and Mental Health

Answer: 1, 2, 5

Rationale: Dysthymia is a chronic depressive disorder lasting for several years. Clinical manifestations of dysthymia include chronic feelings of low self-esteem, poor concentration, and depressed mood. Flight of ideas and increased libido are clinical manifestations found in the manic phase of a bipolar affective disorder. Hallucinations can be found in schizoaffective disorder.

Nursing process: Assessment

Client need: Psychosocial Integrity

Cognitive level: Application

Subject area: Psychiatric and Mental Health

Answer: to ensure that the client remains NPO prior to the treatment

Rationale: Assuring that the client remains NPO prior to the electroconvulsive therapy treatment is a priority nursing action to prevent aspiration during the treatment.

Nursing process: Planning

Client need: Management of Care

Cognitive level: Application

Subject area: Psychiatric and Mental Health

Answer: History and physical

Rationale: It is essential that a history and physical is present in the client's medical record to ensure that the client has been cleared for electroconvulsive treatments.

Nursing process: Assessment

Client need: Management of Care

Cognitive level: Application

Subject area: Psychiatric and Mental Health

23. The nurse is caring for a client who is in the manic state of a bipolar disorder. Which of the following should the nurse prioritize as the most appropriate nursing outcome?

    1. The client will be free of agitation, hyperactivity, and restless behavior.

    2. The client will appropriately verbalize feelings of anger.

    3. The client will be free of aggression and threatened behavior toward others.

    4. The client will demonstrate lessened buying sprees and grandiosity.

24. The nurse is caring for a client with a mood disorder caused by a medical condition. Which of the following are most important for the nurse to assess?

    1. Serum drug screen

    2. ECG

    3. Bowel sounds

    4. Dental hygiene

25. Which of the following clinical manifestations of schizoaffective disorder should the nurse assess the client for?

    Select all that apply:

    [ ] **1.** Flat affect

    [ ] **2.** Hallucinations

    [ ] **3.** Decreased energy

    [ ] **4.** Delusional thinking

    [ ] **5.** Anhedonia

    [ ] **6.** Anorexia

26. The registered nurse is preparing to delegate clinical assignments on a psychiatric unit. Which of the following assignments should the nurse delegate to a licensed practical nurse?

    1. Develop a plan of care for a client with hypomania

    2. Ensure a client is NPO for electroconvulsive therapy

    3. Teach a class on bipolar disorders

    4. Organize the care to be provided to a client with a bipolar disorder

Answer: 3

Rationale: The priority nursing outcome for a client in the manic state of a bipolar disorder is that the client will be free from aggression and threatened behavior toward others.

Nursing process: Evaluation

Client need: Psychosocial Integrity

Cognitive level: Analysis

Subject area: Psychiatric and Mental Health

Answer: 2

Rationale: Approximately 20 to 25% of clients with certain medical conditions, such as myocardial infarction, cancer, stroke, and diabetes mellitus, will develop a major depressive disorder. An ECG would assess the client's cardiac status.

Nursing process: Assessment

Client need: Psychosocial Integrity

Cognitive level: Analysis

Subject area: Psychiatric and Mental Health

Answer: 1, 3, 5

Rationale: Schizoaffective disorder is a disorder characterized by a major depressive, manic, or mixed episode that coincides with a diagnosis of schizophrenia. The clinical manifestations must not be the result of abuse or a medical condition. The main clinical manifestations are flat affect, decreased energy, and anhedonia.

Nursing process: Assessment

Client need: Psychosocial Integrity

Cognitive level: Application

Subject area: Psychiatric and Mental Health

Answer: 2

Rationale: A licensed practical nurse may ensure a client is NPO for electroconvulsive therapy. Developing a plan of care, teaching a class, and organizing care to be provided to a client should be performed by a registered nurse.

Nursing process: Planning

Client need: Management of Care

Cognitive level: Analysis

Subject area: Legal and Ethical Issues

Schizophrenia and Psychotic Disorders

51

1. Because a hospitalized client is disoriented and actively psychotic, plans for nursing intervention should include
   1. requests that the client interact with peers.
   2. encouraging the client to participate in unit programs.
   3. reality orientation.
   4. involvement in the milieu.

2. A male client with schizophrenia is admitted to the hospital for believing that voices are telling him to harm his family because they are evil. The nurse documents this client to be experiencing what? _____

3. A client diagnosed with schizophrenia is displaying a flat affect, slowed thinking, and a lack of motivation. The nurse interprets these as which of the following?
   1. Delusions
   2. Positive symptoms
   3. Hallucinations
   4. Negative symptoms

Answer: 3

Rationale: Requesting a client who is disoriented and psychotic to interact with peers, participate in unit programs, or encourage involvement in the milieu would agitate the client. Reality orientation would orient the client to the surroundings.

Nursing process: Planning

Client need: Psychosocial Integrity

Cognitive level: Application

Subject area: Psychiatric and Mental Health

Answer: Hallucinations

Rationale: Hallucinations pertain to a perceptual distortion of stimuli that is not present or reality based. Hallucinations are a common feature in schizophrenia. It is not uncommon for a client who is out of touch with reality to hear multiple voices at one time, talking to each.

Nursing process: Implementation

Client need: Psychosocial Integrity

Cognitive level: Application

Subject area: Psychiatric and Mental Health

Answer: 4

Rationale: Negative clinical manifestations of schizophrenia are much harder to detect and describe than are positive clinical manifestations. The negative clinical manifestations such as flattened affect, slowed thinking, and lack of motivation are observed and in many ways are more debilitating. Unlike positive clinical manifestations, negative clinical manifestations are behaviors not fundamentally different from behaviors exhibited by many people. They are more common and severe in schizophrenia. They are particularly obvious when contrasted to how the client was before the onset of the disorder. Delusions and hallucinations are positive clinical manifestations because they must be self-reported by the client.

Nursing process: Analysis

Client need: Psychosocial Integrity

Cognitive level: Application

Subject area: Psychiatric and Mental Health

4. Which of the following descriptions of the dopamine hypothesis should the nurse include when educating another nurse about the causes of schizophrenia?

   1. The kidneys cause excessive amounts of dopamine in the body that the kidneys do not readily excrete.

   2. There is an excess of dopamine found at the synaptic clefts in the brain.

   3. Too little dopamine in the brain causes hallucinations.

   4. Abnormal levels of dopamine cause structural brain abnormalities.

5. The family of a client with schizophrenia asks the nurse what the brain imaging study ordered for the client is most likely to find. The most appropriate response by the nurse is

   1. "It would most likely find an absent frontal cortex."

   2. "It would most likely find abnormal auditory and optical nerves."

   3. "It would most likely find overactivity in the center of creativity."

   4. "It would most likely find enlarged lateral and third ventricles."

6. The family of a 25-year-old female client asks the nurse if any of the family members are at risk to get schizophrenia. The nurse anticipates that which of the following individuals is most likely to also suffer from schizophrenia?

   1. The younger brother

   2. The older sister

   3. The monozygotic twin

   4. The 50-year-old maternal aunt

Answer: 2

Rationale: Although the etiology of schizophrenia remains unknown, there is research suggesting the dopamine hypothesis that the functional abnormalities in schizophrenia are the result of excessive amounts of dopamine in the brain. Normally dopamine is produced in the brain and functions as a neurotransmitter.

Nursing process: Analysis

Client need: Psychosocial Integrity

Cognitive level: Analysis

Subject area: Psychiatric and Mental Health

Answer: 4

Rationale: CT scanning may be used to evaluate brain structure in schizophrenic clients. The results have shown that clients with schizophrenia have larger lateral ventricles than nonschizophrenic individuals. This is a well-documented fact, but the meaning behind this finding remains unclear. It remains unknown as to whether the enlargement is the cause or a consequence of the schizophrenia. It also has no bearing on the severity of the clinical manifestations. Some data demonstrate that the ventricular enlargement is related to cerebral atrophy. Although speculative, there is some research that suggests schizophrenia may be a degenerative neurological disorder.

Nursing process: Analysis

Client need: Reduction of Risk Potential

Cognitive level: Application

Subject area: Psychiatric and Mental Health

Answer: 3

Rationale: Schizophrenia is a disorder that has a high genetic component. This conclusion has been reached based on the close incidence of schizophrenia in twins and particularly monozygotic twins. They have a higher concordance rate than any other biological relationship. Although genetics plays a role in the development of schizophrenia, the relationship remains an indecisive one. Some studies indicate that this relationship may be as high as 50%, but other studies indicate that a monozygotic twin has less than a 100% chance of developing schizophrenia when the other twin is affected.

Nursing process: Analysis

Client need: Psychosocial Integrity

Cognitive level: Application

Subject area: Psychiatric and Mental Health

7. Which of the following is the priority nursing intervention in the plan of care for a client with catatonic schizophrenia?

   1. Introduce the client to the other clients
   2. Begin obtaining the client's history
   3. Give the client the prescribed drugs
   4. Settle the client in the room

8. A public health nurse is providing case management for a client who has chronic paranoid schizophrenia. Which of the following is the most appropriate goal for this client? The client will

   1. take public transportation to go shopping.
   2. obtain and hold down a steady job.
   3. attend appointments with health care providers.
   4. socialize with neighbors on a daily basis.

9. A client recently hospitalized for schizophrenia has just returned back to a group home. Although the client's hallucinations have resolved, negative symptoms of schizophrenia continue. Based on this assessment, the nurse should monitor the client for which of the following negative clinical manifestations?

   Select all that apply:

   [ ] 1. Anhedonia
   [ ] 2. Failure to socialize
   [ ] 3. Smiling
   [ ] 4. Strong desire to resume work
   [ ] 5. Alogia
   [ ] 6. Daily hygiene practices

10. A client with acute psychosis is being evaluated in the emergency room to determine the need for hospitalization. During the initial interview, the client became mute and unable to move out of the chair. The nurse appropriately documents this behavior as _____.

Answer: 4

Rationale: Catatonic schizophrenia is a type of schizophrenia in which there is a marked decrease in reactivity to the environment. The client will not likely be able to socialize or adequately communicate secondary to the catatonia. Although administering prescribed drugs may be appropriate, it is not the priority. Decreasing the stimuli in the client's environment is the priority. The client with catatonia will be less stimulated in the client's room.

Nursing process: Planning

Client need: Management of Care

Cognitive level: Application

Subject area: Psychiatric and Mental Health

Answer: 3

Rationale: A function of case management is to coordinate the client's health care needs. The priority goal for a client with paranoid schizophrenia is to encourage the client to regularly attend all the scheduled appointments with health care providers. Although taking public transportation, maintaining a steady job, or socializing with the neighbors may be appropriate interventions, they are not the priority. Clients with paranoid schizophrenia are likely to be socially isolated and have few trusting relationships.

Nursing process: Evaluation

Client need: Psychosocial Integrity

Cognitive level: Analysis

Subject area: Psychiatric and Mental Health

Answer: 1, 2, 5

Rationale: Anhedonia, alogia, and a failure to socialize are all negative clinical manifestations seen in schizophrenia. Anhedonia is the inability to find enjoyment in daily activities. Alogia is a tendency to speak very little or use short empty phrases.

Nursing process: Assessment

Client need: Psychosocial Integrity

Cognitive level: Analysis

Subject area: Psychiatric and Mental Health

Answer: catatonic

Rationale: Catatonia is a state in which there is a large decrease in reactivity to the environment. An extreme degree of immobility and unawareness may result.

Nursing process: Implementation

Client need: Psychosocial Integrity

Cognitive level: Application

Subject area: Psychiatric and Mental Health

11. A client diagnosed with schizophrenia states he is Jesus Christ. The nurse documents this as _____.

12. The nurse caring for a client with schizophrenia evaluates which of the following behaviors as an idea of influence?

1. The belief that a radio can control someone's thoughts

2. Inability to identify person, place, and time

3. Confusion that worsens to the point of delirium

4. Interpreting a shadow as a person

13. The nurse administers which of the following prescribed drugs for the purpose of relieving both the positive and negative clinical manifestations of schizophrenia?

1. Selective serotonin reuptake inhibitor

2. Dopaminergic

3. Anxiolytic

4. Sedative

14. The nurse reviewing the chart of a client who was recently diagnosed with schizophrenia following graduation from college coincides with the client's mother's diagnosis of schizophrenia at the same time. The nurse evaluates the major risk factor contributing to the development of schizophrenia in this client as

1. a recent search for employment.

2. being from a low socioeconomic class.

3. the mother's genetics at the time of diagnosis.

4. being recently divorced.

Answer: grandiose delusion

Rationale: A grandiose delusion is a perception that the individual feels grand importance, has special powers, or is a religious significance that is out of touch with reality.

Nursing process: Implementation

Client need: Psychosocial Integrity

Cognitive level: Application

Subject area: Psychiatric and Mental Health

Answer: 1

Rationale: An idea of influence is a client's false impression that outside activities have a unique meaning for the client. It is an internal thought regarding some content in which the client's thoughts are controlled by an external entity. The client's inability to identify person, place, and time, and confusion to the point of delirium are related to the client's orientation. Interpreting a shadow as a person is an illusion that is an incorrect perception of a sensory stimuli.

Nursing process: Evaluation

Client need: Psychosocial Integrity

Cognitive level: Application

Subject area: Psychiatric and Mental Health

Answer: 2

Rationale: Dopamine has been specifically identified as having an influence on both the positive and negative clinical manifestations of schizophrenia. Selective serotonin reuptake inhibitors treat depression. Anxiolytics treat anxiety, and sedatives are calming agents.

Nursing process: Implementation

Client need: Pharmacological and Parenteral Therapies

Cognitive level: Application

Subject area: Pharmacologic

Answer: 3

Rationale: The mother's genetics at the time of diagnosis of schizophrenia is the major risk factor for the client diagnosed with schizophrenia. Being recently divorced, from a lower socioeconomic status, or a recent search for employment are all environmental influences.

Nursing process: Evaluation

Client need: Psychosocial Integrity

Cognitive level: Analysis

Subject area: Psychiatric and Mental Health

15. The nurse is caring for a client with schizophrenia who is experiencing delusions. Which of the following nursing diagnoses would be appropriate?

1. Impaired verbal communication
2. Ineffective role performance
3. Disturbed thought processes
4. Disturbed sensory perception

16. A newly married client is delusional and believes that his partner is having an affair with the next door neighbor. Which of the following is the priority that will lead the nurse to expect that these delusions will incapacitate this man?

1. He will be consumed by his thoughts.
2. He will predominantly be affected at work.
3. These beliefs will not have any effect on him.
4. These beliefs will affect his social relationships.

17. A well-known substance user is brought to the emergency department at 0200 by the probation officer (P.O.). The P.O. is concerned because the client has been threatening peers with a knife and accusing them of having an affair with the client's partner. While making the assessment, the nurse understands that psychosis is most likely related to

1. using methamphetamine tonight.
2. marijuana use 2 days ago.
3. use of alcohol over the last week.
4. use of a friend's tranquilizers.

Answer: 3

Rationale: Delusions are false ideas that an individual believes to be real despite evidence to the contrary. They are disturbed thought processes, so a nursing diagnosis of disturbed thought processes would be appropriate. A nursing diagnosis of disturbed role performance would be appropriate with a loss of function. Impaired verbal communication would be an appropriate nursing diagnosis for a clinical manifestation of incomprehensible language. Hallucinations are a sensory perception for which there is no reality, and disturbed sensory perception would be an appropriate nursing diagnosis.

Nursing process: Analysis

Client need: Psychosocial Integrity

Cognitive level: Analysis

Subject area: Psychiatric and Mental Health

Answer: 4

Rationale: Paranoid delusions are disturbances in thought processes that generally affect only an individual's social relationships. They do not predominantly impact the work environment or daily functioning.

Nursing process: Analysis

Client need: Management of Care

Cognitive level: Analysis

Subject area: Psychiatric and Mental Health

Answer: 1

Rationale: Methamphetamine causes psychosis and is the most recent drug that was abused so it would be the most plausible explanation for the behavior. Current use of alcohol may cause psychosis but not alcohol taken a week ago. Marijuana used 2 days ago and use of tranquilizers are both unlikely to cause psychosis.

Nursing process: Analysis

Client need: Psychosocial Integrity

Cognitive level: Analysis

Subject area: Psychiatric and Mental Health

18. A nurse using the downtown transportation system in a large city sees a homeless woman sitting on a park bench. The woman is talking to herself and frequently looks over to the empty space on the bench beside her. What is the best explanation for this situation?

   1. The woman is experiencing auditory and visual hallucinations.

   2. The woman is lonely because she is homeless.

   3. She was speaking on her cell phone by using the headset.

   4. She was calling to her friend down the street.

19. The nurse working in an adult inpatient psychiatric unit is admitting a client recently diagnosed with schizophrenia. The nurse notices that this client is constantly drinking water. Which of the following interventions is a priority for this client?

   1. Monitor intake and output

   2. Obtain serum sodium and potassium levels

   3. Restrict the client's oral intake

   4. Educate the client about a low-sodium diet

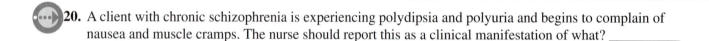 **20.** A client with chronic schizophrenia is experiencing polydipsia and polyuria and begins to complain of nausea and muscle cramps. The nurse should report this as a clinical manifestation of what? _____

21. A client who belongs to a familial religious sect reports seeing "visions." Neither the client nor the family are concerned. The nurse understands that which of the following explanations accounts for the lack of concern about this visualization?

   1. The client is not convinced of the religious sect.

   2. The family believes that the client made it up.

   3. Cultural variations of spiritual beliefs exist.

   4. This is the first time "visions" have been seen.

Answer: 1

Rationale: About 30% of the homeless suffer from schizophrenia. The woman is showing signs of responding to internal stimuli. Auditory and visual hallucinations are precipitated by internal stimuli. Speaking on a cell phone and calling to a friend down the street are both external stimuli.

Nursing process: Analysis

Client need: Psychosocial Integrity

Cognitive level: Analysis

Subject area: Psychiatric and Mental Health

Answer: 2

Rationale: Although monitoring the intake and output may be an appropriate intervention, it is not the priority intervention, because the client is a new admission and the electrolyte levels need to be monitored first to determine if any other nursing interventions are necessary. Educating the client about a low-sodium diet may also be an appropriate intervention but not the priority. The client's oral intake should not be restricted unless there is a medical reason to do so.

Nursing process: Planning

Client need: Management of Care

Cognitive level: Application

Subject area: Psychiatric and Mental Health

Answer: Water intoxication

Rationale: Water intoxication is a major cause of death among clients who have schizophrenia. Polyuria, polydipsia, nausea, and muscle cramps are classic features of water intoxication.

Nursing process: Analysis

Client need: Psychosocial Integrity

Cognitive level: Analysis

Subject area: Psychiatric and Mental Health

Answer: 3

Rationale: Culture variations that exist among spiritual beliefs in family and friends are the most plausible explanation for a lack of concern over seeing "visions."

Nursing process: Analysis

Client need: Psychosocial Integrity

Cognitive level: Analysis

Subject area: Psychiatric and Mental Health

22. Knowing that it is difficult to establish trust with a client experiencing delusions, the nurse who is taking care of a client with delusional disorder should initiate conversation by saying which of the following?

    1. "What happened to make you come here?"
    2. "What is bothering you right now?"
    3. "I'm your nurse; tell me if you need something."
    4. "The other clients want to meet you."

23. The registered nurse on a psychiatric unit is making out clinical assignments. Which of the following assignments should the nurse delegate to a licensed practical nurse?

    1. Plan the medication schedule for a client with schizophrenia
    2. Instruct a client with schizophrenia on the anxiolytic
    3. Document the description of the hallucinations a client is experiencing
    4. Discuss with a client's family the treatment plan for the client

24. A client's family asks the nurse what the primary reason is for conducting a physical exam as part of the diagnostic process for a psychiatric client. Which of the following is the most appropriate response?

    1. "The physical exam is performed to rule out any medical causes for the psychiatric clinical manifestations."
    2. "The physical exam is performed to determine functional status."
    3. "The physical exam is performed to replace the mental status exam."
    4. "The physical exam is performed to test the client's perception of what is happening."

Answer: 3

Rationale: Telling a client who is experiencing delusions that you are the nurse provides the least threatening approach to initiate conversation. The client is most likely experiencing some paranoia along with the delusional content. Asking a client what happened to cause the visit to the hospital has an accusatory tone. Asking what is bothering the client is too intrusive for an initial stage of establishing trust. Telling the client that the other clients want to meet the client is perceived as a socially uncomfortable situation for someone who is experiencing paranoia.

Nursing process: Planning

Client need: Psychosocial Integrity

Cognitive level: Analysis

Subject area: Psychiatric and Mental Health

Answer: 3

Rationale: A licensed practical nurse may document the hallucinations a client is experiencing. Planning a medication schedule, instructing a client on a drug, and discussing a treatment plan with a client's family are all activities that should be performed by a registered nurse.

Nursing process: Planning

Client need: Management of Care

Cognitive level: Analysis

Subject area: Psychiatric and Mental Health

Answer: 1

Rationale: A physical examination is a necessary part of the initial assessment for a client diagnosed to be a psychiatric client, because many clinical manifestations that appear to be psychiatric in nature may in actuality have a medical etiology. Any medical cause must be ruled out before making a definitive psychiatric diagnosis. A physical exam cannot determine functional status. A physical exam cannot replace the mental status exam. Testing the client's perception of what is happening is not the primary reason for conducting a physical exam.

Nursing process: Analysis

Client need: Reduction of Risk Potential

Cognitive level: Analysis

Subject area: Psychiatric and Mental Health

25. A client is admitted to a medical-surgical unit with an infection of the right great toe and temperature of 38.9°C (102°F). The client appears to be becoming psychotic. In determining what action to take next, which of the following factors should the nurse consider?

1. The client is having an acute onset of dementia.

2. The client was postictal.

3. The client's circadian rhythm is unsynchronized.

4. The client is psychotic because of the infection.

26. A client with a bipolar disorder is brought to the emergency department by the spouse after the client pointed a steak knife at the spouse and yelled, "I know that you are jealous of my special gifts from God." The nurse informs the spouse that this behavior is most likely explained by which of the following? The client

1. cannot handle the marital discord.

2. is becoming demented.

3. became psychotic during a manic phase.

4. wants to kill the spouse.

Answer: 4

Rationale: An infection may contribute to a client's distortion of perceptual reality. Dementia does not have an acute onset. There is no evidence that the client had a seizure. It is unlikely that an infection would make someone develop acute dementia.

Nursing process: Analysis

Client need: Psychosocial Integrity

Cognitive level: Analysis

Subject area: Psychiatric and Mental Health

Answer: 3

Rationale: A client may become psychotic during a manic phase of a bipolar disorder. Not handling marital discord or wanting to kill one's spouse do not most likely correlate with a manic episode. Dementia has a slow onset and usually appears in an older client.

Nursing process: Implementation

Client need: Psychosocial Integrity

Cognitive level: Analysis

Subject area: Psychiatric and Mental Health

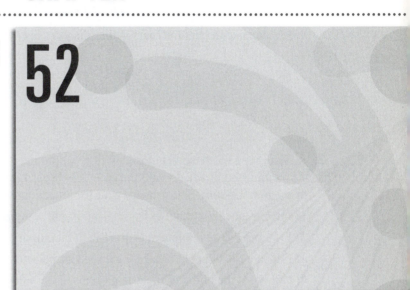

CHAPTER 52

Paranoid Disorders

1. The wife of a client with paranoid personality disorder asks the nurse why the client keeps blaming her for plotting against him. Which of the following is the appropriate response by the nurse?

    1. "A client with paranoid personality disorder suspects others' motives."

    2. "A client with paranoid personality disorder prefers solitary activities."

    3. "A client with paranoid personality disorder lacks interests or hobbies."

    4. "A client with paranoid personality disorder is emotionally detached."

2. A client who has been diagnosed with paranoid personality disorder has been hospitalized because of suspicions and threats toward the company boss. While in the hospital, the client continues to be suspicious of the nursing staff. The primary goal for this client would be which of the following?

    1. Inform the client that the boss has no harmful intentions

    2. Promote the development of trust with the nursing staff

    3. Educate the client about the legal risks of harming the boss

    4. Convince the client of the true motives of the nurses

3. Two staff members are talking and laughing about their weekend activities in the hall outside the room of a client diagnosed with paranoid personality disorder. The client appears annoyed and is suspicious of them while they are talking. Which of the following is the most appropriate intervention?

    1. Encourage the client to engage in the conversation

    2. Report the staff members' inappropriate behavior

    3. Inform the staff members that the talking can be misinterpreted as secretiveness

    4. Close the door to the client's room

4. An important role of the nurse is to facilitate social interactions between a client who is paranoid and the client's peers. The nurse implements this intervention based on the understanding that a client with paranoid personality disorder

    1. is gregarious and outgoing in socialization style.

    2. tends to exhibit loose boundaries when sharing feelings.

    3. likes to be around large groups of people.

    4. tends to be isolated and lacks social skills.

Answer: 1

Rationale: Suspicion of others is a hallmark of paranoid personality disorder. Preferring solitary activities, lacking interest in hobbies or other interests, or becoming emotionally detached are all clinical manifestations of an individual with schizoid personality disorder.

Nursing process: Analysis

Client need: Psychosocial Integrity

Cognitive level: Analysis

Subject area: Psychiatric and Mental Health

Answer: 2

Rationale: Promoting the development of trust with the nursing staff is the best goal for a client who is experiencing paranoia. This will support and encourage the client to make better progress in treatment and begin to trust the staff.

Nursing process: Evaluation

Client need: Psychosocial Integrity

Cognitive level: Analysis

Subject area: Psychiatric and Mental Health

Answer: 3

Rationale: Behavior that can be interpreted as secretive by a client who is paranoid will reinforce the client's feelings of suspiciousness. A client who is paranoid may interpret seeing two staff members talking outside the client's room as being secretive.

Nursing process: Planning

Client need: Psychosocial Integrity

Cognitive level: Application

Subject area: Psychiatric and Mental Health

Answer: 4

Rationale: A client with paranoid personality disorder often becomes socially isolated because of suspiciousness toward others. This client would not be gregarious or outgoing. Such clients do not feel that they have a problem. A client who suffers from paranoia would not have social skills that would be enhanced by being around or sharing with others.

Nursing process: Analysis

Client need: Psychosocial Integrity

Cognitive level: Analysis

Subject area: Psychiatric and Mental Health

5. The nurse encourages a client who is exhibiting paranoid behavior to participate in what type of group? _____

6. A wealthy business owner has been diagnosed with paranoid personality disorder and is listening to the radio. The announcer states that the presidential candidate will be flying into town to meet with the community businesses. The client believes that the presidential candidate had this announcement placed on the radio to specifically make sure that the client attends the meeting. The nurse documents this type of thinking as _____.

7. A client who has been diagnosed with paranoid personality disorder works for airport security and believes that an offer will soon be made to work for the Central Intelligence Agency (CIA). The nurse documents this thought process as what? _____

8. When planning the care of a client who is paranoid, the nurse should include which of the following interventions to increase the sense of trust?
   1. Give the client the nurse's home phone number for support
   2. Spend more time with this client than with other clients
   3. Solicit the client's participation in the development of the treatment plan
   4. Fulfill all of the client's requests to provide assurance of active listening

Answer: Social skills group

Rationale: The most appropriate type of group for a client who is exhibiting paranoid behavior is a social skills group. This client is suspicious of others, and the client's ability to interact with others is most likely impaired.

Nursing process: Implementation

Client need: Psychosocial Integrity

Cognitive level: Application

Subject area: Psychiatric and Mental Health

Answer: ideas of reference

Rationale: Ideas of reference are false ideas in which outside events have special implications for the client. A client who believes that a radio message includes a special personal message indicates that the client is experiencing ideas of reference.

Nursing process: Implementation

Client need: Psychosocial Integrity

Cognitive level: Application

Subject area: Psychiatric and Mental Health

Answer: Delusions of grandeur

Rationale: A delusion is a false belief that the client believes to be true even though there is evidence that it is not. Grandiosity is a belief about one's importance. A client who believes a job offer is coming from the CIA demonstrates a delusion of being more influential than reality supports. The beliefs have given the client a more prominent status than that which really exists.

Nursing process: Implementation

Client need: Psychosocial Integrity

Cognitive level: Application

Subject area: Psychiatric and Mental Health

Answer: 3

Rationale: Soliciting a client's participation in the development of the treatment plan is an effective way to get a client who is paranoid to improve communication and participation in the treatment plan and to develop a trusting relationship. Giving a client a home phone number or spending more time with this client than with other clients violates professional boundaries. Fulfilling all of the client's requests can cause the client to become more suspicious.

Nursing process: Planning

Client need: Psychosocial Integrity

Cognitive level: Application

Subject area: Psychiatric and Mental Health

9. Which of the following interventions would be most appropriate for the nurse to implement for a client in a paranoid state who is having difficulty falling asleep and has tried reading, taking a warm bath, and drinking warm milk, all of which have been unsuccessful?

   1. Instruct the client to try all of these again but for a longer time

   2. Administer a prescribed drug for relaxation

   3. Offer the client a back rub

   4. Encourage the client to listen to the radio

10. A client experiencing paranoid behavior believes that the drugs are poisonous and doesn't want to take them. Which of the following nursing interventions should the nurse include in this client's plan of care?

    1. Administer the drugs intravenously if the client refuses to take them orally

    2. Tell the client that taking the drugs is a part of the treatment

    3. Restrict the client to the room until the client agrees to take the drugs

    4. Inform the client that the doctor ordered the drugs and they are necessary

11. The nurse should instruct a client with paranoid delusions to avoid which of the following beverages? Select all that apply:

    [ ] **1.** Coffee

    [ ] **2.** Ginger ale

    [ ] **3.** Lemonade

    [ ] **4.** Whole milk

    [ ] **5.** Cola

    [ ] **6.** Chocolate milkshake

12. Which of the following does the nurse evaluate as a disturbance in the activities of daily living for a client who is paranoid? The client

    1. goes to the grocery store only when more food is needed.

    2. signs up for the Meals on Wheels service.

    3. refuses to eat any food item that is not prepackaged and can be self-opened.

    4. goes over to the neighbors' for dinner once a week on Friday evenings.

Answer: 2

Rationale: After unsuccessful attempts to sleep, as evidenced by reading, drinking milk, or taking a warm bath, the next appropriate intervention would be to offer a prescribed drug for relaxation. It would be inappropriate to instruct the client to try these measures for a longer time period, to give the client a back rub, or to encourage the client to listen to the radio because the client has already tried nondrug-related measures and continues to be frustrated.

Nursing process: Implementation

Client need: Psychosocial Integrity

Cognitive level: Application

Subject area: Psychiatric and Mental Health

Answer: 2

Rationale: The most appropriate intervention for a client who thinks the drugs are poisonous is to be direct with the client and tell the client that the drugs are an important part of the treatment. Forcing the client to take the drugs, restricting the client to the room until the drugs are taken, or informing the client that the doctor ordered the drugs would not work, because this is a suspicious client who will not respond to reason.

Nursing process: Planning

Client need: Psychosocial Integrity

Cognitive level: Application

Subject area: Psychiatric and Mental Health

Answer: 1, 5, 6

Rationale: A client who has paranoid delusions should be instructed to avoid caffeine-containing beverages because the stimulating effects of caffeine may contribute to feelings of paranoia and anxiety. Coffee, cola, and a chocolate milkshake all contain caffeine.

Nursing process: Planning

Client need: Basic Care and Comfort

Cognitive level: Application

Subject area: Psychiatric and Mental Health

Answer: 3

Rationale: A disturbance in the activities of daily living for a client who is paranoid is to refuse to eat any food that is not prepackaged and can be self-opened. A client with paranoia would not sign up for Meals on Wheels or go to a neighbor's for dinner because the client did not prepare the food and may believe it is contaminated. Going to the grocery store when more food is needed is not an impairment to the activities of daily living.

Nursing process: Evaluation

Client need: Psychosocial Integrity

Cognitive level: Application

Subject area: Psychiatric and Mental Health

13. A client who has been diagnosed with paranoid delusions frequently takes issues to the legal system that result in court hearings. This is most likely due to the fact that

    1. the client initiates legal action due to the persecutory content of the delusions.

    2. other individuals are taking the client to court because of the client's poor decisions.

    3. the client has often been taken advantage of by other individuals.

    4. the client doesn't know how else to get the attention of individuals who hurt the client.

14. A client who has paranoid delusional disorder has been having spousal difficulties but is making good progress at work during this quarter. The nurse identifies which of the following as the most likely cause of the client's behavior?

    1. The client is projecting frustrated energy into work.

    2. The client would rather be at work than at home.

    3. The client's paranoia causes worry about the work situation.

    4. The client's delusions mainly affect relationships.

15. A client who has been diagnosed with paranoid delusional disorder is developing healthier interpersonal relationships. During this development, the nurse encourages the client to

    1. identify people with whom it is safe to talk.

    2. talk about the delusions whenever they occur.

    3. remember the paranoid thoughts until the next therapy session.

    4. seek feedback regarding the realistic nature of the delusion.

Answer: 1

Rationale: A client with persecutory delusions frequently initiates legal action because of the belief that others are attacking. It is through the court actions that the client attempts to remedy these beliefs about the other individuals. Other individuals taking the client to court because of the client's poor decisions is focusing on the thoughts and actions of someone other than the client. The client being taken advantage of also focuses on the other individual's thoughts and actions, rather than the client's. A client with persecutory delusions is not trying to get attention; instead, the issue is about rectification for the wrongs done to the client.

Nursing process: Evaluation

Client need: Psychosocial Integrity

Cognitive level: Analysis

Subject area: Psychiatric and Mental Health

Answer: 4

Rationale: Clients with delusional disorders can generally function adequately when they do not focus on their delusional belief system, which usually affects social and marital relationships. Because of this, the client would be able to manage adequately in the work environment.

Nursing process: Analysis

Client need: Psychosocial Integrity

Cognitive level: Analysis

Subject area: Psychiatric and Mental Health

Answer: 1

Rationale: Establishment of trust and a safe relationship is important and difficult for the client who has paranoid delusions. Talking about the client's delusions whenever they occur, remembering the paranoid thoughts until the next therapy session, and seeking feedback regarding the realistic nature of the delusion all focus on the delusional thoughts.

Nursing process: Implementation

Client need: Psychosocial Integrity

Cognitive level: Application

Subject area: Psychiatric and Mental Health

16. A client is diagnosed with paranoid schizophrenia and has been hospitalized due to auditory hallucinations resulting in verbal threats. These hallucinations are of a persecutory nature. Which of the following is the most appropriate nursing diagnosis?

1. Noncompliance

2. Health maintenance, ineffective

3. Personal identity, disturbed

4. Sensory perception, disturbed

17. A nurse teaching a class on paranoid personality disorder correctly describes the client as appearing angry and argumentative, but in reality the client feels

1. shy and awkward.

2. vulnerable and powerless.

3. depressed and suicidal.

4. secure and confident.

18. A client is being evaluated for headaches and paranoid delusions. A computerized tomography (CT) scan reveals a brain tumor. The diagnosis of paranoid delusional disorder is in question at this point because

1. the clinical manifestations present along with a medical condition.

2. the client is only suspicious of the physician.

3. the client is not experiencing any hallucinations.

4. the clinical manifestations really aren't delusions.

19. A nurse has worked to establish a relationship with a client who has been diagnosed with paranoid personality disorder. It has been difficult to make any progress based on what classic feature of the client's thought pattern? _____

Answer: 4

Rationale: Hallucinations are, by definition, perceptual distortions and are not the effect of deliberate choices. Therefore, the most appropriate nursing diagnosis is disturbed sensory perception. Nursing diagnoses of noncompliance, ineffective health maintenance, and disturbed personal identity would all involve deliberate choices.

Nursing process: Planning

Client need: Psychosocial Integrity

Cognitive level: Analysis

Subject area: Psychiatric and Mental Health

Answer: 2

Rationale: Clients who have paranoid personality disorder use denial and projection as their main defense mechanisms, because in reality they are feeling vulnerable and powerless. Shy, awkward, depressed, suicidal, secure, and confident may co-occur with paranoia, although they do not explain the projection of insecurity into anger.

Nursing process: Analysis

Client need: Psychosocial Integrity

Cognitive level: Analysis

Subject area: Psychiatric and Mental Health

Answer: 1

Rationale: Medical issues must be diagnosed and evaluated as a potential cause of clinical manifestations that may also appear psychiatric in nature.

Nursing process: Analysis

Client need: Psychosocial Integrity

Cognitive level: Analysis

Subject area: Psychiatric and Mental Health

Answer: Mistrust

Rationale: Mistrust accompanies paranoia found in paranoid personality disorder and becomes a barrier to establishing a client-provider relationship.

Nursing process: Analysis

Client need: Psychosocial Integrity

Cognitive level: Analysis

Subject area: Psychiatric and Mental Health

20. A client with paranoid schizophrenia has been seeing a public health nurse every week for drug administration and compliance. The current drugs have been effective in decreasing positive clinical manifestations. The nurse anticipates that the client will report

1. a decrease in motivation to go to church.

2. a week without hearing voices.

3. seeing his or her dead grandmother.

4. a schedule that has become very busy with social outings.

21. A female client hospitalized for paranoid schizophrenia reports to the nursing staff that voices are telling her that a male peer is plotting to kill her. The nurse documents the voices as _____.

22. The registered nurse is preparing to delegate nursing tasks to a licensed practical nurse. Which of the following tasks should the nurse delegate to a licensed practical nurse?

1. Evaluate a client suspected of having paranoid schizophrenia for delusions

2. Document a client's paranoid behavior

3. Assess a client with paranoia for auditory hallucinations

4. Instruct a client's family on the clinical features of paranoid schizophrenia

Answer: 2

Rationale: A client who reports a week without hearing voices demonstrates a decrease in positive clinical manifestations. Lack of motivation is a negative clinical manifestation and a decrease in the motivation to go to church would indicate no improvement in the client's condition. A client who sees one's dead grandmother is having a positive clinical manifestation, clearly demonstrating that the client is still in the throes of paranoid schizophrenia. More social activities is a negative clinical manifestation, indicating an improvement in the client's condition.

Nursing process: Analysis

Client need: Psychosocial Integrity

Cognitive level: Analysis

Subject area: Psychiatric and Mental Health

Answer: persecutory

Rationale: Auditory hallucinations in a client who has paranoid schizophrenia are generally persecutory in nature.

Nursing process: Implementation

Client need: Psychosocial Integrity

Cognitive level: Application

Subject area: Psychiatric and Mental Health

Answer: 2

Rationale: Nursing tasks that involve the skills of evaluating, assessing, and instructing are reserved for the registered nurse. A licensed practical nurse may document a client's paranoid behavior.

Nursing process: Planning

Client need: Psychosocial Integrity

Cognitive level: Analysis

Subject area: Legal and Ethical Issues

23. Which of the following is a priority goal for the nurse to plan in the care of a client who experiences paranoid delusions?

    1. Absence of delusions

    2. Establishment of trust

    3. Participation in all unit activities

    4. Independent activities of daily living

24. A client who suffers from paranoid delusions utilizes denial as a defense mechanism. The nurse wants to foster other ways of dealing with the anxiety that the client experiences. The nurse could best do this by planning for the client to be involved in which of the following activities?

    1. Community mental health support group

    2. Psychodynamic group therapy

    3. Adult education class on emotions

    4. Individualized relaxation therapy

25. A client who has been diagnosed with paranoid delusional disorder is getting ready for an evening discharge. This client has a history of expressing anger by threatening to hurt family members with household objects. In preparation for discharge, the nurse should instruct the family that which of the following is a priority if the client becomes threatening?

    1. Call the client's health care provider in the morning

    2. Encourage the client to go to a quiet room to cool down

    3. Remove any potential weapons from the home

    4. Administer an extra dose of a prescribed drug when the anger surfaces

26. In preparation for practicing new coping skills, the nurse assists the client with paranoia in

    1. asking for the physician's methods.

    2. copying other clients' techniques.

    3. learning by reading books.

    4. identifying personal manifestations of anxiety.

Answer: 2

Rationale: As with many psychiatric disorders, establishing trust is paramount to the success of the nurse-client therapeutic relationship.

Nursing process: Evaluation

Client need: Psychosocial Integrity

Cognitive level: Analysis

Subject area: Psychiatric and Mental Health

Answer: 4

Rationale: A client with paranoid delusions is most likely to deal with the anxiety in situations by getting involved in relaxation therapy. Attempting to get clients involved in group therapy or an education class would foster further paranoia because of the group environment.

Nursing process: Planning

Client need: Psychosocial Integrity

Cognitive level: Analysis

Subject area: Psychiatric and Mental Health

Answer: 3

Rationale: The first action to take when discharging a client who in the past threatened to hurt family members with household items would be to remove any potential weapons from the home. It would not be appropriate to wait to call the health care provider in the morning because the call is too delayed. It would not be particularly helpful for an agitated client to go to a quiet room to cool down. The client should not be unsupervised. Although an extra dose of a drug may be administered, it is not the priority.

Nursing process: Planning

Client need: Management of Care

Cognitive level: Application

Subject area: Psychiatric and Mental Health

Answer: 4

Rationale: Before planning interventions for new coping skills for a client, the nurse needs to consider the client's own manifestations of anxiety. Anxiety is a common emotion with paranoia. Asking the physician for other coping methods, copying other clients' techniques, or reading books focus on sources other than the client. The focus should be on the client and the client's needs.

Nursing process: Implementation

Client need: Psychosocial Integrity

Cognitive level: Application

Subject area: Psychiatric and Mental Health

CHAPTER

Post-Traumatic Stress Disorders

53

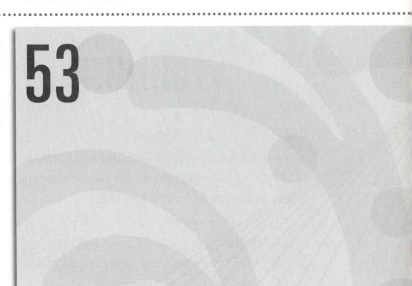

1. A client has been experiencing irritability, difficulty concentrating, difficulty sleeping, and withdrawal for the past 8 weeks since the house burned to the ground after an explosion. The nurse assesses that this client is experiencing

   1. depression.

   2. a panic attack.

   3. post-traumatic stress disorder.

   4. generalized anxiety disorder.

2. A client experiencing post-traumatic stress disorder was started on a monoamine oxidase inhibitor (MAOI). Which of the following should the nurse include in medication teaching?

   Select all that apply:

   [ ] **1.** Sit up slowly when taking an MAOI

   [ ] **2.** Report signs of nausea and vomiting

   [ ] **3.** Avoid foods such as cheese, salami, and smoked fish

   [ ] **4.** Give on an empty stomach

   [ ] **5.** Restrict extra fluids

   [ ] **6.** Monitor for weight loss

3. A client recently started on a monoamine oxidase inhibitor (MAOI) is experiencing severe headache, tachycardia, and cold, clammy skin. Which of the following is the priority nursing intervention?

   1. Assess the client's blood pressure

   2. Instruct the client to lie down

   3. Notify the client's physician

   4. Offer the client a high-carbohydrate snack

Answer: 3

Rationale: Clients may experience clinical manifestations of post-traumatic stress disorder after experiencing a traumatic event, such as a house burning down. Clinical manifestations need to be present for at least 1 month for a diagnosis of post-traumatic stress disorder. The client's clinical manifestations begin abruptly after a traumatic event and last for a period greater than a month.

Nursing process: Assessment

Client need: Psychosocial Integrity

Cognitive level: Application

Subject area: Psychiatric and Mental Health

Answer: 1, 2, 3

Rationale: MAOIs are a classification of drugs used for post-traumatic stress disorder. They act by blocking an enzyme (monoamine oxidase). Clients taking MAOIs should be instructed to sit up slowly to prevent orthostatic hypotension. Nausea, vomiting, and weight gain are all adverse reactions. An MAOI should be administered with food to prevent gastrointestinal upset. Fluids are generally encouraged because constipation is an adverse reaction. Clients must avoid foods that contain tyramine when taking an MAOI. Foods containing tyramine include aged cheese, salami, sauerkraut, beer and wine containing yeast, smoked fish, avocados, fava beans, and caviar. Eating foods containing tyramine when taking an MAOI can lead to a hypertensive crisis, making this the priority intervention.

Nursing process: Planning

Client need: Pharmacological and Parenteral Therapies

Cognitive level: Application

Subject area: Pharmacologic

Answer: 1

Rationale: A toxic and serious adverse reaction to MAOIs is a hypertensive crisis. Clinical manifestations of a hypertensive crisis include severe headache, tachycardia, hypertension, and cold, clammy skin. The nurse's priority would be to assess for an increase in blood pressure. A hypertensive crisis can begin abruptly after taking a contraindicated food or drug. Immediate medical intervention is indicated when a hypertensive crisis is suspected. It is only after assessing the blood pressure and confirming the diagnosis that interventions can begin.

Nursing process: Planning

Client need: Management of Care

Cognitive level: Application

Subject area: Pharmacologic

4. The nurse assesses which of the following clients to be at the highest risk of developing post-traumatic stress disorder?

   1. A client who recently moved to a new city

   2. A client who witnessed a fatal shooting

   3. A client with a family history of depression

   4. A client who has a panic disorder

5. A client reports experiencing nightmares and constant worry about the weather since a tornado destroyed the client's house 1 year ago. The nurse assesses that this client is experiencing

   1. delusions.

   2. panic attacks.

   3. flashbacks.

   4. hallucinations.

6. A client reports having no memory of escaping from a building destroyed in an explosion. The client reports increased difficulty in sleeping, going to work, and interacting with friends. The nurse evaluates this client is using which defense mechanism? _____

7. A client scheduled to begin relaxation therapy as part of treatment for post-traumatic stress disorder asks the nurse what the purpose is of the relaxation therapy. Which of the following is the appropriate response by the nurse?

   1. "It will help you not to be frightened anymore."

   2. "It will help produce effects that are the opposite of those produced by anxiety."

   3. "It will help you learn about your illness."

   4. "It will help you learn calming self-talk."

Answer: 2
Rationale: Experiencing a traumatic event such as a shooting is an event likely to trigger a post-traumatic stress disorder in a person.
Nursing process: Assessment
Client need: Psychosocial Integrity
Cognitive level: Application
Subject area: Psychiatric and Mental Health

Answer: 3
Rationale: A client who repeatedly experiences nightmares and constantly worries about the weather since a tornado destroyed the client's house 1 year ago is experiencing flashbacks. Clients who have flashbacks have recurrent intrusive recollections of the traumatic event. Clients with delusions, hallucinations, and panic attacks would not reexperience the traumatic event in this way.
Nursing process: Assessment
Client need: Psychosocial Integrity
Cognitive level: Application
Subject area: Psychiatric and Mental Health

Answer: Repression
Rationale: Repression is a defense mechanism in which a person unconsciously and automatically pushes unwanted or unpleasant experiences from conscious awareness. Repression is the defense mechanism commonly used by clients experiencing post-traumatic stress disorder. Unless repressed material is resolved, it may result in maladaptive behavior at a later time.
Nursing process: Evaluation
Client need: Psychosocial Integrity
Cognitive level: Application
Subject area: Psychiatric and Mental Health

Answer: 2
Rationale: Relaxation therapy helps the client learn ways to relax the body and reduce the tension produced by anxiety. Relaxation therapy does not guarantee that the client will not be frightened anymore. Helping a client learn about personal illness is the definition of psychoeducation. Helping the client learn calming self-talk defines cognitive restructuring.
Nursing process: Analysis
Client need: Reduction of Risk Potential
Cognitive level: Application
Subject area: Psychiatric and Mental Health

8. The nurse is caring for a client working at a high school who witnessed a bombing at the school and is experiencing sadness, sleeplessness, lack of energy, and appears to be withdrawn. Which of the following interventions should the nurse include in the plan for this client?

   1. Allow the client to talk about the traumatic event in a safe, supportive environment

   2. Assist the client to look at other career choices and work environments

   3. Instruct the client that physical exercise may improve the quality of sleep

   4. Encourage the client to avoid focusing on the event and to make plans for the future

9. When planning the care of a client who is experiencing post-traumatic stress disorder, the nurse identifies which of the following as an appropriate goal? The client will report

   1. spending less time on ritualistic behavior.

   2. a decrease in flashbacks and nightmares.

   3. having more energy.

   4. a decrease in hearing voices.

10. A client tearfully reports having been sexually attacked by a spouse during an argument. The nurse evaluates this situation as

   1. an emotional reaction but not a rape, because the couple is married and has had sexual relations.

   2. the right of the partner to expect sex because they are married.

   3. a rape because sex against one's will is rape.

   4. a reaction to the couple's argument and will most likely not happen again.

11. The client who has been raped tells the nurse, "I am not pressing charges and I'm afraid of seeing my attacker because we live in the same town." Which of the following should the nurse include in the plan of care for this client?

   1. Assess the client's safety and develop a safety plan

   2. Encourage the client to change jobs to avoid future encounters with the perpetrator

   3. Instruct the client not to worry about safety because perpetrators don't attack twice

   4. Support the client's desire to move to a new town and assume a new identity

Answer: 1

Rationale: Allowing clients to talk about traumatic events such as bombings, explosions, and fires enables them to acknowledge their feelings and begin to take control of difficult situations. Assisting the client to consider other career choices, to increase physical exercise, to avoid focusing on the event, and to make plans for the future all discourage the client from acknowledging personal feelings.

Nursing process: Planning

Client need: Psychosocial Integrity

Cognitive level: Application

Subject area: Psychiatric and Mental Health

Answer: 2

Rationale: The target clinical manifestation for a client with post-traumatic stress disorder is flashbacks. Ritualistic behavior is associated with obsessive-compulsive disorder. Having a decreased energy level is associated with depression. Hearing voices is associated with schizophrenia.

Nursing process: Evaluation

Client need: Psychosocial Integrity

Cognitive level: Analysis

Subject area: Psychiatric and Mental Health

Answer: 3

Rationale: Acquaintance rape and marital rape are currently recognized by the court system. The current law allows a person to bring charges against a spouse for rape. Awareness continues to be raised that women are individuals with rights and privileges and not property.

Nursing process: Evaluation

Client need: Psychosocial Integrity

Cognitive level: Analysis

Subject area: Psychiatric and Mental Health

Answer: 1

Rationale: The client may very well be at risk for future attacks if the perpetrator is known. The nurse needs to make a thorough assessment of the client's safety and assist the client in developing a safety plan in the event the perpetrator is encountered. Moving to a new town or changing jobs places the blame and responsibility on the client.

Nursing process: Planning

Client need: Psychosocial Integrity

Cognitive level: Application

Subject area: Psychiatric and Mental Health

12. During an interview, the nurse observes a client becoming increasingly defensive. The client states, "You wouldn't understand what I've been through." Which of the following is the most appropriate response by the nurse?

  1. "You're right, I probably won't understand what you've been through."

  2. "Why are you becoming so defensive?"

  3. "Sometimes it feels like no one else can understand but I would like to try."

  4. "Maybe you will feel better if you concentrate on something else."

13. Which of the following should the nurse include when teaching a class on recognizing post-traumatic stress in children?

  1. Post-traumatic stress disorder is not diagnosed until the age of 18.

  2. Only physically and sexually abused children and adolescents will experience clinical manifestations of post-traumatic stress disorder.

  3. School-age children do not experience clinical manifestations of post-traumatic stress disorder because of their developmental level.

  4. Children and adolescents can develop clinical manifestations of post-traumatic stress disorder after experiencing any traumatic event.

14. The nurse is talking with a client who just had a beautiful bouquet of roses delivered. Suddenly the client becomes tearful and stares out the window. The client has a history of sexual abuse. Which of the following should the nurse include in the plan of care for this client?

  1. Tell the client that the sexual abuse was in the past

  2. Tell the client to relax and enjoy the roses

  3. Give the client some alone time and return later

  4. Assess if the client is having a flashback

15. A client currently taking fluoxetine (Prozac) to decrease clinical manifestations of post-traumatic stress disorder asks the nurse if continuing to take dietary supplements such as Saint John's wort, ginseng, and kava kava is acceptable. The most appropriate response by the nurse is

  1. "If it makes you feel better, continue to take the dietary supplements."

  2. "Dietary supplements may interact negatively with your prescribed drugs; check with your care provider."

  3. "Make sure you take the dietary supplements at a different time."

  4. "Dietary supplements are harmless and won't make any difference in how you feel."

Answer: 3
Rationale: Frequently, clients have experienced things that the nurse has not. By using therapeutic communication skills such as reflecting and empathizing, the nurse can encourage the client to share experiences and begin to understand and develop a therapeutic relationship.
Nursing process: Analysis
Client need: Psychosocial Integrity
Cognitive level: Analysis
Subject area: Psychiatric and Mental Health

Answer: 4
Rationale: Many children and adolescents have experienced natural and man-made disasters in their lives, such as kidnapping, rape, school shootings, peer suicides, fires, and floods. Clinical manifestations of post-traumatic stress disorder may develop in children and adolescents after experiencing these types of traumatic events.
Nursing process: Planning
Client need: Health Promotion and Maintenance
Cognitive level: Application
Subject area: Psychiatric and Mental Health

Answer: 4
Rationale: Clients who have experienced a traumatic event such as sexual abuse may experience flashbacks. The triggers for these flashbacks may be visual, auditory, tactile, or olfactory.
Nursing process: Planning
Client need: Psychosocial Integrity
Cognitive level: Application
Subject area: Psychiatric and Mental Health

Answer: 2
Rationale: Current studies have shown that dietary supplements may have beneficial uses in decreasing clinical manifestations of mild depression, anxiety, and insomnia when not used in conjunction with prescription drugs. Dietary supplements are not controlled by the Food & Drug Administration (FDA). Studies have shown that taking dietary supplements along with prescription drugs may have adverse reactions. The client should be encouraged to discuss the amount and type of supplements being taken with the person who is prescribing the drugs.
Nursing process: Analysis
Client need: Pharmacological and Parenteral Therapies
Cognitive level: Analysis
Subject area: Pharmacologic

16. The registered nurse is preparing the clinical assignments for team members on a psychiatric unit. Which of the following assignments indicates that the nurse has appropriately delegated assignments?

1. Unlicensed assistive personnel attend group therapy with a client.

2. A licensed practical nurse assesses a client suspected of having a post-traumatic stress disorder.

3. Unlicensed assistive personnel sit with a client who is tearful.

4. A licensed practical nurse develops a plan of care for a client who experienced a rape trauma.

Answer: 3

Rationale: Unlicensed assistive personnel may sit with a client who is tearful. A licensed practical nurse should not perform skills of assessing a client or developing a plan of care. These are tasks reserved for the registered nurse. It is not appropriate for unlicensed assistive personnel to attend group therapy with a client.

Nursing process: Planning

Client need: Management of Care

Cognitive level: Analysis

Subject area: Legal and Ethical Issues

Substance Abuse

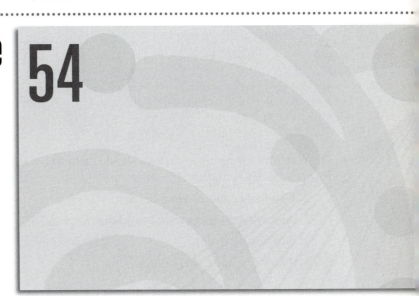

54

1. Which of the following nursing interventions is a priority when planning nursing care for the client experiencing alcohol withdrawal?

   1. Teach techniques to reduce anxiety

   2. Administer a benzodiazepine

   3. Encourage fluid intake

   4. Provide a diet low in fat

2. Which of the following orders should the nurse question when planning the nursing care for a client going into alcohol withdrawal?

   1. Eliminate caffeine from the diet

   2. Assess vital signs every 2 to 4 hours

   3. Nothing by mouth

   4. Teach relaxation techniques

3. After collecting data on a client suspected of being in a narcotic withdrawal, which of the following should the nurse report?

   Select all that apply:

   [   ] **1.** Slurred speech

   [   ] **2.** Decreased blood pressure

   [   ] **3.** Psychomotor retardation

   [   ] **4.** Diarrhea

   [   ] **5.** Muscle aches

   [   ] **6.** Rhinorrhea

4. Which of the following would provide the nurse with the most beneficial assessment data on alcohol abuse?

   1. Complete blood cell count

   2. Chemistry panel

   3. The CAGE questionnaire

   4. Beck Depression Inventory

Answer: 2

Rationale: Because alcohol is a central nervous system depressant, withdrawal will cause the client's central nervous system to be activated. Administering a benzodiazepine takes priority when caring for a client experiencing alcohol withdrawal. It will lower blood pressure and pulse, decrease anxiety, and assist in preventing seizures and death. Encouraging fluids, providing three well-balanced meals, and teaching techniques to reduce anxiety are all appropriate interventions but not the priority.

Nursing process: Planning

Client need: Management of Care

Cognitive level: Application

Subject area: Psychiatric and Mental Health

Answer: 3

Rationale: Fluids should be encouraged for clients experiencing alcohol withdrawal because they often experience dehydration. Fluids would never be withheld. Assessing vital signs, teaching relaxation techniques, and avoiding caffeine in the diet are all appropriate nursing interventions for a client in alcohol withdrawal.

Nursing process: Analysis

Client need: Psychosocial Integrity

Cognitive level: Application

Subject area: Psychiatric and Mental Health

Answer: 4, 5, 6

Rationale: Clinical manifestations of narcotic withdrawal include diarrhea, muscle aches, and rhinorrhea. Slurred speech, decreased blood pressure, and psychomotor retardation are clinical manifestations of opiate intoxication.

Nursing process: Assessment

Client need: Psychosocial Integrity

Cognitive level: Application

Subject area: Psychiatric and Mental Health

Answer: 3

Rationale: A complete blood cell count and a chemistry panel will assist the nurse in identifying medical issues that may be caused by alcohol abuse, but these will not get at the information needed to assess for the alcohol abuse alone. The CAGE questionnaire is the acronym for assessing clients for alcohol abuse. The Beck Depression Inventory assesses a client's severity of depression.

Nursing process: Assessment

Client need: Psychosocial Integrity

Cognitive level: Application

Subject area: Psychiatric and Mental Health

5. The nurse should monitor which of the following for a client experiencing alcohol withdrawal? Select all that apply:

[   ] **1.** Hypertension

[   ] **2.** Tinnitus

[   ] **3.** Pupil constriction

[   ] **4.** Tachycardia

[   ] **5.** Sedation

[   ] **6.** Startles easily

6. The priority nursing intervention in caring for a client experiencing flashbacks from hallucinogenic intoxication include

1. assisting the client with reduction of anxiety.

2. exploring with the client relapse triggers.

3. providing intrapersonal skills training.

4. teaching the client the medical consequences of hallucinogen abuse.

7. The nurse is caring for a client who drank large amounts of alcohol for more than 2 years and abruptly stopped drinking alcohol 30 hours ago. Which of the nursing measures should receive priority in this client's plan of care?

1. Perform a cranial nerve exam

2. Provide adequate nutrition

3. Encourage fluids

4. Monitor vital signs frequently

8. The nurse is admitting a client for alcohol withdrawal. The client states that the last drink of alcohol was at 0800. The nurse should begin to assess this client for clinical manifestations of alcohol withdrawal at _____.

Answer: 1, 4, 6

Rationale: An increased blood pressure and an increased pulse are the most prevalent and first clinical manifestations experienced by the client in alcohol withdrawal. Other clinical manifestations include irritability, a sense of being hyperactive, startling easily, making jerky movements, anxiety, insomnia, and tremors.

Nursing process: Assessment

Client need: Psychosocial Integrity

Cognitive level: Application

Subject area: Psychiatric and Mental Health

Answer: 1

Rationale: Although exploring with the client what triggers a relapse, providing intrapersonal skills, and teaching the client the medical consequences of hallucinogens are important interventions in a client experiencing hallucinogenic intoxication, they are not the priority. Reducing stimuli and the client's anxiety are the priority nursing intervention for a client experiencing flashbacks from hallucinogen intoxication.

Nursing process: Implementation

Client need: Management of Care

Cognitive level: Application

Subject area: Psychiatric and Mental Health

Answer: 4

Rationale: While performing a cranial nerve assessment, providing adequate nutrition, and encouraging fluids are all appropriate interventions, monitoring vital signs is the priority intervention. Monitoring the vital signs frequently will determine when the client goes into alcohol withdrawal.

Nursing process: Planning

Client need: Management of Care

Cognitive level: Application

Subject area: Psychiatric and Mental Health

Answer: 1600 to 2000

Rationale: Alcohol withdrawal clinical manifestations begin between 8 and 12 hours after the last drink of alcohol. If the client had the last drink at 0800, the nurse should begin to assess the client for clinical manifestations of alcohol withdrawal between 1600 and 2000.

Nursing process: Assessment

Client need: Psychosocial Integrity

Cognitive level: Application

Subject area: Psychiatric and Mental Health

9. The nurse is asked to teach a class to a group of clients in a drug rehabilitation clinic on the medical complications of cocaine abuse. Which of the following complications should the nurse include in the class?

1. Hypotension

2. Cardiac arrhythmias

3. Constipation

4. Kidney failure

10. A client comes to an outpatient clinic complaining of an irregular heart rate, restlessness, and nervousness after drinking three cups of coffee and four cola drinks in a 4-hour period. The nurse assesses the client to be experiencing _____.

11. A client repeatedly returns to the hospital with an unsteady gait and slurred speech after several failed inpatient treatment attempts for alcohol dependence. Which of the following nursing interventions is appropriate for the nurse to implement for this client?

1. Promote safety and transition to the hospital

2. Administer a benzodiazepine and a barbiturate

3. Provide a diet high in proteins

4. Administer a nonnarcotic analgesic

12. The nurse notifies the physician that a client admitted for alcohol withdrawal appears jaundiced and has palmar erythema. The nurse suspects this client to be experiencing what complication? _____

Answer: 2

Rationale: Cocaine is a stimulant that works directly on the central nervous system and produces cardiac arrhythmias. Cardiac arrhythmias can lead to death for a client who abuses cocaine. Hypertension is a complication that occurs with toxic levels of cocaine. Constipation does not occur as a result of cocaine. It is actually diarrhea that occurs. Kidney failure is also not a complication of cocaine use.

Nursing process: Planning

Client need: Health Promotion and Management

Cognitive level: Analysis

Subject area: Psychiatric and Mental Health

Answer: caffeine intoxication

Rationale: Intoxication from drugs or substances occurs shortly after use. The effects are felt quickly as a result of the drug's ability to alter the central nervous system. Caffeine is a stimulant and increases cardiac activity, producing cardiac arrhythmias, nervousness, and restlessness.

Nursing process: Assessment

Client need: Psychosocial Integrity

Cognitive level: Application

Subject area: Psychiatric and Mental Health

Answer: 1

Rationale: A client who has an unsteady gait and slurred speech after several failed attempts for alcohol dependence is experiencing alcohol intoxication. Promoting safety and facilitating transition to the hospital is the appropriate intervention for this client. Administering a benzodiazepine, a barbiturate, or a narcotic would actually depress the central nervous system even further and is contraindicated. Increasing protein in the diet is not a standard intervention to be implemented for a client in alcohol intoxication.

Nursing process: Implementation

Client need: Psychosocial Integrity

Cognitive level: Application

Subject area: Psychiatric and Mental Health

Answer: Alcoholic liver cirrhosis

Rationale: Clinical manifestations of alcoholic liver cirrhosis include jaundice and palmar erythema.

Nursing process: Assessment

Client need: Psychosocial Integrity

Cognitive level: Application

Subject area: Psychiatric and Mental Health

13. Which of the following should the nurse include in the plan of care for a client experiencing a morphine sulfate withdrawal?

   1. Provide a cool room

   2. Administer diazepam (Valium)

   3. Administer clonidine (Catapres)

   4. Restrict fluids

14. The nurse documents which of the following clinical manifestations to be present in a client who is experiencing cannabis intoxication?

   Select all that apply:

   [   ] **1.** Anorexia

   [   ] **2.** Dry mouth

   [   ] **3.** Euphoria

   [   ] **4.** Bradycardia

   [   ] **5.** Sensation of slowed time

   [   ] **6.** Drowsiness

15. A client admitted for cannabis intoxication asks the nurse what the average time is for urine drug screens to be positive for cannabis. The appropriate response by the nurse is _____.

16. A client presents to the emergency room complaining of trails of images, moving objects, and flashes of color. The nurse notifies the physician that the client has been abusing which substance? _____

Answer: 3

Rationale: Clonidine (Catapres) blocks opioid receptor sites more effectively than a central nervous system depressant (Valium) in the treatment of opioid withdrawal. Most likely the client would complain of being chilled and require multiple blankets or a warm whirlpool. Fluids are encouraged and not restricted.

Nursing process: Planning

Client need: Pharmacological and Parenteral Therapies

Cognitive level: Application

Subject area: Pharmacologic

Answer: 2, 3, 5

Rationale: The clinical manifestations for cannabis intoxication include dry mouth, euphoria, and a sensation of slowed time. Increased appetite, tachycardia, and anxiety are also experienced.

Nursing process: Implementation

Client need: Psychosocial Integrity

Cognitive level: Application

Subject area: Psychiatric and Mental Health

Answer: 7 to 10 days

Rationale: The average time frame for urine drug screens to be positive for cannabis is 7 to 10 days. Heavy use of cannabis may result in the cannabis being present in the urine for 2 to 4 weeks.

Nursing process: Analysis

Client need: Psychosocial Integrity

Cognitive level: Application

Subject area: Psychiatric and Mental Health

Answer: Hallucinogens

Rationale: The perceptual disturbances of experiencing trails of images, moving objects, and flashes of color occur with hallucinogen use.

Nursing process: Implementation

Client need: Psychosocial Integrity

Cognitive level: Application

Subject area: Psychiatric and Mental Health

17. Which of the following should the nurse include when preparing to teach a nicotine-cessation program?

    1. Nicotine withdrawal clinical manifestations include hot flashes, decreased appetite, and muscle cramps.

    2. The nicotine withdrawal syndrome lasts less than 1 week.

    3. The nurse's personal experience with nicotine withdrawal.

    4. A decreased psychomotor performance, mental dullness, and decreased judgment may be experienced by the client.

18. The nurse is caring for a client who is experiencing cocaine intoxication. Which would indicate to the nurse that the client's condition is deteriorating?

    Select all that apply:

    [ ] **1.** Dyskinesias

    [ ] **2.** Chest pain

    [ ] **3.** Decreased urine output

    [ ] **4.** Hypertension

    [ ] **5.** Anxiety

    [ ] **6.** Tachycardia

19. The nurse is caring for a client admitted with cocaine intoxication who has a fever and is experiencing chest pain, palpitations, and increased blood pressure and pulse. The nursing priority action is to _____.

Answer: 4

Rationale: A decrease in psychomotor performance, mental dullness, and decreased judgment is experienced by the client in a nicotine-cessation program. Hot flashes, decreased appetite, and muscle cramps are not associated with nicotine withdrawal. Nicotine withdrawal lasts several weeks to months. The nurse should keep the focus of the class professional and on educating the participants of the nicotine withdrawal class and not on personal experiences.

Nursing process: Planning

Client need: Health Promotion and Maintenance

Cognitive level: Application

Subject area: Psychiatric and Mental Health

Answer: 2, 4, 6

Rationale: Clinical manifestations of cocaine intoxication include dyskinesias, decreased urine output, anxiety, agitation, chills, weight loss, and anorexia. None of these clinical manifestations are life threatening. Chest pain, palpitation, hypertension, and tachycardia are clinical manifestations that indicate the client's condition is deteriorating. These manifestations indicate that the client is toxic and may experience life-threatening complications such as an arrhythmia, stroke, or myocardial infarction if interventions are not taken.

Nursing process: Analysis

Client need: Psychosocial Integrity

Cognitive level: Analysis

Subject area: Psychiatric and Mental Health

Answer: establish and ensure a patent airway

Rationale: Establishing and ensuring a patent airway is the nursing priority for a client experiencing cocaine intoxication. Fever, chest pain, palpitations, increased blood pressure and pulse are all indications that the client is toxic. If a patent airway is not established first, the client may die from a myocardial infarction, stroke, or life-threatening arrhythmia. As with any emergency situation, the A (airway), B (breathing), and C (circulation) technique must be followed in that order.

Nursing process: Planning

Client need: Management of Care

Cognitive level: Analysis

Subject area: Psychiatric and Mental Health

20. The nurse is preparing to teach a class to a group of new graduate nurses on substance use disorders. Which of the following should the nurse include in the class?

   1. A client with a substance dependence must take the same drug to relieve withdrawal symptoms.

   2. A substance abuse is both a physical and psychological disorder.

   3. A client who is motivated and has a substance dependence can overcome the addiction by stopping the substance.

   4. A substance must be abused over a long period of time before an addiction develops.

21. The nurse should monitor a client who is suspected of having abused dextroamphetamine (Dexedrine) for which of the following?

   Select all that apply:

   [   ] **1.** Constipation

   [   ] **2.** Increased urine output

   [   ] **3.** Chest pain

   [   ] **4.** Pupil dilation

   [   ] **5.** Tachycardia

   [   ] **6.** Increased muscular endurance

22. The registered nurse is preparing the clinical assignments for a psychiatric unit. Which of the following assignments is appropriate for the nurse to delegate to a licensed practical nurse?

   1. Assess a client for cannabis intoxication

   2. Instruct a client on nicotine withdrawal

   3. Provide a safe environment for a client with alcohol dependence

   4. Report the clinical manifestations a client suspected of dextroamphetamine (Dexedrine) is experiencing

Answer: 2

Rationale: A substance use disorder is both physical and psychological. A client with a substance dependence can take a similar substance to relieve withdrawal clinical manifestations. A client cannot overcome a substance use disorder simply by being motivated and stopping the substance. Management of substance use disorders must include professional intervention. Generally, the most effective treatments are in mental health clinics that can provide both physical and psychological assistance. A substance abuse develops shortly after the use of the substance.

Nursing process: Planning

Client need: Health Promotion and Maintenance

Cognitive level: Application

Subject area: Psychiatric and Mental Health

Answer: 3, 4, 5

Rationale: Dextroamphetamine (Dexedrine) is a central nervous stimulant that has a high potential for abuse. Physiological manifestations of Dexedrine abuse include chest pain, tachycardia, pupil dilation, diarrhea, decreased urine output, and muscular weakness.

Nursing process: Assessment

Client need: Pharmacological and Parenteral Therapies

Cognitive level: Application

Subject area: Pharmacologic

Answer: 3

Rationale: A licensed practical nurse may provide a safe environment for a client with alcohol dependence. Assessing, instructing, and reporting are all skills reserved for a registered nurse.

Nursing process: Planning

Client need: Management of Care

Cognitive level: Analysis

Subject area: Psychiatric and Mental Health

23. The nurse is admitting a client who has been abusing phencyclidine (PCP) for several months. In planning this client's care, which of the following should be the priority?

    1. Provide a well-balanced diet

    2. Instruct the client on the medical complications of PCP abuse

    3. Encourage the client to participate in a withdrawal program

    4. Ensure the safety of the client

24. A client who is seeing "pink elephants on the wall," hearing voices, constantly picking at the face and hands, stating "people are out to kill me," and has a blood pressure of 168/90 is admitted. The nurse assesses this client to be experiencing which of the following?

    1. Amphetamine toxicity

    2. Opioid withdrawal

    3. Inhalant side effects

    4. Alcohol dependence

25. A mother brings her adolescent son into a clinic and expresses concerns that the son has been experiencing blurred vision, dizziness, a sense of euphoria, and slurred speech. Which of the following questions is a priority for the nurse to ask?

    1. "How long have you noticed these clinical manifestations and behavior?"

    2. "Has your son's school work declined?"

    3. "Is your son withdrawn and does he seem to spend more time alone?"

    4. "Have you noticed your son inhaling paint or cleaning or aerosol products?"

26. The nurse assesses which of the following in a client with a blood alcohol concentration level of 0.10? Select all that apply:

    [ ] **1.** Impaired balance and movement

    [ ] **2.** Slightly impaired judgment

    [ ] **3.** Inability to make rational decisions

    [ ] **4.** Impaired reaction time

    [ ] **5.** Impaired sense of control

    [ ] **6.** Loss of consciousness

Answer: 4

Rationale: A client who has been abusing PCP experiences distorted perceptions, hallucinations, and delusions that may result in the client becoming violent. Ensuring the client's safety is the priority. The client has the potential to hurt oneself or others. Eating a well-balanced diet, instructing the client on the medical complications of PCP, and encouraging participation in a withdrawal program are all appropriate interventions, but they are not the priority.

Nursing process: Planning

Client need: Management of Care

Cognitive level: Analysis

Subject area: Psychiatric and Mental Health

Answer: 1

Rationale: A client who has a toxic level of amphetamines experiences hallucinations (auditory, visual, and tactile), severe paranoia, picking at the face and extremities, and hypertension.

Nursing process: Assessment

Client need: Psychosocial Integrity

Cognitive level: Application

Subject area: Psychiatric and Mental Health

Answer: 4

Rationale: The priority question to ask the mother of a child suspected of inhaling substances is if she has noticed the child inhaling paint or cleaning or aerosol products.

Nursing process: Assessment

Client need: Management of Care

Cognitive level: Analysis

Subject area: Psychiatric and Mental Health

Answer: 3, 4, 5

Rationale: Inability to make rational decisions occurs with a blood alcohol concentration of 0.06. Impaired reaction time and impaired sense of control occur with a blood alcohol concentration of 0.10. A client with a blood alcohol concentration of 0.10 is legally intoxicated in most states. Slightly impaired judgment occurs with a blood alcohol concentration of 0.06. Impaired balance and movement generally appear with a blood alcohol concentration of 0.15.

Nursing process: Assessment

Client need: Psychosocial Integrity

Cognitive level: Application

Subject area: Psychiatric and Mental Health

Sexual and Gender Identity Disorders

55

1. The nurse is assessing a client with a diagnosis of hypoactive sexual desire. Which of the following characteristics is important for the nurse to assess from the history and physical?
   1. Traumatic brain injury
   2. Hormonal abnormalities
   3. An absence of sexual fantasies
   4. History of substance abuse

2. Which of the following findings would provide the nurse with the most accurate information regarding a client with sexual aversion disorder?
   1. Substance abuse problems
   2. Preoccupation with sexual encounters
   3. Gratification with sexual activity
   4. Marked distress in interpersonal functioning

3. Which of the following assessments would provide the nurse with the most accurate information regarding a client with sexual pain disorder?

   Select all that apply:
   [ ] 1. The disorder does not create distress in the client.
   [ ] 2. The client is void of sexual desire.
   [ ] 3. The disorder is found in females who have been sexually abused.
   [ ] 4. The pain is imagined.
   [ ] 5. The client may experience orgasm without penetration.
   [ ] 6. The client may experience vaginismus.

4. The nurse should instruct a client with a sexual dysfunction about drugs that have a pharmacologic influence on sexual functioning. Which of the following drugs impact sexual functioning and which drugs should the nurse include in this discussion?
   1. Antidepressants
   2. Antibiotics
   3. Analgesics
   4. Anti-inflammatories

Answer: 3

Rationale: The diagnostic criterion for hypoactive sexual drive is the absence of sexual fantasies. Hypoactive sexual desire is diagnosed if there is no substance abuse or medical condition.

Nursing process: Assessment

Client need: Psychosocial Integrity

Cognitive level: Analysis

Subject area: Psychiatric and Mental Health

Answer: 4

Rationale: Marked distress in interpersonal functioning is a criterion for the diagnosis of sexual aversion disorder. Substance abuse alone can cause sexual dysfunction; however, it does not meet the criterion for sexual aversion disorder. Avoidance, rather than preoccupation, with sexual encounters is a characteristic. Frustration, instead of gratification, is seen with sexual aversion disorder.

Nursing process: Evaluation

Client need: Psychosocial Integrity

Cognitive level: Analysis

Subject area: Psychiatric and Mental Health

Answer: 3, 5, 6

Rationale: The disorder occurs most frequently in females with a sexual abuse history. The client may experience orgasm without penetration. Vaginismus is a common clinical manifestation. The disorder creates great anxiety and distress to the client. The client is not void of desire for sexual contact. The client avoids a sexual encounter because it is a painful experience. The pain is real.

Nursing process: Assessment

Client need: Psychosocial Integrity

Cognitive level: Analysis

Subject area: Psychiatric and Mental Health

Answer: 1

Rationale: Antidepressants have a direct effect on sexual performance and result in loss of libido. Antibiotics, analgesics, and anti-inflammatories do not have an effect on sexual functioning.

Nursing process: Planning

Client need: Pharmacological and Parenteral Therapies

Cognitive level: Analysis

Subject area: Pharmacologic

5. A client with orgasmic disorder may have contributing hormonal problems. The nurse should counsel the client that which of the following factors may contribute to the disorder?

   1. Normal aging

   2. Overexercise

   3. Increase in testosterone

   4. Decrease in prolactin

6. The nurse is collecting a nursing history from a client admitted with a sexual dysfunction. Which of the following questions is a priority for the nurse to ask?

   1. "What is your age?"

   2. "What medications do you take?"

   3. "Do you have anxiety about sexual performance?"

   4. "What is your exercise regime?"

7. The nurse is teaching a client with a sexual dysfunction. Which of the following elements would be the most critical for the nurse to teach the client about the disorder?

   1. Mutual respect between partners is crucial.

   2. Gender preference influences sexual dysfunction.

   3. Avoiding drugs will alleviate sexual dysfunction.

   4. Power struggles between partners do not influence sexual dysfunction.

8. Which of the following assessments would provide the nurse with the most accurate information regarding a client with gender identity disorder? Assess and evaluate if the client

   1. is homosexual.

   2. has been sexually abused.

   3. had an early feeling of being trapped in the wrong gender.

   4. has a strong aversion to same-sex individuals.

Answer: 1

Rationale: Normal aging can contribute to the slowing of an orgasm in orgasmic disorder. Exercise is not a factor in orgasmic disorder. Decreases in testosterone may contribute to orgasmic disorder. Increase in prolactin may contribute to orgasmic disorders.

Nursing process: Planning

Client need: Psychosocial Integrity

Cognitive level: Application

Subject area: Psychiatric and Mental Health

Answer: 3

Rationale: Anxiety is the factor that most dramatically affects sexual dysfunction, so it would be a priority to ask if the client has anxiety about sexual performance. The client's age, drugs that the client takes, and the client's exercise regime may contribute to a sexual dysfunction but do not qualify as the priority for it.

Nursing process: Assessment

Client need: Management of Care

Cognitive level: Analysis

Subject area: Psychiatric and Mental Health

Answer: 1

Rationale: Establishing mutual respect is critical between partners being treated for sexual dysfunctions. Preferences of gender do not contribute to sexual dysfunctions. Drugs may precipitate sexual dysfunctions, but they are not the priority. Power struggles between partners do contribute to sexual dysfunctions.

Nursing process: Analysis

Client need: Psychosocial Integrity

Cognitive level: Analysis

Subject area: Psychiatric and Mental Health

Answer: 3

Rationale: An early feeling of being trapped in the wrong gender is the diagnostic criterion for establishing the diagnosis of gender identity disorder. The sexual preference of the individual does not contribute to the disorder. The client's history of abuse also is not a diagnostic criterion for the disorder. Aversion to individuals who are of the same sex is also not a criterion for gender identity disorder.

Nursing process: Assessment

Client need: Psychosocial Integrity

Cognitive level: Application

Subject area: Psychiatric and Mental Health

9. When the nurse is assessing a client for the possibility of gender identity disorder, which of the following clinical manifestations would support the diagnosis?

Select all that apply:

[   ] **1.** Having playmates of the same sex

[   ] **2.** No particular preference for cross-sex role-play

[   ] **3.** Anxiety that accompanies puberty

[   ] **4.** Development of secondary sex characteristics

[   ] **5.** Unconcerned about the disorder

[   ] **6.** Preoccupation with the client's sex

10. A client is admitted to the psychiatric unit with a possible diagnosis of paraphilia. When conducting an assessment, which clinical manifestations would indicate to the nurse that the diagnosis was correct?

1. A disorder with a 3-month duration

2. Recurrent fantasy triggered by stress

3. A persistent disinterest in sex

4. A significant loss of libido

11. The nurse assessing a client with the diagnosis of voyeurism should note which of the following characteristics?

1. Socially skilled individual

2. Peeping becomes compulsive

3. Usually not heterosexual

4. Has many close friends

12. Which of the following assessments would provide the nurse with the most accurate information about a client with transvestism?

1. A desire for a sex change

2. Enjoyment in watching others disrobe

3. Homosexual orientation

4. Develops early in life

Answer: 3, 4, 6

Rationale: Puberty and secondary sex characteristics often produce great anxiety in a client with gender identity disorder. Playmates of the opposite sex are preferred. There is a particular preference for cross-sex role-play. Clients with gender identity disorder are preoccupied with their sex identity and highly concerned about the disorder.

Nursing process: Assessment

Client need: Psychosocial Integrity

Cognitive level: Application

Subject area: Psychiatric and Mental Health

Answer: 2

Rationale: Paraphilia is a disorder of sexual interest, arousal, and orgasm. A recurrent fantasy involving inanimate objects is triggered by stress. The disorder needs to last 6 months in order to meet the diagnostic criterion. There is a persistent interest in sex. There is no loss of libido.

Nursing process: Assessment

Client need: Psychosocial Integrity

Cognitive level: Application

Subject area: Psychiatric and Mental Health

Answer: 2

Rationale: Voyeurism is a sexual disorder that involves watching others disrobe, naked, or engaging in various sexual acts. Peeping becomes compulsive and is preferable to other sexual activities. The individual is usually heterosexual, unskilled, and socially shy. Such individuals usually have few close friends.

Nursing process: Assessment

Client need: Psychosocial Integrity

Cognitive level: Application

Subject area: Psychiatric and Mental Health

Answer: 4

Rationale: Transvestism is a disorder that involves cross dressing or fantasies about cross dressing. It develops early in life. There is no desire for a sex change or for a change in the client's sexual orientation.

Nursing process: Assessment

Client need: Psychosocial Integrity

Cognitive level: Application

Subject area: Psychiatric and Mental Health

13. The nurse treating a client with paraphilia would include which of the following in the care plan?

1. Alternative medicine
2. Residential treatment
3. Short-term therapy
4. Combination therapy

14. The nurse treating a client with sexual addictions should assess for which of the following clinical manifestations when formulating the nursing assessment?

1. The client understands the behavior
2. Patterns of unsuccessful love relationships
3. Need to develop relationship after sexual contact
4. Is not a compulsion

15. When working with the client who has a sexual addiction, the nurse should include which of the following in the nursing care plan?

1. Recommendation for individual and group therapy
2. Avoid groups with similar diagnosis
3. Limit number of friends to small close unit
4. Community support is not a priority

16. The nurse planning care for the client with a sexual addiction would understand that the client is at risk for sexually transmitted disease. What is a priority to include in this client's care plan? _____

Answer: 4

Rationale: The recommended treatment for paraphilia is a combination of therapies. Alternative medicine and residential treatment are not recommended. Therapy should be conducted over an extended period of time.

Nursing process: Planning

Client need: Psychosocial Integrity

Cognitive level: Application

Subject area: Psychiatric and Mental Health

Answer: 2

Rationale: Patterns of unsuccessful love relationships are diagnostic for sexual addictions. The client is bewildered by personal behavior. The client feels a need to escape after sex and is compelled to have frequent sex.

Nursing process: Assessment

Client need: Psychosocial Integrity

Cognitive level: Application

Subject area: Psychiatric and Mental Health

Answer: 1

Rationale: Recommendations for individual and group therapy should be made for clients with sexual addictions. Group therapy is a recommendation. Friendships should not be limited but should be encouraged. A safe and supportive community is essential for client recovery.

Nursing process: Planning

Client need: Psychosocial Integrity

Cognitive level: Application

Subject area: Psychiatric and Mental Health

Answer: Educate the client about safe sex

Rationale: The priority intervention when working with a client who has a sexual addiction is to educate the client about safe sex practice. It is imperative to inform the client about the use of condoms and dental dams and the avoidance of multiple partners. The focus of nursing care should be holistic and preventive rather than disease oriented.

Nursing process: Planning

Client need: Management of Care

Cognitive level: Application

Subject area: Psychiatric and Mental Health

17. The nurse evaluates which of the following disorders to contribute to the severity of a sexual disorder?

    1. Schizophrenia

    2. Bipolar disorder

    3. Diabetes

    4. Anorexia

18. Which of the following drugs does the nurse evaluate to contribute to the development of a sexual disorder? Select all that apply:

    [ ] **1.** Hypertensives

    [ ] **2.** Phenothiazines

    [ ] **3.** Antidepressants

    [ ] **4.** Antibiotics

    [ ] **5.** Cholinergics

    [ ] **6.** Histamine H_2 antagonists

19. The nurse planning for the discharge of a client with sexual dysfunction would take into consideration which of the following measures?

    1. The client will have trusting relationships.

    2. The client's judgment may be clouded by perceptual defenses.

    3. Judgmental thoughts are crucial for recovery.

    4. Power struggles are inevitable and are a key to cure.

20. The most effective treatment tool the nurse should use when working with a client with sexual disorders is

    1. the complete general history.

    2. the sexual disorders history.

    3. drug management.

    4. family therapy.

Answer: 3

Rationale: Diabetes is a physical illness that interferes with sexual functioning. Schizophrenia, bipolar disorder, and anorexia do not contribute to the severity of a sexual disorder.

Nursing process: Evaluation

Client need: Psychosocial Integrity

Cognitive level: Analysis

Subject area: Psychiatric and Mental Health

Answer: 1, 2, 3

Rationale: Hypertensives, phenothiazines, and antidepressants are all drugs that contribute to sexual dysfunction and may result in an impairment such as impotence. Drugs that cause a decrease in androgen levels, such as these, will create problems with sexual functioning.

Nursing process: Evaluation

Client need: Pharmacological and Parenteral Therapies

Cognitive level: Application

Subject area: Pharmacologic

Answer: 2

Rationale: The judgment of a client with a sexual dysfunction may be clouded by perceptual as well as intellectual defenses. The client will need to develop trusting relationships. Recovery is contingent on nonjudgmental thoughts by the nurse and partner. Power struggles with the partner are to be avoided so that recovery can occur.

Nursing process: Planning

Client need: Psychosocial Integrity

Cognitive level: Analysis

Subject area: Psychiatric and Mental Health

Answer: 1

Rationale: The complete general history is crucial to treatment of the whole individual dealing with a sexual disorder. The sexual disorders history will not give clues into underlying or contributing factors. Drug management is not as important as understanding of the whole person. Family therapy alone will not give a full picture.

Nursing process: Planning

Client need: Psychosocial Integrity

Cognitive level: Application

Subject area: Psychiatric and Mental Health

21. When working with a client with hypoactive sexual desire disorder, the nurse should include which of the following recommendations in the treatment plan?

    1. Substance abuse counseling

    2. Treatment for a medical condition

    3. Encourage the client to focus on the disorder

    4. Establish a therapeutic alliance

22. The nurse planning the treatment for a client with aversion disorder considers which of the following in the care plan?

    1. Medical conditions are the etiology.

    2. Interpersonal functioning is a low priority.

    3. Anxiety and disgust contribute to distress.

    4. Aversion is not a part of the disorder.

23. The nurse developing a treatment plan for a client with gender identity disorder would include which of the following measures?

    1. Short-term therapy

    2. Drugs to control dysphoria

    3. Counseling for coping solutions

    4. Legal counseling

24. Which of the following clinical manifestations would the nurse assess as most prevalent in a client suspected of having contracted chlamydia?

    1. Discharge from the genitals

    2. Generalized body aches

    3. Intermittent discomfort when urinating

    4. Spontaneous remission

Answer: 4

Rationale: The most important treatment strategy in working with a client who has hypoactive sexual desire is the establishment of a therapeutic alliance. Substance abuse precludes the client from meeting diagnostic criteria. The existence of a medical condition also precludes the diagnosis of hypoactive sexual disorder. Focusing on the disorder increases anxiety and may exacerbate the clinical manifestations.

Nursing process: Planning

Client need: Psychosocial Integrity

Cognitive level: Application

Subject area: Psychiatric and Mental Health

Answer: 3

Rationale: Anxiety, disgust, or fear for the sexual encounter contributes to extreme psychological distress in a client with aversion disorder. The existence of a medical condition does not meet the diagnostic category. Interpersonal functioning is critical for the remission of the disorder. Aversion and avoidance are classic criteria.

Nursing process: Assessment

Client need: Psychosocial Integrity

Cognitive level: Application

Subject area: Psychiatric and Mental Health

Answer: 3

Rationale: Counseling for coping solutions is essential for the client suffering from gender identity disorder. Therapy is long term. Therapy, rather than drugs, is recommended for control of dysphoria. Legal counseling is appropriate when gender assignment is the only option.

Nursing process: Planning

Client need: Psychosocial Integrity

Cognitive level: Application

Subject area: Psychiatric and Mental Health

Answer: 1

Rationale: Discharge from the genitals is a clinical manifestation of chlamydia. General body aches is not a clinical manifestation. Persistent burning on urination is a clinical manifestation. Treatment involves antibiotics and there is no spontaneous remission.

Nursing process: Assessment

Client need: Physiological Adaptation

Cognitive level: Application

Subject area: Medical-Surgical

25. When assessing a client suspected of having hepatitis B, which of the following clinical manifestations support the diagnosis?

1. Unprotected sexual contact
2. Malnutrition
3. Fecal-oral route
4. Sexual addiction

26. The registered nurse is preparing clinical assignments for a psychiatric unit. Which of the following clinical assignments should the nurse delegate to a licensed practical nurse?

1. Perform a complete general history on a client with gender identity disorder
2. Assess a client with aversion disorder for distress
3. Develop a plan of care for a client with gender identity disorder
4. Document the behavior exhibited by a client with gender identity disorder

Answer: 1

Rationale: Unprotected sexual contact is a route for hepatitis B. Malnutrition does not contribute to hepatitis B. Fecal-oral route relates to hepatitis A. Clients with sexual addiction may or may not contract hepatitis B.

Nursing process: Assessment

Client need: Physiological Adaptation

Cognitive level: Application

Subject area: Medical-Surgical

Answer: 4

Rationale: Documenting the behavior exhibited by a client with gender identity disorder may be delegated to a licensed practical nurse. Performing a complete general history, assessing a client, and developing a plan of care are all assignments that should be performed by a registered nurse.

Nursing process: Planning

Client need: Management of Care

Cognitive level: Analysis

Subject area: Psychiatric and Mental Health

Eating Disorders

56

1. The nurse is teaching a class on eating disorders to a group of nurses. Which of the following should the nurse include in the class?

    1. Eating disorders affect females and males equally.

    2. There is an increased incidence of depression in clients with eating disorders.

    3. There is no mother-daughter connection in eating disorders.

    4. There is a 20% chance of dysthymias in clients with eating disorders.

2. The nurse should monitor a client with an eating disorder for which of the following complications? Select all that apply:

    [ ] 1. Hypertension

    [ ] 2. Dysmenorrhea

    [ ] 3. Parotid swelling

    [ ] 4. Delayed gastric emptying

    [ ] 5. Bradycardia

    [ ] 6. Dysthymias

3. The nurse administers which of the following drugs to a client with an eating disorder who has a delayed gastric emptying time?

    1. Esomeprazole (Nexium)

    2. Metoclopramide (Reglan)

    3. Dicyclomine (Bentyl)

    4. Diphenoxylate with atropine sulfate (Lomotil)

4. The nurse is planning the care for a client with muscle weakness, constipation, a serum potassium of 3.0 mEq/L, and a pulse of 65 bpm. What clinical manifestation should take priority in this client's plan of care? _____

Answer: 2

Rationale: Although the incidence of eating disorders is increasing in male clients, the incidence is much higher in females. There is an increased incidence of depression found in clients with eating disorders. Dysthymias or major depressive episodes have a 50 to 75% incidence of being found. There is a theory of a possible mother-daughter connection.

Nursing process: Planning

Client need: Psychosocial Integrity

Cognitive level: Application

Subject area: Psychiatric and Mental Health

Answer: 3, 4, 5, 6

Rationale: Clients who have eating disorders may experience postural hypotension, amenorrhea, parotid swelling, delayed gastric emptying, bradycardia, and dysthymias.

Nursing process: Assessment

Client need: Psychosocial Integrity

Cognitive level: Application

Subject area: Psychiatric and Mental Health

Answer: 2

Rationale: Esomeprazole (Nexium) is a proton pump inhibitor used in the short-term management of gastroesophageal reflux (GERD). Metoclopramide (Reglan) is a gastrointestinal stimulant used in the treatment of delayed gastric emptying and gastroesophageal reflux. Dicyclomine (Bentyl) is a cholinergic blocking drug used in the treatment of hypermotility and spasms of the gastrointestinal tract associated with irritable colon and spastic colon. Diphenoxylate with atropine sulfate (Lomotil) is an antidiarrheal used in the management of diarrhea.

Nursing process: Implementation

Client need: Pharmacological and Parenteral Therapies

Cognitive level: Application

Subject area: Pharmacologic

Answer: Serum potassium of 3.0 mEq/L

Rationale: Although a client with an eating disorder may have muscle weakness, constipation, and bradycardia, it is the serum potassium of 3.0 mEq/L that should be the priority. Generally a client with a serum potassium level of 3.0 mEq/L would be hospitalized. Severe hypokalemia may lead to dysrhythmias and subsequent death. Normal potassium is 3.5 to 5.0 mEq/L.

Nursing process: Planning

Client need: Management of Care

Cognitive level: Analysis

Subject area: Psychiatric and Mental Health

5. The nurse is admitting a client with bulimia who has been using syrup of ipecac to induce vomiting. What life-threatening complication is a priority for the nurse to monitor this client for? _____

6. The nurse administers which of the following prescribed drugs to a client with anorexia nervosa for the purpose of improving weight gain?

  1. Olanzapine (Zyprexa)

  2. Sertraline (Zoloft)

  3. Fluoxetine (Prozac)

  4. Quetiapine (Seroquel)

7. Which of the following statements would provide the nurse with the most accurate information regarding how successful the treatment has been for a client with a long-standing history of bulimia?

  1. "I take my medicine when I have an urge to binge."

  2. "I try to do other things when I feel I want to eat."

  3. "I have learned to eat a variety of foods."

  4. "I no longer feel the need to see my therapist."

Answer: Cardiomyopathy

Rationale: Syrup of ipecac is sometimes used to induce vomiting after certain types of poisoning. Vomiting generally occurs within 20 minutes of ingestion of the ipecac. Although muscle weakness and hypokalemia are adverse reactions to ipecac abuse, the most serious and life-threatening complication is cardiomyopathy. Cardiomyopathy indicates that the client is suffering from ipecac toxicity.

Nursing process: Assessment

Client need: Management of Care

Cognitive level: Analysis

Subject area: Psychiatric and Mental Health

Answer: 3

Rationale: Olanzapine (Zyprexa) is an antipsychotic used in the management of anorexia nervosa to enhance compliance with treatment and decrease agitation. Sertraline (Zoloft) is a selective serotonin reuptake inhibitor used to decrease binge episodes in clients with a binge eating disorder (obesity). Fluoxetine (Prozac) is a selective serotonin reuptake inhibitor used to improve weight gain in the client with anorexia nervosa. Quetiapine (Seroquel) is an antipsychotic used in the treatment of schizophrenia.

Nursing process: Implementation

Client need: Pharmacological and Parenteral Therapies

Cognitive level: Analysis

Subject area: Pharmacologic

Answer: 3

Rationale: A client who has bulimia and is able to verbalize eating a variety of foods is showing success with treatment. Eating a variety of foods eliminates the myth that there are forbidden foods and the key to success is proportion. A client should not take prescribed medicine only when responding to an urge to binge. Medicine must be taken regularly until the therapist deems it is no longer necessary. Trying to do other things when feeling the urge to binge is a positive step, but it does not indicate success. A client cannot merely try to do other things when feeling the desire to eat. Success would be measured in being successful doing other tasks instead of eating. It is not a positive step for a client to say there is no longer a need to see the therapist. Seeing the therapist should be a regular commitment and not a capricious phenomenon.

Nursing process: Evaluation

Client need: Psychosocial Integrity

Cognitive level: Analysis

Subject area: Psychiatric and Mental Health

8. The nurse is caring for a 25-year-old client with an eating disorder who is in the hospital. The physician ordered periodic laboratory tests to monitor the client's medical status. Which of the following serum laboratory tests should the nurse notify the physician are abnormal?

   1. Calcium of 9.2 mg/dl
   2. Magnesium of 1.8 mEq/L
   3. Potassium of 3.0 mEq/L
   4. Sodium of 128 mEq/L

9. The nurse is collecting data on an 11-year-old client suspected of having anorexia nervosa. Which of the following physical assessment findings should be reported to the client's physician confirming the presence of anorexia nervosa?

   1. A temperature of 37.2°C (99°F)
   2. A pulse of 72 bpm
   3. The presence of lanugo
   4. Dysmenorrhea

10. During an admission interview, a client with anorexia nervosa complains of feeling cold all the time and asks the nurse why. Which of the following is the most appropriate response by the nurse?

    1. "Let me take your temperature."
    2. "You might be getting a cold."
    3. "There is a loss of subcutaneous fat."
    4. "You probably aren't dressing warmly enough."

Answer: 4

Rationale: Routine serum laboratory tests are performed on all clients with eating disorders. Routine tests include calcium, magnesium, potassium, and sodium tests. Normal serum calcium is 9.0 to 10.5 mg/dl. Normal serum magnesium is 1.3 to 2.1 mEq/L. Normal serum potassium is 3.0 to 5.0 mEq/L. Normal serum sodium is 136 to 145 mEq/L.

Nursing process: Analysis

Client need: Psychosocial Integrity

Cognitive level: Analysis

Subject area: Psychiatric and Mental Health

Answer: 3

Rationale: A client with anorexia nervosa generally will exhibit hypothermia, bradycardia, lanugo, and amenorrhea. However, an 11-year-old client with anorexia nervosa may have not started menses and certainly has not had menses long enough to establish a pattern.

Nursing process: Analysis

Client need: Psychosocial Integrity

Cognitive level: Application

Subject area: Psychiatric and Mental Health

Answer: 3

Rationale: Clients who have a history of anorexia frequently complain of feeling cold all the time that is unrelated to weather and clothing. Hypothermia is the result of dehydration or a loss of subcutaneous tissue.

Nursing process: Analysis

Client need: Psychosocial Integrity

Cognitive level: Analysis

Subject area: Psychiatric and Mental Health

11. The nurse should include which of the following interventions in the plan of care for a client with a binge eating disorder?

Select all that apply:

[   ] 1. Encourage the client to keep a diary of food and feelings

[   ] 2. Encourage the client to gain 1/2 pound a week

[   ] 3. Instruct the client to avoid fasting

[   ] 4. Instruct the client that high-calorie foods are to be avoided

[   ] 5. Encourage the client to plan for structured meals

[   ] 6. Instruct the client on well-balanced nutrition

12. The nurse is interviewing a 46-year-old female client with a binge eating disorder who is tearful and admits to the nurse of being depressed. The client states, "I have been fat all my life and I can't lose weight." Which of the following should be the priority response by the nurse?

1. "In order to lose weight, you need to stop binging."

2. "You need to eat a well-balanced diet."

3. "Cognitive behavioral therapy offers the most success."

4. "You will lose weight if you take your sertraline (Zoloft)."

13. The registered nurse is delegating clinical assignments on an eating disorder unit for the day. Which of the following clinical assignments would be appropriate for the nurse to delegate to a licensed practical nurse?

1. Develop a class to be taught on eating disorders

2. Instruct a client with bulimia on the medication

3. Create a meal plan for a client with anorexia nervosa

4. Monitor a client with an eating disorder after meals

Answer: 1, 3, 5, 6

Rationale: Binge eating, also known as obesity, is an eating disorder not otherwise specified. A client with this disorder does not use a compensatory mechanism such as laxatives or diuretics or resort to purging. A client with a binge disorder is overweight and does not need to gain weight. The client should be instructed to avoid fasting because fasting leads to binging. The client should be informed on well-balanced nutrition and that there are no "forbidden foods." Avoiding the concept of "forbidden foods" eliminates the trigger to binge. The client should be instructed that the key to weight maintenance is a balance in the proportion of food and exercise. The client should be encouraged to plan for structured meals.

Nursing process: Planning

Client need: Psychosocial Integrity

Cognitive level: Application

Subject area: Psychiatric and Mental Health

Answer: 3

Rationale: Although a client with a binge eating disorder needs to stop binging and eat a well-balanced diet, the best chance for recovery from a binge eating disorder is cognitive behavioral therapy. Sertraline (Zoloft) is a selective reuptake inhibitor used in binge eating disorders for the purpose of decreasing the binge episodes.

Nursing process: Analysis

Client need: Management of Care

Cognitive level: Analysis

Subject area: Psychiatric and Mental Health

Answer: 4

Rationale: It would be acceptable to delegate monitoring a client with an eating disorder after meals. Only a registered nurse can develop, create, and instruct a client.

Nursing process: Planning

Client need: Management of Care

Cognitive level: Analysis

Subject area: Legal and Ethical Issues

14. A client with anorexia nervosa is crying and tells the nurse, "I just want to die. I can't live like this anymore." In determining what action to take next, which of the following factors is a priority for the nurse to consider?

1. How long the client has been feeling this way

2. The recovery rate with treatment

3. If the client has a suicide plan

4. If the client has a support system

15. The nurse is signing a hospitalized client with bulimia back in after a day pass at home. Which of the following should be the nurse's priority action?

1. Ask the client about any special activities while out on pass

2. Obtain a detailed menu of what was eaten

3. Search the client's belonging for laxatives or diuretics

4. Question the client about any binge and purge behavior at home

16. The nurse is collecting a health history from a 25-year-old client suspected of having an eating disorder. Which of the following questions is a priority question for the nurse to ask the client?

1. "Is your father away from home a lot working?"

2. "Do any siblings have issues with food?"

3. "Does your mother have an eating disorder?"

4. "Do you have a friend who has a body image problem?"

17. The family of a male client suspected of having an eating disorder asks the nurse how their son can have an eating disorder because eating disorders only occur in women. Which of the following is the most appropriate response by the nurse?

1. "Your son is very slender for his height."

2. "Your son has a poor appetite."

3. "The incidence of eating disorders is increasing in males."

4. "Food-related problems in males are different from eating disorders."

Answer: 3

Rationale: The priority action to take with any client who is threatening suicide is to assess the client for a detailed suicide plan. After assessing whether the client is serious and has developed a plan, it would be appropriate to assess how long the client has felt this way and whether the client has a support system. As with any disorder, the chance of recovery is greater with treatment.

Nursing process: Analysis

Client need: Management of Care

Cognitive level: Analysis

Subject area: Psychiatric and Mental Health

Answer: 3

Rationale: The priority action for the nurse to take when signing a client in from a pass at home is to search the client's belongings for laxatives, diuretics, or ipecac that the client can hide and use while in the hospital. Asking what the client did on pass, what was eaten, or if there was any difficulty with binging and purging behavior is relevant, but not the priority.

Nursing process: Planning

Client need: Management of Care

Cognitive level: Application

Subject area: Psychiatric and Mental Health

Answer: 3

Rationale: Although a father who works a lot and is away from home, a sibling with food issues, and a friend with a body image problem may be important for the well-being of a client with an eating disorder, the priority is the mother-daughter connection. Theory exists questioning a possible mother-daughter connection as having the greatest impact on the client's relationship with food.

Nursing process: Assessment

Client need: Management of Care

Cognitive level: Analysis

Subject area: Psychiatric and Mental Health

Answer: 3

Rationale: Although eating disorders are generally the domain of females, the incidence in males is increasing.

Nursing process: Analysis

Client need: Psychosocial Integrity

Cognitive level: Analysis

Subject area: Psychiatric and Mental Health

18. The nurse is caring for a client with anorexia nervosa. Which of the following interventions should the nurse include in this client's plan of care?

Select all that apply:

[   ] **1.** Encourage the client to eat when hungry

[   ] **2.** Limit mealtime to 1 hour

[   ] **3.** Monitor the client for 30 minutes after eating

[   ] **4.** Weigh the client two to three times a week

[   ] **5.** Promote a weight gain of 3 to 5 pounds a week

[   ] **6.** Restrict exercise if the target weight is not maintained

19. The nurse is admitting a client with anorexia nervosa to the hospital based on which of the following criteria?

Select all that apply:

[   ] **1.** A systolic blood pressure of 90 mm Hg

[   ] **2.** A loss of 20% of body weight

[   ] **3.** A temperature of 35.4°C (95.8°F)

[   ] **4.** A serum potassium level of 2.8 mEq/L

[   ] **5.** A pulse of 60 beats per minute

[   ] **6.** Failure to gain weight

20. Which of the nursing diagnoses is appropriate for the nurse to include in the plan of care for a client with a binge disorder?

1. Ineffective thermoregulation

2. Risk for self-mutilation

3. Ineffective health maintenance

4. Anxiety

21. The nurse administers which of the following drugs to a client with a binge eating disorder for the purpose of decreasing the binge episodes?

1. Sertraline (Zoloft)

2. Olanzapine (Zyprexa)

3. Amitriptyline (Elavil)

4. Imipramine (Tofranil)

Answer: 4, 5, 6

Rationale: A highly structured mealtime with scheduled meals is important to include in the plan of care for a client with anorexia nervosa. Mealtime should be limited to 30 minutes. The client should be monitored for up to 1 hour after meals to prevent hoarding of food or purging. Exercise is limited if the target weight is not maintained. The client is generally weighed two to three times a week at a regularly scheduled time and wearing similar clothing. A weight gain of 3 to 5 pounds a week is the goal.

Nursing process: Planning

Client need: Psychosocial Integrity

Cognitive level: Application

Subject area: Psychiatric and Mental Health

Answer: 3, 4, 6

Rationale: Criteria for admission to the hospital for a client with anorexia nervosa include a rapid loss of weight equivalent to 30% of body weight in over 6 months, a failure to gain weight in an outpatient setting, a temperature of less than 36°C (96.8°F), a serum potassium level of less than 3 mEq/L, a systolic blood pressure of less than 70 mm Hg, a pulse of less than 40 beats per minute, and dysrhythmias.

Nursing process: Implementation

Client need: Psychosocial Integrity

Cognitive level: Analysis

Subject area: Psychiatric and Mental Health

Answer: 4

Rationale: An appropriate nursing diagnosis for a client with a binge disorder is anxiety. A client with a binge disorder feels a great deal of distress over the binge behavior. Ineffective thermoregulation and risk for health maintenance are nursing diagnoses appropriate for bulimia.

Nursing process: Planning

Client need: Psychosocial Integrity

Cognitive level: Application

Subject area: Psychiatric and Mental Health

Answer: 1

Rationale: Selective serotonin reuptake inhibitors, such as sertraline (Zoloft), are used to decrease the binge episodes in a client with a binge eating disorder. Olanzapine (Zyprexa) is an antipsychotic that may be used to increase cooperation with treatment and promote weight gain in a client with anorexia nervosa. Amitriptyline (Elavil) and imipramine (Tofranil) are tricyclic antidepressants used in the treatment of depression.

Nursing process: Implementation

Client need: Pharmacological and Parenteral Therapies

Cognitive level: Application

Subject area: Pharmacologic

22. A client with anorexia nervosa who is emaciated is crying and tells the nurse, "I feel so fat when I look in the mirror." Which of the following is the priority response for the nurse?

   1. "You shouldn't look in the mirror if it upsets you."

   2. "You are 30% below your body weight."

   3. "It must be very frightening to feel fat."

   4. "Ask another person for another opinion."

23. The nurse is caring for a client with bulimia who informs the nurse of an unpleasant tingling of the hands and around the mouth and muscular spasms. The nurse should notify the physician of which of the following suspected disorders?

   1. Cushing's syndrome

   2. Addison's disease

   3. Hyperthyroidism

   4. Tetany

24. The nurse is evaluating the medical records of the following four clients. It is essential that the nurse report which of the following clients immediately?

   1. A client with anorexia nervosa who has a pulse of 55 beats per minute

   2. A client with bulimia who has a serum potassium of 3.5 mEq/L

   3. A client with anorexia who has a systolic blood pressure of 90 mm Hg

   4. A client with bulimia who has a serum calcium of 8.6 mg/dl

Answer: 3

Rationale: A client who has anorexia and is emaciated has a body weight of less than 30% of the normal body weight. Telling the client not to look in the mirror serves no purpose, because it is most likely an unrealistic goal. The client is obsessed with body image and frequently checks it in the mirror. Asking another person for another opinion also serves no purpose, because the client is obsessed with body size and most likely won't trust another person's opinion. The most effective intervention is for the nurse to be supportive of the client's self-image and to encourage the client to verbalize a fear of being fat.

Nursing process: Analysis

Client need: Management of Care

Cognitive level: Analysis

Subject area: Psychiatric and Mental Health

Answer: 4

Rationale: Tetany is a neuromuscular excitability associated with a critical decrease in the body's calcium level. An unpleasant tingling of the hands and around the mouth and muscular spasms are characteristic of tetany. If emergency treatment is not begun, laryngospasms may develop.

Nursing process: Analysis

Client need: Psychosocial Integrity

Cognitive level: Analysis

Subject area: Psychiatric and Mental Health

Answer: 4

Rationale: It is essential that the nurse report a client with bulimia who has a serum calcium level of 8.6 mg/dl. Normal serum calcium is 9.0 to 10.5 mg/dl. A client with a low calcium level is at risk for developing tetany, which can be a life-threatening condition. Although a client with anorexia nervosa who has a pulse of 55 beats per minute and a systolic blood pressure of 90 mm Hg has bradycardia and hypotension, reporting these is not as critical as impending tetany. A serum potassium of 3.5 mEq/L is within the normal range.

Nursing process: Analysis

Client need: Psychosocial Integrity

Cognitive level: Analysis

Subject area: Psychiatric and Mental Health

25. The nurse should monitor a client with bulimia for which of the following clinical manifestations of hypokalemia?

Select all that apply:

[   ] **1.** Hypotension

[   ] **2.** Weak, thready pulse

[   ] **3.** Diarrhea

[   ] **4.** Hyperreflexia

[   ] **5.** Decreased urinary output

[   ] **6.** Shallow respirations

Answer: 1, 2, 6

Rationale: Clinical manifestations of hypokalemia include hypotension; a weak, thready pulse; constipation; hyporeflexia; increased urinary output; and shallow respirations.

Nursing process: Assessment

Client need: Psychosocial Integrity

Cognitive level: Application

Subject area: Psychiatric and Mental Health

Gerontologic Nursing

CHAPTER

Health Issues of the Older Adult

57

1. A 92-year-old client with emphysema is experiencing chest pain. The nurse determines with a pulse oximetry that the oxygen saturation is 83%. The nurse understands that it is essential that oxygen be administered by nasal cannula at which of the following rates?

   1. 8 L/minute
   2. 2 L/minute
   3. 5 L/minute
   4. 12 L/minute

2. An 86-year-old client has sustained a fractured femur and has had surgery to repair the fracture. The client is rubbing the surgical site and moaning. Which of the following is the priority nursing intervention?

   1. Administer the prescribed pain medication
   2. Assess the client's pain level
   3. Determine when the client last had pain medication
   4. Inspect the surgical site

3. Which of the following is the appropriate assessment for respiratory depression in the older adult after the administration of an opioid for analgesia? Respiratory depression is

   1. more likely after several doses of the same drug.
   2. most likely after the first dose.
   3. unlikely because the opioid is not prescribed for the older adult in large doses.
   4. unlikely if the drug is given orally.

4. A 73-year-old client has just undergone a colostomy for cancer of the colon. The client tells the nurse the pain is "8" on a scale of 0 to 10. Which of the following is the expected outcome of the nursing care for this client?

   1. The client does not ask for pain medication.
   2. The client self-medicates with an over-the-counter medication.
   3. The client verbalizes satisfaction with the level of pain and pain control.
   4. The client states the pain is "4" on a scale of 0 to 10.

Answer: 2

Rationale: In emphysema, the drive to breathe will be decreased or eliminated if oxygen is administered at a high rate. The best and safest initial rate of oxygen flow is 2 L to 3 L/minute. If higher flow rates are administered, the client may need artificial ventilation.

Nursing process: Analysis

Client need: Reduction of Risk Potential

Cognitive level: Analysis

Subject area: Gerontologic

Answer: 2

Rationale: Older adults may rub or pat a painful area rather than verbalize the pain. The priority intervention is to assess the client's pain level by asking the client. Administering pain medications, determining when the client had the last pain medication, and inspecting the surgical site are all appropriate interventions, but only after the current level of pain is assessed.

Nursing process: Implementation

Client need: Management of Care

Cognitive level: Application

Subject area: Gerontologic

Answer: 2

Rationale: Depending on the pain level, large doses may be prescribed for older adults. If a client is very sensitive to an opioid, the resulting respiratory depression is most likely to occur after the first dose. The route of administration will not decrease the likelihood of respiratory depression.

Nursing process: Assessment

Client need: Pharmacological and Parenteral Therapies

Cognitive level: Analysis

Subject area: Pharmacologic

Answer: 3

Rationale: An older adult in severe pain may not ask for pain medication because of a reluctance to "complain." The nurse cannot determine for the client what is an acceptable level of pain. A good outcome is achieved when the client can verbalize satisfaction with the level of pain and pain control.

Nursing process: Evaluation

Client need: Basic Care and Comfort

Cognitive level: Analysis

Subject area: Gerontologic

5. The nurse assesses which of the following physiological manifestations as indicating that the client is experiencing acute pain?

Select all that apply:

[   ] **1.** Verbalization of pain

[   ] **2.** Crying

[   ] **3.** Hypertension

[   ] **4.** Flushing

[   ] **5.** Tachycardia

[   ] **6.** Moist skin

6. The nurse assesses a 67-year-old client suspected of having a cataract for which of the following clinical manifestations?

Select all that apply:

[   ] **1.** Halos around lights

[   ] **2.** Decrease in vision

[   ] **3.** Eye pain

[   ] **4.** Abnormal color perception

[   ] **5.** Glare

[   ] **6.** Headache

7. The nurse is establishing the goal for the care of a 93-year-old client who experienced a cerebral vascular accident (CVA) two weeks ago and is hospitalized on a rehabilitation unit. What is the appropriate goal associated with rehabilitation? _____

8. The nurse assesses a 92-year-old client who has experienced a recent cerebral vascular accident (CVA) with a cranial nerve VII dysfunction to be exhibiting which of the following manifestations?

1. Loss of sense of smell

2. Ptosis

3. Difficulty in swallowing

4. Asymmetry of facial features

Answer: 3, 5

Rationale: Hypertension and tachycardia are physiological manifestations of acute pain. Crying and verbalizing pain are psychological or emotional manifestations of pain. When a client is in acute pain, the skin is more likely to cool and pale.

Nursing process: Assessment

Client need: Physiological Adaptation

Cognitive level: Application

Subject area: Gerontologic

Answer: 2, 4, 5

Rationale: A decrease in vision, abnormal color perception, and glare are clinical manifestations with cataracts. Halos around lights are common in glaucoma. Eye pain and headaches may be present in a variety of other eye disorders.

Nursing process: Assessment

Client need: Physiological Adaptation

Cognitive level: Application

Subject area: Gerontologic

Answer: Prevent and treat physical deformities

Rationale: Rehabilitation begins when the client enters the health care system. The overall goal of rehabilitation is to prevent and treat physical deformities.

Nursing process: Evaluation

Client need: Physiological Adaptation

Cognitive level: Analysis

Subject area: Gerontologic

Answer: 4

Rationale: An asymmetry of facial features is specific to cranial nerve VII, the facial nerve. A difficulty in swallowing is associated with cranial nerve IX, the glossopharyngeal nerve. Loss of smell is common with injury to cranial nerve I, the olfactory nerve. Ptosis occurs with damage to the cranial nerve III, the oculomotor nerve.

Nursing process: Assessment

Client need: Physiological Adaptation

Cognitive level: Application

Subject area: Gerontologic

9. A nursing intervention for a healthy older adult includes providing an adequate oral intake of fluids daily. The rationale for this activity is that older adults tend to drink less than a normal fluid intake and are prone to what electrolyte imbalance? _____

10. The nurse should include which of the following foods that has the most potassium per serving when instructing a 72-year-old client about foods that are high in potassium?

1. Milk
2. Oranges
3. Colas
4. Chicken

11. Which of the following is a priority for the nurse to assess when evaluating the hydration of an 87-year-old client?

1. Height and weight
2. Previous 24-hour intake
3. Skin turgor on the back of the hand
4. Blood pressure

12. During physical assessment of an older adult, the nurse should report which of the following cardiovascular changes that has occurred as a result of dehydration?

1. Widened pulse pressure
2. Tachycardia
3. Hypertension
4. Decreased respiratory rate

Answer: Hypernatremia

Rationale: Older adults are prone to hypernatremia because of hemoconcentration from a decreased intake of fluids. Hyponatremia may occur from fluid overload, decreased sodium intake, or diuretic use.

Nursing process: Analysis

Client need: Physiological Adaptation

Cognitive level: Analysis

Subject area: Gerontologic

Answer: 2

Rationale: Citrus fruits, such as oranges, have the highest concentrations of potassium.

Nursing process: Planning

Client need: Basic Care and Comfort

Cognitive level: Application

Subject area: Gerontologic

Answer: 4

Rationale: Although weight and previous intake are important in evaluating hydration, blood pressure will give a more accurate indication of current hydration. Skin turgor should be checked in the older adult on the clavicle or forehead. A 24-hour intake of fluids may provide the nurse with additional information about the client's hydration status, but it is not the priority.

Nursing process: Assessment

Client need: Management of Care

Cognitive level: Application

Subject area: Gerontologic

Answer: 2

Rationale: A narrowed pulse pressure and hypotension indicate dehydration and decreased circulating blood volume. Tachycardia and an increased respiratory rate indicate the body is attempting to increase the circulation of oxygen in the blood.

Nursing process: Analysis

Client need: Physiological Adaptation

Cognitive level: Application

Subject area: Gerontologic

13. The nurse evaluates which of the following nursing assessment findings to be consistent with overhydration in a 72-year-old client admitted with congestive heart failure?

1. Periorbital edema

2. Edema of the hands

3. Projectile vomiting

4. Moist rales

14. An 80-year-old client who is confined to bed because of generalized weakness, confusion, and disorientation is admitted to the hospital with dehydration. The family asks the nurse why the client is being turned every two hours. The nurse responds that turning the client every two hours is necessary to prevent decubitus ulcers as a result of _____.

15. A 93-year-old client has been functioning independently in the home but has suddenly become confused. A family member asks the nurse, "Does this mean Dad has Alzheimer's disease?" Which of the following is the most appropriate response?

1. "It is very likely your father has Alzheimer's disease."

2. "Why do you think your father has dementia?"

3. "Confusion can be a sign of an infection in an older adult."

4. "Your father will have to be monitored over time."

Answer: 4

Rationale: Periorbital edema and edema of the hands are related to kidney failure and overhydration. Projectile vomiting in the older adult may be related to increased intracranial pressure. Moist rales indicate left-sided heart failure in a client with congestive heart failure.

Nursing process: Assessment

Client need: Physiological Adaptation

Cognitive level: Application

Subject area: Gerontologic

Answer: pressure

Rationale: Pressure on the tissues and lack of relief from the pressure are the causes of decubiti. Turning the client every two hours alleviates the pressure.

Nursing process: Analysis

Client need: Base Care and Comfort

Cognitive level: Application

Subject area: Gerontologic

Answer: 3

Rationale: An older adult client who suddenly becomes confused may have developed an infection, generally of the lungs and bladder, or may be dehydrated. Confusion that occurs in delirium, Alzheimer's disease, and other forms of dementia develops slowly and over time. Telling a client's family that the client may have dementia and will have to be monitored over time shuts down communication. Telling the family that the acute confusion may be a sign of infection keeps communication open and offers information. Rather than a "why" question, the nurse could ask for more recent history on the client, such as whether the client has experienced a fall or head injury.

Nursing process: Analysis

Client need: Physiological Adaptation

Cognitive level: Analysis

Subject area: Gerontologic

16. A member of an older client's family asks the nurse why medications are ordered at half of the usual dose. Which of the following is the most appropriate response?

    1. "Medications for the older adult are prescribed at a pediatric dose."

    2. "The metabolism of the older adult is much like that of a child of the same weight."

    3. "Medications for the older adult may be at lower doses initially until responses are evaluated."

    4. "Older adults generally take a lower dose of a medication because of the cost."

17. When the nurse is taking a nursing history on a client, the client mentions, "I slipped on a wet spot on the way to the bathroom." Which of the following is a priority for the nurse to ask?

    1. "Have you started on any new medications?"

    2. "Do you drink caffeinated beverages?"

    3. "Have you experienced any incontinent episodes?"

    4. "Have you been feeling excessively weak recently?"

18. Which of the following should the nurse include in the medication instructions for an older adult who has back pain and a mild opioid with codeine has been prescribed?

    1. Assess the respirations three times a day

    2. Increase daily fiber and fluids

    3. Limit the administration of the medication to severe pain

    4. Avoid taking the medication more than two times a day

19. A hospice nurse caring for a terminally ill client should titrate the dose of morphine sulfate given to an older adult based on which of the following assessments?

    1. Blood pressure

    2. Level of consciousness

    3. Level of pain

    4. Request of family

Answer: 3

Rationale: Older adults do not metabolize medications at the same rates as children and younger adults do. The liver and kidneys may have impaired function. Even though a thin older adult may have a body weight similar to that of a child, the dosage of medications must allow for age and comorbid conditions.

Nursing process: Analysis

Client need: Pharmacological and Parenteral Therapies

Cognitive level: Analysis

Subject area: Gerontologic

Answer: 3

Rationale: Although asking clients if they have started on any new medications, drink caffeinated beverages, or are excessively weak are relevant when taking a health history, the possibility of incontinence is significant since the client stated that the fall was the result of "slipping on a wet spot."

Nursing process: Assessment

Client need: Management of Care

Cognitive level: Application

Subject area: Gerontologic

Answer: 2

Rationale: It is difficult for clients to count their own respirations accurately, and that measure is not necessary when taking codeine. The dosing of the medication should be "round the clock" to prevent severe pain. Older adult clients are more prone to constipation than younger clients, and fiber and fluids should be increased in the diet.

Nursing process: Planning

Client need: Physiological Adaptation

Cognitive level: Application

Subject area: Gerontologic

Answer: 3

Rationale: The level of pain acceptable to the client determines the dose of pain medication given to a hospice client. The pain medication is then titrated.

Nursing process: Planning

Client need: Pharmacological and Parenteral Therapies

Cognitive level: Application

Subject area: Pharmacological

20. An older adult asks the nurse why a daily bath is necessary. The nurse should respond that daily bathing

    1. stimulates circulation, provides relaxation, and mobilizes joints.

    2. adds hydration and prevents dry skin.

    3. including combing and brushing of the hair helps to remove excess oil from the scalp.

    4. is necessary to comply with agency policy.

21. Which of the following should the nurse include in the instructions given to an older adult about self-care and hygiene to achieve a positive outcome?

    1. A detailed description of the procedures

    2. A written description of the outcomes

    3. A description of the care center's routines

    4. An article on the importance of hygiene

22. The nurse evaluates which factor as a priority that will adversely affect mobility and self-care in the older adult?

    1. Weakness

    2. Level of consciousness

    3. Disease

    4. Family assistance

23. Older clients have individual preferences in carrying out activities of daily living (ADLs). The nurse should include which intervention as a priority for encouraging independence in ADLs?

    1. Allow the client to decide when to have a bath

    2. Ask the client what ADLs are acceptable to perform

    3. Provide total care for a client who is handicapped

    4. Assess the client's abilities and preferences

Answer: 1

Rationale: Daily bathing may damage fragile skin in the older adult. Daily combing and brushing of the hair helps stimulate the scalp and distribute the oil. Reasons for daily bathing include stimulating circulation, providing relaxation, and mobilizing joints.

Nursing process: Analysis

Client need: Basic Comfort and Care

Cognitive level: Application

Subject area: Gerontologic

Answer: 2

Rationale: By giving the client a written description of the expected outcomes and then explaining the procedures and demonstrating the techniques, the nurse will facilitate learning and mutual goal setting.

Nursing process: Planning

Client need: Health Promotion and Maintenance

Cognitive level: Application

Subject area: Gerontologic

Answer: 1

Rationale: Older adults may have many chronic conditions that do not affect mobility or self-care. Weakness from any cause often means that older adults cannot be mobile and care for themselves.

Nursing process: Evaluation

Client need: Management of Care

Cognitive level: Analysis

Subject area: Gerontologic

Answer: 4

Rationale: It is not advised to ask older clients when they want to take a bath because they may refuse ADLs. Even clients who are handicapped are capable of autonomy and self-care. Asking the client what ADLs are acceptable to perform promotes dependency. Assessing the client's abilities, setting mutual goals, and planning care accordingly promote independence in the client.

Nursing process: Planning

Client need: Management of Care

Cognitive level: Application

Subject area: Gerontologic

24. The nurse finds an 88-year-old client lying on the floor unresponsive. The priority action for the nurse to take is

   1. start CPR.

   2. notify the physician.

   3. place the client back in bed.

   4. assess the respirations and pulse.

25. When planning to interview an older adult for a health history, the nurse should consider which of the following as a priority?

   1. The purpose of the interview is to obtain pertinent historical data from the client.

   2. The interview is directed toward offering solutions to the client's problems.

   3. The interview should be conducted in the client's room.

   4. The goals of the interview vary.

26. The registered nurse is planning clinical assignments for a geriatric nursing unit. Which of the following assignments should the nurse delegate to a licensed practical nurse?

   1. Assess a 67-year-old client after cataract surgery

   2. Monitor the serum electrolytes in an 87-year-old client with renal failure

   3. Take the vital signs of a 71-year-old client following a hip arthroplasty

   4. Perform a physical assessment on a 62-year-old client admitted for abdominal pain

Answer: 4

Rationale: When finding a client unresponsive on the floor, the priority is to assess the respirations and pulse before notifying the physician or starting CPR.

Nursing process: Implementation

Client need: Management of Care

Cognitive level: Application

Subject area: Gerontologic

Answer: 4

Rationale: The interview for a health history should identify past and present problems. It should be conducted in a private environment, and the client's room may not be private. The interview is not for the purpose of offering solutions to the problems. Depending on the setting and the reasons why the nurse is conducting the interview (such as to assess an acutely ill client or to evaluate a client still living at home who has a chronic condition), the goals may vary.

Nursing process: Planning

Client need: Management of Care

Cognitive level: Analysis

Subject area: Gerontologic

Answer: 3

Rationale: A licensed practical nurse may take the vital signs on a client following a hip arthroplasty. Assessing, monitoring, and performing a physical assessment are all skills that require a registered nurse.

Nursing process: Planning

Client need: Management of Care

Cognitive level: Analysis

Subject area: Legal and Ethical Issues

CHAPTER

Delirium and Dementia

58

1. The nurse has determined that a confused older adult client who keeps pulling out the intravenous line and indwelling catheter is in need of soft wrist restraints. Which of the following should the nurse include in this client's plan of care?

   1. Obtain a p.r.n. restraint order

   2. Assess the placement of the wrist restraints, skin, and circulation every hour and document

   3. Place the client in a supine position after applying the restraints and secure the wrist restraints to the side rails when the client is in bed

   4. Remove the restraints once every four hours to perform activities of daily living

2. A family expresses concern to the nurse when their 96-year-old mother with dementia living in a long-term care facility seems more confused and does not remember the activities of daily living. Which of the following is the most appropriate response?

   1. "Don't worry, your mother is safe in the long-term care facility."

   2. "You need to remind your mother how to perform her basic needs."

   3. "Your mother will get worse as time goes on and the dementia progresses."

   4. "This must be frustrating for you."

3. A 77-year-old client expresses concern to a nurse in a walk-in psychiatric clinic of "going crazy or of having Alzheimer's disease" because of feelings of being overwhelmed and sad all of the time, and misplacing things. Which of the following is the priority for the nurse to include in this client's plan of care?

   1. Assist the client to develop areas of strength in coping

   2. Make a psychosocial assessment

   3. Explore the available supports for the client

   4. Assure the client and dispel the idea of "going crazy"

4. Upon admission to a long-term care facility, an 83-year-old client is withdrawn, sitting quietly in a chair with the back to the door of the room. When the nurse speaks to the client, the client says, "Go away and leave me alone. Spend your time on someone who can use it. I just don't want to live if I have to stay here." Which of the following is the priority nursing action?

   1. Create a welcoming and cheerful atmosphere

   2. Encourage the client to discuss the feelings of hopelessness

   3. Allow the client to have periods of solitude as asked for

   4. Assess for depression and suicide potential

Answer: 2

Rationale: The standard of care for restraints is that they can be applied only with a written order from a health care provider. The order must be renewed every 24 hours. A p.r.n. order for restraints is not acceptable. Restraints should be removed once every two hours to perform activities of daily living. The client with wrist restraints should be placed in a lateral position to prevent aspiration. The condition of the skin, circulation, and placement of restraints must be assessed every hour. The assessment must also be documented.

Nursing process: Planning

Client need: Physiological Adaptation

Cognitive level: Application

Subject area: Gerontologic

Answer: 4

Rationale: When a family expresses concern over their mother's confusion and decreased ability to perform her activities of daily living, the most appropriate response to the family is to acknowledge how frustrating it must be for the family. The nurse should not minimize family members' feelings or tell them how to feel. Reminding a client with short-term memory loss may increase agitation. Although the dementia will progress over time, reinforcing that with the family is a negative response and may shut down communication.

Nursing process: Analysis

Client need: Physiological Adaptation

Cognitive level: Analysis

Subject area: Gerontologic

Answer: 2

Rationale: The first step of the nursing process is assessment. Before helping the client deal with a problem or exploring available resources, the nurse should determine if a problem is really present. Assuring the client and dispelling the idea of "going crazy" are negative interventions, and the nature of this client's condition is not yet known.

Nursing process: Planning

Client need: Management of Care

Cognitive level: Application

Subject area: Gerontologic

Answer: 4

Rationale: Although creating a cheerful environment is important in a long-term care facility, the priority intervention is safety. Older adults who express not wanting to live if they have to stay there may be clinically depressed and at risk for self-harm. Encouraging clients to discuss feelings of hopelessness and allowing for periods of solitude may be appropriate interventions, but are not the priorities.

Nursing process: Implementation

Client need: Management of Care

Cognitive level: Analysis

Subject area: Gerontologic

5. An 86-year-old client suddenly becomes confused about time, place, and person. After evaluating the oxygen saturation to be 98%, which of the following should the nurse assess first?

   1. What medications the client is taking
   2. Vital signs
   3. Possibility of a recent fall
   4. The client's pain level

6. A 56-year-old client diagnosed with Stage I (early onset) Alzheimer's disease lives at home with his family. A daughter asks the nurse, "How long will Dad be like this before his memory returns?" The best initial response the nurse can make is

   1. "He may never get better."
   2. "This is just the beginning of a predicted decline."
   3. "Tell me what you know about Alzheimer's disease."
   4. "Is he taking his medicine for Alzheimer's disease?"

7. An older adult is picking at clothing and muttering, "Butterflies are all over me." The nurse does not see any butterflies. Which of the following is the priority for the nurse to perform?

   1. Identify any risk for injury related to altered thought processes
   2. Call for help
   3. Provide a nonstimulating environment
   4. Inform the client there are no butterflies in the room

8. An older adult's cognitive function has declined over the last two years. The family is concerned by the loss of short-term memory and the safety issues posed by the forgetfulness. A complete medical workup including a CT scan of the head has shown no medical cause for the cognitive changes. The nurse explains to the client and family that the medical diagnosis of Alzheimer's disease is based on

   1. the information that no other cause can be found for the changes.
   2. a blood test for C-reactive protein that was positive.
   3. a loss of function seen on the Mini-Mental State Exam.
   4. the results of an x-ray of the skull showing a decrease in the size of the brain.

Answer: 2

Rationale: In the case of delirium and a sudden change in mental status, the nurse should always assess for physiological causes—airway, breathing, and circulation—first. Although medications the client is taking, a recent fall, or the client's pain level may be possible causes of the delirium, the vital signs should be assessed first.

Nursing process: Assessment

Client need: Management of Care

Cognitive level: Analysis

Subject area: Gerontologic

Answer: 3

Rationale: The best response when the family of a client diagnosed with Stage I (early onset) Alzheimer's disease asks when the family member will get better would be to ask family members how much they know about Alzheimer's. This is the best response because it facilitates open communication. Although the disease has a progressive course, telling the family that will close communication. Asking the family member if the client is taking medication for Alzheimer's disease is an inappropriate response, because it changes the subject.

Nursing process: Analysis

Client need: Physiological Adaptation

Cognitive level: Analysis

Subject area: Gerontologic

Answer: 1

Rationale: The first nursing action should be to identify any risks to the client or others because of the alteration in thought processes that the client is experiencing. It may be appropriate to provide a nonstimulating environment, but that is not the priority. Informing the client that there are no butterflies might precipitate a catastrophic reaction.

Nursing process: Implementation

Client need: Management of Care

Cognitive level: Analysis

Subject area: Gerontologic

Answer: 1

Rationale: The definitive diagnosis for Alzheimer's disease is only found on autopsy. When all other possible causes of cognitive decline are ruled out, the medical diagnosis of Alzheimer's disease (or Alzheimer's-like disease) is made. The Mini-Mental State Exam is one of many short tests to measure cognitive function, but it does not actually diagnose dementia. The older adult will show a decrease in the mass of the brain but may not have a corresponding loss of cognitive function. A blood test for C-reactive protein would not be positive for Alzheimer's disease.

Nursing process: Analysis

Client need: Physiological Adaptation

Cognitive level: Analysis

Subject area: Gerontologic

9. When assessing an older adult, the nurse should be alert to the clinical manifestations of depression that may be masked by other chronic conditions. The cardinal and primary behavior exhibited in the depressed older adult is

  1. a loss of interest in previously pleasurable activities.

  2. inactivity.

  3. drinking alcohol.

  4. crying.

10. Donepezil hydrochloride (Aricept) has been prescribed for a client with Alzheimer's disease. Which of the following adverse reactions should the nurse include in the medication instructions given to the family?

  Select all that apply:

  [ ] **1.** Headache

  [ ] **2.** Tachycardia

  [ ] **3.** Insomnia

  [ ] **4.** Hypotension

  [ ] **5.** Constipation

  [ ] **6.** Anorexia

11. Before preparing to use the Mini-Mental State Exam for cognitive function in an older adult, the nurse should consider which of the following limitations of the exam?

  1. The test takes one hour to administer.

  2. The client must be able to see and write.

  3. The exam must take place in a dimly lit room.

  4. The exam is valid only with English-speaking clients.

12. The nurse should consider which of the following medical etiologies in an older adult who has been healthy until recently but has developed dementia?

  1. Sexually transmitted diseases

  2. Electrolyte imbalances

  3. Arthritis

  4. Liver disease

Answer: 1

Rationale: Loss of interest in previously enjoyable activities and withdrawal are indicators to the nurse that the client may be clinically depressed and in need of further assessment. Inactivity, drinking alcohol, and crying may be indicative of depression or other chronic conditions, not just depression.

Nursing process: Assessment

Client need: Management of Care

Cognitive level: Analysis

Subject area: Gerontologic

Answer: 1, 3, 6

Rationale: Donepezil hydrochloride (Aricept) is used in the treatment of mild to moderate Alzheimer's disease. Adverse reactions of Aricept include headache, bradycardia, insomnia, hypertension, diarrhea, and anorexia.

Nursing process: Planning

Client need: Pharmacological and Parenteral Therapies

Cognitive level: Application

Subject area: Pharmacologic

Answer: 2

Rationale: The Mini-Mental State Exam does not require a specially trained individual and requires only 20 to 30 minutes to administer. The client must be able to see and write because the client will be asked to write a sentence as well as to copy a drawn figure.

Nursing process: Analysis

Client need: Reduction of Risk Potential

Cognitive level: Application

Subject area: Gerontologic

Answer: 1

Rationale: The first indication that a client has a sexually transmitted disease such as tertiary syphilis or HIV may be cognitive function changes and dementia.

Nursing process: Analysis

Client need: Physiological Adaptation

Cognitive level: Application

Subject area: Gerontologic

13. Which of the following four older adult clients that the nurse is caring for does the nurse evaluate as most at risk for self-directed violence?

 1. A 76-year-old single man who lives in a retirement center and engages in community activities

 2. A widowed man who is 88 years old, lives alone, and has multiple chronic illnesses

 3. An 83-year-old woman who has type 2 diabetes mellitus and lives with her daughter

 4. A recently widowed woman with multiple chronic illnesses who lives near family

14. An older adult client with chronic depression tells the nurse, "Don't worry about me. I can manage the pain of my arthritis. The way I mix up my medications helps." The best initial response by the nurse is

 1. "Don't mix your medications yourself. Take them only as prescribed."

 2. "That's dangerous. I'll have to take your narcotics from you."

 3. "That's dangerous. I'll have to call your daughter and have her give you your medications."

 4. "Tell me what you take and how you mix them."

15. The nurse is caring for an older adult with situational depression following the death of a spouse. What is the most important outcome for the nurse to plan for?

 1. The client will discuss the spouse and the meaning of the loss.

 2. The client will not cry.

 3. The client will speak of the spouse only positively.

 4. The client will avoid talking about the spouse and engage in social activities.

16. Which of the following is the priority nursing intervention for the nurse to include in the plan of care for a client with behavior problems related to dementia?

 1. Inform the client why the nursing interventions are necessary

 2. Instruct the caregivers on the process of dementia and care to be given

 3. Be consistent by repeating the same intervention as the client's dementia progresses

 4. Assist the client to perform difficult tasks

Answer: 2

Rationale: Older women, even if depressed, tend to be less likely to harm themselves, because they have social support and other interests. Older men without social support who have multiple chronic illnesses and live alone are more likely to commit suicide than older women.

Nursing process: Evaluation

Client need: Reduction of Risk Potential

Cognitive level: Analysis

Subject area: Gerontologic

Answer: 4

Rationale: Clients with chronic illnesses and pain often adjust their own medications or add over-the-counter medications. A client's depression could be a result of the drugs or it could be the reason the client mixes medications. The nurse needs further information to identify risks for injury.

Nursing process: Analysis

Client need: Reduction of Risk Potential

Cognitive level: Analysis

Subject area: Gerontologic

Answer: 1

Rationale: It is most appropriate for the nurse to encourage clients who are experiencing situational depression over the loss of a spouse to verbalize their feelings. Crying is a normal and healthy expression of loss. The relationship with the spouse may not always have been positive, or the client may feel angry about the death. Setting an outcome that the client will speak positively describes how the client should feel and is not necessarily true.

Nursing process: Evaluation

Client need: Physiological Adaptation

Cognitive level: Analysis

Subject area: Gerontologic

Answer: 2

Rationale: Educating the caregivers, whether family members or others, is always the priority when caring for a client with dementia. The caregivers must understand the disease and expected behaviors as well as the interventions for problem behaviors. The same interventions may not be effective as the condition changes. This should be part of the continued evaluation and part of the replanning.

Nursing process: Planning

Client need: Management of Care

Cognitive level: Application

Subject area: Gerontologic

17. A nurse observes a family member continually reminding a client in late Stage II Alzheimer's disease of the date and place. The client is adamant that it is 1922 and the North Pole. The nurse informs the family member that continually reminding the client of the date and place will result in

   1. a return of memory.
   2. increased retention of the information.
   3. a catastrophic reaction.
   4. an interest in having a calendar.

18. An 80-year-old client is admitted to the intensive care unit because of hemorrhaging after a stent is placed in her left femoral artery to improve circulation to the leg. The client is confused, not following instructions, and pulling at the intravenous tubing and indwelling catheter. The client's adult son tells the nurse, "My mom was never like this before. What have you done to her?" The best initial response the nurse can make is

   1. "We've done nothing to her. She must have dementia."
   2. "Older adults will become confused after a bleed to the brain from decreased oxygen."
   3. "Your mother is acting like she is in alcohol withdrawal. Does she drink?"
   4. "You will need to talk to your mother's physician to get information about her condition."

19. An older client in a nursing facility suddenly becomes confused, paranoid, and verbally abusive to the staff. Which of the following is the priority nursing action?

   1. Ask the family members if they had a recent disagreement with the client
   2. Assess the vital signs and obtain a urine specimen
   3. Reorient the client to person, place, and time
   4. Ask whether the client is hearing voices

Answer: 3

Rationale: In late Stage II Alzheimer's disease there is no hope for memory return. Repeating reality orientation for the client whose reality is different may cause anxiety, anger, agitation, and a catastrophic reaction, such as running away or violence.

Nursing process: Implementation

Client need: Physiological Adaptation

Cognitive level: Application

Subject area: Gerontologic

Answer: 2

Rationale: Older adult clients may become confused after a bleed to the brain from decreased oxygen. Telling the family that the medical team has done nothing to the client is a defensive statement and would cut off communication. Dementia is a medical diagnosis, which the nurse does not make. The best initial response by the nurse is to answer the son's question. The nurse may need to know if the client has an alcohol abuse problem, but not until the son's concerns are answered. Passing the son off to the physician at this point would shut down communication with the son.

Nursing process: Analysis

Client need: Management of Care

Cognitive level: Analysis

Subject area: Gerontologic

Answer: 2

Rationale: Assessing the vital signs and obtaining a urine specimen is the priority in an older client who suddenly becomes confused and develops psychotic behavior. A urinary tract infection would be evident from an elevated temperature and bacteria in the urine specimen.

Nursing process: Implementation

Client need: Management of Care

Cognitive level: Analysis

Subject area: Gerontological

20. The nurse assesses which of the following behaviors in a client in early Stage I Alzheimer's disease? Select all that apply:

[   ] **1.** Masks forgetful behavior

[   ] **2.** Has a slow reaction time

[   ] **3.** Repetitive storytelling

[   ] **4.** Inability to follow simple directions

[   ] **5.** Becomes angry when challenged

[   ] **6.** Change in eating patterns

21. An older adult client with dementia becomes increasingly confused and wanders away from a long-term facility. The appropriate nursing action is to

1. call law enforcement officials.

2. restrain the client.

3. follow the client and redirect from a safe distance.

4. offer the client a ride back to the facility.

22. Which of the following should the nurse include in the education provided to a new graduate nurse to protect the nurse from injury when a client with dementia or delirium becomes aggressive?

1. Gently place a hand on the client's shoulder to promote trust

2. Lead the client to the activity area where there are others to distract the client

3. Provide a quiet, calm atmosphere and offer simple directions

4. Offer the client a meal

23. Donepezil hydrochloride (Aricept) is prescribed for an older adult with early dementia, Alzheimer's-like disease (ALD). When reviewing the client's medical conditions and medications, the nurse notifies the physician that there might be a serious interaction because the client has

1. osteoarthritis.

2. cancer of the pancreas.

3. not had a yearly influenza immunization.

4. bradycardia.

Answer: 1, 2, 5

Rationale: A client attempts to mask forgetful behavior, has a slow reaction time, and may become angry when challenged in early Stage I Alzheimer's disease. Repetitive storytelling, an inability to follow simple directions, and a change in eating patterns are behaviors exhibited in Stage II Alzheimer's.

Nursing process: Assessment

Client need: Physiological Adaptation

Cognitive level: Application

Subject area: Gerontologic

Answer: 3

Rationale: When a client with dementia wanders away from a long-term care facility, the nurse should see if the client will return willingly with persuasion and redirection. If the client will not return, notifying law enforcement may be necessary, but the presence of law enforcement officials may also agitate and frighten the client. At no time should the nurse physically restrain the client alone or transport a client.

Nursing process: Implementation

Client need: Physiological Adaptation

Cognitive level: Application

Subject area: Gerontological

Answer: 3

Rationale: Touching an agitated client may increase aggression and precipitate violence against the nurse. The client should be in a quiet, calm atmosphere away from others and simple directions should be offered. Offering a meal may work as a temporary distraction, but the client at this point will be unable to sit and follow instructions about eating.

Nursing process: Planning

Client need: Health Promotion and Maintenance

Cognitive level: Application

Subject area: Gerontologic

Answer: 4

Rationale: Aricept is a cholinesterase inhibitor used in the treatment of Alzheimer's disease, which may cause bradycardia with fainting.

Nursing process: Analysis

Client need: Pharmacological and Parenteral Therapies

Cognitive level: Application

Subject area: Pharmacologic

24. Rivastigmine (Exelon) is prescribed for a client with dementia. Which of the following would be an appropriate outcome of nursing care specific to this drug?

    1. The client will sleep six hours without waking during the night.

    2. The client will eat 50% of all meals and snacks.

    3. The client will maintain a weight within the normal range.

    4. The client will maintain the serum potassium within normal range.

25. The nurse assesses that a deficiency in what nutrient places an older adult with dementia at risk for malnutrition? _____

26. The registered nurse is planning the clinical assignments for a geriatric mental health unit. Which of the following assignments should the nurse delegate to a licensed practical nurse?

    1. Develop a plan of care for a client with dementia

    2. Perform a physical assessment on a client with Alzheimer's disease

    3. Administer donepezil hydrochloride (Aricept) to a client newly diagnosed with Alzheimer's disease

    4. Provide education to the family of a client with dementia

Answer: 3

Rationale: Rivastigmine tartrate is used in the treatment of mild to moderate Alzheimer's disease. Nausea, vomiting, anorexia, and abdominal pain are adverse reactions to Exelon. The nurse should monitor weight weekly. Eating 50% of the food offered may not be sufficient to maintain body weight.

Nursing process: Evaluation

Client need: Pharmacological and Parenteral Therapies

Cognitive level: Analysis

Subject area: Pharmacologic

Answer: Protein

Rationale: The diets of older adults are often deficient in protein. Protein sources may not be chewable or palatable to the client with dementia. Protein should be added to the diet in the form of protein powder or other easily ingested sources, such as ice cream cones.

Nursing process: Assessment

Client need: Basic Care and Comfort

Cognitive level: Application

Subject area: Gerontologic

Answer: 3

Rationale: A licensed practical nurse may administer donepezil hydrochloride (Aricept) to a client with Alzheimer's disease. Developing a plan of care, performing a physical assessment, and providing education to a client's family on dementia are tasks that should be performed by a registered nurse.

Nursing process: Planning

Client need: Management of Care

Cognitive level: Analysis

Subject area: Legal and Ethical Issues

Community Health Nursing

Case Management

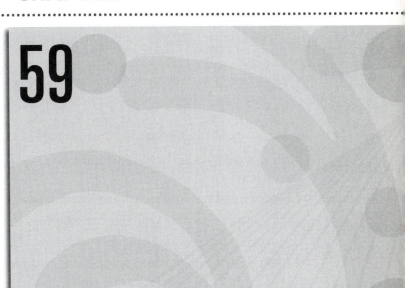

59

1. The nurse working as a case manager understands that case management is often needed when the client
   1. cannot afford to stay in the hospital.
   2. has no one at home to help with the client's care.
   3. has complex acute or chronic health care needs.
   4. is too sick to care for oneself.

2. A client's family asks the nurse what the case manager's primary goal is. The most appropriate response of the nurse is to
   1. save the client money with cheaper care options.
   2. eliminate the need for multiple care providers.
   3. direct the care provided by speech and physical therapists.
   4. promote self-care of the client whenever possible.

3. A nurse has just accepted the position as a case manager at a local hospital. According to the definitions of various professional organizations that work with case managers, case management is
   1. a position in the hospital's social service department.
   2. a cost-effective way to provide direct nursing care.
   3. a collaborative process between various health care providers.
   4. an independent role of the nurse to provide cost-effective care.

4. A nurse is teaching a class about the history and development of case management. The nurse includes the information that case management developed as the result of many factors, such as
   1. the current health system is complex but easily understood.
   2. clients often stay in the hospital until they can care for themselves at home.
   3. health care resources are scarce, so valuable resources must not be wasted.
   4. third-party payers wanted to decrease the costs of hospital stays.

Answer: 3

Rationale: Case management is a process used to assist individuals with complex health care problems, by providing quality care with a cost-effective outcome. It organizes client care through a health care problem meeting, so that specific clinical and financial outcomes are achieved within a designated time period.

Nursing process: Analysis

Client need: Management of Care

Cognitive level: Application

Subject area: Community Health

Answer: 4

Rationale: The goal of case management is to help the client care for oneself. The case manager is responsible for coordinating care and establishing goals, from the admission phase through to discharge. The case manager works with all disciplines to facilitate care.

Nursing process: Analysis

Client need: Management of Care

Cognitive level: Application

Subject area: Community Health

Answer: 3

Rationale: Case managers do not usually work alone, but instead work with various health care team members to provide care for the client. Case management promotes collaboration, communication, and teamwork to provide the best possible care for the client in the most cost-effective manner possible. Case management also promotes timely discharge.

Nursing process: Evaluation

Client need: Management of Care

Cognitive level: Application

Subject area: Community Health

Answer: 3

Rationale: Although health care resources are limited, case managers work to use these resources to provide quality care cost-effectively and to promote timely discharge.

Nursing process: Planning

Client need: Management of Care

Cognitive level: Application

Subject area: Community Health

5. The nurse who has always used the nursing process when planning client care has just taken a position utilizing case management. Based on an understanding of the nursing process and the case management concept, the nurse understands that case management

    1. follows a more complex step-by-step model.

    2. uses care maps, not nursing care plans, for documentation.

    3. follows a process very similar to the nursing process.

    4. is a physician-directed process.

6. When planning a client's care, the nurse uses case management skills to help the client

    1. understand the variety of resources in the community.

    2. understand the importance of keeping appointment times.

    3. save money by always finding the least expensive options.

    4. save time by making phone calls for the client.

7. A nurse applied for a case manager position at the local hospital because the job description of the case manager is to

    1. decide what treatment will be provided.

    2. help clients determine the best care for the least cost.

    3. eliminate the competition from other providers.

    4. provide a service that costs very little to offer.

8. Which of the following would a school nurse perform when functioning as a case manager?

    1. Meet with the newspaper office to run an article on school nursing

    2. Team teach a class on healthy after-school snacks

    3. Contact the school board about the lack of computers in the school

    4. Discipline children in sports who do not adhere to weight maintenance guidelines

Answer: 3

Rationale: Case management follows a process very similar to the nursing process and includes assessment, planning, implementation, and evaluation.

Nursing process: Analysis

Client need: Management of Care

Cognitive level: Application

Subject area: Community Health

Answer: 1

Rationale: With a variety of resources available in the community, the client often needs help to find and use the most appropriate care for personal needs. The nurse may use case management to help the client understand available resources. The case manager usually does not make phone calls for the client and does not make sure the client gets to appointments on time.

Nursing process: Planning

Client need: Management of Care

Cognitive level: Application

Subject area: Community Health

Answer: 2

Rationale: Hospitals needed a mechanism to find high-quality, cost-effective care to meet client needs. Case managers can assist the hospital and the clients to reduce the costs of care and ensure that a high quality of care will be provided.

Nursing process: Evaluation

Client need: Management of Care

Cognitive level: Application

Subject area: Community Health

Answer: 2

Rationale: The focus of case managers in schools is to provide services for the enrolled students that improve health care. Teaching a class on healthy after-school snacks would provide such a service. Meeting with the newspaper office or contacting the school board does not focus directly on improving the health of the students. Disciplining children in sports who do not adhere to weight maintenance guidelines is a punitive action and would not be performed by the nurse.

Nursing process: Planning

Client need: Management of Care

Cognitive level: Application

Subject area: Community Health

9. In evaluating the nurse's role as a case manager, the nurse would determine which of the following skills as most beneficial in caring for clients?

    1. An ability to solve complex problems in a creative way

    2. A legal background, due to an increased atmosphere of lawsuits

    3. Extensive clinical experience as an intensive care nurse

    4. An ability to work according to established protocols and procedures

10. The case manager nurse should be assigned to provide services to which of the following clients?

    1. A mother experiencing her first pregnancy

    2. A client with newly diagnosed diabetes mellitus

    3. A client with a broken arm following a bicycle accident

    4. A group of teenagers who are members of SADD (Students against Drunk Driving)

11. Which of the following should the case manager nurse include in the plan of care for a client injured on the job who is now recovering from a broken leg?

    1. Assist the client with daily exercises to prevent muscle loss

    2. Prevent skin breakdown from limited mobility

    3. Coordinate visits with physical therapy in the home

    4. Provide transportation for the client to medical appointments when needed

12. The nurse is coordinating a case management system of care for which of the following purposes? Select all that apply:

    [   ] **1.** Provides continuity of services

    [   ] **2.** Assists the client with method of payment

    [   ] **3.** Coordinates designated components of health care

    [   ] **4.** Avoids fragmented services

    [   ] **5.** Encourages the client to direct the decision making of the care

    [   ] **6.** Matches the intensity of the services with the client's needs over time

Answer: 1

Rationale: Because the case manager must solve problems for clients in unique situations usually outside of the hospital setting, protocols may not be well established or in written form. The case manager must be flexible and creative in order to solve these problems. Having worked in an environment where established protocols and procedures were closely followed will also help the nurse now working as a case manager.

Nursing process: Evaluation

Client need: Management of Care

Cognitive level: Application

Subject area: Community Health

Answer: 2

Rationale: Case managers usually work with clients who have complex or newly diagnosed conditions, such as a client newly diagnosed with diabetes mellitus.

Nursing process: Planning

Client need: Management of Care

Cognitive level: Analysis

Subject area: Community Health

Answer: 3

Rationale: The case manager coordinates other members of the health care team to provide the multiple services needed by a client, but does not necessarily provide the care directly.

Nursing process: Planning

Client need: Management of Care

Cognitive level: Application

Subject area: Community Health

Answer: 1, 3, 4, 6

Rationale: Case management is a type of delivery of care in which the health care needs of the client are managed by a nurse or physician. The purpose of case management is to ensure continuity of care and avoid fragmented services. It also coordinates all designated components of health care and matches the intensity of the services with the client's needs over time.

Nursing process: Analysis

Client need: Management of Care

Cognitive level: Application

Subject area: Community Health

13. Which of the following is the priority for the nurse case manager planning the discharge of a client who is hospitalized for bone cancer?

1. Establish all physical therapy appointments for the next three months

2. Communicate primarily with the client's family instead of the client

3. Obtain all laboratory records to order the correct medications

4. Transfer the client's care to another case manager in the community setting

14. In caring for a client with a terminal condition, the nurse understands that the case management role in the hospital

1. begins when the client receives the diagnosis of cancer.

2. ends when the client is discharged to a home health service.

3. is not appropriate because a diagnosis of a terminal condition has been made.

4. begins when the order is written to begin chemotherapy.

15. A client has recently been hospitalized for open heart surgery and is going to be transferred to a skilled care facility for additional recovery. Which of the following is the role of the nurse case manager in the hospital?

1. Arrange transportation to the new facility

2. Obtain the necessary equipment to be used in the home

3. Deliver pharmaceutical supplies to the skilled care facility

4. Coordinate volunteers to help the client's spouse at home

Answer: 4

Rationale: Continuity of care is important in the care of clients. Because the hospital case manager may not be able to follow the client at home, it is a priority that the care of the client be transferred to a community case manager upon discharge.

Nursing process: Planning

Client need: Management of Care

Cognitive level: Application

Subject area: Community Health

Answer: 1

Rationale: The case manager should be involved from the time that admission of the client and the process of case management are implemented, shortly after the diagnosis has been made. This ensures that multiple services are provided in an efficient and cost-effective manner.

Nursing process: Analysis

Client need: Management of Care

Cognitive level: Application

Subject area: Community Health

Answer: 1

Rationale: As a case manager, the nurse should help arrange the transition to the new facility, including transportation, transferring orders for medications and activities, and encouraging family involvement in the transfer. Equipment and volunteers needed in the home would not be arranged at the time of transfer. The new facility would be responsible for obtaining any pharmaceutical supplies.

Nursing process: Analysis

Client need: Management of Care

Cognitive level: Application

Subject area: Community Health

Long-Term Care

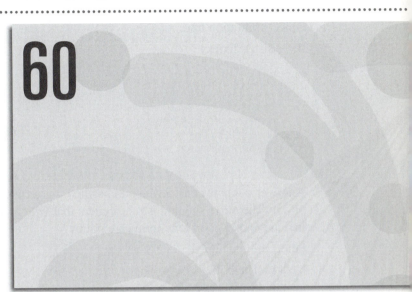

60

1. The nurse is screening a client with mild dementia who is unsafe in the home and needs minimal assistance with activities of daily living. The nurse should recommend which of the following facilities as the most appropriate placement for this client?

   1. Subacute care

   2. Skilled nursing care

   3. Rehabilitation unit

   4. Assisted living

 2. An older client is considering purchasing long-term care insurance and asks the nurse how to select a good policy. The nurse should instruct a client that which of the following are characteristics to consider and are indicative of a good long-term care policy?

   Select all that apply:

   [ ] **1.** The policy is expensive

   [ ] **2.** Annual renewal guaranteed with stable medical condition

   [ ] **3.** $100 daily coverage

   [ ] **4.** Guaranteed lifetime premium

   [ ] **5.** Excludes certain forms of dementia

   [ ] **6.** Includes home care

3. Discharge plans are being made for a 74-year-old client who is widowed, lives alone, and had a left hip arthroplasty after a fall on the ice when volunteering in a day care. Which of the following facilities should the nurse discharge this client to?

   1. Assisted living

   2. Special care unit

   3. Rehabilitation unit

   4. Skilled nursing care facility

Answer: 4

Rationale: An assisted living facility is designed for a client who can no longer stay in the home and who needs only minimal assistance with activities of daily living or medication monitoring. A subacute care unit provides skilled nursing care 24 hours a day for a client with advanced dementia and who needs maximum assistance with activities of daily living. A rehabilitation unit provides specialized therapies, such as speech or physical therapy, for clients with neurological impairments who can return to the home environment after a period of rehabilitation lasting several weeks to months. Skilled nursing care would be necessary if a client needs care 24 hours a day in a structured environment, such as a nursing home facility.

Nursing process: Analysis

Client need: Management of Care

Cognitive level: Application

Subject area: Community Health

Answer: 3, 4, 6

Rationale: A comprehensive long-term care insurance policy would include coverage for Alzheimer's disease and other forms of dementia, home care, a skilled nursing care facility, would have a guaranteed premium and renewal for life, and would allow a minimum of $100 a day coverage.

Nursing process: Planning

Client need: Management of Care

Cognitive level: Application

Subject area: Community Health

Answer: 3

Rationale: It is most appropriate to discharge an older client who had a hip arthroplasty and was independent, living alone, and still working as a volunteer to a rehabilitation unit. The goal of a rehabilitation unit is to return the client to the maximal level of functioning possible and to the home environment.

Nursing process: Planning

Client need: Management of Care

Cognitive level: Application

Subject area: Community Health

4. The registered nurse is preparing the work schedule at a skilled nursing care facility. Which of the following work assignments would be appropriate for the registered nurse to include?

1. Unlicensed assistive personnel will administer drugs to residents.

2. A certified medication aide will perform uncomplicated dressing changes.

3. A licensed practical nurse will be on duty on all three shifts daily.

4. Unlicensed assistive personnel will cut the toenails of residents.

5. The nurse assesses an older client in an assisted living facility who is crying uncontrollably and who tells the nurse, "I am going to be evicted because I ran out of money to live here." Which of the following is the priority response by the nurse?

1. "I am sure something will work out for you."

2. "Can you ask any of your family for money?"

3. "You will qualify for Medicaid now that you have no money."

4. "There are other financial options available to you."

6. Which of the following should receive priority when the nurse is developing the plan of care for an older client in a skilled nursing care facility?

1. The client's age

2. The client's financial resources

3. The client's ethnic origin

4. The client's physical and mental status

Answer: 3

Rationale: A licensed practical or vocational nurse (LP/VN) should be on duty 24 hours a day, seven days a week in a skilled nursing facility. Unlicensed assistive personnel cannot administer drugs. A certified medication aide (CMA) is a certified nurse aide who has taken an additional course on medication administration and may administer medications in some states. It is essential that the nurse making assignments know the law in the resident state. A certified medication aide cannot perform dressing changes and is not allowed to perform nursing care beyond personal care and activities of living.

Nursing process: Planning

Client need: Management of Care

Cognitive level: Analysis

Subject area: Legal and Ethical Issues

Answer: 4

Rationale: The priority response for the nurse to make to a client who has exhausted all personal financial resources in an assisted living facility is that there are other options available. Those other options may include family support or Medicaid. The nurse is not in a position to discuss or advise the client about financial matters. A financial advisor would be the best person to advise the client.

Nursing process: Analysis

Client need: Management of Care

Cognitive level: Analysis

Subject area: Community Health

Answer: 3

Rationale: Although the client's age, ethnic origin, financial resources, and physical and mental status are all important to consider when developing a plan of care for an older client in a long-term care facility, the priority is to consider the client's ethnic origin. Admission to a long-term care facility is viewed differently by people from different cultures, and the client's acceptance and perception of the long term will have a direct impact on the plan of care.

Nursing process: Planning

Client need: Management of Care

Cognitive level: Application

Subject area: Community Health

7. The nurse is teaching a class on long-term care. Which of the following should the nurse include in the lecture?

1. A client has to be financially capable of privately paying to live in an assisted living facility.

2. The cost of assisted living facilities ranges from $500 to $900 per month.

3. The annual cost of a long-term care facility for one client can be $40,000.

4. A client has to be medically and psychologically stable to continue coverage under a long-term care insurance policy.

8. The nurse admits a client with acquired immunodeficiency syndrome (AIDS) to which type of long-term care facility? _____

9. The nurse is planning the new employee orientation and education for an unlicensed assistive personnel aide at a skilled nursing care facility. Which of the following should the nurse include in the orientation and education program?

Select all that apply:

[   ] 1. On-the-job training is better than formal in-service education

[   ] 2. Seventy-five hours of training and education are required within four months of employment

[   ] 3. New unlicensed assistive personnel can only work part-time for the first six months

[   ] 4. The needs of an older client are no different from the needs of a younger client

[   ] 5. Information on elder abuse

[   ] 6. Simulated experiences on aging

Answer: 3

Rationale: The annual expense for long-term care is very costly and may be in excess of $40,000. Approximately two out of every five individuals will need some kind of long-term care at some point in their life. Medicaid and out-of-pocket payments are the primary methods of paying for long-term care. A client does not have to remain medically or psychologically stable to keep one's long-term care insurance. When choosing a long-term care insurance policy, it is essential that the policy include coverage for Alzheimer's disease and other forms of dementia.

Nursing process: Planning

Client need: Management of Care

Cognitive level: Application

Subject area: Community Health

Answer: Special care unit

Rationale: It would be appropriate to admit a client with acquired immunodeficiency syndrome (AIDS) to a special care unit, which is a type of long-term care facility designed to care for clients with special needs. The staff on these units generally have special in-service training to facilitate an understanding of the special needs necessary to care for these clients.

Nursing process: Implementation

Client need: Management of Care

Cognitive level: Application

Subject area: Community Health

Answer: 2, 5, 6

Rationale: Information on aging and elder abuse should be included in the new employee orientation and education for unlicensed assistive personnel. Simulating experiences on aging will assist the new employee to understand aging. Seventy-five hours of training and education are required by the Omnibus Budget Reconciliation Act (OBRA) of 1987 within four months of employment. In-service education is more important than on-the-job training.

Nursing process: Planning

Client need: Management of Care

Cognitive level: Application

Subject area: Community Health

10. An older adult client asks the nurse about the difference between Medicare Part A, Medicare Part B, and Medicaid. The appropriate response by the nurse is

    1. "Medicare Part A covers physician and outpatient services."

    2. "Medicare Part B covers hospitalization."

    3. "Medicaid is granted for low-income clients who receive a social security benefit."

    4. "Medicaid fails to cover preventive services or hospitalization."

Answer: 3

Rationale: Medicare Part A covers hospitalization. Medicare Part B covers outpatient and physician services. Medicaid is a state- and federally funded health care for low-income clients. Physician services, eye and dental care, prescriptions, and preventive services are covered under Medicaid.

Nursing process: Analysis

Client need: Management of Care

Cognitive level: Analysis

Subject area: Community Health

CHAPTER

Home Health Care

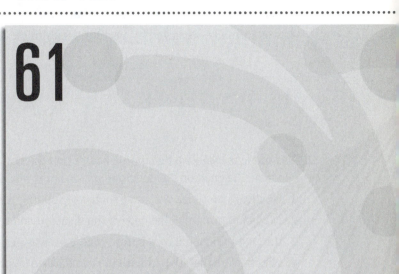

61

1. A nurse has been asked to teach a class about home health care to a local church group. Which of the following points should the nurse include in a class on home health care? Home health care

    1. is a relatively new phenomenon that began with Medicare.

    2. dates back to the beginning of the Red Cross in 1912.

    3. is only provided by charities and churches.

    4. was formally organized by visiting nurses in the late 1800s.

2. The nurse is establishing a home health care agency and knows it is important to understand the influence Medicare has had on the development of home health care because

    1. Medicare provided a regular source of funding for home health care.

    2. Medicare promoted the care of the disabled and the chronically ill.

    3. the cost of hospital care before Medicare was getting too high.

    4. clients were dissatisfied with the standards of home health care prior to Medicare.

3. When meeting with a client for the first time, the nurse working in home health care should include which of the following when describing the services that will be provided for the client?

    1. Care of acute and chronically ill at home

    2. Health promotion activities to individual families in their home

    3. Disease prevention in nursing homes in the community

    4. Care of clients who receive Medicare funding

4. Which of the following should the home health care nurse include when providing home health care for a client?

    1. Custodial care for the client

    2. Charge for each service provided

    3. Receive direct payments from the client

    4. Plan visits based on client needs

Answer: 4

Rationale: Home care was the primary source of care for many years. It began with charities, but was formally organized by visiting nurses in 1877 in New York. Medicare has helped provide a regular source of funding since Medicare began in 1965.

Nursing process: Planning

Client need: Management of Care

Cognitive level: Comprehension

Subject area: Community Health

Answer: 1

Rationale: Medicare is made up of two parts: Part A, or the hospital insurance, and Part B, or the supplemental medical insurance. Prior to Medicare, most home care was provided by voluntary agencies. In 1965, Medicare was passed and provided a source of funding for home care.

Nursing process: Analysis

Client need: Management of Care

Cognitive level: Application

Subject area: Community Health

Answer: 1

Rationale: People are often discharged from the hospital before they are well enough to take care of themselves. Home health care is considered a cost-effective way to provide care to clients with acute or chronic illnesses in their own home.

Nursing process: Planning

Client need: Management of Care

Cognitive level: Application

Subject area: Community Health

Answer: 4

Rationale: The care for each client is planned by the nurse and based on an assessment of each client's individual needs. The home care agency is responsible for billing the client and paying the nurse. The nurse provides skilled nursing care, not custodial care.

Nursing process: Planning

Client need: Management of Care

Cognitive level: Application

Subject area: Community Health

5. Which of the following factors should the home health care nurse consider when planning care for a client in the home?

    1. The client is the only one designated to receive services.

    2. The family should be included in all care rendered in the home.

    3. The nurse will perform physical therapy exercises if needed.

    4. All care should be completed in a designated period of time.

6. A home health care nurse should include which of the following when informing a client about home care service?

    1. A dependency on the home care nurse will develop.

    2. Greater autonomy and control over self-care are fostered.

    3. Home care will cost more than staying in the hospital.

    4. There are limits to advances in technology.

7. When meeting with a client to explain the role of the nurse in home care, which of the following advantages of home care should be explained to the client? Home care

    1. allows the nurse to have primary control over the environment where the client will recover.

    2. saves the client money because the care is provided in a one-to-one situation and is always covered by insurance.

    3. provides a holistic view of the client that helps the nurse to establish appropriate goals and to plan appropriate care.

    4. encourages a dependent relationship between the nurse and the client.

8. The nurse should consider which of the following when interviewing for a position as a home health care nurse at an official agency? The care

    1. is funded by tax dollars at the state or local level.

    2. is governed by a board of directors at the federal level.

    3. is based in the local community hospital.

    4. is certified by Medicare as long as the client is older.

Answer: 2

Rationale: When in the home, the client and family must all be included in any care provided. Working in the home assists the nurse to see how the client functions within the family setting and the home environment.

Nursing process: Analysis

Client need: Management of Care

Cognitive level: Application

Subject area: Community Health

Answer: 2

Rationale: Home care is a cost-effective way of meeting the client's needs in the comfort of the client's home, including the adaptation of high-tech equipment to the home environment. Clients are usually more satisfied and have more control over the care given in their home than the care given in institutions.

Nursing process: Planning

Client need: Management of Care

Cognitive level: Application

Subject area: Community Health

Answer: 3

Rationale: Home care provides a holistic view of the client that influences the client's health. Being in the home environment provides an opportunity for the client to exercise more autonomy and control over personal care and encourages the client to function at the highest level of independence possible.

Nursing process: Planning

Client need: Management of Care

Cognitive level: Application

Subject area: Community Health

Answer: 1

Rationale: Official agencies are publicly funded by taxes and operate in state or local health departments that fall under the control of local health departments. Being an official agency does not guarantee certification by Medicare. The agency must still qualify for Medicare certification.

Nursing process: Analysis

Client need: Management of Care

Cognitive level: Application

Subject area: Community Health

9. When a client calls a nurse who has established a private nonprofit home care agency in his or her community, the nurse should explain that nurses at the agency

   1. are paid a salary exempt from federal income tax.

   2. work for an agency that is governed by the local board of health.

   3. are concerned about saving money for the stockholders of the corporation.

   4. may receive funding from voluntary agencies, such as United Way.

10. A nurse working in a hospital-based home care agency is presenting the annual report to the hospital board. The nurse states, "In order for the hospital to operate this home care agency,

    1. the hospital must be a nonprofit agency."

    2. third-party payers will reimburse all costs."

    3. the primary source of referrals comes from the inpatient population."

    4. funding is determined by the state board of health."

11. The home care nurse is assigned to change the dressing of a 78-year-old client following an emergency gallbladder surgery. The client asks the nurse if the home services will be covered by Medicare reimbursement. The most appropriate response by the nurse is

    1. "Reimbursement of services is based on the financial need of each client."

    2. "Your home care will be covered because your physician certified you as homebound."

    3. "I will update your plan of care every six months to maintain your coverage."

    4. "Your care will be covered as a nonskilled nursing service."

12. The local hospital has contacted a new home health agency in the community to identify what services the agency can provide. Which of the following services would be appropriate for the nurse to include in the examples given to the hospital of care that is available?

    1. Follow-up on three cases of tuberculosis in the local community

    2. Teaching prenatal classes in the local hospital

    3. Screening older people at a meal site for nutritional problems

    4. Running a hospice at the local hospital

Answer: 4

Rationale: Private nonprofit agencies are governed by a board of directors and often receive funding from voluntary agencies. The agency, not the employees, has a tax exempt status. Proprietary agencies have stockholders who are concerned about making a profit.

Nursing process: Planning

Client need: Management of Care

Cognitive level: Application

Subject area: Community Health

Answer: 3

Rationale: Most institutional-based agencies are operated and funded by hospitals and are governed by the hospital's board of directors. The hospital expects the home care agency to serve as a source of revenue by providing home care for inpatients after discharge.

Nursing process: Implementation

Client need: Management of Care

Cognitive level: Analysis

Subject area: Community Health

Answer: 2

Rationale: In order to qualify for reimbursement of home health care, the physician must certify that the client is homebound and requires skilled nursing care. Medicare only covers a client over the age of 65 years or a client who is permanently disabled. Outcome and Assessment Information Set (OASIS) is a mandated federal requirement for all home health agencies. Its purpose is to measure outcomes for outcome-based quality improvement. Data must be collected at admission and every 60 days until discharge.

Nursing process: Analysis

Client need: Management of Care

Cognitive level: Analysis

Subject area: Community Health

Answer: 1

Rationale: The home health care nurse might be involved in case finding and follow-up that may impact the health in the community. The home health care nurse is usually not involved in screening, teaching, or managing in specific organizations.

Nursing process: Planning

Client need: Management of Care

Cognitive level: Application

Subject area: Community Health

13. A public health nurse and a home health care nurse are meeting to discuss their roles in the community. The home health care nurse states that the nurse's role in home health care focuses on

    1. health promotion in the home.

    2. disease prevention in the home.

    3. illness care in the hospital.

    4. illness care in the home.

14. When planning the home care for a client who has returned home after suffering a stroke, the home health care nurse should plan to supervise which of the following?

    1. The speech therapist who works with the client

    2. The discharge planner who works with the client and family

    3. The home care aide who assists the client with personal cares

    4. The physical therapist who helps the client regain mobility

15. During an initial home visit to assess the client's needs, the nurse should inform the client

    1. about the physician's orders that mandate care.

    2. about the client's rights at the start of care.

    3. what must be paid by the client directly to Medicare.

    4. that advanced medical directives do not apply in the home setting.

Answer: 4

Rationale: Home health care focuses on illness care in the home and posthospital follow-up. Public health focuses on health promotion and prevention in the community.

Nursing process: Implementation

Client need: Management of Care

Cognitive level: Application

Subject area: Community Health

Answer: 3

Rationale: Although the home health care nurse may coordinate and collaborate with the discharge planner and the speech and physical therapists, the only supervisory responsibility will be with the home care aide.

Nursing process: Planning

Client need: Management of Care

Cognitive level: Application

Subject area: Community Health

Answer: 2

Rationale: The Home Care Bill of Rights expects the nurse to obtain informed consent at the start of care, to detail what can be expected from the home care services, and to explain the rights of the client under those services, including the option for advanced medical directives.

Nursing process: Implementation

Client need: Management of Care

Cognitive level: Application

Subject area: Community Health

Hospice

62

1. The daughter of a client asks the nurse how her mother can become a hospice client. Which of the following is the appropriate response by the nurse?

   1. "Anyone can make a hospice referral."
   2. "Your mother's physician must refer your mother."
   3. "The hospital discharge planner must make the referral from the hospital."
   4. "Your mother must start with home health first and then move to hospice."

2. The nurse assesses a hospice client to be unresponsive and incontinent, with limbs that are cool and mottling, and with a blood pressure of 80/48. The nurse evaluates this client and determines the client

   1. is experiencing a drug overdose.
   2. should go to the hospital.
   3. is moribund.
   4. needs a home health aide.

3. When preparing for stabilization of a client with end-stage breast cancer who develops a gastrointestinal bleed, it would be essential for the nurse to explain which of the following?

   1. Stabilization at home because there is no hospitalization or hospice
   2. Stabilization at home because the client is terminal
   3. Hospitalization for stabilization paid by the client
   4. Hospitalization for stabilization paid by hospice

4. A nurse in the pediatric infectious disease unit should give which of the following information about hospice to the family of a child with acquired immunodeficiency syndrome (AIDS)?

   1. Hospice will pay for all the child's drugs.
   2. Hospice provides an interdisciplinary team to support families.
   3. Hospice means that the physician has given up on caring for the child.
   4. Hospice means there is no longer hope for the child.

Answer: 1

Rationale: Hospice is a palliative program of coordinated care designed to deliver care to terminally ill clients and their families. Hospice relieves pain and other clinical manifestations without the intention of curing the client. Anyone can refer clients to hospice.

Nursing process: Analysis

Client need: Management of Care

Cognitive level: Analysis

Subject area: Community Health

Answer: 3

Rationale: Although drug overdose may produce some of the clinical manifestations, a client who is moribund, or nearing death, will exhibit cool mottled limbs, be unresponsive and incontinent, and have a low blood pressure.

Nursing process: Evaluation

Client need: Management of Care

Cognitive level: Application

Subject area: Community Health

Answer: 4

Rationale: Medicare hospice will pay for the hospitalization to stabilize the client's clinical manifestations for respite, long-term, and short-term care.

Nursing process: Analysis

Client need: Management of Care

Cognitive level: Analysis

Subject area: Community Health

Answer: 2

Rationale: Medicare is the only insurance that guarantees medication payment. Medicare does not cover children. A decision to choose hospice care means that the family and caregivers switch from trying to cure to intensive caring, which includes control of the clinical manifestations. Trying to improve the family's quality of life becomes the goal.

Nursing process: Planning

Client need: Management of Care

Cognitive level: Application

Subject area: Community Health

5. A hospice nurse is caring for a client in the hospital with congestive heart failure who has problems of impaired mobility, skin alteration, impaired breathing, alteration in oral mucous membranes, and impaired nutrition. The client develops a new abdominal pain. The nurse should prepare the client for which of the following treatment modalities?

   1. Hospitalization to determine the etiology of the abdominal pain

   2. Laparoscopy to diagnose the etiology for the abdominal pain

   3. Aggressive relief of the clinical manifestations

   4. No change in the treatment for the abdominal pain

6. The nurse informs the family of a client in hospice that which of the following services are available for Medicare coverage?

   Select all that apply:

   [ ] 1. Diagnostic services

   [ ] 2. Surgery

   [ ] 3. Medications

   [ ] 4. Curative radiation

   [ ] 5. Durable medical equipment

   [ ] 6. Psychiatrist

7. The nurse should include which of the following priority considerations to determine a client's readiness to learn?

   Select all that apply:

   [ ] 1. The client's medications

   [ ] 2. The nurse's teaching ability

   [ ] 3. The client's stress level

   [ ] 4. The client's level of wellness

   [ ] 5. The lesson plan

   [ ] 6. The client's medical diagnosis

8. A client in the moribund state is experiencing periods of dyspnea followed by periods of apnea, then rapid breathing. The nurse documents this as _____.

Answer: 3

Rationale: Hospice provides for aggressive relief of the clinical manifestations even within the hospital setting. It does not provide for surgery of other ailments, or for diagnosis of new conditions.

Nursing process: Planning

Client need: Management of Care

Cognitive level: Application

Subject area: Community Health

Answer: 3, 5

Rationale: Hospice expenses covered under Medicare include medications and durable medical equipment. Diagnosis, curative treatments, and curative medications are not part of the hospice benefit.

Nursing process: Implementation

Client need: Management of Care

Cognitive level: Application

Subject area: Community Health

Answer: 1, 3, 4, 6

Rationale: Learning readiness is defined as how prepared the client is to learn when the educator first addresses learning. Medications, level of wellness, medical diagnosis, stress, desire to change, and many other conditions affect learning readiness. The nurse's teaching ability and the lesson plan both focus on the nurse and not the client's readiness.

Nursing process: Planning

Client need: Management of Care

Cognitive level: Analysis

Subject area: Community Health

Answer: Cheyne-Stokes

Rationale: Breathing that begins normally, slows to apnea, and then begins again with rapid breathing is called Cheyne-Stokes respiration and is common just before death.

Nursing process: Implementation

Client need: Management of Care

Cognitive level: Comprehension

Subject area: Community Health

9. After receiving a terminal diagnosis of congestive heart failure, a client is hostile to family members and hospice staff. The family is very upset by this and asks the nurse why the client is so hostile. The most appropriate response by the nurse is which of the following?

   1. "A terminal disease causes a sudden change in personality."

   2. "The lack of oxygen to the brain causes the client to act angry."

   3. "Drugs like digoxin (Lanoxin) can cause sudden mood shifts."

   4. "This is a temporary stage, as the client prepares for an imminent death."

10. The hospice team has not been able to relieve the client's pain after repeated tries. One caregiver expresses concern to another caregiver that the pain is not real. The nurse tells the caregiver that pain is

    1. an unpleasant sensory and emotional experience arising from tissue damage.

    2. a cry for attention when clients do not cope with their mortality.

    3. the result of an emotional reaction.

    4. associated with all physical and mental illnesses.

11. A student nurse caring for a hospice client who is moribund and has not had a bowel movement for five days asks the nurse about giving the client an enema. Which of the following is the priority response by the nurse?

    1. "Mineral oil is more effective than an enema."

    2. "Maintaining a bowel program is essential to avoid pain and impactions."

    3. "A stool softener may be administered."

    4. "The body is slowing down and constipation is expected."

12. The nurse should prepare to administer which of the following drugs to a hospice client experiencing mild pain?

    1. Codeine

    2. Meperidine (Demerol)

    3. Hydromorphone (Dilaudid)

    4. Morphine

Answer: 4

Rationale: Hostility can be a reaction to the realization that one will soon die. The period is usually a short one, as the person generally adjusts to the facts and moves on to completing life's cycle.

Nursing process: Analysis

Client need: Management of Care

Cognitive level: Analysis

Subject area: Community Health

Answer: 1

Rationale: Pain is defined as an unpleasant sensory and emotional experience arising from tissue damage.

Nursing process: Implementation

Client need: Management of Care

Cognitive level: Application

Subject area: Community Health

Answer: 4

Rationale: The body slows down just before death and constipation is a common condition. Giving an enema or a stool softener would stress the body further. The caregiver can be directed to care in other ways that meet the client's needs during the last few hours before death.

Nursing process: Analysis

Client need: Management of Care

Cognitive level: Analysis

Subject area: Community Health

Answer: 1

Rationale: Codeine is the drug commonly given to ease the mild discomfort of a hospice client. Morphine, meperidine (Demerol), and hydromorphone (Dilaudid) are drugs used to treat moderate to severe pain.

Nursing process: Planning

Client need: Pharmalogic and Parenteral Therapies

Cognitive level: Application

Subject area: Pharmalogic

13. Which of the following drugs would be most appropriate for the nurse to administer to a client with end-stage carcinoma who has a recent diagnosis of uncontrollable pain?

    1. Loratab with nonsteroidal anti-inflammatory drugs

    2. Codeine with nonsteroidal anti-inflammatory drugs

    3. Fentanyl

    4. Morphine

14. Which of the following clients should the nurse refer to a hospice program?

    1. A client recently diagnosed with breast cancer

    2. A client scheduled for a bone marrow transplant

    3. A client who has terminal ovarian cancer

    4. A client who has pancreatic cancer

Answer: 4

Rationale: Morphine is appropriate for severe pain. Fentanyl is administered after a client has been on morphine sulfate for an extended period.

Nursing process: Implementation

Client need: Pharmacological and Parenteral Therapies

Cognitive level: Application

Subject area: Pharmacologic

Answer: 3

Rationale: Although diagnoses of breast and pancreatic cancers or a client who is to have a bone marrow transplant carry uncertain courses of treatment and prognoses, the client must already be determined to be terminal before a referral to hospice can be made.

Nursing process: Implementation

Client need: Management of Care

Cognitive level: Application

Subject area: Community Health

UNIT VIII

Legal and Ethical Issues

Cultural Diversity

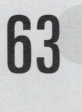

63

1. The outpatient care nurse is discussing postoperative dismissal teaching with an Asian-American client. During the discussion, the client looks at the floor, smiles at times, and nods his head. The nurse interprets this nonverbal behavior as

   1. an acceptance of the dismissal instructions.

   2. an understanding of the material taught.

   3. a reflection of cultural values.

   4. an ability to follow through with instructions.

2. The nurse in the emergency room is evaluating a head laceration on an 8-year-old Asian-American client. Prior to the physical assessment, the nurse should

   1. ask the parents to step out of the room.

   2. ask permission to examine the head.

   3. touch the child gently, explaining the procedure.

   4. discuss the dismissal care of a laceration.

3. The admission nurse is gathering family information on an Asian-American client. The client mentions the term "clan." The nurse understands this term to mean

   1. a group of friends and relatives that accompanied the client.

   2. the client's spouse.

   3. a sacred symbol the client wishes to keep nearby at all times.

   4. a recognized group of families with the same last name and line of ancestors.

4. The nursing instructor is describing the Chinese-American philosophy of *yin* and *yang* to a group of nursing students. The instructor describes how foods are classified using this belief system. Which of the following statements should the nursing instructor include that correctly describes the *yin* and *yang* food correlation?

   1. *Yin* foods are hot.

   2. *Yin* and *yang* deals with energy, not food.

   3. *Yang* foods are cold.

   4. Cold foods are consumed when a hot illness is present.

Answer: 3

Rationale: In the Asian-American culture, eye contact is avoided with authority figures. Head nodding does not necessarily reflect agreement. Direct eye contact is frequently viewed as rude. The Asian-American culture typically avoids confrontation. The word "no" is avoided because it would show disrespect.

Nursing process: Analysis

Client need: Management of Care

Cognitive level: Analysis

Subject area: Legal and Ethical Issues

Answer: 2

Rationale: In the Asian-American culture, the head is considered sacred. Touching the head is seen as disrespectful. Permission must be sought to touch the client. The parents should remain with the child to offer comfort and support.

Nursing process: Planning

Client need: Management of Care

Cognitive level: Application

Subject area: Legal and Ethical Issues

Answer: 4

Rationale: In the Asian-American culture, a clan is a family structure that includes a group of individuals considered ancestors and who have the same last name.

Nursing process: Analysis

Client need: Management of Care

Cognitive level: Application

Subject area: Legal and Ethical Issues

Answer: 4

Rationale: In the Chinese-American culture, foods are classified as hot or cold and are transformed into *yin* and *yang* energy when metabolized by the body. *Yin* and *yang* represent a balance between positive and negative forces. *Yin* foods are cold and *yang* foods are hot. Cold foods are eaten when a hot illness is present. Hot foods are eaten when a cold illness is present.

Nursing process: Planning

Client need: Management of Care

Cognitive level: Analysis

Subject area: Legal and Ethical Issues

5. The nurse in the urgent care center is assessing an Asian-American adolescent with complaints of a sore throat. When auscultating lung sounds, the nurse notices round bluish marks along each side of the client's back. The nurse reports this as which of the following?

   1. A potential skin infection
   2. A sign of abuse
   3. The practice of cupping
   4. An allergy to a medication

6. During a care conference involving the nurse, physician, social worker, Asian-American client, and Asian-American family members, some suggestions for further care are being discussed. The client is sitting in a chair at the edge of the room. The client looks only at the family and does not speak during the conference. The nurse assesses the client's behavior as

   1. a withdrawal from the situation.
   2. a sign of denial regarding the condition.
   3. a lack of understanding of the discussion.
   4. a sign of respect for members of the health care team.

7. The nurse is reviewing follow-up instructions with an African-American client. The nurse notices that the client has missed two follow-up appointments in the last week. The client states "something else came up." The nurse interprets this as

   1. a lack of understanding of the follow-up routine.
   2. uncertainty of the willingness of the client to pursue further care.
   3. a sense of noncommitment toward the plan of care.
   4. a cultural value of a flexible time frame.

8. An African-American client with hypertension is attending a class on ways to take control of hypertension. The nurse explains dietary measures that can be used to help control blood pressure. Which of the following indicates the client has understood the material presented?

   1. "I love fried chicken, but will choose broiled skinless chicken as my entrée."
   2. "It is okay to use table salt, just not too much."
   3. "I can still drink wine or beer with my dinner; these fluids don't interfere with blood pressure."
   4. "I've never been a big vegetable eater; I don't suppose I need to start now."

Answer: 3

Rationale: In the Asian-American culture, cupping involves applying a glass over the skin to create a suction that causes the skin to swell and turn bluish. This practice is believed to let the unhealthy air currents out of the body. If an allergy to a medication existed, the rash typically would be located in more areas than just the back. Further investigation and discussion would be necessary before abuse could be suspected.

Nursing process: Analysis

Client need: Management of Care

Cognitive level: Analysis

Subject area: Legal and Ethical Issues

Answer: 4

Rationale: The Asian-American culture is typically viewed as quiet, polite, avoiding direct eye contact. Silence is valued and maintaining a distance is respected. Nonverbal communication is very important.

Nursing process: Assessment

Client need: Management of Care

Cognitive level: Application

Subject area: Legal and Ethical Issues

Answer: 4

Rationale: A characteristic of African-American culture is the concept of time as flexible. The present takes precedent over the future. Members of the cultural group avoid rigidly scheduled appointments.

Nursing process: Analysis

Client need: Management of Care

Cognitive level: Analysis

Subject area: Legal and Ethical Issues

Answer: 1

Rationale: In the African-American culture, clients typically enjoy fried, fatty foods. They slow-cook foods in added fat. The client has made an appropriate alteration to this food choice by choosing broiled skinless chicken over fried chicken. Salt and alcohol should be avoided. Encouraging fresh fruits and vegetables is also appropriate.

Nursing process: Evaluation

Client need: Management of Care

Cognitive level: Application

Subject area: Legal and Ethical Issues

9. An older adult African-American client has just received a diagnosis of prostate cancer. During a discussion with the family and nurse, the client states, "This is all in God's hands now; there's not much more I can do." The nurse interprets this statement as the client

   1. accepts the diagnosis.

   2. gives up on a possible cure.

   3. expresses feelings of loss of control.

   4. expresses a cultural belief in the connectedness of God, health, and illness.

10. The nurse is caring for an African-American client who recently had a hysterectomy. The client requests certain herbs from the dietician to be included with meals. When the meals arrive, the client and the faith healer perform a ritual over the herbs. The nurse assesses this as

    1. an unacceptable event and reports it to the charge nurse.

    2. a common practice to combine herbs, faith healing, and Western medicine.

    3. a way for the client to think she has control.

    4. a way for the client to individualize her own care.

11. The nurse in the diagnostic imaging center is preparing an African-American client with a history of headaches for a CT scan. Which of the following questions should the nurse avoid asking during the initial assessment?

    1. "Do you experience vision changes?"

    2. "Do you experience shortness of breath?"

    3. "Do you have a close relationship with your family?"

    4. "Do you typically experience headaches daily?"

12. The nurse is involved in discharge planning for an older Hispanic-American client with a terminal illness. The nurse offers services, such as Meals on Wheels, nursing care, and hospice. The client's family insists on providing all the care. The nurse identifies this situation as

    1. an unrealistic expectation for members of the family.

    2. an inability to accept other forms of help.

    3. a common practice, since it is often seen as a privilege when family members care for older adults.

    4. a way for family to stay in control of the older adult client.

Answer: 4

Rationale: In the African-American culture, there is a strong belief in God. They view God, health, and illness as being interconnected.

Nursing process: Evaluation

Client need: Management of Care

Cognitive level: Analysis

Subject area: Legal and Ethical Issues

Answer: 2

Rationale: It is common in the African-American culture to combine Western medicine with other traditions. An herbalist or folk healer may be consulted before an individual seeks traditional medicine. Certainly the patient has a right to request herbs and a faith healer. This activity would not warrant the charge nurse being notified.

Nursing process: Assessment

Client need: Management of Care

Cognitive level: Analysis

Subject area: Legal and Ethical Issues

Answer: 3

Rationale: In the African-American culture, it is considered intrusive to ask personal questions during the initial assessment. Asking a client about having vision changes, shortness of breath, or headaches is physiologically based; these questions take priority during the admission process.

Nursing process: Assessment

Client need: Management of Care

Cognitive level: Application

Subject area: Legal and Ethical Issues

Answer: 3

Rationale: In the Hispanic-American culture, older adults are respected and honored. Extended families typically live together and provide care as necessary. This is seen as a privilege, not an obligation. Family members encourage involvement of the extended family.

Nursing process: Analysis

Client need: Management of Care

Cognitive level: Analysis

Subject area: Legal and Ethical Issues

13. A home health care nurse is visiting a Hispanic-American client who does not speak English. A translator is not available at the time of the visit. The best approach for the nurse to overcome the language barrier is to

   1. discuss one issue at a time.

   2. write the medical terms down.

   3. offer to return at a different time.

   4. use simple words, gestures, and pictures.

14. A Hispanic-American client arrived at the emergency room complaining of severe stomach pains and cramps. Upon evaluation, the client described to the nurse a home remedy that included massage, prayer, rubbing, and gently pinching the spine. The nurse interpreted this behavior as

   1. an extreme attempt to avoid visiting a physician.

   2. an example of traditional folk remedies accepted by the Hispanic-American culture.

   3. a denial of the seriousness of the medical condition.

   4. an alternative approach with no scientific basis.

15. The nurse informs another nurse that which of the following statements best describes American Indians' beliefs about health?

   1. "The earth gives food, shelter, and medicine to humankind, and all things of the earth belong to human beings and nature."

   2. "Health is believed to reflect internal harmony."

   3. "Traditional health beliefs focus on illness and achieving health through nature."

   4. "The human body is viewed as several parts working together to attain health."

16. The nurse is explaining preoperative information to an American Indian client. The nurse observes the client to be quiet, looking at the picture on the wall, and not readily responding to the nurse's questions. This behavior would indicate the client

   1. is not accepting the information.

   2. has a hearing impairment.

   3. is listening to the nurse.

   4. is focusing on the environment.

Answer: 4

Rationale: If a translator is not present with a client who does not speak English, communication will take more time. The nurse must be creative and patient. Using simple words, gestures, and pictures may prove helpful. Written medical terms will not be effective if the client doesn't understand English. Discussion of one issue at a time does not overcome the language barrier. Rescheduling home visits is not generally acceptable.

Nursing process: Planning

Client need: Management of Care

Cognitive level: Application

Subject area: Legal and Ethical Issues

Answer: 2

Rationale: Folk remedies are widely accepted practices in the Hispanic-American culture. At times, a combination of folk remedies and Western medicine are utilized. Many Hispanic-American clients will not discuss folk remedies with their physician.

Nursing process: Analysis

Client need: Management of Care

Cognitive level: Analysis

Subject area: Legal and Ethical Issues

Answer: 1

Rationale: Traditional American Indian health beliefs reflect a bond between person and nature. Health is believed to reflect harmony with the surrounding environment and family. Traditional beliefs focus on wellness, not illness. The body is divided into two halves that are seen as plus and minus or two energy poles, one positive and one negative.

Nursing process: Implementation

Client need: Management of Care

Cognitive level: Analysis

Subject area: Legal and Ethical Issues

Answer: 3

Rationale: Typical nonverbal behavior of American Indians is quiet listening. Silence is respected and eye contact is considered disrespectful. Communication style is often slow with a low tone of voice and reflection between statements.

Nursing process: Analysis

Client need: Management of Care

Cognitive level: Analysis

Subject area: Legal and Ethical Issues

17. The nurse admitting an American Indian client is working on the admission forms. The nurse has asked the client to speak louder and to repeat several comments. The client gets frustrated and won't continue the interview. Which of the following best describes this interaction?

1. The nurse was unaware of acceptable forms of communication with Indian clients.

2. The client was feeling rushed during the interview process.

3. The nurse was seeking clarification during the interview.

4. The client was uncertain about the interview process.

18. A nurse teaching a class on the characteristics of an Arab-American family unit uses the term "patrilineal." The nurse should include which of the following statements to best describe patrilineal?

1. A concept of honor or shame in the family

2. A philosophy of time orientation specific to the Arab culture

3. A special bond evident in most Arab families

4. A family group consisting of family members on the father's side

19. A nurse is reviewing a diet with an Arab-American client. The nurse understands which of the following foods are typical in the Arab diet?

Select all that apply:

[   ] **1.** Fried foods

[   ] **2.** Rice

[   ] **3.** Canned processed foods

[   ] **4.** Soup

[   ] **5.** Chicken

[   ] **6.** Lamb

20. The nurse is teaching a class on the cultural aspects of the Arab-American client. Which of the following should the nurse include in this class?

1. Friends are the strongest social unit in the Arab-American culture.

2. The majority of Arabs immigrating to the United States are Muslims.

3. Following Islam has no effect on the lifestyles of Arab Americans.

4. Mealtime is a social time of long duration.

Answer: 1

Rationale: During an interview, asking an American Indian to speak louder and repeat responses is seen as rude and disrespectful.

Nursing process: Evaluation

Client need: Management of Care

Cognitive level: Analysis

Subject area: Legal and Ethical Issues

Answer: 4

Rationale: Patrilineal descent is typical of Arab-American families and means a family group consisting of family members on the father's side.

Nursing process: Planning

Client need: Management of Care

Cognitive level: Application

Subject area: Legal and Ethical Issues

Answer: 2, 4, 5, 6

Rationale: The Arab diet is rich in rice, soup, chicken, and lamb. Fried and canned foods are usually avoided. Pork is prohibited and meat is slaughtered in a specific fashion.

Nursing process: Analysis

Client need: Basic Care and Comfort

Cognitive level: Application

Subject area: Legal and Ethical Issues

Answer: 2

Rationale: The majority of Arab Americans immigrating to the United States are Muslims. Family members, not friends, are the strongest social unit. Following Islam is the pillar of the Arab-American lifestyle. Meals are often consumed very quickly and in silence.

Nursing process: Planning

Client need: Management of Care

Cognitive level: Analysis

Subject area: Legal and Ethical Issues

21. An Arab-American client is referred for continuing care related to dizziness and vision changes. The nurse understands that an Arab-American client would prefer which of the following therapies as a treatment of the condition?

1. Continued monitoring of the clinical manifestations

2. CT scan of the head

3. Blood work to check electrolytes

4. Vision screening

22. A nurse caring for an Arab-American client is assessing the client's pain following angiography. The client is lying in bed, eyes tightly closed, and continually asks for more pain medication. The client states, "I asked for pain medication right away and I need it now!" Which of the following nursing actions would be most appropriate at this time?

1. Check to see when the pain medication was last given

2. Explain to the client that the nurse was not aware of the discomfort

3. Try to obtain more information regarding the pain

4. Inform the client that the pain medication will be administered after assisting another client

23. Which of the following should the nurse include in a class on the health belief system associated with clients of the Russian-American culture?

1. A belief that man has little control over nature

2. A belief that God's will is the only will

3. A belief that nature, environment, and man are directly linked to health and wellness

4. A belief that eating right will maintain health

24. A nurse educator is working with staff on cultural diversity issues related to nonverbal communication. The educator explains to another nurse that appropriate nonverbal communication in the Russian-American culture includes which of the following?

1. Nodding is a gesture of approval.

2. Handshakes are avoided.

3. Direct eye contact is avoided.

4. Touch is considered an invasion of privacy.

Answer: 2

Rationale: Generally, Arab-American clients prefer highly technical, even invasive, procedures over noninvasive treatment modalities.

Nursing process: Analysis

Client need: Management of Care

Cognitive level: Analysis

Subject area: Legal and Ethical Issues

Answer: 1

Rationale: It is typical of the Arab-American culture that immediate pain relief is expected and may be persistently requested. Trying to obtain more information or explaining that the nurse was unaware of the discomfort is not appropriate at this time. Assisting another client should be delegated to another staff member.

Nursing process: Planning

Client need: Management of Care

Cognitive level: Application

Subject area: Legal and Ethical Issues

Answer: 1

Rationale: Russian-American cultural belief regarding health is very much the idea that one has little or no control over health and illness. Nature, environment, God's will, and eating right have no part in the belief system.

Nursing process: Planning

Client need: Management of Care

Cognitive level: Analysis

Subject area: Legal and Ethical Issues

Answer: 1

Rationale: Direct eye contact is used and appreciated in the Russian-American culture. Eye contact indicates trustworthiness and honesty. Touch and handshaking are used for formal greetings. Nodding is a gesture of approval.

Nursing process: Implementation

Client need: Management of Care

Cognitive level: Application

Subject area: Legal and Ethical Issues

25. A care conference is scheduled to discuss the prognosis of a terminally ill Russian-American client. The family members insist the client not be told the diagnosis. The nurse interprets this behavior as

1. unacceptable because every client has a right to personal medical information.

2. an ethical violation on the part of the family.

3. a typical response in Russian-American cultural tradition dealing with terminal illness.

4. a dishonest way of communicating.

Answer: 3

Rationale: In the case of a terminal illness, a common Russian-American cultural practice is to only disclose the medical condition to nearest relatives. It is believed the client will do better if the client continues to have hope for recovery.

Nursing process: Analysis

Client need: Management of Care

Cognitive level: Analysis

Subject area: Legal and Ethical Issues

Leadership and Management

64

1. A family has recently moved to a new metropolitan area and is looking for a health care delivery system that will serve the needs of all family members, including a father who is an older adult and recently had a stroke and is in need of rehabilitative services. The nurse informs the family that which of the following agencies would be the best health care choice?

   1. A home health care service
   2. A university medical center and outpatient services
   3. A suburban community hospital
   4. Health promotion services for the entire family

2. A family selected population-based health care practice of America. The nurse manager teaching this family about the health care services available would include which of the following statements?

   1. "We have an asthma clinic specifically for clients of all ages."
   2. "The major initiative of our care delivery system is restorative care."
   3. "The main advantage to families is that palliative care is the main priority."
   4. "If specialty care is needed, the health care provider will make a referral to a tertiary care system."

3. Based on an understanding of evidence-based client care, the nurse manager should include which of the following instructions for the staff on how to address the home care needs of a group of clients who have had knee replacements?

   1. "I know from experience that these clients will need a concrete exercise plan."
   2. "Most clients exhibit anxiety when describing the stairs within their homes."
   3. "Knee replacement care is complex because of the age of these clients."
   4. "Dietary instructions at home are based on common standards of practice and the most recent research for promoting healing."

Answer: 2

Rationale: Tertiary health care services include restorative and rehabilitative services for clients of all ages. A university medical center with outpatient services is best equipped to deliver care across the continuum for this family. A home health care service, suburban community, and health promotion services for the entire family are limited to a specific level of care.

Nursing process: Implementation

Client need: Management of Care

Cognitive level: Application

Subject area: Legal and Ethical Issues

Answer: 1

Rationale: Population-based health care practice is the development, provision, and evaluation of multidisciplinary health care services to population groups experiencing an increased risk in partnership with consumers of health care and the community, in order to improve the health of the community and its diverse population groups. Population-based care is a managed care approach for a specific group of clients, not just individuals. The goal of care in a population-based system is to maintain and promote wellness, not restorative care. Specialty care and palliative care can be a part of the services, but may not be the priority; nor is referral necessary to a larger system.

Nursing process: Planning

Client need: Management of Care

Cognitive level: Analysis

Subject area: Legal and Ethical Issues

Answer: 4

Rationale: Evidence-based practice is a combination of knowledge and expertise in clinical practice, as well as the most recent research findings with each specific client. While clients usually understand the exercise plan needed to strengthen overall muscle and joints, anxiety can be minimized with teaching and practice dealing with steps. Knee replacement care is complex, but the age of the client is not relevant. Dietary instructions, such as increase protein, are important for healing following a knee replacement.

Nursing process: Planning

Client need: Management of Care

Cognitive level: Analysis

Subject area: Legal and Ethical Issues

4. A new graduate nurse is interviewing for a staff position in a health care delivery system that has agencies in five different states. Which of the following statements indicates that the new nurse understands the legalities of nursing practice, if hired by this company?

   1. "Standards of practice are established by the governing agency, so practice issues will be covered at each agency site."

   2. "A registered nurse license is acknowledged in all of the 50 states without additional paperwork."

   3. "The nurse practice act in each state will provide the legal guidelines for professional nursing practice."

   4. "The nurse will practice nursing at any of the five agencies based on the nurse practice act in the nurse's home state."

5. After reviewing incident reports for one month, a nurse working in the risk management department at a local health care facility determines which of the following violations of client care is most common?

   1. Physical abuse

   2. Substance abuse

   3. Malpractice actions

   4. Negligence of care

6. Which of the following laws require a nurse to report a peer who is keeping a portion of narcotics ordered for a client?

   1. Reporting laws

   2. Malpractice laws

   3. Jurisdiction laws

   4. Civil court laws

7. Which of the following should the nurse manager include in staff development classes related to ethical decision making?

   1. The practice of ethics is the philosophy of individual opinion and values.

   2. Ethical decisions made in client care are based on the opinion of the client and family.

   3. Ethical decision making is based on knowledge, facts, and a strong commitment to right and wrong.

   4. Ethical decision making in client care can only be made by an interdisciplinary team.

Answer: 3

Rationale: Nurse practice acts may differ from state to state. The state board of nursing for each state monitors the legal practice of nursing in each state. While standards of care may be policy at each agency, they do not override the standards outlined in the nurse practice act for each agency's state. Once an RN license has been obtained, reciprocity to practice in other states must be granted by each state board.

Nursing process: Evaluation

Client need: Management of Care

Cognitive level: Analysis

Subject area: Legal and Ethical Issues

Answer: 4

Rationale: Negligence is the most common violation of client care in health care facilities. Negligence is a deviation from the appropriate standard of care, usually due to carelessness. Physical abuse, substance abuse, and malpractice actions are all criminal acts and occur less frequently.

Nursing process: Analysis

Client need: Management of Care

Cognitive level: Application

Subject area: Legal and Ethical Issues

Answer: 1

Rationale: Reporting laws in each state require a professional to report incompetent practice, client abuse, and professional impairment. Malpractice laws, jurisdiction laws, and civil court laws may vary from state to state.

Nursing process: Analysis

Client need: Management of Care

Cognitive level: Analysis

Subject area: Legal and Ethical Issues

Answer: 3

Rationale: Making ethical decisions requires skill in analyzing knowledge, facts, rules of care, and a strong personal distinction between what is right and wrong in a specific client situation. Opinion is not the driving force in decision making. Ethical decision making in client care made by an interdisciplinary team is ultimately possible when ethics committees meet to discuss individual client cases. It is important to remember that every nurse practices as an individual professional and incorporates ethical decision making into everyday practice.

Nursing process: Planning

Client need: Management of Care

Cognitive level: Analysis

Subject area: Legal and Ethical Issues

8. The nursing manager on the orthopedic unit evaluates a new staff nurse on the night shift as a born "leader," based on which of the following true leadership qualities?

   1. Having incomplete intake and output records on the night shift was a problem; records have been consistently complete since the new staff nurse arrived.

   2. The new staff nurse has scheduled staff journal club discussions once a month to increase current knowledge about client care issues.

   3. The new staff nurse always works overtime when asked by the nurse manager.

   4. Incomplete shift counts for medications were first noticed by the new staff nurse.

9. The nurse manager who wishes to empower the nurses on the unit recognizes that strategies must be found to promote their leadership ability. Which of the following supports the nurse manager's knowledge of leadership?

   1. Leadership qualities are demonstrated by those in formal and informal management positions.

   2. Nurses at all levels of the organizational chart are not responsible for leadership traits.

   3. Leadership characteristics are not measurable on performance appraisals.

   4. Only top-level managers have the vision, passion, and integrity to demonstrate leadership.

10. The nurse leader who empowers the staff to participate in decision-making activities is exhibiting which of the following leadership styles?

    1. Laissez-faire

    2. Situational

    3. Autocratic

    4. Democratic

11. The nurse describes which of the following leadership models as an integral part of the democratic leadership style?

    1. Transactional

    2. Transformational

    3. Transdepartmental

    4. Transprofessional

Answer: 2

Rationale: Knowing the importance of keeping up-to-date on practice issues and having the confidence to implement a strategy to discuss client care issues as a new staff member both demonstrate leadership quality in this staff nurse.

Nursing process: Evaluation

Client need: Management of Care

Cognitive level: Analysis

Subject area: Legal and Ethical Issues

Answer: 1

Rationale: Leadership qualities and an ability to influence others to achieve goals can be exhibited by any employee in an organization. Individuals with good management skills may not demonstrate leadership ability.

Nursing process: Evaluation

Client need: Management of Care

Cognitive level: Analysis

Subject area: Legal and Ethical Issues

Answer: 4

Rationale: Democratic leaders seek participation in decision-making activities by all levels of staff affected at the unit level. Laissez-faire leadership is a passive and permissive style of leadership that defers decision making. An autocratic leadership style involves decision making that is centralized with the leader making decisions and using power to command and control others. Situational leadership confirms that there is not one best leadership style, but rather that effective leadership is matched to the group's level of task-relevant readiness.

Nursing process: Evaluation

Client need: Management of Care

Cognitive level: Application

Subject area: Legal and Ethical Issues

Answer: 2

Rationale: Transformational leadership theory includes explicitly seeking collaboration, consultation, and consensus building among team members. Transactional leadership model is aligned with transactional leadership. Transdepartmental and transprofessional are strategies, not leadership models, for gathering information across departments within an organization or within the profession as a whole.

Nursing process: Implementation

Client need: Management of Care

Cognitive level: Application

Subject area: Legal and Ethical Issues

12. The management process is incorporated in many job descriptions, such as head nurse, staff nurse, nutritionist, and therapist. Which of the following managerial activities are common to all health care positions?

Select all that apply:

[   ] **1.** Budgeting

[   ] **2.** Planning

[   ] **3.** Organizing

[   ] **4.** Liaison

[   ] **5.** Coordinating

[   ] **6.** Spokesperson

13. Which of the following are priorities for the nurse manager to incorporate into the nurse manager role of guiding and directing goal achievement?

Select all that apply:

[   ] **1.** Collaborator

[   ] **2.** Caregiver

[   ] **3.** Negotiator

[   ] **4.** Delegator

[   ] **5.** Communicator

[   ] **6.** Liaison

14. The nurse manager introduces to the staff the new organizational policy and procedural changes for administering blood products. According to Lewin's model for implementing change, which of the following steps of the change process is the nurse manager addressing?

1. Unfreeze

2. Move

3. Refreeze

4. Evaluate

15. A staff nurse has been assigned to the Standards of Care Committee in which the standard of care for wound care and dressing changes is going to be refined. As an effective change agent, the staff nurse will need to exhibit which of the following characteristics?

1. Quality interpersonal skills

2. Respect from clients and families

3. Expertise in clinical therapeutics

4. High ethical decision making

Answer: 2, 3, 5

Rationale: Managers of human resources, client care, and other health-related disciplines include role functions of planning, organizing, and coordinating client care activities. Not all personnel have the responsibilities of budgeting, department liaison, or director and spokesperson.

Nursing process: Analysis

Client need: Management of Care

Cognitive level: Application

Subject area: Legal and Ethical Issues

Answer: 1, 3, 4, 5

Rationale: While functioning as a caregiver and liaison is possible, the functions that are the priority for the nurse manager are collaborator, negotiator, delegator, and communicator. Nurse managers may have to assume the duties of caregiver in certain circumstances, but usually they do not have a client care assignment. The liaison role is usually carried out by the nursing staff, on behalf of the client. The nurse manager would function as spokesperson to speak on behalf of the staff of a department.

Nursing process: Planning

Client need: Management of Care

Cognitive level: Analysis

Subject area: Legal and Ethical Issues

Answer: 1

Rationale: The first step for implementing change, or unfreezing, is to assist others to understand the need for change and the steps necessary to implement the change. Communication and information sharing are essential in this step. Actual implementation of the change and accepting the change as the standard of care are activities that occur with moving and refreezing. Evaluating is necessary for overall quality management, but is not a part of the change process as described by Lewin's change theory.

Nursing process: Evaluation

Client need: Management of Care

Cognitive level: Analysis

Subject area: Legal and Ethical Issues

Answer: 1

Rationale: Although respect from clients and families, expertise in clinical therapeutics, and high ethical decision making are admirable for the staff nurse, the change process related to procedure of wound care and dressing changes will need to be discussed hospitalwide, unit by unit, utilizing quality interpersonal skills. Teaching and information sharing are essential when a change affects so many people, and these require quality interpersonal skills.

Nursing process: Analysis

Client need: Management of Care

Cognitive level: Analysis

Subject area: Legal and Ethical Issues

16. The nurse manager and staff of a 25-bed surgical unit have decided to change the client care delivery model from primary nursing to team nursing. The nurse manager prepares which of the following statements for the administration that is most appropriate to support this change?

    1. "No transition period will be necessary because all staff have experience working in teams."

    2. "The staffing goal is to have four teams, with a total of 3 to 4 RNs, 2 to 3 LPNs, and 2 nursing assistants for each shift."

    3. "The nursing assistants, who are also senior nursing students, have the knowledge and skill to lead a staffing team."

    4. "The registered nurses on the unit will be assigned 24 hours of responsibility for client care planning."

17. Based on an understanding of the differentiated nursing practice model, nurses on the burn and trauma unit have decided to assign certain client care activities because

    1. nurses have client care rounds and discuss differences in client outcomes.

    2. there is a pay differential for registered nurses who work overtime.

    3. all unit staff are accountable for annual validation of CPR, safety precautions, and client confidentiality guidelines.

    4. bachelor of science nurses (BSN) and master of science nurses (MSN) are expected to plan and implement education and research-based staff development sessions.

18. Based on an understanding of the nurse manager role, the nurse manager was notified at home of a staffing issue for the night shift because

    1. the nurse manager must be an autocratic leader.

    2. the nurse manager has 24-hour, seven-day-a-week accountability for nursing care.

    3. the regular staff members do not have managerial responsibility for problem-solving outcomes of staffing issues.

    4. the nurse manager is responsible for all staff decisions, including staffing changes.

Answer: 2

Rationale: A staffing goal of having four teams with a total of 3 to 4 RNs, 2 to 3 LPNs, and 2 nursing assistants is the best staffing option for implementing care based on flexibility and acuity of client care for a 25-bed unit. Transition in staffing and operational issues will be necessary even if all staff members have previously worked using a team nursing model. Assuming that all nursing assistants are senior nursing students is not a legally sound staffing assignment. Assigning a registered nurse to be responsible for 24-hour client care is indicative of a primary nursing model.

Nursing process: Planning

Client need: Management of Care

Cognitive level: Analysis

Subject area: Legal and Ethical Issues

Answer: 4

Rationale: Expectations to plan and implement education and research-based staff development sessions by bachelor of science nurses (BSN) and master of science nurses (MSN) are best, considering that the assignment of educational sessions is based on the education level of the nursing staff. Differentiated practice includes the assignment of duties based on education level, competence, and certification. Nurses who have client care rounds, staff nurses who work overtime, and unit staff members who are held accountable for violation of unit requirements all require nurses to do similar activities regardless of education, clinical expertise, and competence levels.

Nursing process: Analysis

Client need: Management of Care

Cognitive level: Analysis

Subject area: Legal and Ethical Issues

Answer: 2

Rationale: The nurse manager has 24-hour, seven-day-a-week accountability for nursing care. Nursing staff members are participative decision makers because of their position in the organization. Staff members should have input into the overall decision-making process.

Nursing process: Analysis

Client need: Management of Care

Cognitive level: Analysis

Subject area: Legal and Ethical Issues

19. Which of the following roles is the charge nurse applying when assigning unlicensed assistive personnel (UAP) to tasks of custodial care, vital sign monitoring, and intake and output measurement for all the clients on the unit?

   1. Delegation
   2. Accountability
   3. Responsibility
   4. Outcome measurement

20. The nurse manager incorporates which of the following functional roles of the team members when planning to conduct a class on effective team building and group process?

   1. There will always be one person who wants to dominate the discussion using personal examples.
   2. Every group needs a person in the role of creator, coordinator, and record keeper.
   3. An effective team always rallies around the leadership traits demonstrated by the group or team spokesperson.
   4. Some teams are motivated to get the job done in spite of dysfunctional behavior of a few team members.

21. The communication process is essential to the leader or manager role and to the role of the manager of client care. It is essential for all managers, including the manager of client care, to be effective communicators. The nurse who effectively analyzes the communication process understands that messages are

   1. synchronous and asynchronous.
   2. coded and encoded.
   3. verbal and nonverbal.
   4. native and foreign.

Answer: 1

Rationale: Delegation is the assignment of tasks to others who are competent and skilled to perform them. Accountability and responsibility are qualities that all caregivers must demonstrate, regardless of level of position. While the unlicensed assistive personnel (UAP) may collect data to carry out a nursing task, a nurse at a higher education level would be responsible for the overall evaluation and reporting.

Nursing process: Analysis

Client need: Management of Care

Cognitive level: Analysis

Subject area: Legal and Ethical Issues

Answer: 2

Rationale: Every group needs a person in the role of creator and coordinator as well as a record keeper. This description contains the functional roles of members of a team. A dominator is a person who wants to dominate. Some teams always rally around the leadership traits of a member of the group or team, but it takes all team members working together collaboratively to be an effective team. Some teams are motivated to get the job done in spite of the dysfunctional behavior of a few team members, but to be a more effective group all team members need to work together.

Nursing process: Planning

Client need: Management of Care

Cognitive level: Analysis

Subject area: Legal and Ethical Issues

Answer: 3

Rationale: The most effective communication process includes both verbal and nonverbal cues. The terms "synchronous" and "asynchronous" and "coded" and "encoded" describe communication concepts within computer technology. Native and foreign describe language as being one's first, or native, language or a language learned later, that is, a foreign language.

Nursing process: Analysis

Client need: Management of Care

Cognitive level: Application

Subject area: Legal and Ethical Issues

22. Which of the following communication skills should the nurse include when planning to manage client care? Select all that apply:

    [   ] 1. Observation
    [   ] 2. Attending
    [   ] 3. Teaching
    [   ] 4. Responding
    [   ] 5. Clarifying
    [   ] 6. Focusing

23. The nurse should consider which of the following sources of power to be most effective within an organization?

    1. Expert
    2. Referent
    3. Connection
    4. Legitimate

24. The nurse should include which of the following in the discharge instructions given to a client who was recently diagnosed with diabetes mellitus to promote dietary compliance?

    1. Empowerment
    2. Authority
    3. Connectedness
    4. Charisma

Answer: 2, 4, 5, 6

Rationale: Facilitating communication requires more than verbal and nonverbal cues. Strategies to enhance understanding of the message communicated by the client and others will assist the nurse to provide quality, accurate feedback. Communication skills that should be used to manage client care include attending, responding, clarifying, and focusing. Observation and teaching are skills needed by the nurse in planning client care, but are not necessarily strategies for accurate and effective communication.

Nursing process: Planning

Client need: Management of Care

Cognitive level: Application

Subject area: Legal and Ethical Issues

Answer: 4

Rationale: Legitimate power is the minimum source of power, derived by merely holding a position of authority. Expert, referent, and connection are all sources of power that are derived in ways other than by holding a position. Expert power is power derived from the knowledge and skills the nurse possesses. Referent power, also known as charismatic power, is power conferred by others, based on their respect and liking for an individual, group, or organization. Connection power is the connection between nurses having power, such as networking between positions of authority.

Nursing process: Analysis

Client need: Management of Care

Cognitive level: Analysis

Subject area: Legal and Ethical Issues

Answer: 1

Rationale: Empowerment involves the ability to facilitate the participation of others to action and appropriate decision making. In the case of a client with diabetes mellitus and the need for dietary compliance, the nurse facilitates empowerment and compliance by teaching the client what the correct choices are. Authority and charisma do not ensure compliance. For some older clients, these traits of authority and charisma might be negative influences. Connectedness is a possible influence on the client, but because it would require that the nurse connect often with the client to assess compliance, it would not be a realistic motivator.

Nursing process: Planning

Client need: Management of Care

Cognitive level: Analysis

Subject area: Legal and Ethical Issues

25. The nurse manager called a meeting with one of the unit team leaders because clients have complained that they are not receiving their medication on time. The nurse manager should include which of the following time management strategies during the meeting with the unit team leader?

    1. The nurse manager wants all team leaders to take the first hour of each shift to set client care priorities.

    2. The nurse manager realizes that time management strategies are unrealistic when staffing is too low.

    3. All team leaders must look at the overall work to be done and set appropriate priorities.

    4. Optimal outcomes can only be achieved by implementing essential physical tasks.

26. The charge nurse must transfer a client from a medical-surgical unit to a maternity unit in order to make a bed available. It would be most appropriate for the charge nurse to transfer which client?

    1. A 55-year-old client with tonic-clonic seizures

    2. A 22-year-old client with a gastrointestinal bleed on a vasopressin (Pitressin) drip

    3. A 40-year-old client who had a knee replacement with a continuous motion device

    4. A 30-year-old mastectomy client who will be discharged

Answer: 3

Rationale: All team leaders must look at the overall work to be done and set appropriate priorities. Time management can be accomplished by knowing the overall needs of the clients and then setting appropriate priorities. Team leaders who take the first half hour of every shift to set priorities are lacking time management skills; the tasks could be handled by efficient shift reporting. During a nursing shortage, time management skills are essential and should be realistic.

Nursing process: Planning

Client need: Management of Care

Cognitive level: Analysis

Subject area: Legal and Ethical Issues

Answer: 1

Rationale: Obstetrical nurses would have the appropriate knowledge and skills to care for a client having seizures because they routinely care for pregnant women who have hypertension and experience eclampsia (seizures).

Nursing process: Analysis

Client need: Management of Care

Cognitive level: Analysis

Subject area: Legal and Ethical Issues

Ethical Issues

65

1. A student nurse asks the nurse, "Why did my advisor recommend an ethics class for me?" Which of the following is the best response by the nurse?

    1. "It is the responsibility of nurses to recognize ethical dilemmas in clinical situations."

    2. "Ethics must be learned in order to obey the law."

    3. "You must have misunderstood because nurses do not have to study ethics."

    4. "You may find studying ethics interesting."

2. The nurse tells another nurse that which of the following best describes the purpose of the American Nurses Association Code for Nurses?

    1. To communicate the values of the profession

    2. To defend the actions of nurses in lawsuits

    3. To develop the good character of nurses

    4. To help recognize nurses for their ethical behavior

3. Which of the following is the best example of an ethical dilemma faced by the nurse?

    1. Deciding whether or not to place a client in a private room

    2. Deciding whether or not to tell a client about the client's diagnosis

    3. Deciding the order in which staff members should take their breaks

    4. Deciding whether or not to ask another nurse to care for a very complex patient

Answer: 3

Rationale: Utilitarianism is a moral theory that holds an action is judged as good or bad in relation to the consequences. It attempts to maximize the greatest good for the greatest number, giving equal weight to all parties involved. The nurse must consider the feelings of the client, family members, and all others potentially affected by the sharing of the diagnosis. According to the theory of utilitarianism, the nurse must suspend the principle of veracity in order to fulfill the wishes of the client and sustain the happiness that is sure to come to the family members through the wedding celebration. While obtaining support from one's family does support coping, there is no indication that the client is not coping well at this time, and there will be time for coping after the wedding. The nurse must also consider the obligation to uphold the client's confidentiality.

Nursing process: Evaluation

Client need: Management of Care

Cognitive level: Analysis

Subject area: Legal and Ethical Issues

Answer: 2

Rationale: Kantianism, also called deontology, is based on the rationalist view that the rightness or wrongness of an act depends on the nature of the act. The theory of Kantianism uses the categorical imperative to test actions. This imperative states that a person should act as one would wish everyone to act (as if it were a universal law) in that situation. It also says that persons should be treated as ends rather than as means to an end. Pressuring the client treats the client as a means to the end, with which the nurse feels more comfortable and avoids conflict. Keeping the disease progression secret supports the client in treating the spouse as a means to an end by being dishonest. Neither truth telling nor confidentiality alone always applies under this theory, but what is important is a consideration of how one ought to behave if one's actions were to become a universal law. Since sharing the cancer diagnosis with the family is known to support coping of the client and family, it would be generally accepted to support this behavior in most situations in order to uphold principles of beneficence, autonomy, and rule of veracity. Therefore, the nurse should not take the responsibility of telling, but should provide guidance, education, and support to the client's behavior of telling.

Nursing process: Evaluation

Client need: Management of Care

Cognitive level: Analysis

Subject area: Legal and Ethical Issues

Answer: 4

Rationale: The principle of autonomy is upheld when sufficient information and guidance are provided by the nurse so that the client may freely give informed consent. Beneficence is doing good, while nonmaleficence is not doing harm. Truth telling is an ethical rule rather than a principle, and relates to the nurse's obligation to be truthful out of respect for the client.

Nursing process: Evaluation

Client need: Management of Care

Cognitive level: Analysis

Subject area: Legal and Ethical Issues

7. The nurse informs a young, healthy client that the scarce amount of flu vaccine will be given to older clients and those with immunosuppressed responses first. Which of the following ethical principles is best described by the nurse's statement?

   1. Beneficence

   2. Autonomy

   3. Justice

   4. Nonmaleficence

8. The nurse chooses to delay taking a break so that pain medication could be administered on time rather than making the client wait until the nurse's break is complete. Which of the following ethical principles is best described by the nurse's action?

   1. Beneficence

   2. Justice

   3. Nonmaleficence

   4. Autonomy

9. A mentally ill client with an order for a general diet requests a vegetarian meal. Which of the following actions by the nurse best demonstrates the nurse's understanding of the principle of autonomy?

   1. Tell the client that a vegetarian meal cannot be substituted for a general diet

   2. If necessary, obtain an order from the physician for a vegetarian meal; otherwise, provide a vegetarian meal per the client's request

   3. Contact the client's family and obtain their consent to provide a vegetarian meal to the client

   4. Contact the client's medical power of attorney for permission to make a diet change

10. The nurse returns to the client's room in exactly four hours to administer the next dose of pain medication as promised. Which of the following ethical rules is best demonstrated by the nurse?

    1. Justice

    2. Nonmaleficence

    3. Fidelity

    4. Confidentiality

Answer: 3
Rationale: Equitable distribution of resources is described by the principle of justice. Beneficence is doing good, and nonmaleficence is not doing harm. Autonomy is providing the freedom to act.
Nursing process: Analysis
Client need: Management of Care
Cognitive level: Analysis
Subject area: Legal and Ethical Issues

Answer: 1
Rationale: Beneficence is described as doing what one ought to do to promote good. Nonmaleficence is not causing intentional harm. Justice is the equitable distribution of resources. Autonomy is upholding a client's right to make informed choices.
Nursing process: Analysis
Client need: Management of Care
Cognitive level: Analysis
Subject area: Legal and Ethical Issues

Answer: 2
Rationale: Limited autonomy, such as what type of meal to eat, may be granted to those clients who are not deemed competent for other medical decisions. Neither the client's family nor the power of attorney needs to be contacted to make a diet change, even if they make other types of medical decisions for the client.
Nursing process: Analysis
Client need: Management of Care
Cognitive level: Analysis
Subject area: Legal and Ethical Issues

Answer: 3
Rationale: Justice and nonmaleficence are ethical principles dealing with fair distribution of services and doing no harm. These are principles, not rules. Confidentiality is an ethical rule emphasizing the importance of respecting the client's right to privacy of information. Fidelity is the rule demonstrated by this nurse by keeping the promise made and returning with the pain medication.
Nursing process: Analysis
Client need: Management of Care
Cognitive level: Application
Subject area: Legal and Ethical Issues

CHAPTER

Legal Issues for Older Adults

66

1. A nurse admitted an older adult with a history of alcohol abuse. The client asked for assurance that leather restraints would not be used under any circumstances during alcohol withdrawal after surgery. The nurse promised that no restraints would be used. After surgery, the client was very agitated, delirious, and combative. Although restraints were indicated to preserve the client's safety, the nurse opposed using them because of the promise made. This action by the nurse was

   1. appropriate because of the nurse's promise.
   2. inappropriate because the promise was not safe.
   3. a violation of the American Nurses Association Code of Ethics for Nurses.
   4. a violation of the American Nurses Association Nursing Standards.

2. A staff member observes a nurse assigned to a postoperative nursing unit reading the chart of a friend's grandmother who is a client on the unit. The nurse is not assigned to this client and does not have a responsibility for this client's care. The client was just diagnosed with terminal cancer and the family does not know. The staff member evaluates the action by the nurse as

   1. appropriate because the nurse is a health care worker and assigned to the unit.
   2. inappropriate because the grandmother is not assigned to the nurse.
   3. not being a violation of the client's privacy because the nurse does not tell anyone what is in the chart.
   4. gaining information to assist a friend through a difficult time.

3. The nurse is concerned about the medical care a long-term care resident is receiving. The nurse asks an opinion about the medical care from a physician who is not responsible for the client. The nurse has

   1. violated the principle of confidentiality.
   2. acted appropriately to gain information on the client's behalf.
   3. gone to the appropriate chain of command.
   4. followed institutional policy.

4. A nursing home resident is offered the opportunity to participate in research on a new drug therapy to treat pressure ulcers. The resident decides after signing the consent form not to participate in the research project. Based on an understanding of the legal issues related to nursing homes, which of the following is appropriate in this situation? The client

   1. cannot withdraw from the study after the consent is signed.
   2. can withdraw at any time from the study.
   3. cannot participate in a study because of being incompetent.
   4. can withdraw only if the family requests withdrawal.

Answer: 2

Rationale: The nurse should not have made a promise that would possibly compromise the client's safety. The client could also receive some medication for the agitation, delirium, or combative behavior.

Nursing process: Evaluation

Client need: Management of Care

Cognitive level: Application

Subject area: Legal and Ethical Issues

Answer: 2

Rationale: Nurses only have the right to health care information that involves the clients for whom they are responsible and to whom the nurses have a duty.

Nursing process: Evaluation

Client need: Management of Care

Cognitive level: Application

Subject area: Legal and Ethical Issues

Answer: 1

Rationale: A resident of a long-term facility, as other clients, has the right to confidentiality about personal health care information. If the nurse has a concern, the matter should be discussed with the primary physician.

Nursing process: Analysis

Client need: Management of Care

Cognitive level: Application

Subject area: Legal and Ethical Issues

Answer: 2

Rationale: Even though living in a long-term care facility, the older adult is considered competent unless legally declared otherwise. A client can withdraw from a research study at any time.

Nursing process: Analysis

Client need: Management of Care

Cognitive level: Analysis

Subject area: Legal and Ethical Issues

5. The nurse is eating lunch in a nursing home cafeteria. Two nurse aides can be heard at the next table talking about a resident by name. Which of the following is the priority nursing action?

    1. Talk to the nurse aides privately later about this inappropriate behavior

    2. Tell the nurse aides they are being overheard and should talk quietly

    3. Report them to their supervisor

    4. Tell the nurse aides that they are breaching confidentiality

6. The nurse is working in an outpatient same day surgery unit. An 86-year-old client signs the surgical consent form and asks the nurse, "What did I just sign? My wife always takes care of the paperwork." Which of the following is the priority nursing action?

    1. Assess what the client understands about the surgery

    2. Notify the surgeon that the client does not understand the surgery

    3. Ask the client's wife to explain the consent for surgery

    4. Ask the client's wife to sign the consent form because the client is not competent

7. Which of the following is the appropriate nursing action when a nursing student assigned to the surgery suite for observation asks the nurse for permission to photocopy the surgical record from a client's chart for an assignment the student must write?

    1. Photocopy the pages for the student

    2. Allow the student to photocopy the pages without the client's name

    3. Allow the student to write down pertinent but no identifying information

    4. Ask the physician for permission to photocopy the pages

8. The nurse working in a long-term care facility is orientating a new nurse to the facility. The nurse tells the new nurse that which of the following is the priority reason that health care issues of older adults become an ethical dilemma?

    1. The choices for health care options do not seem to be clearly right or wrong.

    2. Decisions are made based on value systems.

    3. Decisions are made quickly.

    4. The legal rights of the client coexist with the health professional's obligation to provide care for the client.

Answer: 4

Rationale: Residents of a nursing home, as all clients, have the right to confidentiality. The priority action is to deal with this inappropriate behavior as soon as it occurs. The nurse has the responsibility to protect the resident's privacy.

Nursing process: Planning

Client need: Management of Care

Cognitive level: Analysis

Subject area: Legal and Ethical Issues

Answer: 1

Rationale: Assessment of the client's understanding of the surgery is essential. If a client has signed a surgical consent form then questions what was signed, it is a priority to assess what the client understands. After assessing what the client understands, or if the client is incompetent, then it would be appropriate to notify the physician.

Nursing process: Planning

Client need: Management of Care

Cognitive level: Analysis

Subject area: Legal and Ethical Issues

Answer: 3

Rationale: When a nursing student wants to photocopy a client's medical record, nonidentifying information may be written down. The client has the right to confidentiality and any information that could be linked to the client, such as names or addresses, cannot be shared.

Nursing process: Planning

Client need: Management of Care

Cognitive level: Analysis

Subject area: Legal and Ethical Issues

Answer: 4

Rationale: Although health care options do not seem clearly right or wrong and decisions in a long-term care facility are made quickly, the priority reason health care issues in older adults become highly charged ethical dilemmas is that the client's rights to care and for a dignified death are managed in the context of the health professional's obligations to provide care.

Nursing process: Implementation

Client need: Management of Care

Cognitive level: Analysis

Subject area: Legal and Ethical Issues

9. The nurse informs a nursing student that the document that permits an older adult to list the medical treatment refused if unable to make decisions is called _____.

10. The temporary nurse from a registry is working on the night shift in a long-term care facility. This nurse has had little experience working with the older adult. Which of the following is an appropriate assignment for the charge nurse to give the nurse from the registry?

  1. An 83-year-old hospice client who is expected to die soon

  2. Administration of medication to 18 clients

  3. Six clients who are stable

  4. Two clients with fevers of unknown origin

11. The nurse is planning care for a group of older adult clients. Which of the following clients is a priority for the nurse to care for first?

  1. An 87-year-old client in need of a dressing change

  2. An 83-year-old client with an infected total knee replacement incision

  3. A 92-year-old client who has a temperature of 38.3°C, or 101°F

  4. A 90-year-old client who has potassium of 6.7 mEq/L

Answer: advance directive

Rationale: An advance directive is a document that outlines the medical treatments a person chooses to refuse if unable to make decisions.

Nursing process: Implementation

Client need: Management of Care

Cognitive level: Application

Subject area: Legal and Ethical Issues

Answer: 3

Rationale: A nurse who is not familiar with the agency or the clients should be assigned to the most stable clients. Assigning a nurse to a hospice client, to clients with fevers of unknown etiology, or to administering medication to clients all require knowledge of the particular clients.

Nursing process: Planning

Client need: Management of Care

Cognitive level: Analysis

Subject area: Legal and Ethical Issues

Answer: 4

Rationale: Although a client with an infected knee replacement, a temperature of 38.3°C, or 101°F, and a client in need of a dressing change all need an assessment by the nurse, the client with a potassium level of 6.7 mEq/L is the most acute and at risk.

Nursing process: Analysis

Client need: Management of Care

Cognitive level: Analysis

Subject area: Legal and Ethical Issues

12. A nurse is teaching a class of new graduate nurses on negligence. Which of the following situations is a priority for the nurse to include in the class as an example of negligence?

1. Not giving a prescribed medication to an older adult

2. Not turning off the oxygen at the bedside when a client at home wants to smoke in bed

3. Not allowing a family member to awaken an older adult client who is sleeping

4. Talking about a client outside of the long-term care facility

13. One of the unlicensed assistive personnel (UAPs) caring for an older adult with fragile skin reports to the nurse a red, painful, and swollen IV site in the hand. Which of the following requests by the nurse does the UAP interpret as inappropriate and illegal?

1. "Tell the client I'll be there as soon as I can."

2. "Carefully take the IV out."

3. "Put a cool washcloth on the IV site."

4. "Elevate the client's hand on a pillow."

14. After reviewing the records of four older clients in a long-term care facility, which of the following situations does the nurse recognize as violating the client's right to privacy?

1. Administering a medication to a client in the presence of other clients

2. Placing the client's name on the client's bed

3. Placing a photograph of the client in the medication administration record

4. Placing a photograph of the client in the medical record

Answer: 2

Rationale: Negligence is the result of either omitting to do something that another reasonable person, guided by those ordinary considerations that ordinarily regulate human affairs, would do, or of doing something another reasonable or prudent person would not do. If there is imminent danger to a client, the nurse must take every measure to protect the client. It may be appropriate in the case of a client with a sudden rash that the nurse withholds a prescribed antibiotic, which may contribute to the development of the rash. It is inappropriate to talk about a client outside of a long-term care facility because it violates the client's right to privacy, but it is not negligence.

Nursing process: Planning

Client need: Management of Care

Cognitive level: Analysis

Subject area: Legal and Ethical Issues

Answer: 2

Rationale: Unlicensed assistive personnel cannot legally perform a nursing function such as removing an IV. This would be interpreted as inappropriate and illegal.

Nursing process: Evaluation

Client need: Management of Care

Cognitive level: Application

Subject area: Legal and Ethical Issues

Answer: 1

Rationale: The medications that a client receives are private. The medications should not be administered where someone else, such as another client, can see what the client is receiving. Placing the client's name on the client's bed, and placing a photograph in the client's medical record or medication administration record are for the client's safety and do not violate the right to privacy. Only authorized personnel have access to that information.

Nursing process: Evaluation

Client need: Management of Care

Cognitive level: Analysis

Subject area: Legal and Ethical Issues

15. A 66-year-old client is admitted to a long-term care facility for rehabilitation following a total hip replacement. The client refuses to stay in the facility and tells the nurse, "I am going to walk home." Which of the following is the appropriate action by the nurse?

   1. Tell the client that rehabilitation is necessary and leaving is not possible

   2. Restrain the client to prevent the client from leaving

   3. Call security to restrain the client

   4. Do not prohibit the client from leaving

16. The older adult client in a long-term care facility is soiled with feces. The client calls out, "Stop, don't hurt me. Help!" while being bathed by the nurse. Because the nurse did not have the client or the client's guardian's expressed permission to bathe the client, the nurse is at risk for being accused of

   1. assault.

   2. battery.

   3. malpractice.

   4. negligence.

17. A 66-year-old client with developmental disabilities and schizophrenia living in a long-term care facility develops pneumonia and is seriously ill. There are no advance directives and no legal guardian. Which of the following is the appropriate nursing intervention as the client's condition worsens?

   1. Do not resuscitate because of the impairment of the client

   2. Do not resuscitate because of the age of the client

   3. Provide all possible medical treatment including resuscitation

   4. Call the client's physician for a do not resuscitate order

Answer: 4

Rationale: A client who is in a long-term care facility for rehabilitation and who wants to go home is competent and able to make decisions, even if those decisions may endanger the client's health. It would be inappropriate to prevent the client from leaving, because the client can make health care decisions unless incompetence has been declared. Restraining the client would be false imprisonment or battery.

Nursing process: Planning

Client need: Management of Care

Cognitive level: Analysis

Subject area: Legal and Ethical Issues

Answer: 2

Rationale: Because the client is protesting the bathing, the nurse could be accused of battery without the permission of the guardian. Battery is the unlawful touching of another person. Assault is an unjustifiable attempt or a threat to touch a person without consent that results in fear of immediate harm. The touching may not actually occur. Malpractice is a type of negligence in which any unreasonable act or professional misconduct results in injury to the client. Negligence is the failure to do something that a reasonable person, led by those ordinary considerations that ordinarily regulate human affairs, would do, or the doing of something another reasonable person would not do.

Nursing process: Analysis

Client need: Management of Care

Cognitive level: Analysis

Subject area: Legal and Ethical Issues

Answer: 3

Rationale: In the absence of advance directives by the client or a guardian, the nurse must provide all appropriate care.

Nursing process: Planning

Client need: Management of Care

Cognitive level: Application

Subject area: Legal and Ethical Issues

18. A nurse observes a staff member telling an older adult client that if the client does not take prescribed oral medications, dessert will be withheld. The nurse reports the behavior of the staff member as

    1. assault.

    2. battery.

    3. malpractice.

    4. negligence.

19. A new employee to a long-term care facility asks the nurse if pictures of the residents may be taken. The appropriate response is, "Pictures

    1. cannot be published without the resident's or guardian's permission."

    2. may only be taken by the family."

    3. can be published if the residents are not identified."

    4. will not violate the right to privacy when taken discreetly."

20. An older adult client receives a gift of boxed chocolate candy. The client has dementia and does not understand that the candy is the client's and what it is. The nurse should

    1. tell the client the candy is the client's and offer a piece.

    2. offer the candy to the other clients.

    3. send the candy home with the client's family.

    4. throw the candy away, since the client is unable to eat it.

Answer: 1

Rationale: Assault is a deliberate threat that the client believes could be carried through, or an unjustifiable attempt or threat to touch a person without consent that results in fear of immediate harm. Battery is unlawful touching of another person. Malpractice is a type of negligence in which any unreasonable act or professional misconduct results in injury to the client. Negligence is the omission of doing something that a reasonable person, led by those ordinary considerations that ordinarily regulate human affairs, would do or doing something another reasonable person would not do.

Nursing process: Analysis

Client need: Management of Care

Cognitive level: Application

Subject area: Legal and Ethical Issues

Answer: 1

Rationale: The right to privacy includes the publishing of pictures or any other information about a client without the client's or guardian's permission. The nurse has the responsibility to advocate for and protect the client's privacy. Pictures may be taken in a long-term care facility for the purpose of placing the photograph in the client's medical record or on the medication administration record.

Nursing process: Analysis

Client need: Management of Care

Cognitive level: Analysis

Subject area: Legal and Ethical Issues

Answer: 1

Rationale: When a client with dementia does not recognize that the candy gift belongs to the client, the nurse should take every opportunity to get the client to enjoy it. The candy is a gift and the personal property of the client. The nurse cannot take the candy. This could constitute larceny.

Nursing process: Planning

Client need: Management of Care

Cognitive level: Application

Subject area: Legal and Ethical Issues

21. Based on an understanding of the legal liability in health care, a nurse who fails to monitor the bowel movement pattern of an older adult client, which leads to an impaction, has committed _____.

22. A nurse allowed an older adult who is confused to hold onto her purse. Later, the client was receiving oxygen by nasal prongs and attempted to light a cigarette with a cigarette lighter from the purse. An explosion, fire, and injury subsequently resulted. The case goes to court and the nurse is charged with _____.

23. An older adult client tells the nurse that the client has human immunodeficiency virus (HIV). The nurse should

   1. document this information in the client's chart.

   2. tell the client's physician.

   3. inform the health care team who will come in contact with the client.

   4. encourage the client to disclose this information to the client's physician.

Answer: negligence

Rationale: Negligence is the omission or commission of an act that departs from the acceptable and reasonable standards of practice. The nurse is expected to monitor the elimination patterns of clients.

Nursing process: Analysis

Client need: Management of Care

Cognitive level: Application

Subject area: Legal and Ethical Issues

Answer: criminal negligence

Rationale: Criminal negligence is the disregard of protecting the safety of another person. The nurse has the responsibility to protect the client. In this case, the nurse failed to protect the client with oxygen from lighting cigarettes with a lighter and sustaining injury.

Nursing process: Analysis

Client need: Management of Care

Cognitive level: Application

Subject area: Legal and Ethical Issues

Answer: 4

Rationale: The nurse must protect the client's right to privacy of health care information. Documenting a client's HIV status in the client's chart, telling the client's physician, and informing the health care team who will come in contact with the client all violate the client's right to privacy.

Nursing process: Planning

Client need: Management of Care

Cognitive level: Application

Subject area: Legal and Ethical Issues

24. The nurse caring for an older adult tears the skin of the client while removing a piece of tape. The skin is attached to the upper arm and to the tape. The nurse cuts the attached part of the skin with a scissors in order to remove the tape. The nurse fails to understand that if harm comes to the client during the act of cutting the skin with the scissors, which of the following could the nurse be charged with?
    1. Malpractice
    2. Negligence
    3. Acceptable practice
    4. Assault

25. The nurse caring for an older adult client soiled with feces fails to clean and bathe the client, leaving the client for another staff member to care for. Another nurse reports this nurse as guilty of
    1. nonmaleficence.
    2. negligence.
    3. malpractice.
    4. assault.

26. Which of the following should the nurse include when teaching a class on restraint application in the older adult?
    1. Restraints should be removed and reapplied every four hours.
    2. Place a client with extremity restraints in a prone position to ensure safety.
    3. A physician must evaluate a client within one hour after restraints are applied in an emergency situation.
    4. A client should have a belt restraint on at all times as a safety precaution.

Answer: 1

Rationale: Cutting the skin of a client with a scissors could be considered a medical procedure and not within the scope of nursing practice. A charge of malpractice could result. Malpractice is a type of negligence in which any unreasonable act or professional misconduct results in injury to the client. Negligence is the omission or commission of an act that departs from the acceptable and reasonable standards of practice. Assault is an unjustifiable attempt or threat to touch a person without consent that results in fear of immediate harm. The touching may not actually occur.

Nursing process: Analysis

Client need: Management of Care

Cognitive level: Analysis

Subject area: Legal and Ethical Issues

Answer: 2

Rationale: The nurse is failing to perform an expected action, keeping the client clean and safe from harm. This is negligence. Negligence is the omission or commission of an act that departs from the acceptable and reasonable standards of practice. Malpractice is a type of negligence in which any unreasonable act or professional misconduct results in injury to the client. Assault is an unjustifiable attempt or threat to touch a person without consent that results in fear of immediate harm. The touching may not actually occur. Nonmaleficence is a principle that requires the nurse to act in such a way as to prevent harm to a client.

Nursing process: Analysis

Client need: Management of Care

Cognitive level: Application

Subject area: Legal and Ethical Issues

Answer: 3

Rationale: The least restrictive type of restraint should be used. If restraints are used in an emergency situation, a physician must evaluate the client within one hour after the restraint is applied. Restraints should be reassessed every hour and removed every two hours. Wrist and ankle restraints should not be applied with the client in a prone position because there is an increased risk for aspiration. The client should be placed in a supine position. A belt restraint should not be used just because the client is an older adult and without justification. This is considered false imprisonment.

Nursing process: Planning

Client need: Health Promotion and Maintenance

Cognitive level: Planning

Subject area: Legal and Ethical Issues

27. The nurse should include which of the following in the plan of care for a client who is confused, combative, bedridden, and has a vest restraint?

    1. Securely tie the straps of the vest restraint to the side rails of the bed
    2. Crisscross the vest in the front and tie the vest with a quick-release knot
    3. Remove the client's gown before applying the vest to ensure a snug fit
    4. Provide hygienic care around the vest, taking care not to untie or remove the vest

28. The nurse is caring for an older adult client who is very combative and is constantly hitting the staff at a long-term care facility. The decision was made that extremity restraints are temporarily necessary. Which of the following is most appropriate to include in this client's plan of care?

    1. Place the client in a lateral position
    2. Insert one finger between the restraint and the client's extremity
    3. Secure the restraint to the nonmovable part of the bed
    4. Remove the restraint after four hours to assess the skin

29. The nurse appropriately applies a mummy restraint to which of the following clients?

    1. An older adult client who is confused
    2. A screaming child prior to an eye irrigation
    3. An adolescent who is having a drug reaction
    4. An older adult client who is combative and scratching the staff

30. The registered nurse is preparing to delegate nursing tasks. Which of the following should the nurse delegate to unlicensed assistive personnel?

    1. Perform a neurovascular assessment on an older adult client who has a jacket restraint
    2. Assess the skin integrity of an older adult client with a belt restraint
    3. Perform range-of-motion exercises on an older adult client with an extremity restraint
    4. Assess the oxygenation status of an older adult client with a vest restraint

Answer: 2

Rationale: A vest restraint should be crisscrossed in the front and tied with a quick-release knot. The restraint should be applied over the client's clothes to prevent friction on the skin. A restraint should never be tied to the side rails of the bed. This poses the risk of strangulation.

Nursing process: Planning

Client need: Physiological Adaptation

Cognitive level: Application

Subject area: Medical-Surgical

Answer: 1

Rationale: A client who has an extremity restraint should be placed in the lateral position. Placing this client in a supine position would place the client at risk for aspiration. Two fingers should be inserted under a restraint to prevent it from being too tight. The restraint should never be applied to the nonmovable part of the bed, to avoid the restraint from becoming too tight when the bed is raised or lowered. The skin under a restraint must be assessed every hour and the restraint must be removed every two hours.

Nursing process: Planning

Client need: Physiological Adaptation

Cognitive level: Application

Subject area: Medical-Surgical

Answer: 2

Rationale: A mummy restraint is most generally used with a small child during some kind of short-term examination or treatment. Older adult clients should never be restrained because they are confused or combative. An adolescent would never be restrained just because of a drug reaction.

Nursing process: Implementation

Client need: Physiological Adaptation

Cognitive level: Application

Subject area: Medical-Surgical

Answer: 3

Rationale: Performing specific assessments, such as a neurovascular or an oxygenation assessment, or checking for skin integrity should not be delegated to unlicensed assistive personnel. These tasks require the skills of a nurse. Unlicensed assistive personnel may perform range-of-motion exercises on a client who has a restraint.

Nursing process: Planning

Client need: Management of Care

Cognitive level: Analysis

Subject area: Legal and Ethical Issues

31. The registered nurse is preparing the client assignments for the day in a long-term care facility. Which of the following client assignments would be appropriate for the registered nurse to delegate to unlicensed personnel?

   1. Application of a prescribed restraint

   2. Administration of medications through a nasogastric tube

   3. Assessment of a postoperative stoma

   4. Irrigation of a Foley catheter

Answer: 1

Rationale: Although unlicensed assistive personnel should not perform any assessments on a client with a restraint, they have been trained to apply the restraint. Administration of medications through a nasogastric tube, assessment of a postoperative stoma, and irrigation of a Foley catheter should be performed by a nurse.

Nursing process: Planning

Client need: Management of Care

Cognitive level: Analysis

Subject area: Legal and Ethical Issues

CD-ROM to Accompany Practice Questions for NCLEX-RN®

IMPORTANT! READ CAREFULLY: This End User License Agreement ("Agreement") sets forth the conditions by which Thomson Delmar Learning, a division of Thomson Learning Inc. ("Thomson") will make electronic access to the Thomson Delmar Learning-owned licensed content and associated media, software, documentation, printed materials, and electronic documentation contained in this package and/or made available to you via this product (the "Licensed Content"), available to you (the "End User"). BY CLICKING THE "I ACCEPT" BUTTON AND/OR OPENING THIS PACKAGE, YOU ACKNOWLEDGE THAT YOU HAVE READ ALL OF THE TERMS AND CONDITIONS, AND THAT YOU AGREE TO BE BOUND BY ITS TERMS, CONDITIONS, AND ALL APPLICABLE LAWS AND REGULATIONS GOVERNING THE USE OF THE LICENSED CONTENT.

1.0 SCOPE OF LICENSE

1.1 <u>Licensed Content</u>. The Licensed Content may contain portions of modifiable content ("Modifiable Content") and content which may not be modified or otherwise altered by the End User ("Non-Modifiable Content"). For purposes of this Agreement, Modifiable Content and Non-Modifiable Content may be collectively referred to herein as the "Licensed Content." All Licensed Content shall be considered Non-Modifiable Content, unless such Licensed Content is presented to the End User in a modifiable format and it is clearly indicated that modification of the Licensed Content is permitted.

1.2 Subject to the End User's compliance with the terms and conditions of this Agreement, Thomson Delmar Learning hereby grants the End User, a non-transferable, nonexclusive, limited right to access and view a single copy of the Licensed Content on a single personal computer system for noncommercial, internal, personal use only. The End User shall not (i) reproduce, copy, modify (except in the case of Modifiable Content), distribute, display, transfer, sublicense, prepare derivative work(s) based on, sell, exchange, barter or transfer, rent, lease, loan, resell, or in any other manner exploit the Licensed Content; (ii) remove, obscure, or alter any notice of Thomson Delmar Learning's intellectual property rights present on or in the Licensed Content, including, but not limited to, copyright, trademark, and/or patent notices; or (iii) disassemble, decompile, translate, reverse engineer, or otherwise reduce the Licensed Content.

2.0 TERMINATION

2.1 Thomson Delmar Learning may at any time (without prejudice to its other rights or remedies) immediately terminate this Agreement and/or suspend access to some or all of the Licensed Content, in the event that the End User does not comply with any of the terms and conditions of this Agreement. In the event of such termination by Thomson Delmar Learning, the End User shall immediately return any and all copies of the Licensed Content to Thomson Delmar Learning.

3.0 PROPRIETARY RIGHTS

3.1 The End User acknowledges that Thomson Delmar Learning owns all rights, title and interest, including, but not limited to all copyright rights therein, in and to the Licensed Content, and that the End User shall not take any action inconsistent with such ownership. The Licensed Content is protected by U.S., Canadian and other applicable copyright laws and by international treaties, including the Berne Convention and the Universal Copyright Convention. Nothing contained in this Agreement shall be construed as granting the End User any ownership rights in or to the Licensed Content.

3.2 Thomson Delmar Learning reserves the right at any time to withdraw from the Licensed Content any item or part of an item for which it no longer retains the right to publish, or which it has reasonable grounds to believe infringes copyright or is defamatory, unlawful, or otherwise objectionable.

4.0 PROTECTION AND SECURITY

4.1 The End User shall use its best efforts and take all reasonable steps to safeguard its copy of the Licensed Content to ensure that no unauthorized reproduction, publication, disclosure, modification, or distribution of the Licensed Content, in whole or in part, is made. To the extent that the End User becomes aware of any such unauthorized use of the Licensed Content, the End User shall immediately notify Thomson Delmar Learning. Notification of such violations may be made by sending an e-mail to delmarhelp@thomson.com.

5.0 MISUSE OF THE LICENSED PRODUCT

5.1 In the event that the End User uses the Licensed Content in violation of this Agreement, Thomson Delmar Learning shall have the option of electing liquidated damages, which shall include all profits generated by the End User's use of the Licensed Content plus interest computed at the maximum rate permitted by law and all legal fees and other expenses incurred by Thomson Delmar Learning in enforcing its rights, plus penalties.

6.0 FEDERAL GOVERNMENT CLIENTS

6.1 Except as expressly authorized by Thomson Delmar Learning, Federal Government clients obtain only the rights specified in this Agreement and no other rights. The Government acknowledges that (i) all software and related documentation incorporated in the Licensed Content is existing commercial computer software within the meaning of FAR 27.405(b)(2); and (2) all other data delivered in whatever form, is limited rights data within the meaning of FAR 27.401. The restrictions in this section are acceptable as consistent with the Government's need for software and other data under this Agreement.

7.0 DISCLAIMER OF WARRANTIES AND LIABILITIES

7.1 Although Thomson Delmar Learning believes the Licensed Content to be reliable, Thomson Delmar Learning does not guarantee or warrant (i) any information or materials contained in or produced by the Licensed Content, (ii) the accuracy, completeness or reliability of the Licensed Content, or (iii) that the Licensed Content is free from errors or other material defects. THE LICENSED PRODUCT IS PROVIDED "AS IS," WITHOUT ANY WARRANTY OF ANY KIND AND THOMSON DELMAR LEARNING DISCLAIMS ANY AND ALL WARRANTIES, EXPRESSED OR IMPLIED, INCLUDING, WITHOUT LIMITATION, WARRANTIES OF MERCHANTABILITY OR FITNESS FOR A PARTICULAR PURPOSE. IN NO EVENT SHALL THOMSON DELMAR LEARNING BE LIABLE FOR: INDIRECT, SPECIAL, PUNITIVE OR CONSEQUENTIAL DAMAGES INCLUDING FOR LOST PROFITS, LOST DATA, OR OTHERWISE. IN NO EVENT SHALL THOMSON DELMAR LEARNING'S AGGREGATE LIABILITY HEREUNDER, WHETHER ARISING IN CONTRACT, TORT, STRICT LIABILITY OR OTHERWISE, EXCEED THE AMOUNT OF FEES PAID BY THE END USER HEREUNDER FOR THE LICENSE OF THE LICENSED CONTENT.

CD-ROM to Accompany Practice Questions for NCLEX-RN®
System Requirements

- Operating System: Microsoft® Windows™ 98SE, Microsoft® Windows™ 2000, or Microsoft® Windows™ XP

- RAM: 32 MB for Windows 98SE, 64 MB for Windows 2000, and 128 MB for Windows XP

- Hard drive disk space: 40MB

- Display: 800x600 with 16-bit color

- PDA Operating System Requirements: Windows Mobile 2003 or newer or Palm OS 3.0 or newer. Devices must have a minimum of 6MB of available memory for the full question database.

Set-up Instructions

1. Insert disk into CD-ROM drive. The program should automatically begin installing. You will be prompted by installation instructions. Follow through to end. If it does not automatically start, go to step 2.

2. From My Computer, double-click the icon for the CD drive.

3. Double-click on "NCLEX-RN" and the program should begin installing.

4. PDA downloads are accessible from the CD menu screen once program has been installed.

Technical Support

Telephone: 1-800-477-3692, 8:30 A.M.-5:30 P.M. Eastern Time

Fax: 1-518-881-1247

E-mail: delmarhelp@thomson.com

StudyWare™ is a trademark used herein under license.

Microsoft® and Windows® are registered trademarks of the Microsoft Corporation.

Pentium® is a registered trademark of the Intel® Corporation.